The must-have handbook on occupational health psychology fo. scholars and practitioners. I thoroughly recommend this comprehensive collection brought to you by renowned experts in the field.

—Sharon Clarke, PhD, Professor, Alliance Manchester Business School,
University of Manchester, Manchester, England

This updated handbook is a must-have resource for students, researchers, and practitioners working in occupational health psychology and Total Worker Health®. The in-depth topical summaries provided in each chapter of this volume come from an all-star cast of researchers and practitioners in these domains.

—Christopher J. L. Cunningham, PhD, University of Tennessee at Chattanooga,
Chattanooga, TN, United States; Past President, Society for Occupational Health Psychology

As too many jobs continue to wreak havoc on our lives, this book presents the state of the science on health and well-being at work.

—Adam Grant, PhD, organizational psychologist, The Wharton School,
University of Pennsylvania, Philadelphia, PA, United States;
#1 *New York Times* bestselling author of *Think Again*

More than ever, occupational health is at the center of employees' well-being and organizations' success. This book is a wonderful resource along this route. A set of leading scholars provide their insights into the models, causes, consequences, evaluation, and interventions related to occupational stress. Brilliant work that anyone concerned about health in the workplace should read.

—Christian Vandenberghe, PhD, FRSC, Management Department,
HEC Montréal, Montréal, Québec, Canada

This handbook offers a rich knowledge base for students who are brand new to the field, as well as for the seasoned occupational health psychology professional who wants to understand the state of the research. The excellent team of authors features scientist-practitioners who are leading experts in their areas. The added material acquainting readers with allied areas of research and practice is incredibly helpful for scholars and practitioners who desire to embrace an interdisciplinary approach.

—Kristen Jennings Black, PhD, Associate Professor of Psychology,
University of Tennessee at Chattanooga, Chattanooga, TN, United States

HANDBOOK OF

Occupational
Health
Psychology

THIRD EDITION

HANDBOOK OF

Occupational Health Psychology

THIRD EDITION

EDITED BY
Lois E. Tetrick, Gwenith G. Fisher,
Michael T. Ford, and James Campbell Quick

AMERICAN PSYCHOLOGICAL ASSOCIATION

Published by
American Psychological Association
750 First Street, NE
Washington, DC 20002
https://www.apa.org

Order Department
https://www.apa.org/pubs/books
order@apa.org

Typeset in Meridien and Ortodoxa by Circle Graphics, Inc., Reisterstown, MD

Printer: Lake Book Manufacturing, Melrose Park, IL
Cover Designer: Anne C. Kerns, Anne Likes Red, Inc., Silver Spring, MD

Library of Congress Cataloging-in-Publication Data

Names: Tetrick, Lois E., editor. | Fisher, Gwenith G., editor. |
 Ford, Michael, 1961 June 18- editor. | Quick, James C., editor.
Title: Handbook of occupational health psychology / edited by Lois E.
 Tetrick, Gwenith G. Fisher, Michael T. Ford, and James Campbell Quick.
Description: Third edition. | Washington, D.C. : American Psychological
 Association, [2024] | Revised edition of: Handbook of occupational
 health psychology / edited by James Campbell Quick and Lois E. Tetrick.
 2nd ed. c2011. | Includes bibliographical references and index.
Identifiers: LCCN 2022036045 (print) | LCCN 2022036046 (ebook) |
 ISBN 9781433837777 (paperback) | ISBN 9781433837784 (ebook)
Subjects: LCSH: Industrial psychiatry--Handbooks, manuals, etc. | Clinical
 health psychology--Handbooks, manuals, etc. | Psychology,
 Industrial--Handbooks, manuals, etc. | BISAC: PSYCHOLOGY / Industrial &
 Organizational Psychology | MEDICAL / Occupational & Industrial Medicine
Classification: LCC RC967.5 .H358 2024 (print) | LCC RC967.5 (ebook) |
 DDC 616.89--dc23/eng/20220829
LC record available at https://lccn.loc.gov/2022036045
LC ebook record available at https://lccn.loc.gov/2022036046

https://doi.org/10.1037/0000331-000

Printed in the United States of America

10 9 8 7 6 5 4 3 2 1

CONTENTS

CONTRIBUTORS

Joyce A. Adkins, PhD, MPH, Founder, President, and CEO, VALoR Institute, Hampton, VA, United States

Zofia Bajorek, PhD, MSc, Senior Research Fellow, Institute for Employment Studies, Brighton, England, United Kingdom

Peter A. Bamberger, PhD, Professor, Simon I. Domberger Chair in Organization and Management, Coller School of Management; Vice President and Program Chair, Academy of Management, Tel Aviv University, Ramat Aviv, Israel

Cristina Banks, PhD, Director of the Interdisciplinary Center for Healthy Workplaces, University of California, Berkeley, Berkley CA, United States

Larissa K. Barber, PhD, Associate Professor, Department of Psychology, San Diego State University, San Diego, CA, United States

Joel Bennett, PhD, Founder, Organizational Wellness and Learning Systems, Fort Worth, TX, United States

Leonard Bickman, PhD, Professor, Florida International University, Miami, FL; Ontrak Health, Henderson, NV, United States

Thomas W. Britt, PhD, Professor of Psychology, College of Behavioral, Social and Health Sciences, Clemson University, Clemson, SC, United States

Carol Brown, PhD, Deputy Director, Center for Health, Work, and Environment, Colorado School of Public Health, Aurora, CO, United States

Christopher J. Budnick, PhD, Associate Professor, Department of Psychology, Southern Connecticut State University, New Haven, CT, United States

Tim Bushnell, PhD, MPA, Economist, National Institute for Occupational Safety and Health, Centers for Disease Control and Prevention, Cincinnati OH, United States

Pascale Carayon, PhD, Professor Emerita, Department of Industrial and Systems Engineering, University of Wisconsin–Madison, Madison, WI, United States

Wendy J. Casper, PhD, Associate Editor, *Journal of Applied Psychology*; Associate Dean for Research, Peggy E. Swanson Endowed Chair of Management, University of Texas at Arlington, Arlington, TX, United States

Jennifer Cavallari, ScD, CIH, Associate Professor, Occupational and Environmental Epidemiology, University of Connecticut, Farmington, CT, United States

Aldrich Chan, Research Assistant, Organizational Wellness and Learning Systems, Arlington, TX, United States

Chu-Hsiang Chang, PhD, Professor of Organizational Psychology, Michigan State University, East Lansing, MI, United States

BongKyoo Choi, ScD, MPH, RPh, Director, Center for Work and Health Research, Irvine, CA, United States

Cary L. Cooper, PhD, Professor of Organizational Psychology, University of Manchester, Manchester, England, United Kingdom

Tori L. Crain, PhD, Assistant Professor, Department of Psychology, Portland State University, Portland, OR, United States

Bryan J. Dik, PhD, Professor, Department of Psychology, Colorado State University, Fort Collins, CO, United States

Marnie Dobson Zimmerman, PhD, Assistant Adjunct Professor, University of California Irvine, Irvine, CA; Director, Healthy Work Campaign, Culver City, CA, United States

Susan Douglas, PhD, Associate Professor, Vanderbilt University, Nashville, TN, United States

Alicia G. Dugan, PhD, Assistant Professor of the Practice of Human Development, University of Connecticut School of Medicine, Farmington, Connecticut, United States

Mark G. Ehrhart, PhD, Professor of Industrial/Organizational Psychology, University of Central Florida, Orlando, FL, United States

Gwenith G. Fisher, PhD, Associate Professor, Department of Psychology, Colorado State University, Fort Collins, CO, United States

Michael T. Ford, PhD, Associate Professor, Department of Management, University of Alabama, Tuscaloosa, AL, United States

Stefanie Fox, MS, Doctoral Candidate, Graduate Research Assistant in Applied Industrial/Organizational Psychology, Portland State University, Portland, OR, United States

Charlotte Fritz, PhD, Associate Professor, Industrial and Organizational Psychology, Portland State University, Portland, OR, United States

Michael R. Frone, PhD, Research Professor, University of Buffalo, State University of New York, Buffalo, NY, United States

Javier García Rivas, PhD, MA, Researcher, Centro Interamericano de Estudios de Seguridad Social (Inter-American Center for Social Security Studies), Mexico City, Mexico

Jennifer Garza, ScD, Assistant Professor, University of Connecticut School of Medicine, Farmington, CT, United States

David Gilkey, PhD, Associate Professor, Science and Engineering, Montana Technological University, Butte, MT, United States

Viviola Gomez Ortiz, PhD, Associate Professor, Department of Psychology, Universidad de Los Andes, Bogotá, Colombia

Leslie B. Hammer, PhD, Professor, Oregon Institute of Occupational Health Sciences; Co-Director, Oregon Healthy Workforce Center, Oregon Institute of Occupational Health Sciences, Oregon Health and Science University, Portland, OR, United States

Alexis Hanna, PhD, Assistant Professor of Management, Management Department, College of Business, University of Nevada, Reno, NV, United States

M. Blake Hargrove, PhD, Professor, Shippensburg University, Shippensburg, PA, United States; and Profesor ad Honorem, Universidad Politécnica de Madrid, Madrid, Spain

Catherine A. Heaney, PhD, MPH, Associate Professor of Psychology and Medicine, Stanford University, Stanford, CA, United States

Peter Hoonakker, PhD, Distinguished Scientist, Wisconsin Institute for Health Systems Engineering, University of Wisconsin–Madison, Madison, WI, United States

John Howard, MD, MPH, JD, LLM, MBA, Director, National Institute for Occupational Safety and Health, Centers for Disease Control and Prevention, Washington, DC, United States

Jinyu Hu, PhD, Assistant Professor, Management Department, College of Business, University of Nevada, Reno, Reno, NV, United States

Joseph J. Hurrell, Jr., PhD, National Institute for Occupational Safety and Health (Retired), Batavia, OH, United States

Shelia A. Hyde, PhD, SHRM-SCP, Assistant Professor, College of Business, Texas Woman's University, Denton, TX, United States

Arturo Juárez-García, PhD, Professor, School of Psychology, Psychological and Research Services Unit (UNISEP in Spanish), Universidad Autónoma del Estado de Morelos, Cuernavaca, Morelos, México

Göran Kecklund, PhD, Deputy Head, Department of Psychology, Stockholm University, Stockholm, Sweden

E. Kevin Kelloway, PhD, Professor of Psychology, Saint Mary's University, Halifax, Nova Scotia, Canada

Andrew Kinder, MsC, Professional Head of Mental Health Services, Optima Health, Headley, England, United Kingdom

Niklas Krause, PhD, Professor, Director of the Southern California Education and Resource Center (ERC), University of California Los Angeles, Los Angeles, CA, United States

Maribeth Kuenzi, PhD, Associate Professor of Management and Organizations, Southern Methodist University, Dallas, TX, United States

Paul Landsbergis, PhD, EdD, MPH, Associate Professor, Department of Environmental and Occupational Health Sciences, School of Public Health, Downstate Health Sciences University, State University of New York, Brooklyn, NY, United States

Michael P. Leiter, PhD, Honorary Professor of Organizational Psychology, School of Psychology, Deakin University, Geelong, Victoria, Australia

Jian Li, PhD, Professor, Department of Environmental Health Sciences, University of California Los Angeles, Los Angeles, CA, United States

Christina Maslach, PhD, Professor of the Graduate School, University of California, Berkeley, CA, United States

Charn P. McAllister, PhD, Director, NAU Institute for Public and Professional Ethics in Leadership, Assistant Professor of Management, Northern Arizona University, Flagstaff, AZ, United States

Katharine McMahon, PhD, Prevention Program Assistant, U.S. Center for SafeSport, Boston, MA, United States

Zachary A. Mercurio, PhD, Professor, Center for Meaning and Purpose, Colorado State University, Fort Collins, CO, United States

Jane Mullen, PhD, MSc, Professor, Department of Commerce, Mount Allison University, Sackville, New Brunswick, Canada

Lee S. Newman, MD, MA, Distinguished Professor; Director, Center for Health, Work, and Environment; Interim Department Chair, Environmental and Occupational Health, Colorado School of Public Health, University of Colorado Anschutz Medical Campus, Aurora, CO, United States

Karina Nielsen, PhD, Chair in Work Psychology, Institute of Work Psychology, Sheffield University Management School, University of Sheffield, Sheffield, England, United Kingdom

Regina Pana-Cryan, PhD, Chief Economist, National Institute for Occupational Safety and Health, Centers for Disease Control and Prevention, Washington, DC, United States

Pamela L. Perrewé, PhD, Professor Emerita, Florida State University, Tallahassee, FL, United States

Richard Pompei, DO, MPH, Senior Clinical Instructor, Family Medicine, Colorado School of Public Health, University of Colorado Anschutz Medical Campus, Aurora, CO, United States

James Campbell Quick, PhD, Colonel, United States Air Force (Retired); Distinguished University Professor, Academy of Distinguished Scholars, and Professor Emeritus, The University of Texas at Arlington, Arlington, TX, United States

Cora Roelofs, ScD, Research Professor, University of Massachusetts Lowell; Research Scholar, Ronin Institute, Boston, MA, United States

Steven L. Sauter, PhD, Academy of Senior Professionals at Eckerd College, Saint Petersburg, FL, United States

Peter Schnall, PhD, Professor Emeritus, University of California at Irvine at UCI Health, Irvine, CA, United States

Natalie V. Schwatka, PhD, MS, Assistant Professor, Center for Health, Work, and Environment, Colorado School of Public Health, Aurora, CO, United States

William Scott, BS, Organizational Psychology, Michigan State University, East Lansing, MI, United States

William S. Shaw, PhD, Associate Professor of Medicine, University of Connecticut School of Medicine, Farmington, CT, United States

Bret L. Simmons, PhD, Associate Professor and Chair of Management, Management Department, College of Business, University of Nevada, Reno, NV, United States

Robert R. Sinclair, PhD, Professor, College of Behavioral, Social and Health Sciences, Clemson University, Clemson, SC, United States

Michael J. Smith, PhD, Professor Emeritus, College of Engineering, University of Wisconsin–Madison, Madison, WI, United States

Paul E. Spector, PhD, Adjunct Professor and Distinguished Emeritus Professor, School of Information Systems and Management, University of South Florida; Organizational Development Consultant, Tampa General Hospital, Tampa, FL, United States

Amanda Sonnega, PhD, Associate Research Scientist, Survey Research Center of the Institute for Social Research at the University of Michigan, Ann Arbor, MI, United States

John Sonnega, PhD, Associate Professor, School of Health Promotion and Human Performance, Eastern Michigan University, Ypsilanti, MI, United States

Michael F. Steger, PhD, Professor, Department of Psychology, Colorado State University, Fort Collins, CO, United States

Liliana Tenney, DRPh, MPH, Assistant Professor, Associate Director of Outreach and Programs, Center for Work, Health, and Environment, Colorado School of Public Health, Aurora, CO, United States

Lois E. Tetrick, PhD, Professor Emerita, College of Humanities and Social Sciences, George Mason University, Fairfax, VA, United States

Tabatha Thibault, PhD, Research Associate, the Conference Board of Canada, Ottawa, Ontario, Canada

Philip Tucker, PhD, Associate Professor of Psychology, Swansea University, Swansea, England, United Kingdom

Hoda Vaziri, PhD, Assistant Professor, Department of Management, G. Brint Ryan College of Business, University of North Texas, Denton, TX, United States

Patrick Voorhies, EdD, Learning Experience Architect, Chevron, Houston, TX, United States

Gwendolyn Paige Watson, PhD, Research Assistant, Clemson University, Clemson, SC, United States

Julie H. Wayne, PhD, David C. Darnell Presidential Chair of Principled Leadership; Area Chair of Strategy, Management, IS, Law, & Entrepreneurship, Professor, Wake Forest University, Winston-Salem, NC, United States

Brian Williams, MD, MPH, Clinical Assistant Professor; Associate Director (OEM Residency & Fellowship), Colorado School of Public Health, University of Colorado Anschutz Medical Campus, Aurora, CO, United States

Liu-Qin Yang, PhD, Associate Professor, Department of Psychology, Portland State University, Portland, OR, United States

Len Zwack, ScD, Environmental and Occupational Health Professional, West Haven, CT, United States

MISSION AND HISTORY

INTRODUCTION: MISSION AND HISTORY

Part I of this handbook provides an overview of occupational health psychology (OHP) to present pertinent background information and a description of the history of the field. Chapter 1 includes a description of the organization of this volume, which may help readers locate topics of interest to them. This third edition of the handbook has considerable breadth and covers a wide range of topics. In fact, the content in the third edition was significantly expanded due to the growing and expanding nature of OHP over the last decade. Thus, readers may want to consult multiple chapters to gain an appreciation of the scope of OHP from a theoretical and practice perspective. Chapter 2 describes the historical development of OHP primarily from a North American perspective, although the chapter also recognizes the parallel developments in Europe.

1

Introduction

Public Health and Prevention in Occupational Settings

Lois E. Tetrick, Gwenith G. Fisher, Michael T. Ford, and
James Campbell Quick

People spend a significant proportion of their lives at work, and often their jobs bring meaning and structure to their lives (Jahoda, 1982; Warr, 2007). Because work is a central aspect of many people's lives, societies generally recognize that workers should have a safe and healthy work environment. Employees should not have to worry about injury or illness, and governments in many industrialized countries, including the United States, the Netherlands, Sweden, and European Union, have introduced legislation to help ensure this (Kompier, 1996; Tetrick, 2008). The focus of much of the early work on occupational safety and health was on occupational medicine and workers' exposures to physical hazards in the work environment. Over time, scholars and practitioners have recognized the workplace is also a logical, appropriate context for health and well-being promotion, not just the prevention of injuries and illness (Cooper & Quick, 2017). This broader perspective is concerned with healthy people and healthy organizations (Nelson & Quick, 2019). Since the second edition of the handbook, the National Institute for Occupational Safety and Health (NIOSH) has developed and proliferated the science and practice of *Total Worker Health*® (Hudson et al., 2019), integrating safety and health protection with health promotion. Alongside this broadened focus, occupational health psychology researchers have theorized about and delved into how work-related experiences affect workers and their families outside of work (Carlson et al., 2019; Grzywacz & Marks, 2000).

https://doi.org/10.1037/0000331-001
Handbook of Occupational Health Psychology, Third Edition, L. E. Tetrick, G. G. Fisher,
M. T. Ford, and J. C. Quick (Editors)

In this chapter, we first describe the conceptualization of health and the purpose and origins of occupational health psychology (OHP) as a catalyst in bringing together research from multiple disciplines to promote healthy workers and healthy organizations. Next, we review the context in which work today is performed and examine changes in the nature of work. This context plays a role in the optimal functioning of individuals and organizations and drives many key issues in occupational health. We then offer a model for integrating a public health perspective on OHP with a more psychological perspective. Finally, we describe the organization of the rest of the book.

HEALTHY ORGANIZATIONS, HEALTHY WORKERS, AND HEALTHY COMMUNITIES

Regarding the health of workers, in 1946 the World Health Organization defined *health* as not just the absence of disease but also a state of complete physical, mental, and social well-being (WHO, 1948). Health has also been conceptualized more broadly as the ability to have and reach goals, meet personal needs, and cope with everyday life (Raphael et al., 1999). Scholars have, accordingly, taken an expansive view of individual health to include the absence of illness or injury and restoration of health, as well as optimal functioning and flourishing (Hofmann & Tetrick, 2003; Macik-Frey et al., 2007; Schaufeli, 2004). For example, Chari and colleagues (2018) developed a broad, multidimensional model of worker well-being that not only includes workers' physical and mental health but also considers workers' job and life satisfaction, positive emotional experiences, sense of meaningfulness, social support and relationships, as well as a healthy and safe workplace culture and climate as part of worker well-being. NIOSH et al. (2021) recently developed the Worker Well-Being Questionnaire (WellBQ) to assess worker well-being based on this broad conceptualization. In accordance with this framework, this handbook takes an expansive view of worker health.

OHP studies the health of the organization itself, the health of its people, and the impact of organizational practices on the public health of the surrounding community. Regarding the organization itself, Miles (1965) defined a healthy organization as one that survives and continues to cope adequately over the long haul, continuously developing and expanding its coping abilities. Abraham Maslow called for healthy work environments characterized by high productivity, high employee satisfaction, good safety records, few disability claims and union grievances, low absenteeism, low turnover, and the absence of violence (Quick, 1999, 2021b). Nelson and Quick (2019) used a systems view of a healthy organization, arguing that such an organization is able to sustain a healthy and satisfying work environment, even in times of market turbulence. Across these perspectives is the view that a healthy organization has an internal work environment that facilitates the health and productivity of its workers while sustaining itself and adapting to changes in its external environment.

With regard to worker health, the first edition of the handbook had a work–life system view that explicitly acknowledged workers' multiple roles to include roles at work, in the family, and in other nonwork arenas, such as religious, civic, and leisure activities. The boundaries and interfaces that link these multiple systems are instrumentally important to organizational well-being, which of course includes the well-being of the worker (Chari et al., 2018; Quick, 2021a).

Finally, OHP also takes a public health perspective in considering the implications of work for the health of the surrounding community and society at large. Public health aims to maximize the benefit for the greatest number of people and addresses health, safety, and well-being for the entire population. This public health perspective of OHP focuses on the role of organizations as being critical in preventing ill health and in promoting well-being in the general population, which includes workers and their families. By extension, organizations can have a positive influence on the health of the communities within which they operate. Taking a public health perspective, communities can have healthier citizens when their organizations use policies and practices that prevent injury and illness and promote health and well-being.

PURPOSE AND ORIGINS OF OCCUPATIONAL HEALTH PSYCHOLOGY

The purpose of OHP is to develop, maintain, and promote the safety, health, and well-being of employees and that of their families. Worker safety, health, and well-being are important both from economic and humanitarian perspectives. Estimates suggest the health care costs and lost productivity due to employee injuries and distress are substantial (Hassard et al., 2018). Meanwhile, working conditions and work-related stress and injuries are a significant factor in the length and quality of life for workers. The primary focus of OHP is the prevention of illness or injury by creating safe and healthy working environments (Quick et al., 2013; Sauter et al., 1999). Key areas of concern are work organization factors that place individuals at risk of injury, disease, and distress. At the least this requires a multidisciplinary approach with experts from multiple disciplines working together, or an interdisciplinary approach that integrates knowledge and methods from multiple disciplines. An ideal goal is a transdisciplinary approach that extends beyond a multi- or interdisciplinary perspective by developing a unified framework across multiple disciplines within and beyond psychology (Maclean et al., 2000). For example, psychology specialties such as industrial and organizational, human factors, cognitive, social, health, clinical, counseling and developmental psychology inform OHP, as do other disciplines such as public health, preventive medicine, occupational medicine, ergonomics, industrial hygiene, and industrial engineering (Schneider et al., 1999). OHP aims to integrate these disciplines with a primary focus on prevention. Therefore, the main focus of OHP is on organizational interventions that reduce the risk of injury and ill health, promote health and well-being, and help employees cope with stressors or rehabilitate rather than rely upon individual interventions such as counseling (Quick, 1999).

OHP emerged from psychology, engineering, and the practice of preventive and occupational medicine to be uniquely recognized in the 1990s, with a particular focus on the prevention of stress and related health issues. These scientific origins are also the foundations for occupational medicine and occupational safety (Macik-Frey et al., 2007, 2009). Since its original recognition in the 1990s, OHP has progressed to focus on worker well-being; positive work experiences including meaningfulness of work; the behavioral factors in occupational safety and injury; organizational climate; social support and fair treatment; healthy leadership practices; the work–nonwork interface; recovery from work; and a renewed concern for equity and fair treatment, workplace interventions, healthy work design, job resources, healthy boundaries between work and nonwork, among other things. These positive advances demonstrate some of the promise that OHP holds for the future.

The challenges to OHP in promoting healthy organizations and healthy people can be more fully appreciated by considering contextual issues and changes that are occurring in workplaces and in the workforce. These changes shape the nature of occupational risks to which people are exposed and the context within which they work. Key changes that relate to OHP are described in the following sections.

THE EVOLVING CONTEXT OF WORK

Since the second edition of the *Handbook of Occupational Health Psychology* was published in 2011, there are many profound ways in which work and workers' experiences have shifted. Examples include macrolevel factors such as continued globalization, an increase in service-oriented jobs and "knowledge" work, changing workforce demographics and increased diversity, labor supply and demand, unemployment, job insecurity, continual technological advantages (e.g., AI, automation), more variability and a higher prevalence of alternative work arrangements (e.g., contract work and new forms of contingent work, including "gig" work, and telework), and more recently the global COVID-19 pandemic. These contextual shifts in the nature and organization of work have implications for the experiences of workers and their families, with potential effects on well-being and health.

Amid the contextual shifts described above, OHP researchers have made considerable theoretical and empirical advances. During the early emergence of OHP as an area of study, researchers paid the greatest attention toward understanding occupational stress. Since the publication of the second edition of the handbook, there have been important advances in our understanding of the work stress process and work stress theories (such as further refinement and extensions of the job demands–resources model and more acknowledgment of allostatic load regarding chronic stressors; see Chapter 3, this volume). As a field we have made great strides in our understanding of the effects of organizational policies and practices on the safety, health, and well-being of employees, their families, and their organizations (see, for example, the special issue of the

Journal of Occupational Health Psychology in 2017 that reviewed 20 years of research). Research findings in recent years have also increased our knowledge about a variety of important workplace stressors (e.g., multiple forms of interpersonal mistreatment, telepressure) and positive experiences (e.g., meaningfulness, recovery) that had previously received limited attention. Additionally, there is a growing recognition of and attention to the inter- and multidisciplinary nature of the field of OHP and a need for more empirical studies to evaluate the effectiveness of occupational health interventions (Burgess et al., 2020). As a result, the third edition of the *Handbook of Occupational Health Psychology* has been expanded to cover these developments to the greatest extent possible. This book has added chapters to cover additional topics and developments in the field (e.g., recovery, sleep, meaningfulness of work, mistreatment, and nonstandard work arrangements). It has also been restructured to include other important areas of occupational health research and practice that overlap with occupational health psychology, including public health, occupational medicine, occupational ergonomics, and industrial hygiene.

One of the more notable and sweeping changes to the nature of work over the past 2 decades concerns the process of globalization, which has increased the international competition for organizations, increased stressors for companies and individuals alike, and decreased people's job security. Globalization has been accompanied by greater global interdependencies. For example, advances in the high-technology sectors helped fuel job creation in Europe during the late 1990s. However, because of subsequent downturns in the global economy, national economic swings, and organizational restructuring, these interdependencies have created uncertainty for organizations and employees. Organizational structures, organizational policies and practices, and work arrangements, collectively referred to as the *organization of work*, have become much more dynamic. Additionally, the workforce has become increasingly diverse in relation to many characteristics of employees, including age, gender, sexual orientation, and disabilities, to name a few.

Changes in Employment Context

Especially as a result of the global COVID-19 pandemic that triggered the "Great Resignation" (in which large numbers of workers quit their jobs, many seeking work with better working conditions) and a wide range of other economic impacts, world economies are seeing a substantial shift in the number of jobs in various sectors. In the United States, continued growth in service-oriented jobs is projected, whereas jobs in manufacturing have continued to decline due to productivity enhancements and international competition. Among the service-oriented occupations, health care, social assistance, and hospitality are expected to show the greatest increases, while substantial increases are also expected in professional, management, and business services. By contrast, declines are expected in office support, retail, and sales occupations. Meanwhile there is continued growth in jobs related to information technology, and significant increases are also expected in mining, oil, and gas extraction. These changes have implications for the types of hazards and stressors that workers will be increasingly exposed to in the coming years.

In addition to these industry and occupational changes, employment arrangements have also shown increasing variability in recent years. Alternative work arrangements such as contract work, temporary or agency work, and on-call work have drawn greater attention (Spreitzer et al., 2017). There has also been a rapid increase in remote work in some occupations, further accelerated by changes in response to the COVID-19 pandemic. In some cases, alternative work arrangements can provide flexibility for employees and employers, which may enhance employees' well-being (Broschak et al., 2008) and organizational effectiveness. However, these arrangements also may lead to underemployment, fewer employment benefits, lower job security, and less control over predictability in one's schedule. Further research is needed to fully understand the potential benefits and risks of alternative work arrangements for employee health.

Changes in the Organization of Work

In addition to the changes in work context, the organization of work has undergone significant changes. *Organization of work* refers to the management systems, supervisory practices, production processes, and their influence on the way work is performed (Sauter et al., 1999). Among these changes are continued globalization and increased competition; other economic pressures and technological innovations; complexity of organizational structures and task interdependence; and higher prevalence of nonstandard work arrangements such as on-demand, gig employment:

- Globalization may result in relocation, displacement, unemployment, and fear of unemployment, and these in turn can result in stress and negative health effects among workers and their families. The increased diversity resulting from globalization may also be stressful, perhaps as a result of difficulty in communication or conflict among cultural values or norms (Brislin, 2008).

- Increased competition and economic pressures have resulted in new practices (e.g., lean production, agile HR systems) designed to help organizations respond more quickly and efficiently to environmental pressures and uncertainty (McMackin & Heffernan, 2021). Such practices may result in work intensification to the detriment of employees' health (Polanyi & Tompa, 2004).

- Technological innovations, such as the need to keep up with advances in technology, may also intensify work demands in these instances, increase employees' responsibilities to the detriment of employees' well-being. Increased automation and AI may contribute to work under- or overload, fatigue, unemployment, or increased job insecurity (Cham et al., 2021; Gagné et al., 2021).

- Increased complexity of organizational structures and environmental pressures have resulted in the downsizing and restructuring of many organizations

(Burke & Nelson, 1998; Tetrick, 2000). The health and safety effects of down-sizing and restructuring have been found to be negative for the victims, the survivors, and the managers who implemented the downsizing efforts (de Jong et al., 2016; Vinokur & Price, 2015).

- Growth of the gig economy, which comprises on-demand work and other nonstandard work arrangements (Chapter 11, this volume; Tran & Sokas, 2017).

Changes in Workforce Characteristics

Age

Most developed and many developing countries have aging populations and workforces. This has implications for a variety of factors related to occupa-tional health, including the influence of work on healthy physical and mental development, the potential for age discrimination and associated health effects, and changes in worker skills and abilities as individuals grow older. The design of work and other management practices can potentially improve the health, safety, and/or well-being of older workers (Rudolph & Zacher, 2021; Truxillo et al., 2014). For example, increasing autonomy and designing jobs to foster generativity and provide opportunities for older workers with extensive job knowledge to mentor others may be beneficial. There is also evidence sug-gesting that positive working conditions and job characteristics such as job complexity are beneficial for workers' cognitive functioning (Fisher et al., 2014, 2017; Parker et al., 2021). Findings on the effects of work on successful and healthy aging are now beginning to accrue (e.g., Zacher et al., 2019).

Gender

Labor force participation among women across the world is 47%, ranging from 17% in the Middle East and North Africa to 61% in Sub-Saharan Africa (The World Bank, 2021). With the continued high rate of labor force participation among working mothers, flexible working arrangements (e.g., flexibility in location and time/work schedule) have been implemented to reduce the work–family conflict associated with competing work and family demands. However, such arrangements are not accessible to all workers (Bulger & Fisher, 2012) and can also result in blurred work–family boundaries (Allen et al., 2021; Lewis & Cooper, 1999) and difficulty detaching from work. The positive and negative effects of the work–family interface for the health, safety, and well-being of working men and women have been studied extensively over the past couple of decades and will be discussed in this handbook.

Race and Ethnicity

Paralleling globalization, the U.S. labor force has experienced a shift in the racial and ethnic composition of the workforce, mirroring changes in the population. According to the U.S. Bureau of Labor Statistics, in 2020 12.1% of the U.S. labor force age 16 or older was Black and 6.4% was Asian. Additionally, 17.6% of the labor force was of Hispanic or Latino ethnicity. This increased diversity in the workforce has implications for OHP (Bell, 2017). Research has documented differential disease rates across racial and ethnic groups, some of which may be related to working conditions and exposures (Barr, 2019). Recent years have also seen an increased emphasis on workforce diversity as well as a focus on the need for equity and inclusion of workers from underrepresented racial and ethnic groups.

The American Psychological Association has undertaken a broad initiative to address the issues of diversity, equity, and inclusion. A joint task force of the Publications and Communications Board and the Board of Scientific Affairs was established in 2020 and worked into 2021 to chart out initiatives to be undertaken in the scientific research and publications directorates of the association. These initiatives are echoed in the broad range of leading universities and colleges as well as Fortune 500 organizations.

Disabilities

According to the U.S. Department of Labor in December 2021, the labor participation rate for individuals aged 16+ with a disability was 22.3%, and 36.7% for individuals aged 16 to 64. OHP research during the last decade has recognized unique stressors (e.g., stigma) and other challenges for workers with chronic health conditions (Beatty & McGonagle, 2018; McGonagle et al., 2020) and those with invisible disabilities (Santuzzi & Keating, 2020).

Between 30% and 50% of adults in the United States experience mental illness at some point during their lifetime (Goetzel et al., 2018). Recent studies highlighted the negative effects of the COVID-19 pandemic on workers' mental health (Khajuria et al., 2021). With poor mental health being a highly prevalent issue and costly problem for society, organizations, and workers, there continues to be an urgent need for research and interventions to improve workers' mental health.

THE PATH MODEL

Considering these changes in workers and the workplace, as well as the resulting risks for physical, emotional, and mental health, it is no surprise that psychologists are giving increased attention to creating and maintaining healthy workplaces. Grawitch and colleagues (2006) reviewed the literature that had been discussed and/or demonstrated to be responsible for psychologically healthy workplaces. The resulting model is the Practices for Achieving Total Health (PATH) model.

The PATH model has five categories of healthy workplace practices: work–life balance, employee growth and development, health and safety, recognition, and employee involvement. These categories are designed to result in employee well-being and organizational improvement. Employee well-being includes the physical, mental, and emotional facets of employee health, as indicated by physical health, mental health, stress, motivation, commitment, job satisfaction, and morale. Organizational improvement includes competitive advantage, performance and productivity, reduced absenteeism and turnover, reduced accident and injury rates, increased cost savings, hiring selectivity, improved service and product quality, and better customer service and satisfaction. The model promises to be a useful framework for organizing approaches to individual and organizational health.

Macik-Frey et al. (2009) cited the PATH model as an underpinning of the American Psychological Association's psychologically healthy workplace agenda and awards. For example, in 2019 a nonprofit organization in Maine was recognized for their workplace flexibility and transition program for older employees. Other organizations were recognized for their commitment to employees, a culture of collaboration, and support from leadership. The model is useful for both challenging organizations to achieve healthy workplace practices and recognizing and rewarding those who achieve success and meet the challenge.

PREVENTION AND THE PUBLIC HEALTH MODEL

The public health model classifies interventions into three categories: primary interventions, secondary interventions, and tertiary interventions (Schmidt, 1994). Figure 1.1 presents a prevention and public health model showing interventions at different targets within the population. Primary interventions focus

FIGURE 1.1. A Prevention and Public Health Model

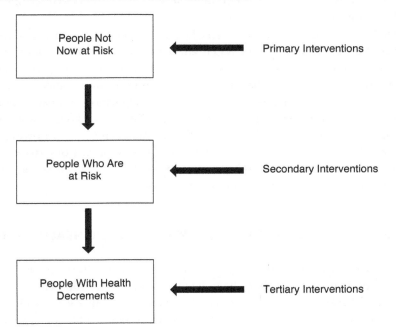

on prevention among people regardless of risk level or health status. The goal of primary interventions is generally to eliminate or reduce the exposure to, or severity of, health hazards. This is essentially a population-based model in which the intervention is applied to entire populations or groups. Within OHP, a primary intervention might involve redesigning the job to reduce or eliminate work stressors, and/or provide additional job resources such as autonomy or support, offering increased worker flexibility, or developing a positive organizational climate.

Secondary interventions focus on people who are suspected to be at risk of illness, injury, or other strain. Secondary interventions may be administered to groups or individuals and are aimed at reducing the negative health effects of stressors and other hazards. Examples include providing social support, team building, and coping strategies to workers and work groups.

Tertiary interventions focus on those who have experienced a loss in their well-being and attempt to restore well-being. Tertiary interventions are largely therapeutic and curative in nature. These interventions are typically individual based, although they can also be group based. Examples include employee assistance programs, psychotherapy, and counseling.

As previously stated, a great deal of OHP focuses on primary interventions and the factors those interventions target. From a public health and preventive medicine perspective, primary prevention is always the preferred point of intervention (Boulton & Wallace, 2021). A prevention model is highly appropriate in OHP because it is systemic in nature, accounts for work stress as a process that unfolds over time, and recognizes the life history and multifaceted complexity of many health problems (Ilgen, 1990; Quick et al., 2013). Chronic health problems stand in contrast to the infectious and contagious illnesses for which the traditional public health model was developed, originally to prevent disease epidemics.

OHP interventions extend the public health model of prevention by addressing changes to organizations or systems, groups, and individuals. For example, changing the organizational culture to value learning and foster psychological safety would reduce strain that occurs from a fear of making mistakes. Because the organizational culture affects everyone in the population, or organization in this case, it could change groups and individuals. The resultant decrease in strain at the individual level would improve the health of employees. However, as Quick (1999) pointed out, there may be times when secondary or tertiary interventions are needed because primary prevention was not feasible or individual factors create health concerns for only some people.

INTEGRATING THE PATH MODEL WITH THE PUBLIC HEALTH MODEL

The OHP literature has not integrated the PATH model with the public health model, perhaps because there have been relatively few empirical interventions and because the most frequent interventions focus on the individual level (Bellarosa & Chen, 1997; Parks & Steelman, 2008; Richardson & Rothstein, 2008). However, epidemiology and public health are essential for

TABLE 1.1. Example Interventions Integrating the PATH Model With the Public Health Model

Area of intervention	Intervention		
	Primary	**Secondary**	**Tertiary**
Work–life balance	Benefits such as flextime, personal days off that are applicable to all employees	Work–family benefits that are applicable to those with family responsibilities	Employee assistance programs for individuals who are experiencing difficulties with nonwork responsibilities
Employee growth and development	Training both job-related (skills) and interpersonal for all employees	Training aimed at employees' needs for development of skills	Remedial training for those who have experienced illness and/or injury
Health and safety	General education campaigns relative to risk factors	Safety tips for individuals working in hazardous situations	Smoking cessation; weight-loss programs for those who are experiencing health declines
Recognition	Rewards for safe behavior	Rewards for lack of accidents (which have been shown to be susceptible to negative consequences)	Incentives/ disincentives for weight loss/gain
Employee involvement	Quality-of-life circles	Health and safety committees for employees in hazardous environments	Peer counseling relative to substance use

Note. PATH = Practices for Achieving Total Health.

understanding healthy organizations (see Goh et al., 2016) and for the science and practice of OHP (see Boulton & Wallace, 2021). To illustrate how these two models could be integrated, we have included in Table 1.1 examples of the types of interventions that might fit within a matrix, crossing the dimensions of the PATH model (rows) with the types of interventions of the public health model (columns).

TOTAL WORKER HEALTH®

Total Worker Health® (TWH) is a comprehensive, transdisciplinary approach to improving worker health that integrates worker safety and protection from work-related injuries and illnesses with health promotion (Hudson et al., 2019). It was developed and launched by NIOSH in 2011 as a

strategy integrating occupational safety and health protection with health promotion to *prevent* worker injury and illness and to *advance* health and well-being.

This approach eliminates the either/or proposition, overcomes the disconnect-edness that exists in many organizations, and provides comprehensive tools and approaches to creating environments where employees thrive. (Schill & Chosewood, 2013, S8)

The TWH approach aims to support organizational efforts to take a systematic approach for addressing and improving worker health and well-being rather than perpetuating a siloed or narrow approach.

Empirical evidence thus far indicates that there are benefits to and success with a TWH approach for addressing worker health and well-being (Anger et al., 2019; Hudson et al., 2019; Lemke, 2021). Although TWH was created in the United States, successful organizational interventions have taken place in other countries. For example, Jaramillo and colleagues (2021) recently applied a TWH approach in a multinational Latin American agribusiness, and Hoge et al. (2019) described a similar approach in Germany called "Workplace Health Management." However, Lemke (2021) recommended taking a complex systems approach (Diez-Roux, 2011; Kaplan et al., 2017) to help ensure success with the *Total Worker Health*® approach. Additional chapters in the handbook describe *Total Worker Health*® and its applications.

ORGANIZATION OF THIS VOLUME

In revising this third edition of the handbook, we have added several chapters to better address advances in the field and a risk-problem-prevention-intervention model. Part I offers an overview of occupational health and its history. Part II provides several models and frameworks employed in OHP, including occupational stress, safety, health hazards, savoring, organizational wellness, models of the work–nonwork interface, and cross-cultural perspectives. Part III contains information on causes of and risk factors for ill health and injury, discussing organizational climate, nonstandard work schedules and nonstandard work arrangements, as well as sleep and fatigue, and mistreatment in organizations. Part IV focuses on symptoms and disorders, including burnout, cardiovascular disease, pain and musculoskeletal injuries, return to work, substance use and abuse, psychological well-being, recovery from work, and meaningful work. Part V discusses interventions and treatment, including job stress interventions, worksite health interventions, employee assistance programs, leadership, and policies and practices relative to the work–nonwork interface. Part VI addresses methodology and evaluation. Part VII presents brief descriptions of several allied occupational health disciplines that relate to and in some ways overlap with OHP. The allied disciplines include occupational ergonomics, industrial hygiene, public health, and occupational medicine. In the concluding section, Part VIII, the coeditors aim to integrate some important aspects of the developments in the field of OHP covered in this volume, discuss issues for graduate training, and predict how OHP will advance in the next decade or so.

CONCLUSION

The practice of OHP requires a sound scientific basis for developing healthy organizations and healthy people. To this end, more theoretical development and supporting research are needed to define health not just as the absence of illness but as something more. Perhaps the efforts of positive psychology to understand optimum human functioning and happiness (Csikszentmihalyi & Seligman, 2000) have implications for occupational safety and health and the design of primary interventions to promote health in the workplace. Seligman (1998) chided psychology for focusing on disease to the exclusion of working toward building strength and resilience in people. It appears that OHP has heard this call, and as indicated in several of the chapters in this third edition of the handbook, there is growing recognition that OHP is concerned with creating and sustaining healthy people and healthy organizations, not just the prevention of injury and illness.

REFERENCES

Allen, T. D., Merlo, K., Lawrence, R. C., Slutsky, J., & Gray, C. E. (2021). Boundary management and work–nonwork balance while working from home. *Applied Psychology, 70*(1), 60–84. https://doi.org/10.1111/apps.12300

Anger, W. K., Rameshbabu, A., Olson, R., Bodner, T., Hurtado, D. A., Parker, K., Wan, W., Wipfli, B., & Rohlman, D. S. (2019). Effectiveness of Total Worker Health® interventions. In H. L. Hudson, J. A. S. Nigam, S. L. Sauter, L. C. Chosewood, A. L. Schill, & J. Howard (Eds.), *Total Worker Health* (pp. 61–89). American Psychological Association. https://doi.org/10.1037/0000149-005

Barr, D. A. (2019). *Health disparities in the United States: Social class, race, ethnicity, and the social determinants of health.* JHU Press.

Beatty, J. E., & McGonagle, A. K. (2018). Chronic health conditions and work identity from a lifespan development frame. In S. Werth & C. Brownlow (Eds.), *Work and identity* (pp. 9–22). Palgrave Macmillan, Cham.

Bell, M. P. (2017). *Diversity in organizations* (3rd ed.). South-Western/Cengage.

Bellarosa, C., & Chen, P. Y. (1997). The effectiveness and practicality of occupational stress management interventions: A survey of subject matter expert opinions. *Journal of Occupational Health Psychology, 2,* 247–262. https://doi.org/10.1037/1076-8998.2.3.247

Boulton, M. L., & Wallace, R. B. (2021). *Maxcy-Rosenau-Last: Public health and preventive medicine* (16th ed.). McGraw Hill Medical.

Broschak, J. P., Davis-Blake, A., & Block, E. S. (2008). Nonstandard, not substandard: The relationship among work arrangements, work attitudes, and job performance. *Work and Occupations, 35,* 3–43. https://doi.org/10.1177/0730888407309604

Brislin, R. (2008). *Working with cultural differences: Dealing effectively with diversity in the workplace.* Praeger/Greenwood.

Bulger, C. A., & Fisher, G. G. (2012). Ethical imperatives of work/life balance. In N. P. Reilly, M. J. Sirgy, & C. A. Gorman (Eds.), *Work and quality of life: Ethical practices in organizations* (pp. 181–200). Springer.

Burgess, M. G., Brough, P., Biggs, A., & Hawkes, A. J. (2020). Why interventions fail: A systematic review of occupational health psychology interventions. *International Journal of Stress Management, 27*(2), 195–207. https://doi.org/10.1037/str0000144

Burke, R. J., & Nelson, D. (1998). Mergers and acquisitions, downsizing, and privatization: A North American perspective. In M. K. Gowing, J. D. Kraft, & J. C. Quick (Eds.), *The new organizational reality: Downsizing, restructuring, and revitalization* (pp. 21–54). American Psychological Association. https://doi.org/10.1037/10252-001

Carlson, D. S., Thompson, M. J., & Kacmar, K. M. (2019). Double crossed: The spillover and crossover effects of work demands on work outcomes through the family. *Journal of Applied Psychology, 104*(2), 214–228. https://doi.org/10.1037/apl0000348

Cham, B. S., Andrei, D. M, Griffin, M. A., Grech, M., & Neal, A. (2021). Investigating the joint effects of overload and underload on chronic fatigue and wellbeing. *Work and Stress, 35*(4), 344–357. https://doi.org/10.1080/02678373.2021.1888822

Chari, R., Chang, C. C., Sauter, S. L., Sayers, E. L. P., Cerully, J. L., Schulte, P., Schill, A. L., & Uscher-Pines, L. (2018). Expanding the paradigm of occupational safety and health: A new framework for worker well-being. *Journal of Occupational and Environmental Medicine, 60*(7), 589–593. https://doi.org/10.1097/JOM.0000000000001330

Cooper, C. L., & Quick, J. C. (2017). *The handbook of stress and health: A guide to research and practice.* Wiley Blackwell.

Csikszentmihalyi, M., & Seligman, M. (2000). Positive psychology. *American Psychologist, 55*(1), 5–14.

de Jong, T., Wiezer, N., de Weerd, M., Nielsen, K., Mattila-Holappa, P., & Mockallo, Z. (2016). The impact of restructuring on employee well-being: A systematic review of longitudinal studies. *Work & Stress, 30*, 91–114. https://doi.org/10.1080/02678373.2015.1136710

Diez-Roux, A. V. (2011). Complex systems thinking and current impasses in health disparities research. *American Journal of Public Health, 101*, 1627–1634. https://doi.org/10.2105/AJPH.2011.300149

Fisher, G. G., Stachowski, A., Infurna, F. J., Faul, J. D., Grosch, J., & Tetrick, L. E. (2014). Mental work demands, retirement, and longitudinal trajectories of cognitive functioning. *Journal of Occupational Health Psychology, 19*(2), 231–242. https://doi.org/10.1037/a0035724

Fisher, G. G., Chaffee, D. S., Tetrick, L. E., Davalos, D. B., & Potter, G. G. (2017). Cognitive functioning, aging, and work: A review and recommendations for research and practice. *Journal of Occupational Health Psychology, 22*(3), 314–336. https://doi.org/10.1037/ocp0000086

Gagné, M., Parker, S. K., & Griffin, M. A. (2021). How does future work need to be designed for optimal engagement? In J. P. Meyer & B. Schneider (Eds.), *A research agenda for employee engagement in a changing world of work* (pp. 137–154). Edward Elgar Publishing.

Goetzel, R. Z., Roemer, E. C., Holingue, C., Fallin, M. D., McCleary, K., Eaton, W., Agnew, J., Azocar, F., Ballard, D., Bartlett, J., Braga, M., Conway, H., Crighton, K. A., Frank, R., Jinnett, K., Keller-Greene, D., Rauch, S. M., Safeer, R., Saporito, D., . . . Mattingly, C. R. (2018). Mental health in the workplace: A call to action proceedings from the mental health in the workplace—Public health summit. *Journal of Occupational and Environmental Medicine, 60*(4), 322. https://doi.org/10.1097/JOM.0000000000001271

Goh, J., Pfeffer, J., & Zenios, S. A. (2016). The relationship between workplace stressors and mortality and health costs in the United States. *Management Science, 62*(2), 608–628. https://doi.org/10.1287/mnsc.2014.2115

Grawitch, M. J., Gottschalk, M., & Munz, D. C. (2006). The path to a healthy workplace: A critical review linking healthy workplace practices, employee well-being, and organizational improvements. *Consulting Psychology Journal: Practice and Research, 58*, 129–147. https://doi.org/10.1037/1065-9293.58.3.129

Grzywacz, J. G., & Marks, N. F. (2000). Reconceptualizing the work–family interface: An ecological perspective on the correlates of positive and negative spillover between work and family. *Journal of Occupational Health Psychology, 5*(1), 111–126. https://doi.org/10.1037/1076-8998.5.1.111

Hassard, J., Teoh, K. R. H., Visockaite, G., Dewe, P., & Cox, T. (2018). The cost of work-related stress to society: A systematic review. *Journal of Occupational Health Psychology, 23*(1), 1–17. https://doi.org/10.1037/ocp0000069

Hofmann, D. A., & Tetrick, L. E. (2003). The etiology of the concept of health: Implications for "organizing" individual and organizational health. In D. A. Hofmann & L. E. Tetrick (Eds.), *Health and safety in organizations* (pp. 1–28). Jossey-Bass.

Hoge, A., Ehmann, A. T., Rieger, M. A., & Siegel, A. (2019). Caring for workers' health: Do German employers follow a comprehensive approach similar to the Total Worker Health concept? Results of a survey in an economically powerful region in Germany. *International Journal of Environmental Research and Public Health, 16*(5), 726. https://doi.org/10.3390/ijerph16050726

Hudson, H. L., Nigam, J. A., Sauter, S. L., Chosewood, L., Schill, A. L., & Howard, J. E. (2019). *Total Worker Health*. American Psychological Association.

Ilgen, D. R. (1990). Health issues at work: Opportunities for industrial organizational psychology. *American Psychologist, 45*, 273–283. https://doi.org/10.1037/0003-066X.45.2.273

Jahoda, M. (1982). *Employment and unemployment: A social psychological analysis*. Cambridge University Press.

Jaramillo, D., Krisher, L., Schwatka, N. V., Tenney, L., Fisher, G. G., Clancy, R. L., Shore, E., Asensio, C., Tetreau, S., Castrillo, M. E., Amenabar, I., Cruz, A., Pilloni, D., Zamora, M. E., Butler-Dawson, J., Dally, M., & Newman, L. S. (2021). International Total Worker Health: Applicability to agribusiness in Latin America. *International Journal of Environmental Research and Public Health, 18*(5), 2252. https://doi.org/10.3390/ijerph18052252

Kaplan, G. A., Diez-Roux, A. V., Simon, C. P., & Galea, S. (Eds.). (2017). *Growing inequality: Bridging complex systems, population health, and health disparities*. Westphalia Press.

Khajuria, A., Tomaszewski, W., Liu, Z., Chen, J.-H., Mehdian, R., Fleming, S., Vig, S., & Crawford, M. J. (2021). Workplace factors associated with mental health of healthcare workers during the COVID-19 pandemic: An international cross-sectional study. *BMC Health Services Research, 21*(1), 262. https://doi.org/10.1186/s12913-021-06279-6

Kompier, M. A. J. (1996). Job design and well-being. In M. J. Schabracq, J. A. M. Winnubst, & C. L. Cooper (Eds.), *Handbook of work and health psychology* (pp. 349–368). Wiley.

Landsbergis, P. A., Schnall, P. L., Belkic, K. L., Baker, D., Schwartz, J. E., & Pickering, T. G. (2011). Workplace and cardiovascular disease: Relevance and potential role for occupational health psychology. In J. C. Quick & L. E. Tetrick (Eds.), *Handbook of occupational health psychology* (2nd ed., pp. 243–264). American Psychological Association.

Lemke, M. K. (2021). Is the Total Worker Health program missing its mark? Integrating complex systems approaches to unify vision and epistemology. *Journal of Occupational and Environmental Medicine, 63*(5), e304–e307. https://doi.org/10.1097/JOM.0000000000002183

Lewis, S., & Cooper, C. L. (1999). The work–family research agenda in changing contexts. *Journal of Occupational Health Psychology, 4*, 382–393. https://doi.org/10.1037/1076-8998.4.4.382

Macik-Frey, M., Quick, J. C., & Nelson, D. L. (2007). Advances in occupational health: From a stressful beginning to a positive future. *Journal of Management, 33*, 809–840. https://doi.org/10.1177/0149206307307634

Macik-Frey, M., Quick, J. D., Quick, J. C., & Nelson, D. L. (2009). Occupational health psychology: From preventive medicine to psychologically healthy workplaces. In A.-S. G. Antoniou, C. L. Cooper, G. P. Chrousos, C. D. Spielberger, & M. W. Eysenck (Eds.), *Handbook of managerial behavior and occupational health* (pp. 3–19). Edward Elgar.

Maclean, L. M., Plotnikoff, R. C., & Moyer, A. (2000). Transdisciplinary work with psychology from a population health perspective: An illustration. *Journal of Health Psychology, 5,* 173–181. https://doi.org/10.1177/13591053000050020

McGonagle, A. K., Schmidt, S., & Speights, S. L. (2020). Work-health management interference for workers with chronic health conditions: Construct development and scale validation. *Occupational Health Science, 4*(4), 445–470. https://doi.org/10.1007/s41542-020-00073-2

McMackin, J., & Heffernan, M. (2021). Agile for HR: Fine in practice, but will it work in theory? *Human Resource Management Review, 31*(4), 100791. https://doi.org/10.1016/j.hrmr.2020.100791

Miles, M. B. (1965). Planned change and organizational health: Figure and ground. In F. D. Carver & T. J. Sergiovanni (Eds.), *Organizations and human behavior: Focus on schools* (pp. 375–391). McGraw-Hill.

Nelson, D. L., & Quick, J. C. (2019). *ORGB⁶: Organizational Behavior.* Cengage/South-Western.

NIOSH, Chari, R., Chang, C. C., Sauter, S. L., Petrun Sayers, E. L., Huang, W., & Fisher, G. G. (2021). NIOSH worker well-being questionnaire (WellBQ) (DHHS [NIOSH] Pub. No. 2021–110, Rev. 5/2021). U.S. Department of Health and Human Services, Centers for Disease Control and Prevention, National Institute for Occupational Safety and Health. https://doi.org/10.26616/NIOSHPUB2021110

Parker, S.K., Ward, M.K., & Fisher, G.G. (2021). Can high-quality jobs help adults learn new tricks? A multi-disciplinary review of work design for cognition. *Academy of Management Annals, 15*(2), 406–454. https://doi.org/10.5465/annals.2019.0057

Parks, K. M., & Steelman, L. A. (2008). Organizational wellness programs: A meta-analysis. *Journal of Occupational Health Psychology, 13,* 58–68. https://doi.org/10.1037/1076-8998.13.1.58

Polanyi, M., & Tompa, E. (2004). Re-thinking work-health models for the new global economy: A qualitative analysis of emerging dimensions of work. *Work: Journal of Prevention, Assessment and Rehabilitation, 23,* 3–18.

Quick, J. C. (1999). Occupational health psychology: The convergence of health and clinical psychology with public health and preventive medicine in an organizational context. *Professional Psychology: Research and Practice, 30,* 123–128. https://doi.org/10.1037/0735-7028.30.2.123

Quick, J. C. (2021a). Organizational stress in the United States of America: Research and practice. In K. A. Sharma, C. L. Cooper, & D. M. Pestonjee (Eds.), *Organizational stress around the world* (pp. 303–317). Routledge/Taylor & Francis Group.

Quick, J. C. (2021b). Wellbeing and work–life boundaries/interfaces. In T. Wall, C. L. Cooper, & P. Brough (Eds.), *The SAGE handbook of organizational wellbeing* (pp. 89–103). Sage Publications.

Quick, J. C., Wright, T. A., Adkins, J. A., Nelson, D. L., & Quick, J. D. (2013). *Preventive stress management in organizations* (2nd ed.). American Psychological Association.

Raphael, D., Steinmetz, B., Renwick, R., Rootman, I., Brown, I., Sehdev, H., Phillips, S., & Smith, T. (1999). The Community Quality of Life Project: A health promotion approach to understanding communities. *Health Promotion International, 14*(3), 197–209. https://doi.org/10.1093/heapro/14.3.197

Richardson, K. M., & Rothstein, H. (2008). Effects of occupational stress management intervention programs: A meta-analysis. *Journal of Occupational Health Psychology, 13,* 69–93. https://doi.org/10.1037/1076-8998.13.1.69

Rudolph, C. W., & Zacher, H. (2021). Age inclusive human resource practices, age diversity climate, and work ability: Exploring between- and within-person indirect effects. *Work, Aging and Retirement, 7*(4), 387–403. https://doi.org/10.1093/workar/waaa008

Santuzzi, A. M., & Keating, R. T. (2020). Managing invisible disabilities in the workplace: Identification and disclosure dilemmas for workers with hidden impairments. In S.L. Fielden, M.E. Moore, & G.L. Bend (Eds.) *The Palgrave handbook of disability at work* (pp. 331–349). Palgrave Macmillan, Cham. https://doi.org/10.1007/978-3-030-42966-9

Sauter, S. L., Hurrell, J. J., Fox, H. R., Tetrick, L. E., & Barling, J. (1999). Occupational health psychology: An emerging discipline. *Industrial Health, 37,* 199–211. https://doi.org/10.2486/indhealth.37.199

Schaufeli, W. B. (2004). The future of occupational health psychology. *Applied Psychology: An International Review, 53,* 502–517.

Schill, A. L., & Chosewood, L. C. (2013). The NIOSH Total Worker Health program. *Journal of Occupational and Environmental Medicine, 55*(12), S8-S11. https://www.jstor.org/stable/48500336

Schmidt, L. R. (1994). A psychological look at public health: Contents and methodology. In S. Maes, H. Leventhal, & M. Johnston (Eds.), *International review of health psychology* (Vol. 3, pp. 3–36). Wiley.

Schneider, D. L., Camara, W. J., Tetrick, L. E., & Stenberg, C. R. (1999). Training in occupational health psychology: Initial efforts and alternative models. *Professional Psychology: Research and Practice, 30,* 138–142. https://doi.org/10.1037/0735-7028.30.2.138

Seligman, M. E. P. (1998, January). Building human strength: Psychology's forgotten mission. *APA Monitor, 29*(1), 2. https://doi.org/10.1037/e529932010-003

Spreitzer, G. M., Cameron, L., & Garrett, L. (2017). Alternative work arrangements: Two images of the new world of work. *Annual Review of Organizational Psychology and Organizational Behavior, 4,* 473–499. https://doi.org/10.1146/annurev-orgpsych-032516-113332

Tetrick, L. E. (2000). Linkages between organizational restructuring and employees' wellbeing. *Journal of Tokyo Medical University, 58,* 357–363.

Tetrick, L. E. (2008). Prevention: Integrating health protection and health promotion perspectives. In M. Sverke, K. Näswall, & J. Hellgren (Eds.), *The individual in the changing work life* (pp. 403–418). Cambridge University Press.

Tetrick, L. E., & Quick, J. C. (2003). Prevention at work: Public health in occupational settings. In J. C. Quick & L. E. Tetrick (Eds.), *Handbook of Occupational Health Psychology* (pp. 3–17). American Psychological Association.

Tran, M., & Sokas, R. K. (2017). The gig economy and contingent work: An occupational health assessment. *Journal of Occupational and Environmental Medicine, 59*(4), e63–e66. https://doi.org//10.1097/JOM.0000000000000977

Truxillo, D. M., Cadiz, D. M., & Rineer, J. R. (2014). The aging workforce: Implications for human resource management research and practice. In M. A. Hitt, S. E. Jackson, S. Carmona, L. Bierman, C. E. Shalley, & M. Wright (Eds.), *The Oxford handbook of strategy implementation* (pp. 179–238). https://doi.org/10.1093/oxfordhb/9780190650230.013.004

Vinokur, A. D., & Price, R. H. (2015). Promoting reemployment and mental health among the unemployed. In J. Vuori, R. Blonk, & R. H. Price (Eds.), *Sustainable working lives* (pp. 171–186). Springer, Dordrecht.

Warr, P. (2007). *Work, happiness and unhappiness.* Erlbaum.

The World Bank. (2021). *Labor force participation rate, female (% of female population ages 15+) (modeled ILO estimate).* https://data.worldbank.org/indicator/SL.TLF.CACT.FE.ZS

World Health Organization. (1948). Preamble to the Constitution of the World Health Organization as adopted by the International Health Conference, New York, 19–22 June 1946; signed on 22 July 1946 by the representatives of sixty-one states (Official Records of the World Health Organization, no. 2, p.100) and entered into force on 7 April 1948.

Zacher, H., Esser, L., Bohlmann, C., & Rudolph, C. W. (2019). Age, social identity and identification, and work outcomes: A conceptual model, literature review, and future research directions. *Work, Aging, and Retirement, 5,* 24–43. https://doi.org/10.1093/workar/way005

The Origins of Occupational Health Psychology

Another Look

Joseph J. Hurrell, Jr., and Steven L. Sauter

Occupational health psychology (OHP) concerns the application of psychology to improving the quality of work life and to protecting and promoting the safety, health, and well-being of workers (Sauter & Hurrell, 1999). This broad definition of OHP was formulated by the National Institute for Occupational Safety and Health (NIOSH) and the American Psychological Association (APA) in 1993 (Sauter & Hurrell, 1999) and has since guided the field's development. It is worthwhile to briefly consider the "NIOSH definition" of OHP to fully appreciate the field's inherent purview. *Application* of psychology clearly implies the notions of both research (theoretical and applied) and professional practice. The expression *quality of working life* refers to worker perceptions of the overall "acceptability" of employment and is thought to be determined by numerous and diverse working conditions and worker characteristics. The expression *protecting and promoting* refers to actions aimed at both the elimination of work-related hazards (health protection) and the promotion of resistance to work- and nonwork-related risks (health promotion). Such actions encompass primary, secondary, and tertiary prevention as practiced in the field of occupational safety and health, as well as efforts—in the spirit of positive psychology—to improve the capacity of workers to thrive. The terms *safety* and *health* are inclusive of a wide array of physical and mental conditions and

Portions of this chapter are adapted from "Occupational Health Contributions to the Development and Promise of Occupational Health Psychology," by S. L. Sauter and J. J. Hurrell, Jr., 2017, *Journal of Occupational Health Psychology, 22*(3), pp. 251–258 (https://doi.org/10.1037/ocp0000088). Copyright 2017 by the American Psychological Association.

https://doi.org/10.1037/0000331-002
Handbook of Occupational Health Psychology, Third Edition, L. E. Tetrick, G. G. Fisher, M. T. Ford, and J. C. Quick (Editors)

injuries.[1] Finally, the term *well-being* is rich in implied meaning. It connotes both physical and psychological health and safety and incorporates a holistic view of human experience whereby multiplicities of factors, including those outside of work environments, affect individual welfare (see Chari et al., 2018 for a discussion of this topic).

Despite the relatively recent emergence of the OHP field, its historical origins have been the subject of numerous journal articles, book chapters, and other published materials. In addition to our own works (Sauter & Hurrell, 1999, 2017; Sauter et al., 1999), there have been various other scholarly discussions of the topic (e.g., Barling & Griffiths, 2003, 2011; Houdmont & Leka, 2010; Quick, 1999a, 1999b; Quick et al., 1997; Schonfeld & Chang, 2017). The present chapter acknowledges the antecedents and contributions to development of the OHP field as described in these prior works, but it augments this material by drawing attention to contributions from the field of occupational health with the goal of providing a fuller picture of the origins the OHP field as we know it today—that is, as a recognized and distinctive field of study and application. The chapter is informed by our involvement as psychologists working, for nearly 50 years respectively, directly in the field of occupational health and safety, primarily at NIOSH, as well as our ongoing efforts to develop and promote the field of OHP. However, in the end, it's "a history and not *the* history" of OHP (see Barling & Griffiths, 2003, p. 20), and, given the sweeping breadth of the field, a truly comprehensive history is beyond the scope of a single book chapter or journal article.

With few exceptions, the principal focus of previous histories (outside our own) is on research and practical contributions by the field of psychology to occupational health and to what would later become OHP. In reading them, one might get the impression that OHP emerged organically and almost passively from the field of psychology. But our perspective is that OHP as we know it today, especially with regard to development in the United States, is the product of deliberate efforts and initiatives in the fields of occupational health and government organizations in combination with contributions from the field of psychology. We will attempt to highlight many of these efforts. We acknowledge (like all other OHP histories) that academic research by behavioral scientists focusing on occupational health problems has helped define the field. However, we will devote more substantial attention to focused efforts by institutions (government, professional, and academic) that have received less attention in prior OHP chronicles (Sauter & Hurrell, 2017). Further, previous histories have tended to place emphasis on contributions of industrial and organizational (I/O) psychology and I/O psychologists, perhaps leading to a perception that OHP evolved directly from I/O psychology. The histories of OHP and I/O psychology overlap in places, but they are not

---

[1]The NIOSH and APA authors of the definition discussed the merits of entitling the emerging field "occupational health and safety psychology" or "occupational safety and health psychology." It was concluded that the term *health* was inclusive of "injuries" and therefore "occupational health psychology" entailed the concept of safety.

inextricably intertwined. For a detailed and critical treatment of the history of I/O psychology specifically, and where it may converge with that of OHP, interested readers should see Vinchur and Koppes (2007, 2011) and Viteles (1932). Finally, others (e.g., Cooper & Dewe, 2004) have suggested that a history of OHP is a history of stress. However, while job stress is a foundational theme in OHP, nearly all conceptualizations of OHP encompass a broad array of health and safety concerns and endpoints.

Past accounts of OHP's history generally follow a common script, usually beginning with the 19th-century social and economic philosophies that took exception to capitalism and the industrial organization of work. They then turn to scientific management and to early industrial psychology (e.g., Münsterberg, 1913). However, it is noteworthy and not explicit in previous histories that the major concerns of industrial psychology of the day were *not* principally health and safety. While factors such as fatigue, monotony, and accidents were of interest, they were most often considered in the context of productivity enhancement, personnel selection, and placement for productivity purposes. Furthermore, interest in fatigue by early industrial psychologists was preceded by others' work. For example, British industrialist William Mather conducted an elaborate experiment in the early 1890s that sought to determine the relationship between working hours, fatigue, productivity, health, and well-being (McIvor, 1987). Past OHP histories note that the early industrial psychology era was followed by the human relations movement (in management), originating in Elton Mayo and Fritz Roethlisberger's Hawthorne studies in the mid-1920s and early 1930s. This movement drew important attention to social aspects of the working environment and job satisfaction (Kompier, 2006). Although perhaps again underplayed in previous histories, much of the interest in job satisfaction appears to have been driven by a presumed relationship between job satisfaction and performance/productivity (Lawler & Porter, 1967), not its direct relevance to health, safety, or well-being. Previous histories then continue with more contemporary interests of psychology in occupational stress, work organization, and the well-being of working people.

MISSING PERSPECTIVE

We contend that absent the field of occupational health's interest and investment in OHP, there would likely be no field of OHP as we know it. To our knowledge, the expression *occupational health psychology* and its analogs (e.g., *occupational health psychologist*) arose originally in occupational health contexts. As we will show, the vision in occupational health for OHP foreshadowed the widely held contemporary paradigm for the field—that is, training in psychology that crosses into the field of occupational health, and participation of psychologists with occupational health professionals in occupational health and safety research and practice. This view was proffered almost concurrently, yet independently, in Australia, Scandinavia, and the United States in the 1970s and early 1980s, creating the impression of a zeitgeist in occupational health that fostered the creation of OHP.

OCCUPATIONAL HEALTH AND EARLY OHP

OHP and the Australian Connection

A 1977 essay, "The Psychologist and Occupational Health," by David Ferguson, MD, a founder of the Australian College of Occupational Medicine, is likely the first formal articulation and embrace in occupational health for what are the tenets and interests of present-day OHP (Ferguson, 1977). Although Feldman was credited with the first use of the expression *occupational health psychology* in 1985 (Feldman, 2010; Schonfeld & Chang, 2017), Ferguson in fact used a variant of this expression (*occupational health psychologist*) in 1977, and the actual expression *occupational health psychology* specifically in 1981 (Ferguson, 1981) in reference to the role in occupational health for psychologists "who combine some of the skills of clinical, social, occupational, organizational and applied experimental psychology with some knowledge of occupational health, ergonomics and safety" (p. 41). As discussed later in this chapter, the expression *occupational health psychologist* was likely in use, too, in Scandinavian occupational health services in the early 1980s or before.

There is little difference between Ferguson's 1977 vision for OHP and the framework today. As characterized by Ferguson (1977), occupational health psychologists work together with physicians as "part of a variable multidisciplinary group that may include the engineer, designer, manager and others" (p. 44) in applications that span the areas of research, education, consultation, and intervention. Ferguson noted that these applications "relate not just to occupational disease and injury but to the total health and safety of the worker" (p. 44) by extending to community risk factors; and that they bridge the areas of primary, secondary, and tertiary intervention. Ferguson explained, for example, that occupational health psychologists follow

> the classic twin person–environment occupational approach; that is, they are directed both towards identifying and influencing the health related behaviors of workers and groups of workers, and towards inculcating health and safety factors in the design of tasks and of the physical and social work environment. (p. 44)

Ferguson identified numerous topics of research and practice for occupational health psychologists. Notable among them are topics of prime interest in OHP today, including labor market risk factors, health education, work design, organizational climate, individual differences, and high-risk occupations.

Early OHP in Scandinavia

Partnership between occupational health and psychology also arose in the context of the Occupational Health Services (OHS) in Sweden and Finland.

Westlander (1994) described a program of advanced training of behavioral scientists employed within Sweden's OHS to serve as *occupational psychologists* or *OHS psychologists* in multiprofessional OHS teams in providing services to employers. Training of psychologists in this capacity began in 1983. A full (academic) year of training was provided by researchers in what was then the Swedish National Institute of Occupational Health. Training content included topics of work and organizational psychology, behavioral science methodology relevant to OHS applications, and physical hazards at work (e.g., noise, vibration). Training was also provided on practical aspects of OHS interventions and teamwork with OHS professionals such as occupational physicians and nurses, engineers, industrial hygienists, and physiotherapists. According to Westlander (1994), approximately 300 OHS psychologists had been trained under this program by 1993. In 2007, it was estimated that 250 to 300 psychologists were employed in the Swedish occupational health service organizations (European Agency for Safety and Health at Work, 2017).

Psychologists were similarly trained and employed as occupational health psychologists in the context of Finnish OHS as early as the 1970s (Kivistö, 2002). As described by Kivistö (2002), occupational health psychologists working in Finnish OHS received 7 weeks of training in occupational health and participated in multiprofessional teams with occupational health physicians, nurses, physiotherapists, hygienists, ergonomists, and other professionals in applications ranging from crisis and trauma care to organizational interventions.

Parallel to these training developments in Finland, the Finnish Institute for Occupational Health (FIOH) began to shift away from occupational neurobehavioral research (examining the neurobehavioral consequences of occupational exposures) and move toward research that focused on work-related psychosocial factors and their relationships to health and safety. In 1982, FIOH and NIOSH entered into a cooperative agreement to explore future opportunities for collaboration in 10 occupational health and safety areas that included "work psychology." This agreement, and subsequent ones, led to six joint institute symposia, exchange visits of psychological researchers, and jointly authored publications. Occupational health's interest in OHP at FIOH was clearly acknowledged at FIOH's 50th anniversary in 1995 by long-time FIOH scientific director and renowned occupational epidemiologist Sven Hernberg, MD:

> Much has happened in 50 years. Today we face new challenges. The emphasis of occupational health is now clearly moving towards "softer" problems, such as the psychosocial work environment, musculoskeletal disorders, work with computers, teachers' and health care personnel's problems and so forth. This shift in direction requires a new kind of competence and new research approaches. (Hernberg, 1995, p. 163)

OHP and the Johns Hopkins School of Public Health

In 1985, Robert H. Feldman used the expressions *occupational health psychology* and *occupational health psychologist*, albeit sparingly and concomitantly with *occupational health educator*, in a book chapter ("Promoting Occupational Safety and Health") that addressed roles for psychologists in the occupational safety and health field (Feldman, 1985). Feldman coedited this book with George Everly, Jr., who subsequently authored a chapter titled "An Introduction to Occupational Health Psychology" in another volume (Everly, 1986). Of relevance to the present discussion, Feldman explained that his inspiration for what he would later call OHP arose from his joint appointment in 1978 in the Division of Health Education and Division of Occupational Health at the Johns Hopkins School of Public Health (Feldman, 2010). As described by Feldman, this appointment resulted in extensive interaction with occupational medicine faculty while he helped to develop what he termed "the discipline of occupational health education" under the auspices of a newly funded NIOSH training center in occupational health at the school. Feldman noted that, during his tenure at the school, he also cotaught a course titled "Social and Psychological Aspects of Occupational Safety and Health," which he characterized as possibly the first course in OHP.

Consistent with Ferguson (1977), the Scandinavian model, and contemporary thinking in OHP, Feldman envisioned that occupational health psychologists would participate in a teamwork arrangement with industrial hygienists, occupational physicians, and occupational health educators to prevent occupational illness and injury. However, Feldman did not clearly differentiate applications in OHP from health education, and the applications described by both Feldman and Everly are quite narrow. The principal emphasis in both chapters is on individual-level (behavioral and educational) interventions, such as health promotion, behavioral safety, and efforts to improve worker awareness and assessment of safety and health risks at work. Training and training venues for occupational health psychologists were not discussed.

OHP AND NIOSH

NIOSH is the U.S. federal agency responsible for conducting occupational health and safety research and making recommendations for the prevention of work-related injury and illness. In the following sections, we describe the role NIOSH has and continues to play in OHP

Setting the Stage for OHP

Occupational Safety and Health Act Mandates

It could be said that OHP is in the DNA of NIOSH. By virtue of stipulations of the Occupational Safety and Health Act of 1970 that created NIOSH, psychologists and psychological factors had an important place in occupational safety and health research at NIOSH since the inception of the institute. In the mandate for federal agency research in occupational safety and health, the Act specified that this research shall include the study of psychological, behavioral, and motivational factors involved (Sections 2b5, 20a1, and 20a4). In its first year, NIOSH cosponsored (along with the U.S. Department of Labor) the University of Michigan's Quality of Employment Survey and added specific questions to assess potential sources of stress at work and their physical and psychological consequences (Quinn & Shepard, 1974). Conducted in 1972 and 1973, this landmark survey helped establish work-related psychosocial hazards as an important area of concern for the field of occupational health and safety (see Margolis et al., 1974). In this same period (1971), Elliot Richardson, then secretary of the U.S. Department of Health Education and Welfare, commissioned a task force inclusive of NIOSH consultants to examine health, education, and welfare problems in relation to work life. The highly influential report of the task force (Work in America, 1973) concluded that workers and society are bearing medical costs that have their genesis in preventable workplace stressors and that the institution of work was "a point where considerable leverage could be exerted to improve the quality of life" (p. xv). Other very early NIOSH efforts included sponsoring and collaborating in the conduct of the University of Michigan's *Job Demands and Worker Health* study (Caplan et al., 1975). Published as a NIOSH technical report, this seminal epidemiological investigation examined occupational differences in job stress and health and provided one of the first large-scale tests of person–environment fit job stress theory. Also, in 1971 efforts at NIOSH were initiated to determine the status of psychological research into occupational safety. Concluding that knowledge was scattered and applications were haphazard, NIOSH developed what may have been the first comprehensive text on the subject. Entitled *The Human Side of Accident Prevention* (Margolis & Kroes, 1975), this book presented information in the form of guidelines for accident reduction in the areas of organizational psychology, engineering psychology, training and behavior modification. Cohen and Margolis (1973), writing in *American Psychologist*, reported on the initial program of psychological research at the institute. Of special note relative to the Act and contemporary interests in OHP, they commented that collaboration between psychologists and occupational medicine, industrial hygiene, and other relevant disciplines was the hallmark of this work. (See Murphy, 2002, and Smith et al., 1980, for descriptions of early NIOSH intramural and sponsored extramural research in the behavioral sciences.)

Recommendations to the U.S. Public Health Service

While the requirements of the Occupational Safety and Health Act and subsequent NIOSH activities were foundational to the development of OHP in NIOSH and beyond, the pathway to OHP in the United States stretches back almost a decade earlier to concerns and recommendations arising in the Public Health Service (PHS) that likely influenced the Act. In 1962, for example, a subcommittee of the PHS Committee on Environmental Health Problems was convened to address the PHS program on occupational health. The report from the subcommittee expressed needs for a more holistic and integrated approach to occupational health—an approach that directly implicated psychology:

> Methods, disciplines, and approaches not now common in studies of occupational health must be introduced. Psychology, sociology, and economics must enter, not only into the implementation of preventive measures but also into the basic study of how man—the total man—reacts to environmental stressors, and how his reactions affect his realization as a member of society. (U.S. Department of Health, Education, and Welfare, 1962, p. 179)

A similar message was heard from a working group appointed in 1964 under the PHS National Advisory Environmental Health Committee to develop a new charter for the PHS Division of Occupational Health (U.S. Department of Health, Education, and Welfare, 1966). The working group foresaw many of the changes in the organization of work that are at the center of attention in OHP today and expressed apprehension about the potential physical and mental health effects of these developments. Among the prescient concerns cited were potential risks associated with increasing workforce diversity, automation and job loss, growth in nonstandard employment practices, and the shift to a service economy and knowledge work. Of special note relative to the present-day emphasis in OHP on interdisciplinary training and research, The working group declared an urgent need for cross-disciplinary training and research in occupational and mental health to better address the mental health of workers.

The NIOSH–OHP Initiative

The NIOSH-Proposed Strategy for Prevention of Work-Related Psychological Disorders

Although the handprint of OHP was clearly visible at NIOSH from the beginning of the institute, the formal OHP initiative at NIOSH awaited further developments in the workplace and in occupational health that brought job-stress-related disorders and worker mental health in particular to the forefront of the NIOSH agenda. In the 1980s, for example, state worker compensation bureaus were beset with runaway claims for what was termed *gradual mental stress*, referring to the cumulative psychological effects of chronic exposure to workplace stressors (see National Council on Compensation Insurance, 1985). At the same time, job stress and the organization of work were increasingly implicated in the etiology of a variety of occupational health problems, such as a dramatic increase in the prevalence of upper-extremity musculoskeletal disorders in sectors of the workforce (Moon & Sauter, 1996).

Against this backdrop, NIOSH elevated psychological disorders to the "NIOSH-Suggested List of Ten Leading Work-Related Diseases and Injuries" (Millar, 1984). This action triggered the formation of a multidisciplinary working group consisting of psychologists and occupational health specialists from NIOSH, APA, academia, labor, and industry to develop a national prevention strategy to address work-related risks to the mental health of workers. Of the four recommendations featured in the working group report *Prevention of Work-Related Psychological Disorders: A National Strategy Proposed by the National*

Institute for Occupational Safety and Health (Sauter et al., 1990), the recommendation for increased training and information dissemination pertaining to the causes and prevention of work-related psychological disorders was most actionable within the purview of NIOSH. In many ways it was this recommendation, strongly endorsed by NIOSH stakeholders, that became the wellspring for the formalization of OHP in the United States.

The NIOSH–APA Training Collaborative in OHP

In response to the recommendation for training and information dissemination for prevention of work-related psychological disorders, NIOSH entered into a cooperative agreement with APA in 1992 to establish university-based, postdoctoral training programs in OHP via a competitive funding mechanism that was managed by APA.[2] This activity was similarly guided by a multidisciplinary advisory body that was populated with professionals from psychology, occupational health, employee assistance, management, health education, and industrial engineering. Notably, the stated purpose for the cooperative agreement went beyond the narrow focus on psychological disorders in the NIOSH-proposed national strategy. Rather, the specified purpose was to "to establish necessary expertise to advance the knowledge of psychosocial and job stress factors in the workplace, and their effects on the mental and physical health, performance, and well-being of workers, and ways for preventing such problems" (U.S. Department of Health and Human Services Centers for Disease Control, 1992, p. 1). Behind this statement of purpose, however, was an even more generic agenda—to improve the capacity of psychologists for research and practice in occupational safety and health.

Formal academic training in OHP was without precedent in the United States in 1992, and OHP itself was an uncommon expression, let alone a well-defined concept. Most familiar was the vision by Raymond and colleagues (1990) for training in OHP. As stated, OHP would deal with "more than psychological disorders and stress in the workplace" (p. 1159), and that it "would integrate and synthesize insights, frameworks, and knowledge from a diverse number of specialties" (p. 1159) in psychology and occupational health, as well as from other areas such as sociology and business (Raymond et al., 1990). Absent an established paradigm for OHP or OHP

---

[2]APA representatives who championed and were integral to OHP training and other activities to promote OHP under this cooperative agreement included former APA CEO Raymond Fowler, former APA Presidents Joseph Matarazzo, Charles Spielberger, Jack Wiggins and Patrick DeLeon, former Executive Directors of the APA Science Directorate, Wayne Camera and Christine Hartel and their representatives, Heather Roberts Fox and Dianne Schneider, and former Executive Director of APA Public Interest Directorate, Gwendolyn Puryear Keita and her associate, Wesley Baker. In addition to former NIOSH Director J. Donald Millar, NIOSH principals included the present authors and also Alex Cohen, all of whom occupied leadership positions in behavioral science at NIOSH.

training in the United States at the outset of this project, NIOSH and APA were not overly prescriptive in steering the design of OHP training programs supported under the cooperative agreement. NIOSH, APA, and the advisory body all recognized that both need and opportunity existed in occupational health for many specialties in psychology, such as health, social, I/O, and clinical psychology. And two dozen topics for training (e.g., health promotion, job stress, disability management, occupational safety) were enumerated in the application for funding to support postdoctoral training. But however broad this training framework, instructions to applicant organizations were very specific in asking for evidence of interdisciplinary links between psychology and occupational health at proposed university training sites. (See Schneider et al., 1999, for further detail regarding the concept and development of postdoctoral training under the NIOSH–APA cooperative agreement.)

In the period 1994 to 1998, two university health programs (Duke University Medical Center and the Johns Hopkins School of Public Health) and one psychology program (Department of Psychology at Wayne State University) were awarded funding for postdoctoral training under the cooperative agreement. In 1997, a follow-up cooperative agreement between NIOSH and APA redirected funding toward the startup of graduate-level training programs in OHP. And in the period 1997 to 2003, competition for funds to seed graduate training in OHP resulted in awards to psychology departments at 10 universities and a school of medicine at one university. Similar to stipulations in the application package for postdoctoral funding, applications for funding OHP training at the graduate level specifically stated that "training experiences should draw upon and integrate knowledge and faculty from several relevant areas such as psychology, management, public health, human factors, occupational medicine, occupational health nursing, and epidemiology" (APA, 1997, p. 3).

Today, nearly 30 years after NIOSH launched its OHP training initiative, training activities in OHP are prolific. Working with graduate students and faculty from Northern Kentucky University, we orchestrated an online international survey of the prevalence of college and university coursework in OHP utilizing lists of colleges and universities with possible OHP trainings that were provided by the APA, the Society for Occupational Health Psychology (SOHP), and the European Academy of Occupational Health Psychology (Ullrich et al., 2016, 2017). Individuals ($N = 301$) representing 29 different countries, across six continents responded. Results suggested that coursework termed *occupational health psychology* existed at as many as 81 distinct universities across 24 countries and six continents. The concentration of OHP training was greatest in the United States, with universities in 26 states reporting formal coursework titled "Occupational Health Psychology." A follow-up survey (Moberg, 2019) was conducted to better understand the nature of the OHP training at these 81 institutions. Forty-six (mostly from North America and Europe) provided complete questionnaires. Of these 46, twelve offered formal programs in OHP, six offered training programs with a primary focus on OHP, and 28 offered OHP-related coursework but not within a formal OHP program or a training program with a primary focus on OHP.

The Society for Occupational Health Psychology

NIOSH separately funded, helped organize, and participated in three working meetings of OHP graduate training programs in 2001 (University of South Florida) and 2003 (Toronto Work, Stress, and Health conference, and Portland State University) to consider ways to further shape, strengthen, and promote the field of OHP. Much discussion was given at these meetings to further conceptualizing OHP and defining its intellectual territory, as well as to training curricula and research and practice applications appropriate to OHP. But perhaps most important, the November 2003 Portland State University meeting concluded with a resolution and plan to explore the formation of a professional society to help cement the identity of OHP as a distinctive discipline, and to draw recognition to the field and nurture its growth. By March 2004, this exploratory work was completed under the guidance of Leslie Hammer with funding support from NIOSH, and in October 2004 the SOHP was founded at a follow-up working meeting at APA headquarters in Washington, DC.

NIOSH-Supported OHP Training Programs Today

NIOSH continues with sustained support of graduate training programs in OHP at the University of Connecticut, Portland State University, the University of South Florida, and Colorado State University. At the University of South Florida and Colorado State University, the OHP training programs are embedded in NIOSH Education and Research Centers, which are the primary venues in the United States for professional training in industrial hygiene, occupational medicine, nursing, and safety. NIOSH Training Project Grants support OHP training programs in departments of psychology at the University of Connecticut and Portland State University. Faculty members from occupational health participate in all of these programs.

The Work, Stress, and Health Conference Series and *JOHP*

Beyond OHP training programs, the NIOSH-proposed national strategy had yet further implications for OHP. Beginning in 1990, NIOSH partnered with APA to cosponsor the Work, Stress, and Health conference series, which was organized by Gwendolyn Keita and the present authors and continues today. And in 1999, NIOSH established the first OHP website and worked with APA to create the OHP listserv (ohplist@lists.apa.org). Additionally, NIOSH conceived of what would be the original North American journal *Journal of Occupational Health Psychology* (*JOHP*) for communication of scholarly research in OHP. After vetting the concept of the journal with senior colleagues and exploratory discussions with publishing houses, NIOSH invited Jim Quick to serve as the inaugural editor. NIOSH subsequently provided startup support for the journal and collaborated in remaining developmental activities for the journal, which was formally launched at the University of Texas at Arlington in February 1994. Under the successive editorships of Jim Quick, Julian Barling, Lois Tetrick, Joseph Hurrell, and Peter Chen, the 5-year impact factor of *JOHP* has risen to 7.36 in 2021 with a 1-year impact factor exceeding that of the *Journal of Applied Psychology* (https://www.apa.org/pubs/journals/apl).

OCCUPATIONAL HEALTH AND OHP TODAY AND TOMORROW

Sustained Interest From Occupational Health

Need and enthusiasm in occupational health for partnership with psychology have been strengthened as the occupational health field faces new challenges in the 21st century. So, too, have opportunities for research and practice in OHP increased.

According to a report from the Future of Occupational Health project at the University of Washington, profound changes in the organization of work, changing workforce demographics, globalization, and the blurring of lines between work and nonwork risks necessitate a reenvisioning of occupational health (Peckham et al., 2017). The report expressed that the lines of interest in occupational health needed to be redrawn across academic disciplines, including the social sciences, management, and economics to better understand and address determinants of workers' health in today's economy. To accomplish this, the report remarks, "it is critical that universities with worker health programs seek opportunities to develop academic collaborations for interdisciplinary teaching and research on work-related determinants of health" (Peckham et al., 2017, p. 10). Among the disciplines highlighted for collaboration were social sciences, occupational psychology, and social epidemiology. Similar issues surfaced in a 2015 survey of global trends in occupational medicine across 21 countries (Loeppket et al., 2017). Attention to "psychosocial and mental health issues" (p. e15) arose as one of the most prevalent responses to a question on future demands in occupational medicine.

Concerns expressed by national and international authorities who participated in the Future of Occupational Health project and Global Trends survey add weight and urgency to earlier recommendations from a report by the Institute of Medicine (IOM) regarding future training needs in occupational safety and health. The IOM (2000) report noted that occupational health personnel "need to be able to recognize and react to effects of these work organization factors on cognitive and behavioral functioning, including stress-related conditions and their link to health, safety, and performance" (p. 7). The report specifically recommended enlargement of training in occupational health to include work organization and work-related stress.

Affinity for OHP is seen also in the ever-growing OHP content in scholarly journals in occupational health (Hurrell, 2011). A NIOSH title and keyword search for the terms *stress, psychosocial factors,* and *work organization* in four prominent international occupational health journals (*Journal of Occupational and Environmental Medicine, American Journal of Industrial Medicine, Industrial Health, Scandinavian Journal of Work Environment and Health*) yielded fewer than two dozen articles in the period 1990 to 1991, preceding the NIOSH–APA OHP training initiative. In the years immediately following the training collaborative (2004–2005), the article count had increased sevenfold (Sauter, 2006). Even casual perusal of these journals today reveals that OHP subject matter comprises core journal content. Of interest in this regard is that one leading occupational health journal *Annals of Industrial Hygiene* reinvented itself in 2016 as the *Annals of Work Exposure and Health*, and specifically cites psychosocial factors and work organization as exposures of concern and interest to the journal (see Annals of Work Exposure and Health, https://academic.oup.com/annweh/pages/About).

Last, progressive uptake of OHP in occupational health is evidenced in growing, albeit still nascent, demand for employment in the United States of occupational health psychologists in occupational health contexts. The 2011 (NIOSH-sponsored) National Assessment of the Occupational Safety and Health Workforce investigated the current employment and anticipated hiring of occupational safety and health professionals in 470 establishments nation-wide (McAdams et al., 2011). Among the types of professionals targeted in this survey, occupational health psychologists were specifically named. Survey results revealed that the number of occupational health psychologists employed at the time of the survey was not large ($n = 22$), as would be expected given the emergent status of academic training programs in OHP. More impressive, however, was the expressed intent of establishments for future employment of occupational health psychologists. Consistent with IOM recommendations to expand the occupational health knowledge base in behavioral science, establishments reported that they expected more than a fourfold ($n = 92$) increase in new hires in OHP within the next 5 years. For none of the remaining eight categories of occupational health professions targeted by the survey were the numbers for anticipated new hires in excess of base employment.

The Promise for Psychology

Much has been said here about the contemporary interests of occupational health in OHP, but the literature says comparatively little about the promise for psychology except in general terms. We continue our discussion of occupational health and OHP with a brief look at tangible benefits and opportunities of OHP training for psychologists, building on input from an informal survey of the four OHP training programs presently supported by NIOSH. Directors of these programs, all I/O psychologists, were asked to comment on the perceived benefits to psychology students and faculty from the tight interface with occupational health in their OHP programs.

As might be expected, there was complete agreement that this interface resulted in substantial collaboration across disciplinary lines for both faculty and students. Staff from three of the OHP programs pointed to a competitive advantage in attracting students to their graduate programs in psychology. Respondents from three of the programs commented that the interfaced OHP programs strengthened funding support for students by way of scholarships, teaching and research assistantships, internships, or grant funding from new sources, including the private sector. Additionally, three programs indicated that graduate training in OHP has made their students more competitive in the job market, including academic and both public- and private-sector placements. Evidence of success in the job market for OHP graduates comes, too, from the 2011 National Assessment of the Occupational Safety and Health Workforce, which also surveyed providers of professional training in occupational safety and health (McAdams et al., 2011). This survey found that OHP training programs were more likely than training programs for all other occupational safety and health professionals to report that 95% of their students with graduate degrees obtained positions within their disciplines within 2 years of graduation (64% for OHP training programs vs. 15%–63% for training programs for other professionals).

Other positive outcomes were attributed to these tightly interfaced OHP programs. Three programs, for example, commented that the programs drew increased recognition to their departments and faculty, resulting in new research funding or faculty promotion. Perhaps most important, however, was uniform agreement that the integrated programs broadened interests and research pursuits in occupational health for both faculty and students. Engagement with occupational health programs is a conduit for exposure of psychologists to new concerns and developments in occupational health and is thus a gateway to new research and practice possibilities. By virtue of their interface with occupational health programs, for example, psychologists in three of the four NIOSH-supported OHP programs (Colorado State, Portland State University, and University of Connecticut) are now heavily invested in *Total Worker Health*® research and application (see NIOSH, 2018). The NIOSH *Total Worker Health*® (TWH) approach denotes a paradigm shift in the occupational health field from a focus on occupational or workplace health to *worker* health—one that more prominently acknowledges the collective influence of individual, social, and occupational determinants of worker health, as well as the importance of interventions that address these determinants in a comprehensive and integrated capacity (https://www.cdc.gov/niosh/twh/default.html; Hudson et al., 2019; Hymel et al., 2011; Institute of Medicine, 2005).

While still emerging, TWH's holistic framework's influence on the field of occupational health has been both rapid and widespread (Lemke, 2021) and offers enormous opportunities for psychologists with interests in occupational health. LaMontagne and colleagues (2014), for example, provided a conceptual model for integrated interventions to safeguard the mental health of workers (reduction of organizational risk factors + promotion of positive aspects of work and personal strengths + promotion of mental health literacy in organizations) that yielded positive outcomes in feasibility studies. Numerous opportunities exist within the TWH framework for further uptake and integration of OHP in occupational health. For example, in a recent *Journal of Occupational and Environmental Medicine* article describing the establishment of core competencies for training of professionals entering the field of TWH, Newman et al. (2020) clearly articulated a need for OHP training for

occupational medicine physicians and nurses, industrial hygienists, ergonomists, safety engineers, and others, as well as a need to train OHP professionals in core competencies of TWH.

MAKING THE MOST OF OCCUPATIONAL HEALTH INTERESTS IN OHP

As we have shown, a well-articulated vision for OHP was tendered in occupational health as early as the 1970s. And there is every indication that interest in
OHP within the occupational health field has strengthened progressively since
then. This interest has opened new opportunities for research, research funding,
and practice for psychologists in occupational health. But close engagement of
OHP with the occupational health field is needed to capitalize on this interest.
Accounts of OHP widely embrace an interdisciplinary model of OHP—one of
partnership with occupational health and commitment to interdisciplinary
training that crosses from psychology into occupational health and other relevant disciplines (Chen et al., 2005; Houdmont & Leka, 2010; Raymond et al.,
1990; Sauter & Hurrell, 1999, 2017; Sauter et al., 1999; Schneider et al., 1999;
Sinclair, 2009; Tetrick & Quick, 2011). SOHP (2017) described OHP in terms of
"the interdisciplinary partnerships of psychological and occupational health
science professionals." In practice, some level of engagement with occupational
health is evident. Professionals from occupational safety and health institutes
participate on the *JOHP* Editorial Board, and NIOSH joins with APA and SOHP
in coordinating the biennial Work, Stress, and Health conferences. Also, as
noted, occupational health professionals work closely with psychologists in
conduct of NIOSH-supported OHP and TWH programs. Especially encouraging,
SOHP recently launched the Multidisciplinary Collaborative for Occupational
Health Professionals as a hub to improve collaboration among OHP professionals and other occupational health and safety–focused professionals to identify common interests, share knowledge, and develop joint opportunities for
collaborative research and practice—an initiative consistent with Ferguson's
1977 conceptualization of OHP in action. Various mechanisms for OHP to
achieve closer engagement with occupational health can be envisioned. At
NIOSH, strategic planning for issues relevant to OHP is governed jointly by
professionals from the fields of occupational medicine, psychology, and economics under the auspices of the NIOSH Healthy Work Design and Well-Being
Cross-Sector Program (https://www.cdc.gov/niosh/nora/crosssectors.html).
Governing bodies for professional organizations, journals, and training programs
in OHP could emulate this leadership model via multidisciplinary participation
in their executive structures.

In sum, after nearly 25 years of formal investment, the psychology adven-
ture in OHP has proven remarkably productive. Ever-expanding enthusiasm
for OHP within the occupational health field portends an even brighter future.
With this in mind, we believe that it's useful for OHP to take stock of its relationship with occupational health and consider ways to further strengthen

and expand it, not just for the good of the field but also for the welfare of working people.

REFERENCES

American Psychological Association. (1997). *Application to develop graduate training programs in occupational health psychology* [Funding application package]. NIOSH–APA OHP Cooperative Agreement Document Collection, National Institute for Occupational Safety and Health Library.

Barling, J., & Griffiths, A. (2003). A history of occupational health psychology. In J. C. Quick & L. E. Tetrick (Eds.), *Handbook of occupational health psychology* (pp. 19–31). American Psychological Association.

Barling, J., & Griffiths, A. (2011). A history of occupational health psychology. In J. C. Quick & L. E. Tetrick (Eds.), *Handbook of occupational health psychology* (2nd ed., pp. 21–34). American Psychological Association.

Caplan, R. D., Cobb, S., French, J. R., Jr., Harrison, R.V., & Pinneau, S.R., Jr. (1975), *Job demands and worker health: Main effects and occupational differences* (DHEW NIOSH Pub. No. 75-160). U.S. Government Printing Office.

Chari, R., Chang, C. C., Sauter, S. L., Petrun Sayers, E. L., Cerully, J. L., Schulte, P., Schill, A. L., & Uscher-Pines, L. (2018). Expanding the paradigm of occupational safety and health: A new framework for worker well-being. *Journal of Occupational and Environmental Medicine, 60*(7), 589–593. https://doi.org/10.1097/JOM.0000000000001330

Chen, P. Y., Huang, Y. H., & DeArmond, S. (2005). Occupational health psychology: Opportunities and challenges for psychologists in the 21st century. *Research in Applied Psychology, 27,* 43–56.

Cohen, A., & Margolis, B. (1973). Initial psychological research related to the Occupational Safety and Health Act of 1970. *American Psychologist, 28*(7), 600–606. https://doi.org/10.1037/h0034997

Cooper, C. L., & Dewe, P. (2004). *Stress: A brief history.* Blackwell Publishing. https://doi.org/10.1002/9780470774755

European Agency for Safety and Health at Work. (2017). *European Agency for Safety and Health at Work WIKI. OSH system at national level—Sweden.* https://oshwiki.eu/wiki/OSH_system_at_national_level_-_Sweden

Everly, G. S., Jr. (1986). An introduction to occupational health psychology. In P. A. Keller & L. G. Ritt (Eds.), *Innovations in clinical practice: A source book* (Vol. 5, pp. 331–338). Professional Resource Exchange.

Feldman, R. H. (2010, June). Occupational health psychology—Beginnings. *Society for Occupational Health Psychology Newsletter, 8,* 19. https://sohp-online.org/wp-content/uploads/2019/04/sohpnewsletterv08-june2010.pdf

Feldman, R. H. L. (1985). Promoting occupational safety and health. In G. Everly & R. H. L. Feldman (Eds.), *Occupational health promotion: Health behavior in the workplace* (pp. 188–207). Wiley.

Ferguson, D. (1977). The psychologist and occupational health. *Proceedings of the Annual Conference, Ergonomics Society of Australia and New Zealand* (pp. 41–50). Department of Psychology, University of Adelaide, Adelaide, S. Australia.

Ferguson, D. (1981). Occupational health in Australia: Debit and credit. *Community Health Studies, 5*(1), 53–70.

Hernberg, S. (1995). Research, prevention, and impact. *Scandinavian Journal of Work, Environment & Health, 21*(3), 161–163. https://doi.org/10.5271/sjweh.24

Houdmont, J., & Leka, S. (2010). An introduction to occupational health psychology. In S. Leka & J. Houdmont (Eds.), *Occupational health psychology* (pp. 1–30). Wiley-Blackwell.

Hudson, H., Nigam, J. A. S., Sauter, S. L., Chosewood, L. C., Schill, A. L., & Howard, J. (2019). *Total Worker Health.* American Psychological Association. https://doi.org/10.1037/0000149-000

Hurrell, J. J., Jr. (2011). Editorial. *Journal of Occupational Health Psychology, 16*(1), 1–2. https://doi.org/10.1037/a0022004

Hymel, P. A., Loeppke, R. R., Baase, C. M., Burton, W. N., Hartenbaum, N. P., Hudson, T. W., McLellan, R. K., Mueller, K. L., Roberts, M. A., Yarborough, C. M., Konicki, D. L., & Larson, P. W. (2011). Workplace health protection and promotion: A new pathway for a healthier—and safer—workforce. *Journal of Occupational and Environmental Medicine, 53*(6), 695–702. https://doi.org/10.1097/JOM.0b013e31822005d0

Institute of Medicine. (2000). *Safe Work in the 21st Century: Education and Training Needs for the Next Decade's Occupational Safety and Health Personnel.* The National Academies Press. https://doi.org/10.17226/9835

Institute of Medicine. (2005). *Integrating employee health: A model program for NASA.* The National Academies Press.

Kivistö, S. (2002, July). Finnish psychologists in occupational health services. *European Academy of Occupational Health Psychology Newsletter, 3,* 10–11.

Kompier, M. A. (2006). The "Hawthorne effect" is a myth, but what keeps the story going? *Scandinavian Journal of Work, Environment & Health, 32*(5), 402–412. https://doi.org/10.5271/sjweh.1036

LaMontagne, A. D., Martin, A., Page, K. M., Reavley, N. J., Noblet, A. J., Milner, A. J., Keegel, T., & Smith, P. M. (2014). Workplace mental health: Developing an integrated intervention approach. *BMC Psychiatry, 14*(131). https://doi.org/10.1186/1471-244X-14-131

Lawler, E. E., III, & Porter, L. W. (1967). The effect of performance on job satisfaction. *Industrial Relations: A Journal of Economy and Society, 7*(1), 20–28. https://doi.org/10.1111/j.1468-232X.1967.tb01060.x

Lemke, M. K. (2021). Is the Total Worker Health program missing its mark? Integrating complex systems approaches to unify vision and epistemology. *Journal of Occupational and Environmental Medicine, 63*(5), e304–e307. https://doi.org/10.1097/JOM.0000000000002183

Loeppke, R., Heron, R., Bazas, T., Beaumont, D., Spanjaard, H., Konicki, D. L., Eisenberg, B., and Todd, H. (2017). Global trends in occupational medicine: Results of the International Occupational Medicine Society Collaborative Survey. *Journal of Occupational and Environmental Medicine, 59,* e13–e16. https://doi.org/10.1097/JOM.0000000000000974

Margolis, B. L., & Kroes, W. H. (Eds.). (1975). *The human side of accident prevention: Psychological concepts and principles which bear on industrial safety.* Charles C Thomas.

Margolis, B. L., Kroes, W. H., & Quinn, R. P. (1974). Job stress: An unlisted occupational hazard. *Journal of Occupational Medicine, 16*(10), 659–661.

McAdams, M. T., Kerwin, J. J., Olivo, V., & Goksel, H. (2011). *National assessment of the occupational safety and health workforce.* Westat.

McIvor, A. J. (1987). Employers, the government, and industrial fatigue in Britain, 1890–1918. *British Journal of Industrial Medicine, 44*(11), 724–732. https://doi.org/10.1136/oem.44.11.724

Millar, J. D. (1984). The NIOSH-suggested list of the ten leading work-related diseases and injuries [Letter to the editor]. *Journal of Occupational Medicine, 26*(5), 340–341. https://doi.org/10.1097/00043764-198405000-00002

Moberg, P. (2019, November). *Academic training in OHP: A preliminary summary of international resources.* Paper presented at "Work, Stress, and Health 2019—What does the future hold?" Philadelphia, PA, United States.

Moon, S. D., & Sauter, S. L. (Eds.). (1996). *Beyond biomechanics: Psychosocial aspects of musculoskeletal disorders in office work.* Taylor & Francis.

Münsterberg, H. (1913). *Psychology and industrial efficiency.* Houghton Mifflin. https://doi.org/10.1037/10855-000

Murphy, L. R. (2002). Job stress research at NIOSH: 1972–2002. In P. L. Perrewé & D. C. Ganster (Eds.), *Historical and current perspectives on stress and health* (pp. 1–55). Elsevier Science/JAI Press. https://doi.org/10.1016/S1479-3555(02)02001-2

National Council on Compensation Insurance. (1985). *Emotional stress in the workplace— New legal rights in the eighties.*

National Institute for Occupational Safety and Health. (2018). *NIOSH Centers of Excellence for Total Worker Health.* Centers for Disease Control and Prevention. https://www.cdc.gov/niosh/twh/centers.html

Newman, L. S., Scott, J. G., Childress, A., Linnan, L., Newhall, W. J., McLellan, D. L., Campo, S., Freewynn, S., Hammer, L. B., Leff, M., Macy, G., Maples, E. H., Rogers, B., Rohlman, D. S., Tenney, L., & Watkins, C. (2020). Education and training to build capacity in Total Worker Health®: Proposed competencies for an emerging field. *Journal of Occupational and Environmental Medicine, 62*(8), e384–e391. https://doi.org/10.1097/JOM.0000000000001906

Occupational Safety and Health Act of 1970, Pub. L. No. 91-596, 84 Stat. 1590 (1970).

Peckham, T. K., Baker, M. G., Camp, J. E., Kaufman, J. D., & Seixas, N. S. (2017). Creating a future for occupational health. *Annals of Work Exposures and Health, 61*(1), 3–15.

Quick, J. C. (1999a). Occupational health psychology: Historical roots and future directions. *Health Psychology, 18*(1), 82–88. https://doi.org/10.1037/0278-6133.18.1.82

Quick, J. C. (1999b). Occupational health psychology: The convergence of health and clinical psychology with public health and preventive medicine in an organizational context. *Professional Psychology: Research and Practice, 30*(2), 123–128. https://doi.org/10.1037/0735-7028.30.2.123

Quick, J. C., Camara, W. J., Hurrell, J. J., Jr., Johnson, J. V., Piotrkowski, C. S., Sauter, S. L., & Spielberger, C. D. (1997). Introduction and historical overview. *Journal of Occupational Health Psychology, 2*(1), 3–6. https://doi.org/10.1037/1076-8998.2.1.3

Quinn, R. P., & Shepard, L. D. (1974). *The 1972–73 Quality of Employment Survey: Descriptive statistics with comparison data from the 1969–70 Survey of Working Conditions.* University of Michigan. https://files.eric.ed.gov/fulltext/ED117414.pdf

Raymond, J. S., Wood, D. W., & Patrick, W. K. (1990). Psychology doctoral training in work and health. *American Psychologist, 45*(10), 1159–1161. https://doi.org/10.1037/0003-066X.45.10.1159

Sauter, S. L. (2006, March). *Conference welcome address.* Presented at "Work, Stress, and Health 2006—Making a Difference in the Workplace," Miami, FL, United States.

Sauter, S. L., & Hurrell, J. J., Jr. (1999). Occupational health psychology: Origins, content, and direction. *Professional Psychology: Research and Practice, 30*(2), 117–122. https://doi.org/10.1037/0735-7028.30.2.117

Sauter, S. L., & Hurrell, J. J., Jr. (2017). Occupational health contributions to the development and promise of occupational health psychology. *Journal of Occupational Health Psychology, 22*(3), 251–258. https://doi.org/10.1037/ocp0000088

Sauter, S. L., Hurrell, J. J., Jr., Fox, H. R., Tetrick, L. E., & Barling, J. (1999). Occupational health psychology: An emerging discipline. *Industrial Health, 37*(2), 199–211. https://doi.org/10.2486/indhealth.37.199

Sauter, S. L., Murphy, L. R., & Hurrell, J. J., Jr. (1990). Prevention of work-related psychological disorders: A national strategy proposed by the National Institute for Occupational Safety and Health (NIOSH). *American Psychologist, 45*(10), 1146–1158. https://doi.org/10.1037/0003-066X.45.10.1146

Schneider, D. L., Camara, W. J., Tetrick, L. E., & Sternberg, C. R. (1999). Training in occupational health psychology: Initial efforts and alternative models. *Professional Psychology: Research and Practice, 30*(2), 138–142. https://doi.org/10.1037/0735-7028.30.2.138

Schonfeld, I., & Chang, C. (2017). *Occupational health psychology.* Springer Publishing.

Sinclair, R. R. (2009, January). The future of OHP: The experts speak. *Society for Occupational Health Psychology Newsletter, 5*, 11–13. https://sohp-online.org/about/newsletter/sohpnewsletterv05-january2009/

Smith, M., Colligan, M., & Hurrell, J. J. Jr. (1980). A review of psychological stress research carried out by NIOSH, 1971–1976. In R. M. Schwartz (Ed.), *New developments in occupational stress* (Proceedings of a conference held in Los Angeles, CA, November 13, 1978; DHHS Publication No. 81-102, pp. 2–9). https://files.eric.ed.gov/fulltext/ED201822.pdf

Society for Occupational Health Psychology. (2017). *Field of OHP: What is occupational health psychology?* https://sohp-online.org/field-of-ohp/

Tetrick, L. E., & Quick, J. C. (2011). Overview of occupational health psychology: Public health in occupational settings. In J. C. Quick & L. E. Tetrick (Eds.), *Handbook of occupational health psychology* (2nd ed., pp. 3–20). American Psychological Association.

Ullrich, N. A., Lysaght, H., Erickson, K., Romero-Lazaro, M., & Zepeda, D. (2016, Fall). An international investigation of training in occupational health psychology. *Society for Occupational Health Psychology Newsletter, 16*, 9–10. https://sohp-online.org/about/newsletter/sohpnewsletterv16-fall2016/

Ullrich, N. A., Zepeda, D., Erickson, K., Lysaght, H., Romero-Lazaro, M., & Moberg, M. J. (2017, June). *International prevalence of coursework and training in occupational health psychology (OHP)* [Paper presentation]. Work, Stress, and Health 2017—Contemporary Challenges and Opportunities, Minneapolis, MN, United States.

U.S. Department of Health and Human Services Centers for Disease Control. (1992, June 15). Announcement number 246. Program announcement and availability of funds program guidance. Cooperative agreement for developing/implementing postdoctoral specialty training programs in occupational health psychology. *Federal Register, 57*, 26662.

U.S. Department of Health, Education, and Welfare. (1962). *Report of the committee on environmental health problems to the Surgeon General.* U.S. Government Printing Office.

U.S. Department of Health, Education, and Welfare. (1966). *Protecting the health of eighty million Americans: A national goal for occupational health.* U.S. Government Printing Office.

Vinchur, A. J., & Koppes, L. L. (2007). Early contributors to the science and practice of industrial psychology. In L. L. Koppes (Ed.), *Historical perspectives in industrial and organizational psychology* (pp. 37–58). Lawrence Erlbaum Associates Publishers.

Vinchur, A. J., & Koppes, L. L. (2011). A historical survey of research and practice in industrial and organizational psychology. In S. Zedeck (Ed.), *APA handbook of industrial and organizational psychology: Vol. 1. Building and developing the organization* (pp. 3–36). American Psychological Association. https://doi.org/10.1037/12169-001

Viteles, M. S. (1932). *Industrial psychology.* W. W. Norton & Co.

Westlander, G. (1994). Training of psychologists in occupational health work: Ten years of course development—Experience and future perspectives. *European Work and Organizational Psychology, 4*(2), 189–202. https://doi.org/10.1080/13594329408410483

Work in America. (1973). *Work in America, report of a special task force to the Secretary of Health, Education, and Welfare.* MIT Press.

II

MODELS AND FRAMEWORKS

INTRODUCTION: MODELS AND FRAMEWORKS

Part II of this handbook covers basic theoretical approaches and models for core areas of occupational health psychology (OHP). The purpose of Part II is to discuss fundamental constructs, processes, theories, and methods for understanding stress, well-being, safety, and the work–family interface. Chapter 3 reviews fundamental theories of stress, covering concepts such as the fight-or-flight response, the allostatic load model, and the transactional model of stress. The chapter then discusses theories specific to occupational stress, including conservation of resource theory, the effort–reward imbalance model, the job demand–control and job demands–resources models, and the person–environment fit approach. Chapter 4 expands upon Chapter 3 by delving into distinctions between eustress and distress and the ways they are managed and studied. Shifting gears, Chapter 5 describes the causes of occupational accidents alongside frameworks and methods for measuring and controlling hazards and promoting safe behavior. Chapter 5 also describes the Systems Engineering Initiative for Patient Safety, a systems approach to occupational safety and health, and applies this approach to key examples. Chapter 6 moves from the individual to the organizational level to discuss organizational wellness, describing themes and trends in organizational well-being, key competencies for OHP practice, and OHP's interface with other business functions. Chapter 7 reviews the latest in theory on the work–nonwork interface and presents an integrative model of work–nonwork balance that incorporates strain and motivation pathways through which demands and resources spill over across life domains. Finally, Chapter 8 reviews cross-cultural research on occupational stress, safety, and the work–family interface, assessing the generalizability of many of OHP's core findings.

Collectively, the chapters in Part II address concepts and areas that recur in more specific forms throughout this handbook. For example, Chapter 7 covers theory on the work–nonwork interface, whereas Chapter 26 discusses research on work–family policies, practices, and interventions, which are not covered in Chapter 7. Chapter 3 addresses basic theories of stress that also come up in later chapters on stress, well-being, and health (e.g., Chapters 16 and 19). Chapter 5 focuses on some issues in occupational safety that are discussed in more detail in later chapters (e.g., Chapter 17). The concept of job crafting is discussed in Chapter 4, and it comes up again in Chapter 15 when discussing job burnout. The purpose of Part II is to introduce some of the theories, frameworks, and concepts most fundamental to OHP, whereas chapters in later sections apply and discuss many of these issues as they relate to more specific antecedents, outcomes, and contexts.

3

Examining the Dynamics of Major Theories of Occupational Stress

Pamela L. Perrewé and Charn P. McAllister

In this chapter, we review the work stress theories that have had the most prominent impact on the field of work and occupational health psychology (OHP). The importance of theories should not be underestimated, as they provide thoughtful and insightful explanations for the relationships among phenomena. In general, *theories* are broadly accepted principles that explain why and how different variables and concepts relate to one another. Theories are particularly important to the study of occupational stress because they can provide explanations of how and why occupational stressors, experienced stress, and health are linked together.

We begin with a review of basic stress theory from the physiology literature, as this work provides the conceptual substrate for most of the work-based theory and research in OHP. In this realm of basic research, the allostatic load model (McEwen, 1998) has taken center stage and represents the latest in an evolution of models proposed by Cannon (1932) and Selye (1955). Our review provides a brief overview of this model and its related research as a backdrop to occupationally based research. We then discuss some of the more influential job stress theories, including the transactional model (Lazarus, 1966), demand–control model (Karasek, 1979), and job demands–resources model (Demerouti et al., 2001), conservation of resources theory (Hobfoll, 1989), challenge and hindrance stressors, and the person–environment fit approach.

The authors would like to thank Daniel C. Ganster for his work on an earlier draft of this chapter.

https://doi.org/10.1037/0000331-003
Handbook of Occupational Health Psychology, Third Edition, L. E. Tetrick, G. G. Fisher, M. T. Ford, and J. C. Quick (Editors)

BASIC CONCEPTUALIZATIONS OF STRESS AND PHYSIOLOGY

The concept of homeostasis—the body maintaining steady states in various physiological systems—has been at the core of explanations for how individuals react to environmental demands. According to Cannon (1932), experienced stress results from an external environmental demand that was disturbing to individuals' natural homeostatic balance. Cannon's early writings provided the groundwork for the *fight-or-flight response* and thus presented experienced stress as a survival response to environmental threats. When confronted with an environmental demand (e.g., threat), the fundamental decision that individuals must make is to either defend against it (i.e., fight) or to flee from it (i.e., flight). This conceptualization placed stress within a reactive stimulus–response framework and emphasized the importance of outside demands external to the person. Upon the removal or defeat of the perceived threat, the autonomic system should recover and eventually return to normal. However, when individuals cannot overcome a perceived threat, they are likely to experience chronic stress and the recovery process may not occur, leading to deleterious health outcomes.

Selye (1955) conceptualized the stress experience as a process of adaptation, which he termed the *general adaptation syndrome* (GAS). His initial inspiration for the GAS came from a series of endocrinology experiments in which he injected mice with extracts of various organs to discover a new hormone. Initial results suggested support for a new hormone; the first injection resulted in several physical changes to the rats. Yet, with each new extract he introduced, including a toxic substance now classified as a stressor agent, the mice experienced the same physiological changes. This discovery, paired with his observation that people with different diseases exhibited similar symptoms, led to his description of how the body physiologically reacts to the introduction of "noxious agents." He later termed this response as *stress*, a term now accepted into the lexicon of languages around the world.

Selye (1955) argued that the human body goes through three stages (i.e., GAS) when confronted with an intense demand. The first stage is the alarm reaction, characterized by hormonal changes in the body (i.e., production of cortisol and adrenaline), analogous to Cannon's fight-or-flight response. The resistance stage follows and represents the body's attempts to diminish the effects of the changes brought about during the alert stage. However, prolonged exposure to a stressor can inhibit this return to normal, and exhaustion begins to set in. Selye argued that because the adaptability of an organism is finite, this last stage would lead to death unless there was some aid from an outside source.

Selye (1955) recognized and argued that stress is the nonspecific response of the body to a demand, regardless of whether the demand results in pleasant or unpleasant conditions. When demands result in unpleasant conditions, people experience *distress*; when demands result in pleasant conditions, people experience *eustress*. Although eustress is positive, it does often cause physiological reactions similar to distress because the hormones released are the same for both forms of stress; yet it is important to note that most of the damage occurs when individuals are under distress rather than eustress (Selye, 1974). Selye's nonspecific, or stereotyped, model of responses to stress has been challenged by subsequent research that demonstrated a great variety in physiological responses depending on the different cues and situations facing the individual (Goldstein & Eisenhofer, 2000).

Allostatic Load Model

Despite the groundbreaking work of Cannon and Selye, physiologists have rejected the notion of homeostasis as a universal physiological imperative. The initial thinking that the body maintains homeostasis—a stable internal environment—through predictable physiological reactions to external factors was deemed too simple and not illustrative of the body's actual function. There are certain physiological systems, like blood oxygen levels, that require the body to maintain relevant values within a very narrow range (i.e., homeostasis). However, most physiological systems (e.g., immune, cardiovascular) operate within a wide range of acceptable levels that vary with any number of internal and external demands (McEwen, 1998). Thus, it is not surprising that just as organisms exhibit a broad range of physical responses to demands, they also exhibit a broad range of behavioral responses. This more permissive, wide range of responses moved stress research away from the homeostatic models and toward those based on allostasis.

The concept of allostasis was first proposed by Sterling and Eyer (1988). Frequently described as "stability through change," *allostasis* refers to physiological response systems that supplement the basic homeostatic systems and respond to environmental demands and anticipated demands (Sterling, 2012). Whereas such systems, such as the hypothalamic–pituitary–adrenal (HPA) axis, operate around certain set points, some of which are subject to diurnal or even seasonal rhythms, these set points can also be reset after exposure to chronic demands that continually push them beyond their normal ranges. Another important distinction of the allostasis model is the critical role played by the central nervous system, which controls physiological reactions, often directly, by using prior knowledge and experience in conjunction with environmental events, to anticipate the need for adaptation. The transactional model, discussed later, is entirely consistent with this allostatic perspective.

Allostasis, then, refers to the process of adjustment of various effector systems (cardiovascular, neuroendocrine, and others) to cope with real or imagined challenges to homeostatic systems (Goldstein & McEwen, 2002). *Allostatic state* refers to a chronic overactivation of allostatic regulatory systems and the alteration of set points. Finally, *allostatic load* refers to various symptoms of pathology caused by a chronic allostatic state. This perspective highlights two points that are especially salient to work stress and health. First, unlike in Selye's (1955) model, which defines stress as a nonspecific response of the body (primarily the HPA axis) to challenge a threat, the allostasis model allows for a greater diversity of physiological responses. Often, multiple effectors are used to control values for a given homeostatic variable. For example, insulin, adrenaline, cortisol, glucagon, and growth hormones can affect blood glucose levels. This is an example of the diversity of responses that the body can make to correct perturbations in internal homeostatic systems. Similarly, there can be a variety of different physiological responses to environmental demands. This variety of allostatic mechanisms makes stress research more complicated because it argues against a simple reliance on single indicators. Likewise, the operationalization of allostatic load, which is a pathological state caused by chronic stress, also requires a consideration of different indicators. Singer and colleagues (2004) provided a detailed review of allostatic load measurement models. The criteria for assessing operationalizations of allostatic load ultimately depend on their value as risk factors that presage morbidity and mortality.

A second implication of the allostatic load model comes from the key role that the central nervous system plays in orchestrating the array of allostatic responses and in initially triggering these responses. Compared to Selye's perspective, the allostasis model very much stresses the mind–body connection in the stress process. For stress researchers this means, of course, that many of the stressors of interest in the workplace, and probably all of the psychosocial ones, exert their effects on the body through cognitive processing. Compared with earlier conceptualizations of homeostasis, the allostatic perspective views the individual (human or otherwise) not solely as a reactive organism but as one who perceives aspects of the environment and initiates allostatic responses in *anticipation* of predicted needs. This perspective is very much in accordance with the transactional model of stress as developed by Lazarus (1966).

Transactional Model

One of the most popular frameworks for understanding psychosocial stress remains the transactional model (Folkman & Lazarus, 1990; Lazarus, 1966), which suggests that stress stems from the person or the environment as well as the interaction between the two. The transactional model views stressors subjectively, meaning that what is stressful to one individual may not be stressful to another. Stress is therefore cognitively determined. Lazarus was more concerned about the appraisal and cognitive components of stress as opposed to the medical and physiological approaches of earlier researchers. Like Cannon and Selye, Lazarus saw experienced stress as a response to an environmental demand; however, Lazarus emphasized the person's cognitive *appraisal* of events. The primary role of cognition (i.e., the central nervous system) in the stress process bridges the allostatic and transactional models. Curiously, the allostatic model developed in the biological literature seems to have evolved independently of the transactional model in psychology. Lazarus's work is rarely cited in the former.

Based on Lazarus's (1991) belief in the primacy of cognition, the transactional model posits that two processes (i.e., cognitive appraisal and coping) mediate between environmental stressors and resulting responses. According to the model, an event in the work environment engages the cognitive appraisal process: the *primary* appraisal. This consists of an evaluation of whether the event is a threat to individuals' well-being or whether they can dismiss it as benign or perhaps challenging. If the primary appraisal results in the individual perceiving the event as a threat to their well-being, the *secondary* appraisal process is engaged to determine whether they can do anything to handle (i.e., cope with) the situation. In this secondary appraisal stage, individuals evaluate their available options for coping with the stressor. An individual may use either *emotion-focused* or *problem-focused* coping (Lazarus & Folkman, 1984). Emotion-focused coping occurs when individuals believe they cannot ameliorate the source of stressor; this results in a more internally focused attempt at coping (e.g., meditation) to help alleviate the negative effects of the situation on their well-being. If they deem the stressor controllable, the model predicts that individuals engage in problem-focused coping, whereby they attempt to alter the stressor itself.

Sterling (2004), of the biological allostasis position, might refer to emotion-focused coping as analogous to intervening at the level of physiological perturbation of homeostatic systems. An analogy from the medical perspective would be the different ways to intervene to control hypertension or chronically elevated blood pressure. Treating hypertension at the low level of homeostasis involves the use of drugs such as diuretics to reduce blood volume or heart rate antagonists to reduce cardiac output. Alternatively, problem-focused interventions at a higher level involve modifying the environmental demands that triggered the allostatic load (expressed as hypertension) in the first place. In the work stress domain, this distinction is analogous to the difference between intervention approaches (e.g., through mindfulness, taking stock of one's feelings, or expressing emotions: see Eatough & Chang, 2018, cognitive behavior modification, or relaxation) aimed at helping stressed individuals deal with their stress symptoms and those aimed at changing the characteristics of the work environment that are driving the allostatic state (e.g., through job crafting: see Bruning & Campion, 2018).

The transactional model is not without its critics. In a published academic debate, Zajonc (1984) refuted Lazarus's belief that cognitive processes were necessary for affective processes to occur, arguing instead that affect often occurs without any temporally antecedent cognitive processing. This might also occur for gradual threats to health. For example, some stressors in the workplace, such as rotating shift schedules, might affect stress responses with no significant cognitive mediation. Although the transactional approach is still a prominent theoretical approach to psychosocial stress, it does not enumerate specific workplace events or characteristics that are apt to be interpreted as stressors. Explaining the conditions of work that produce stress responses is the province of occupational stress theories.

OCCUPATIONAL STRESS THEORIES

Work contexts and the people within those contexts are anything but static. It follows then that stressors experienced in the workplace vary greatly and can manifest in a multitude of ways. Thus, at the heart of work stress research is a series of robust, flexible theories that can be leveraged to assess and provide recommendations to ameliorate workplace stressors. The following represents an overview of the most important work stress theories.

Conservation of Resources Theory

According to the conservation of resources theory (COR), *resources* are the objects, energies, personal characteristics, and conditions that are valued by the individual or that assist the individual in obtaining these resources. Hobfoll (1989) argued that stress results from an actual or threatened net loss of resources, or from a lack of resource gain following the investment of resources. The theory posits that the effects of stressful situations may be buffered or attenuated if the individual perceives that he or she has the resources to cope with the stressor. Like the transactional model, the COR model views control, or the ability to cope, in subjective terms.

COR theory proposes that experienced stress is most likely to occur when there is a perceived resource loss. More directly, it posits four primary resource categories. Resources can be (a) object or material resources, such as cars or homes; (b) conditional or environmental resources, such as socioeconomic status or being valued at work; (c) personal or individual resources, such as self-efficacy and self-esteem; and (d) energy resources, such as time and money. These are resources that are valued by individuals and that serve to meet their goals. Thus, situations can become stressful to the extent that they threaten or result in the actual loss of critical resources (Treadway et al., 2005).

Perceived resource losses can come from numerous sources. Specifically, a resource loss can be an actual loss or simply a perceived threat of a loss of resources. Further, perceived resource losses can include a work situation in which individuals perceive they do not have adequate resources to meet their work demands (e.g., quantitative or qualitative overload) or when individuals invest a lot of their own resources and do not believe their returns on these investments will be realized (Hobfoll, 1989, 2001). Specifically, COR theory states that individual resources are needed and used to meet demands; experienced stress occurs when there is a resource loss and when events create demands that outstrip individual resources.

Negative conditions within the workplace, such as abusive supervision or perceptions of organizational politics, may threaten or reduce employee personal resources, such as self-esteem and workplace status. Importantly, research suggests that the loss of resources can be cumulative (Hobfoll, 2001). After initial resource losses, fewer resources are available to individuals to resist stress. In essence, these losses can lead to individuals becoming less resilient and more vulnerable to stressors.

Hobfoll and Shirom (2000) offered four corollaries of the COR theory. First, individuals must already have resources to prevent a loss of resources. Second, individuals with greater resources are more capable of gaining resources and less susceptible to losing resources. Third, individuals who do not have strong resources are more likely to experience increased resource losses because initial losses lead to more losses down the road. Finally, individuals with strong resources are more likely to seek opportunities to risk resources for increased resource gains.

Hobfoll (2001) connected these corollaries to workplace stress research. He argued that factors such as individual optimism, self-efficacy, and self-esteem should be considered as resources in reducing stress. Specifically, Hobfoll and Shirom (2000) argued that personality traits that made individuals more resilient and that led to feelings of control over their environment seemed to buffer these individuals from experienced stress. Finally, previous research has used the COR theory as a potential explanation for the job stress–performance linkage. More directly, emotional exhaustion represents a condition in which employees are drained of resources (Wright & Cropanzano, 1998). Thus, the authors argued that emotionally exhausted individuals are unable to gather the personal resources needed to resist organizational stressors and maintain their performance.

COR theory has influenced work stress research primarily in the areas of burnout (e.g., De Cuyper et al., 2012), work–family conflict (Che et al., 2017), and respites from work (e.g., vacations; Sonnentag & Fritz, 2007). A review by Westman et al. (2005) concluded that studies in these areas demonstrate the utility of the COR conceptualization of stress in terms of resource losses and gains. It is unclear, however, whether the tenets of COR theory provide a superior explanation for the results in many of these studies. Even though much of the research utilizing COR theory identifies relationships between strain outcomes and various demands, it does not effectively demonstrate that COR theory makes different predictions from those made by other models, or that it can account for empirical results that other conceptualizations cannot. What distinguishes COR theory from most other approaches to work stress are propositions such as (a) "resource loss is disproportionately more salient than resource gain" (Westman et al., 2005, p. 169), and (b) resource losses will trigger loss spirals. Elaborating on the loss spiral prediction, Westman et al. (2005) described it as "a critical aspect of the theory, because it predicts that loss cycles will occur quickly and powerfully. Further, at each iteration of loss in the sequence, the cycle will gain in strength and momentum" (p. 169). The theoretical strength of these propositions is that their specificity enhances the falsifiability of the model. But the model can also be criticized for its lack of specificity in enumerating what constitutes a resource; for whereas COR theory lays out broad categories of resources such as *objects, conditions, personal characteristics,* and *energies,* it is conceivable that almost any positive construct in the context of the work environment could be considered a resource. This lack of specificity renders the model less falsifiable. The critical research needed to test the COR model in the work setting must overcome the challenge of defining resources in an a priori way such that the theoretical propositions can be falsified. Such specificity will allow researchers to critically test the central propositions of loss versus gain salience and loss spirals. To adequately test these propositions, moreover, longitudinal designs—in which investigators can capture both gains and losses of resources over multiple measurement occasions—are needed.

Effort–Reward Imbalance Theory

The model of effort–reward imbalance (ERI) at work is derived from a more general approach toward examining the psychosocial dimension of human health and well-being. Siegrist (2001, 2002) proposed that personal self-regulation is important for health and well-being in adult life and that this well-being is largely contingent on experiencing or perceiving social exchanges at work and at home as balanced or successful. The ERI approach focuses on social reciprocity and is characterized by mutual cooperative investments based on the norm of return expectancy. More succinctly, individuals' efforts are balanced by the anticipated rewards they will gain in return. Thus, failed reciprocity (i.e., high efforts spent and low rewards received) is likely to elicit recurrent negative emotions and sustained stress responses in exposed individuals because it threatens the fundamental reciprocity and exchange principle. Conversely, positive emotions evoked by appropriate social rewards and exchanges promote well-being, health, and survival.

The ERI model maintains that availability of a work role is associated with recurrent options of contributing and of performing as well as of being rewarded and of belonging to some meaningful group (e.g., work colleagues). Yet these potentially beneficial effects are contingent on a basic prerequisite of exchange (i.e., reciprocity). Effort at work is part of a socially organized exchange process to which society contributes in terms of rewards. Rewards are distributed by three systems: money, esteem, and career opportunities. The ERI model claims that lack of reciprocity between the costs and gains (i.e., high-cost/low-gain conditions) elicits negative emotions with a propensity to sustained autonomic and neuroendocrine activation (Siegrist, 1996).

The following three hypotheses are derived from the ERI model. First, an imbalance between effort and reward (i.e., nonreciprocity) increases the risk of reduced health over and above the risk associated with each one of the components. Second, overcommitted people are at increased risk of reduced health, regardless of whether work characteristics reinforce this pattern of coping. Third, the relatively highest risks of reduced health are expected in people characterized by the first and second conditions. Imbalances often results from the fact that the social exchange between employee and employer is based on an incomplete contract. In incomplete contracts, both parties make assumptions of trust regarding mutual commitments. However, under certain conditions it is likely that incomplete contracts result in high-cost/low-gain conditions for employees. The risk of nonreciprocity in exchange is particularly high if employees have no other reasonable options in the labor market. Further, if employees' skills are poor or if they subscribe to short-term contracts, nonreciprocity may occur.

Employees themselves may also contribute to high-cost/low-gain conditions at work, either intentionally or unintentionally. For example, for a short period and for strategic reasons, they may accept job assignments that are considered unfair, as they tend to improve their opportunities for career promotion or other rewards later. Finally, there are psychological reasons for a continued mismatch between efforts and rewards at work. People characterized by a motivational pattern of excessive overcommitment to work and a high need for approval may incorrectly assess the perceived demands facing them as well as the coping resources needed more often than their less-involved colleagues (Siegrist, 1996, 2002). Perceptual distortion prevents the overcommitted individuals from accurately assessing cost–gain relations. Therefore, they underestimate the demands and overestimate their own coping resources while not being aware of the actual value of their own contribution to nonreciprocal exchange. In summary, the ERI model is based on the sociological hypothesis that structured social exchange, as mediated through core work roles, is rooted in contracts of reciprocity. In addition to its importance to basic social functioning, this reciprocal contractual exchange has been shown to produce beneficial effects for individual health and well-being (Griep et al., 2020; Siegrist & Li, 2017).

Job Demand–Control Model

The job demands–resources model began with the demand–control model of job stress introduced by Karasek (1979) about 45 years ago, and it has had a dominant role in shaping the research agenda within the fields of work stress and health. Unlike earlier models, the *demand–control model* can be classified as a content model because it specifies the job characteristics that are thought to be the primary stressors in the workplace. The model conceptualizes *demands* as the task requirements at work and includes issues such as role conflict and time pressure (Karasek & Theorell, 1990). The *control* (i.e., decision latitude) portion of the model includes both workers' authority to make decisions and the breadth of skills they can employ (Verhoeven et al., 2003). Based on the dimensions of demands and control, Karasek (1979) posited four types of job situations: low strain, high strain, passive, and active. Workers experience *low strain* when control is high and demands are low; they experience *high strain* when control is low and demands are high. Similarly, low demands and control result in a *passive* job, whereas both high control and demands results in an *active* job.

In an update to the original model, Karasek and Theorell (1990) proposed the demand–control-support model, adding the component of social support as another critical factor in determining responses to job demands. Several researchers tested the moderating effects of social support in the job demand-control (JDC) model. However, although the demand–control-social support conceptualization demonstrated relationships with strain outcomes, only modest support has been found for the buffering effect of control, at most demonstrating that in order for control to have a buffering effect, it needs to correspond to the types of demands placed on the individual (Van der Doef & Maes, 1998, 1999). Concerning the strain hypothesis of the JDC model, some researchers have suggested that the effects of demands and control could be either additive or interactive, and that more research to date supports an additive rather than interactive model (Turner et al., 2005). Relatively little research has been conducted regarding the *activity-level* hypothesis; however, some evidence suggests that high control promotes learning and that high demands are harmful to these same outcomes (Taris et al., 2003). Furthermore, the demand–control-support model has been criticized by some researchers (e.g., Verhoeven et al., 2003) as being too simplistic for explanations of individual health and well-being, at least for certain populations.

Research suggests that the mixed results found by the JDC model indicate the importance of individual difference variables. Schaubroeck and Merritt (1997) found that individuals with high self-efficacy benefited from increased control, whereas those with low self-efficacy did not. Similarly, the results of another study (de Rijk et al., 1998) indicated that individuals high in active coping benefited from greater control, but those low in active coping were more likely to suffer burnout from increased control. In addition, Parker and Sprigg (1999) found general support for both the strain and learning (active) aspects of the demand–control model for those high in proactive personality.

Like any theory, the demand–control model also has critics. For example, Taris (2006) discussed the limited research support for the interaction of job demands and decision latitude. Although researchers generally find that high job demands and low decision latitude independently predict strain, studies on the interaction of the two are not always supportive. Specifically, Taris argued that although the variables of demands and control are effective predictors of work stress and poor health, this does not mean that the statistical interaction between demands and control affects stress and health. Further, Taris contended that the assumptions about the curvilinear relations among job demands, control, and social support to employee health have not been well documented.

Perhaps the greatest contribution of the demand–control model has been its heuristic value for the field of stress research. It clearly has stimulated a large body of research and importantly, has had a significant influence on the thinking and research of those in epidemiology and medicine. The demand–control model should also be credited with bringing the construct of control, which has been so fundamental to psychology, to the forefront in work stress research.

Job Demands–Resources Model

One of the most comprehensive approaches based on job-demands models is the job demands–resources (JD-R) model (Demerouti et al., 2001). The JD-R model elegantly classifies all job characteristics as either job demands or job resources (Bakker & Demerouti, 2017). Although the various job demands first noted by Karasek (1979) and expanded upon by later research remain, the JD-R model defines *resources* more broadly, thus allowing it to subsume both control and social support under this umbrella, while also including a host of varied job characteristics. By drawing a single bright line between job demands and resources, the model itself proves more versatile than previous demand–control iterations. As such, the JD-R model is flexible and expansive, capable of providing context for any number of stressors and resources that individuals may experience in the workplace.

At its most basic level, the JD-R model assumes experienced job stress occurs when job demands are high; however, motivation occurs when resources are high (Demerouti et al., 2001). As in earlier models, resources neutralize the negative effects (e.g., experienced stress) of job demands (Bakker et al., 2007). Of note is that resources include traditional job-based resources (e.g., autonomy) in addition to personal resources such as optimism and self-efficacy. This nuance paved the way for extensive research into how personal resources can affect experienced stress in the workplace and provided additional context for why certain individuals may cope with certain job demands better than their colleagues.

This perspective—that employees can experience the same job demands present in their workplace differently than their colleagues—enshrines the agency of individuals. Job demands are not a monolith, and individuals retain the ability to combat or cope with them as they see fit. Likewise, rather than solely being reactive to the environment, the JD-R model assumes that individuals can be *proactive* when anticipating job demands and marshaling resources (Bakker et al., 2007). For example, JD-R demonstrates that individuals often will engage in *job crafting* (Wrzesniewski & Dutton, 2001) to improve their work experience (Demerouti et al., 2015). The result of behaviors like job crafting is that individuals who proactively work to make their job demands more challenging than stressful while simultaneously working to increase their resources experience *gain spirals;* these spirals manifest as reduced stress and increased work outcomes such as engagement. However, the inverse is also true: Those individuals who are overburdened with job demands and bereft of the resources to cope with them are likely to experience *loss spirals.*

Interestingly, there are also approaches to examining the pros and cons of organizational stressors, and researchers have distinguished between challenge and hindrance stressors. *Challenge stressors* are job demands such as job scope, responsibility, and workload; *hindrance stressors* are those job demands such as organizational politics, role conflict, role ambiguity, resource inadequacy, and job insecurity (LePine et al., 2005). In general, challenge stressors are associated positively with motivation and performance, whereas hindrance stressors are associated negatively with motivation and performance. Although both challenge and hindrance stressors can be strain provoking, challenge stressors create high-performance opportunities and feelings of accomplishment, while hindrance stressors interfere with the attainment of personal goals, leading to a lack of feelings of accomplishment (Webster et al., 2011). In an interesting "point–counterpoint" research debate, O'Brien and Beehr (2019) argued that the distinction between challenge and hindrance stressors can provide an interesting framework from which to examine organizational stressors and should give impetus to invaluable and innovative stress research programs. However, other researchers (e.g., Mazzola & Disselhorst, 2019) have argued that there are limited organizational variables from which challenge and hindrance stressors make differential predictions. Thus, it seems clear that additional research is needed to make more specific recommendations regarding the usefulness of this model in organizational research.

Person–Environment Fit Approach

The idea that the psychological outcomes that workers experience stem from the degree of correspondence between their personal characteristics and the outcomes and demands of their jobs has been central in the work psychology literature for at least 50 years (e.g., Lofquist & Dawis, 1969). Caplan and colleagues (1975) elaborated and operationalized the person–environment (P-E) fit model in the field of job stress and conducted much of the early research testing. The *P-E fit model* theorizes that the stressfulness (or strain) experienced at work is caused by a lack of fit between (a) outcomes provided by the job and the needs, motives, and preferences of the worker, and (b) the requirements of the job and the skills and abilities of the worker. Some large-scale tests of the P-E fit model have been conducted, including the study of 23 occupations by Caplan et al. (1975). In his review of this literature, Harrison (1985) concluded that fit scores, generally operationalized as the differences between self-reported E and P components, often, but not always, predicted strain outcomes better than did the components themselves.

The evidence supporting P-E fit theory has been subjected to some significant criticism. Edwards and Cooper (1990), for example, articulated four major shortcomings of this research. First, researchers generally did not specify their models in terms of how the two types of fit related to different kinds of outcomes. Second, there are theoretically distinct mathematical forms of fit, including discrepancy, interactive, and proportional models, but investigators failed to statistically model these different forms. Third, researchers often used inappropriate measures of the P and E components and relied exclusively on self-report approaches. Finally, statistical models of fit most often relied on simple difference score measures that yielded mostly uninterpretable results. Later work by Edwards (1995) addressed the statistical problems arising from the use of difference scores to assess fit and proposed polynomial regression in addition to response surface analysis strategies for testing theoretically specified fit models. Edwards's critique of the use of difference scores, generally, calls into question most of the P-E fit findings reported in the work stress literature.

Although P-E fit theory addressed the phenomenon of stress in the workplace, the theory itself does not necessarily specify the components of the person and the work environment that should be most salient. In this sense it is a process theory, much as Lazarus and Folkman's (1984) more general transactional model, and it does not enumerate those features of the work environment that should be the key constructs generating a stress response. Most investigators of P-E fit have used the same small set of eight components used in Caplan and colleagues' (1975) study. The P-E fit model has played a much less prominent role in the work stress and health literature in recent years, although the basic notion of fit undergirds, at least implicitly, many conceptualizations of stress in the workplace. Upcoming research in this area will almost certainly be affected by the COVID-19 pandemic. A renewed focus on how changing or evolving work environments result in employees becoming misfits is of the utmost importance—particularly after workers around the globe found themselves in the same job but in quite different environments.

SUMMARY AND SUGGESTIONS FOR FUTURE RESEARCH

Each of the work stress models discussed in this chapter contributes unique perspectives to the understanding of the role of work experiences on health and general well-being. However, they are not competing theories, and efforts to pit them against one another in critical experiments are unlikely to be successful. Each of these stress theories has played an important heuristic function in the field of work stress. Even though they represent complementary rather than competing approaches, each has stimulated a line of investigation into factors that predict health outcomes that might have otherwise been neglected. We encourage investigators to continue to combine elements of the different models in prospective studies of work stress and well-being (e.g., Trougakos et al., 2020), while expanding their research strategy to better incorporate both measures of the objective environment and physiological measures of the allostatic state.

We also need to further develop ways of measuring the allostasis process in the context of work stress, for this is the process that is generally theorized to intervene between the workplace conditions described by work stress theories and the health outcomes that they are hypothesized to cause. It is unlikely that investigators studying work stress and health can make strong causal inferences, based on experimental interventions, regarding the effects of work stressors on health, or even on the allostatic load markers that are predictive of health outcomes. Disease endpoints, at least those believed to be related to psychosocial stress, generally develop slowly, reflecting chronic exposures to allostatic states that may span years. It is difficult to relate work stressors to such endpoints in prospective designs that have high internal validity because exposure to stressors can vary significantly over the years of the study. Linking stressors to health outcomes in experimental intervention studies is virtually impossible for much the same reason: The integrity of the experimental design would need to be maintained for perhaps years. Thus, a focus on the relatively short-term markers of the allostatic state holds much promise for bridging this gap.

Research is also needed to examine the physical and psychological effects of work stress on the individual and their family outside of work. Research is just now beginning to examine how one's personality may change because of experienced workplace stress (Smallfield & Kluemper, 2022)—a line of research that, if supported, will represent a massive shift in our understanding of the long-term implications of experiencing stress at work. In terms of the family, although much has been written about the spillover effects from work to home and home to life (e.g., Leiter & Durup, 1996) as well as the crossover effects from one person to another (e.g., Westman, 2001), less is known about the effects of work stress on family members besides the spouse. Recently, researchers examined the effect of perceived pregnancy discrimination on the health and well-being of pregnant mothers and their children (Hackney et al., 2021). The authors found that perceptions of pregnancy discrimination led to perceived stress, which led to increased levels of postpartum depressive symptoms for the mothers as well as lower birth weights, lower gestational ages, and increased number of doctors' visits for the babies. We feel these findings are important as they highlight the effects that workplace stress can have not only on the employee and the spouse but on the entire family.

Another promising area of workplace stress research involves the examination of self-regulation. Defined as "the capacity for altering one's own responses, especially to bring them into line with standards such as ideals, values, morals, and social expectations, and to support the pursuit of long-term goals" (Baumeister et al., 2007, 351), *self-regulation* has remained a mostly overlooked variable with the workplace stress literature. Recent findings focus primarily on state self-regulation (e.g., willpower) and the role that workplace stressors play in depleting individuals' stores of self-regulatory resources. For example, employees perceiving their supervisors as abusive are likely going to lose self-regulatory resources and be more likely to retaliate (Lian et al., 2014). Additional findings suggest the more nuanced role that trait self-regulation plays in the workplace stress process. Consider how self-regulation relates to lashing out in retaliation against an abusive supervisor: Those with high levels of trait self-regulation should be better at holding their tongue. As such, it follows that these same people who excel at self-regulating are likely to experience increased levels of job tension (McAllister et al., 2018). One explanation for this finding is that these excellent self-regulators never reach that moment of catharsis (even if temporary) that comes with speaking their mind, instead choosing to keep their feelings bottled up. Self-regulation is a variable worthy of future investigation because it can be explored as a stand-alone mechanism affecting experienced stress, or it can be paired with existing theories of stress (e.g., Bakker & de Vries, 2021) to provide additional context to the work stress process.

CONCLUSION

In conclusion, we have reviewed the work stress theories that have had the most prominent effect on the field of work and OHP. We began with a review of early stress theories from the physiology literature and then examined some of the most influential stress theories, namely, the allostatic load model (McEwen, 1998), the transactional model (Lazarus, 1966), the demand–control model (Karasek, 1979), the job-resources model (Demerouti et al., 2001), COR theory (Hobfoll, 1989), challenge and hindrance stressors (LePine et al., 2005), and the P-E fit approach (Lofquist & Dawis, 1969). We also updated this earlier literature and highlighted the more recent research on occupational stress that utilized these theories as the backdrop. The theories we reviewed here have all had a significant impact on the course of work stress research.

It is important to understand that although these theories may focus on different concepts and terms, they are more alike than they are different. Rather than offering competing perspectives, we view them more as complementary approaches, such as the model presented in Mackey and Perrewé (2014). Their model is an integrative conceptualization of occupational stress that combines research from multiple models and theories. We must account for the complexities that ensue when employees experience organizational demands. Utilizing a multitheory approach might be the best way to better understand the complexities stemming from occupational stress. It is unlikely that one or the other of the theories will "win out" over the others from head-to-head empirical competition. But we believe that our understanding of how work experiences affect health and well-being will be advanced by combining elements of these theories in more comprehensive examinations of working conditions and health.

REFERENCES

Bakker, A. B., & de Vries, J. D. (2021). Job demands–resources theory and self-regulation: New explanations and remedies for job burnout. *Anxiety, Stress, and Coping, 34*(1), 1–21. https://doi.org/10.1080/10615806.2020.1797695

Bakker, A. B., & Demerouti, E. (2017). Job demands–resources theory: Taking stock and looking forward. *Journal of Occupational Health Psychology, 22*(3), 273–285. https://doi.org/10.1037/ocp0000056

Bakker, A. B., Hakanen, J. J., Demerouti, E., & Xanthopoulou, D. (2007). Job resources boost work engagement, particularly when job demands are high. *Journal of Educational Psychology, 99*(2), 274–284. https://doi.org/10.1037/0022-0663.99.2.274

Baumeister, R. F., Vohs, K. D., & Tice, D. M. (2007). The strength model of self-control. *Current Directions in Psychological Science, 16*(6), 351–355. https://doi.org/10.1111/j.1467-8721.2007.00534.x

Bruning, P. F., & Campion, M. A. (2018). A role–resource approach–avoidance model of job crafting: A multimethod integration and extension of job crafting theory. *Academy of Management Journal, 61*(2), 499–522. https://doi.org/10.5465/amj.2015.0604

Cannon, W. B. (1932). *The wisdom of the body* (2nd ed.). Norton. https://doi.org/10.1097/00000441-193212000-00028

Caplan, R. D., Cobb, S., French, J. R. P., Harrison, R. V., & Pinneau, S. R. (1975). Job demands and worker health (Pub. No. 75-158). National Institute for Occupational Safety and Health.

Che, X. X., Zhiqing, Z. E., Kessler, S. R., & Spector, P. E. (2017). Stressors beget stressors: The effect of passive leadership on employee health through workload and work–family conflict. *Work and Stress, 31*(4), 338–354. https://doi.org/10.1080/02678373.2017.1317881

De Cuyper, N., Raeder, S., Van der Heijden, B. I. J. M., & Wittekind, A. (2012). The association between workers' employability and burnout in a reorganization context: Longitudinal evidence building upon the conservation of resources theory. *Journal of Occupational Health Psychology, 17*(2), 162–174. https://doi.org/10.1037/a0027348

de Rijk, A. E., Le Blanc, P. M., Schaufeli, W. B., & de Jonge, J. (1998). Active coping and need for control as moderators of the job demand–control model: Effects on burnout. *Journal of Occupational and Organizational Psychology, 71*(1), 1–18. https://doi.org/10.1111/j.2044-8325.1998.tb00658.x

Demerouti, E., Bakker, A. B., & Halbesleben, J. R. B. (2015). Productive and counterproductive job crafting: A daily diary study. *Journal of Occupational Health Psychology*, *20*, 457–469.

Demerouti, E., Bakker, A. B., Nachreiner, F., & Schaufeli, W. B. (2001). The job demands-resources model of burnout. *Journal of Applied Psychology*, *86*, 499–512. https://doi.org/10.1037/0021-9010.86.3.499

Eatough, E. M., & Chang, C. H. (2018). Effective coping with supervisor conflict depends on control: Implications for work strains. *Journal of Occupational Health Psychology*, *23*(4), 537–552. https://doi.org/10.1037/ocp0000109

Edwards, J. R. (1995). Alternatives to difference scores as dependent variables in the study of congruence in organizational research. *Organizational Behavior and Human Decision Processes*, *64*(3), 307–324. https://doi.org/10.1006/obhd.1995.1108

Edwards, J. R., & Cooper, C. L. (1990). The person-environment fit approach to stress: Recurring problems and some suggested solutions. *Journal of Organizational Behavior*, *11*(4), 293–307. https://doi.org/10.1002/job.4030110405

Folkman, S., & Lazarus, R. S. (1990). Coping and emotion. In N. L. Stein, B. Leventhal, & T. Trabasso (Eds.), *Psychological and biological approaches to emotion* (pp. 313–332). Lawrence Erlbaum.

Goldstein, D. S., & Eisenhofer, G. (2000). Sympathetic nervous system physiology and pathophysiology in coping with the environment. In B. S. McEwen (Ed.), *Handbook of physiology, coping with the environment* (pp. 21–43). Oxford University Press.

Goldstein, D. S., & McEwen, B. (2002). Allostasis, homeostats, and the nature of stress. *Stress*, *5*(1), 55–58. https://doi.org/10.1080/102538902900012345

Griep, Y., Bankins, S., Vander Elst, T., & De Witte, H. (2020). How psychological contract breach affects long-term mental and physical health: The longitudinal role of effort–reward imbalance. *Applied Psychology. Health and Well-Being*, *13*(2), 263–281. https://doi.org/10.1111/aphw.12246

Hackney, K. J., Daniels, S. R., Paustian-Underdahl, S. C., Perrewé, P. L., Mandeville, A., & Eaton, A. A. (2021). Examining the effects of perceived pregnancy discrimination on mother and baby health. *Journal of Applied Psychology*, *106*(5), 774–783. https://doi.org/10.1037/apl0000788

Harrison, R. V. (1985). The person–environment fit model and the study of job stress. In T. A. Beehr & R. S. Bhagat (Eds.), *Human stress and cognition in organizations* (pp. 23–55). Wiley.

Hobfoll, S. E. (1989). Conservation of resources: A new attempt at conceptualizing stress. *American Psychologist*, *44*(3), 513–524. https://doi.org/10.1037/0003-066X.44.3.513

Hobfoll, S. E. (2001). The influence of culture, community, and the nested-self in the stress process: Advancing conservation of resources theory. *Applied Psychology*, *50*(3), 337–421. https://doi.org/10.1111/1464-0597.00062

Hobfoll, S. E., & Shirom, A. (2000). Conservation of resources theory: Application to stress and management in the workplace. In R. T. Golembiewski (Ed.), *Handbook of organizational behavior* (pp. 57–81). Dekker.

Karasek, R. A., Jr. (1979). Job demands, job decision latitude, and mental strain: Implications for job redesign. *Administrative Science Quarterly*, *24*(2), 285–307. https://doi.org/10.2307/2392498

Karasek, R. A., & Theorell, T. (1990). *Healthy work: Stress, productivity, and the reconstruction of working life*. Basic Books.

Lazarus, R. S. (1966). *Psychological stress and the coping process*. McGraw-Hill.

Lazarus, R. S. (1991). Psychological stress in the workplace. *Journal of Social Behavior and Personality*, *6*(7), 1–13.

Lazarus, R. S., & Folkman, S. (1984). *Stress, appraisal, and coping*. Springer.

Leiter, M. P., & Durup, M. J. (1996). Work, home, and in-between: A longitudinal study of spillover. *The Journal of Applied Behavioral Science*, *32*(1), 29–47. https://doi.org/10.1177/0021886396321002

LePine, J. A., Podsakoff, N. P., & LePine, M. A. (2005). A meta-analytic test of the challenge stressor–hindrance stressor framework: An explanation for inconsistent relationships among stressors and performance. *Academy of Management Journal, 48*(5), 764–775. https://doi.org/10.5465/amj.2005.18803921

Lian, H., Brown, D. J., Ferris, L., Liang, L. H., Keeping, L. M., & Morrison, R. (2014). Abusive supervision and retaliation. *Academy of Management Journal, 57*(1), 116–139. https://doi.org/10.5465/amj.2011.0977

Lofquist, L. H., & Dawis, R. B. (1969). *Adjustment to work.* Appleton-Century-Crofts.

Mackey, J. D., & Perrewé, P. L. (2014). The triple "A" (appraisals, attributions, adaptation) model of job stress: The critical role of self-regulation. *Organizational Psychology Review, 4*(3), 258–278. https://doi.org/10.1177/2041386614525072

Mazzola, J. J., & Disselhorst, R. (2019). Should we be "challenging" employees? A critical review and meta-analysis of the challenge-hindrance model of stress. *Journal of Organizational Behavior, 40*(8), 949–961. https://doi.org/10.1002/job.2412

McAllister, C. P., Mackey, J. D., & Perrewé, P. L. (2018). The role of self-regulation in the relationship between abusive supervision and job tension. *Journal of Organizational Behavior, 39*(4), 416–428. https://doi.org/10.1002/job.2240

McEwen, B. S. (1998). Stress, adaptation, and disease: Allostasis and allostatic load. *Annals of the New York Academy of Sciences, 840*(1), 33–44. https://doi.org/10.1111/j.1749-6632.1998.tb09546.x

O'Brien, K. E., & Beehr, T. A. (2019). So far, so good: Up to now, the challenge–hindrance framework describes a practical and accurate distinction. *Journal of Organizational Behavior, 40*(8), 962–972. https://doi.org/10.1002/job.2405

Parker, S. K., & Sprigg, C. A. (1999). Minimizing strain and maximizing learning: The role of job demands, job control, and proactive personality. *Journal of Applied Psychology, 84*(6), 925–939. https://doi.org/10.1037/0021-9010.84.6.925

Schaubroeck, J., & Merritt, D. E. (1997). Divergent effects of job control on coping with work stressors: The key role of self-efficacy. *Academy of Management Journal, 40*, 738–754. https://doi.org/10.5465/257061

Selye, H. (1955). Stress and disease. *Science, 122*(3171), 625–631. https://doi.org/10.1126/science.122.3171.625

Selye, H. (1974). *Stress without distress.* JB Lippincott.

Siegrist, J. (1996). Adverse health effects of high-effort/low-reward conditions. *Journal of Occupational Health Psychology, 1*(1), 27–41. https://doi.org/10.1037/1076-8998.1.1.27

Siegrist, J. (2001). A theory of occupational stress. In J. Dunham (Ed.), *Stress in the workplace: Past, present, and future* (pp. 52–66). Whurr Publishers.

Siegrist, J. (2002). Effort-reward imbalance at work and health. In P. L. Perrewé & D. C. Ganster (Eds.), *Research in occupational stress and well-being: Vol. 2. Historical and current perspectives on stress and health* (pp. 261–291). Elsevier/JAI. https://doi.org/10.1016/S1479-3555(02)02007-3

Siegrist, J., & Li, J. (2017). Work stress and altered biomarkers: A synthesis of findings based on the effort–reward imbalance model. *International Journal of Environmental Research and Public Health, 14*(11), 1–18. https://doi.org/10.3390/ijerph14111373

Singer, B., Ryff, C. D., & Seeman, T. (2004). Operationalizing allostatic load. In J. Schulkin (Ed.), *Allostasis, homeostasis, and the costs of physiological adaptation* (pp. 113–149). Cambridge University Press. https://doi.org/10.1017/CBO9781316257081.007

Smallfield, J., & Kluemper, D. H. (2022). An explanation of personality change in organizational science: Personality as an outcome of workplace stress. *Journal of Management, 48*(4), 851–877. https://doi.org/10.1177/0149206321998429

Sonnentag, S., & Fritz, C. (2007). The Recovery Experience Questionnaire: Development and validation of a measure for assessing recuperation and unwinding from work. *Journal of Occupational Health Psychology, 12*(3), 204–221. https://doi.org/10.1037/1076-8998.12.3.204

Sterling, P. (2004). Principles of allostasis: Optimal design, predictive regulation, patho-physiology, and rational therapeutics. In J. Schulkin (Ed.), *Allostasis, homeostasis, and the costs of physiological adaptation* (pp. 17–64). Cambridge University Press. https://doi.org/10.1017/CBO9781316257081.004

Sterling, P. (2012). Allostasis: A model of predictive regulation. *Physiology & Behavior, 106*(1), 5–15. https://doi.org/10.1016/j.physbeh.2011.06.004

Sterling, P., & Eyer, J. (1988). Allostasis: A new paradigm to explain arousal pathology. In S. Fisher & J. Reason (Eds.), *Handbook of life stress, cognition, and health* (pp. 629–649). Wiley.

Taris, T. W. (2006). Bricks without clay: On urban myths in occupational health psychology. *Work and Stress, 20*(2), 99–104. https://doi.org/10.1080/02678370600893410

Taris, T. W., Kompier, M. A. J., De Lange, A. H., Schaufeli, W. B., & Schreurs, P. J. G. (2003). Learning new behaviour patterns: A longitudinal test of Karasek's active learning hypothesis among Dutch teachers. *Work and Stress, 17*(1), 1–20. https://doi.org/10.1080/0267837031000108149

Treadway, D. C., Ferris, G. R., Hochwarter, W., Perrewé, P., Witt, L. A., & Goodman, J. M. (2005). The role of age in the perceptions of politics–job performance relationship: A three-study constructive replication. *Journal of Applied Psychology, 90*(5), 872–881. https://doi.org/10.1037/0021-9010.90.5.872

Trougakos, J. P., Chawla, N., & McCarthy, J. M. (2020). Working in a pandemic: Exploring the impact of COVID-19 health anxiety on work, family, and health outcomes. *Journal of Applied Psychology, 105*(11), 1234–1245. https://doi.org/10.1037/apl0000739

Turner, N., Chmiel, N., & Walls, M. (2005). Railing for safety: Job demands, job control, and safety citizenship role definition. *Journal of Occupational Health Psychology, 10*(4), 504–512. https://doi.org/10.1037/1076-8998.10.4.504

Van der Doef, M., & Maes, S. (1998). The job demand–control (–support) model and physical health outcomes: A review of the strain and buffer hypotheses. *Psychology & Health, 13*(5), 909–936. https://doi.org/10.1080/08870449808407440

Van der Doef, M., & Maes, S. (1999). The job demand–control (–support) model and psychological well-being: A review of 20 years of empirical research. *Work and Stress, 13*(2), 87–114. https://doi.org/10.1080/026783799296084

Verhoeven, C., Maes, S., Kraaij, V., & Joekes, K. (2003). The job demand–control–social support model and wellness/health outcomes: A European study. *Psychology & Health, 18*(4), 421–440. https://doi.org/10.1080/0887044031000147175

Webster, J. R., Beehr, T. A., & Love, K. (2011). Extending the challenge-hindrance model of occupational stress: The role of appraisal. *Journal of Vocational Behavior, 79*(2), 505–516. https://doi.org/10.1016/j.jvb.2011.02.001

Westman, M. (2001). Stress and strain crossover. *Human Relations, 54*(6), 717–751. https://doi.org/10.1177/0018726701546002

Westman, M., Hobfoll, S., Chen, S., Davidson, O., & Laski, S. (2005). Organizational stress through the lens of Conservation of Resources (COR) Theory. In P. L. Perrewé & D. C. Ganster (Eds.), *Research in occupational stress and well-being: Vol. 4. Exploring interpersonal dynamics* (pp. 167–220). Elsevier/JAI. https://doi.org/10.1016/S1479-3555(04)04005-3

Wright, T. A., & Cropanzano, R. (1998). Emotional exhaustion as a predictor of job performance and voluntary turnover. *Journal of Applied Psychology, 83*(3), 486–493. https://doi.org/10.1037/0021-9010.83.3.486

Wrzesniewski, A., & Dutton, J. E. (2001). Crafting a job: Revisioning employees as active crafters of their work. *Academy of Management Review, 26*(2), 179–201. https://doi.org/10.2307/259118

Zajonc, R. B. (1984). On the primacy of affect. *American Psychologist, 39*(2), 117–123. https://doi.org/10.1037/0003-066X.39.2.117

The Holistic Model of Stress

Savoring Eustress While Coping With Distress

Bret L. Simmons, Alexis Hanna, and Jinyu Hu

Most employees have a love–hate relationship with work: A job often consists of a mixed bag of things we find both exciting and exhausting. For example, the COVID-19 pandemic necessitated a switch to working remotely for many employees around the globe, which often meant working from home. As a result of this sudden transition, people experienced the uncertainty of learning new ways of communicating with team members and clients, the fatigue of spending countless hours in online meetings, the anxiety of being away from coworkers, and the frustration of not knowing when, or if, there would ever be a return to the office. Simultaneously, this experience brought the satisfaction of learning new skills, the freedom of spending more time with friends and family, the meaningfulness of helping team members or clients with challenges they were experiencing, and the hope of knowing things would change again, even if they might never return to "normal." This mix of positive and negative attitudes and emotions resulted from individual interpretations of a single event. We found strategies to cope with the bad, and we explored ways to enjoy and extend the good. Ultimately, many employees experienced changes in their own work performance behaviors, and maybe even their mental and physical health.

Although quite a lot is known about distress, or the negative response to stressors, as well as dysfunctional outcomes that typically follow from distress, the positive outcomes that arise from stress at work merit increased attention. The extension of the positive psychology movement into the realm of

https://doi.org/10.1037/0000331-004
Handbook of Occupational Health Psychology, Third Edition, L. E. Tetrick, G. G. Fisher, M. T. Ford, and J. C. Quick (Editors)

occupational health psychology allows us to study the positive side of the stress experience: eustress. We assert that the proper way to advance the study of eustress is to add the positive aspect of the stress experience to the well-developed psychology of disease and dysfunction. Thus, we propose a holistic theoretical model that integrates our vast knowledge of negative causes, consequences, and outcomes with current developments in stress research and positive psychology. As shown in Figure 4.1, this conceptual framework captures both positive (eustress) and negative (distress) psychological responses to job demands. As an extension of Simmons and colleagues' work on eustress (Nelson & Simmons, 2003; Simmons, 2000), the current holistic model of stress draws upon the principles of the job demands–resource (JD-R) theory (Demerouti et al., 2001) and emphasizes the role of person–environment (P-E) fit in distress and eustress responses (Edwards et al., 1998; Kristof, 1996).

The demands, distress response, coping, and outcomes portion of the model are well known in the occupational stress literature, so they are discussed only briefly. The unique aspects of this model—the demands, eustress, savoring, and outcomes pathway—are the main focus of discussion. In particular, we explore in detail the indicators of eustress and savoring of eustress. We close by considering some of the methodological challenges in the study of eustress.

THE CONCEPT OF EUSTRESS

We believe that eustress can best be conceptualized as capturing the positive aspects of the stress response itself. Building on Simmons and Nelson's (2007) eustress model, our central tenets are as follows:

- Demands/stressors are inherently neutral.

- Demands are cognitively appraised to the degree to which they are both challenging and hindering.

- This cognitive appraisal produces a simultaneous positive and negative response. It is this response that has positive and/or negative valence based on the degree of attraction and/or aversion the individual experiences toward the event or object.

- Job resources, personal resources, and the match between a person and their work environment each affect the ways in which demands are appraised; therefore, they moderate the relationship between demands and appraisals.

- Positive and negative responses are complex and mixed; therefore, they manifest themselves in a variety of distinct physiological, psychological, and behavioral indicators. Degrees of both positive and negative indicators of responses will be present for any given demand. (Note: Our model does not focus on physiological indicators because they are less observable by managers interacting with employees, and therefore are less subject to

FIGURE 4.1. Holistic Model of Work Stress

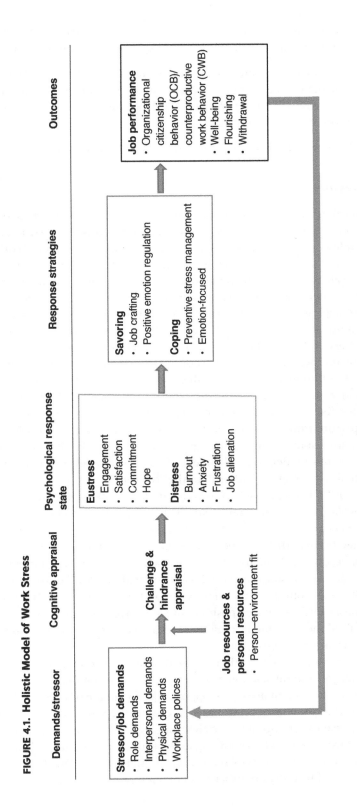

managerial intervention. Nonetheless, we acknowledge that these physiological indicators do exist and are experienced by employees.)

- Individuals select strategies to either eliminate or alleviate negative responses to demands (i.e., coping) and/or to accentuate or extend positive responses (i.e., savoring). These strategies can be focused either on the perceived demand or on the stress response.

- Positive and negative responses differentially affect valued outcomes at work.

Stressors

The physical or psychological stimuli to which an individual responds are commonly referred to as *stressors* or *demands*. Stressors at work take the form of role demands, interpersonal demands, physical demands, workplace policies, and job conditions (Quick et al., 1997). Some of these demands will be less salient for certain individuals while producing significant responses in others. Because knowledge of demands has typically been embedded in the pathological perspective of stress and health, some work refers to these demands as *distressors*. Other stress researchers have distinguished between *challenge stressors* and *hindrance stressors*, which place positive or negative valence on both the demand and the response (Podsakoff et al., 2007). In this framework, hindrance stressors produce strain, as indicated by burnout, anxiety, frustration, and exhaustion; but challenge stressors facilitate positive job attitudes like satisfaction and commitment. However, our model presents a departure from these perspectives. We suggest that to be consistent with the cognitive appraisal of *neutral* stressors, which provides the theoretical foundation of our model, the assignment of valence should be reserved for the individual stress *response* rather than the stressor.

Our holistic approach to stress is squarely rooted in the transactional model articulated by Lazarus and Folkman (1984) and further built upon by the more recent JD-R theory (Demerouti et al., 2001). The transactional model of stress suggests that stress can be conceived of as an imbalance between demands and resources. Similarly, the JD-R theory proposes that different demands interact with resources to produce an individual's level of well-being at work. Following from these theories, we expect that most work situations simultaneously elicit a mix of positive and negative responses in individuals as a result of the individual's cognitive appraisal of a particular demand given their particular set of resources.

For example, a recently promoted individual should be expected to experience joy and satisfaction associated with the recognition of achievement, as well as excitement about the opportunity to pursue new goals and challenges at work. At the same time, and as a result of the same situation, the individual may also experience anxiety about moving to a new department away from their usual coworkers or having to tell friends, family, and colleagues that the new promotion involves relocation to another city. On the other hand, an individual recently downsized out of a job can be expected to experience loss and anxiety about having to find a new position. Yet at the same time, they may feel relieved to be leaving a stressful job on a sinking ship or may see the job loss as an opportunity to spend more coveted time with family.

Indeed, empirical work supports the notion that stressors simultaneously elicit positive and negative stress responses. For instance, one of the most significant sources of stress for hospital nurses is the death of a patient (Gray-Toft & Anderson, 1981). It is easy to understand how the loss of a patient could result in distress for a nurse; but along with that distress, the death of a patient may also be appraised as positive. One study found that contrary to expectations, the variable "death–dying" had a significant positive relationship with eustress and a nonsignificant relationship with distress. One interpretation of this finding was that when nurses were faced with the demand of death–dying in their patients, they became significantly more engaged in their work (Simmons, 2000).

A meta-analysis of challenge stressors and hindrance stressors also reports this pattern of simultaneous positive and negative responses (Podsakoff et al., 2007). Our model proposes that for any given demand, individual cognitive appraisals will typically identify aspects of both challenges and hindrances. As an illustration for a particular type of stressor, situational constraints will certainly be appraised as a hindrance by most individuals. Yet individuals with a positive core self-evaluation and access to other job resources might simultaneously find a motivational challenge in the same constraint.

Furthermore, workers can be engaged in their work and experience positive benefits even when confronted with extremely demanding stressors. A study of female and male soldiers participating in the U.S. peacekeeping mission in Bosnia found that soldiers who were engaged in meaningful work during the deployment found it to be a positive experience (Britt et al., 2001). Even such an extreme factor as witnessing the destruction caused by warring factions was associated with reporting positive benefits of the peacekeeping mission. In this context, destruction was likely seen as justification for the mission, which added meaning to the soldiers' work.

Indicators of Eustress

Positive and negative stress responses are separate, distinct, multidimensional, and potentially interactive in nature. To assume the presence of the positive by simply observing the absence of the negative, or vice versa, is an unacceptably simplistic approach to understanding the sources, responses, and consequences of stress. In other words, the full range of the stress response cannot be appreciated without a strategy to assess eustress and distress concurrently. Thus, each positive and negative stress response will have its own associated indicators or subdimensions.

Indicators of the stress response could be physiological, behavioral, or psychological, though our model focuses only on psychological indicators. As Edwards and Cooper (1988) suggested, indicators of the positive response to stressors will be positive psychological states, and indicators of the negative response will be negative psychological states. Thus, consistent with the holistic representation of stress, eustress can be operationally defined as a positive psychological response to a stressor, as indicated by the presence of positive psychological states; distress can be operationally defined as a negative psychological response to a stressor, as indicated by the presence of negative psychological states (Simmons, 2000).

Because psychological states must be subject to change according to cognitive appraisals of stressors, stable dispositional variables are not acceptable indicators of eustress (or distress). Thus, work attitudes and emotions are preferable indicators. Specifically, attitudes and emotions such as positive affect, meaningfulness, manageability, hope, and vigor may be good indicators of eustress (Simmons, 2000; Simmons & Nelson, 2001; Simmons et al., 2001). For example, positive affect reflects the extent to which a person feels enthusiastic, active, and alert (Watson et al., 1988) and is associated with seeing opportunity in an issue (Mittal & Ross, 1998), which could be an indicator of eustress following exposure to an event. Likewise, manageability is the extent to which a person perceives that resources at their disposal are adequate to meet the demands posed by a work situation (Simmons, 2000), which corresponds to a positive evaluation of that situation.

Although conceptually distinct, these constructs all represent aspects of engagement, which itself includes another promising indicator of eustress. Job engagement is the simultaneous investment of cognitive, emotional, and physical presence into performing a work role (Kahn, 1990). Example items from Rich et al.'s (2010) measure of job engagement include: "At work, I focus a great deal of attention on my job" (cognitive), "I feel energetic at my job" (emotional), and "I try my hardest to perform well on my job" (physical). Antecedents of engagement include core self-evaluation, perceived organizational support, and value congruence (an aspect of P-E fit); and engagement predicts job performance and organizational citizenship behavior (Rich et al., 2010). Our model suggests that individual differences, job resources, and P-E fit moderate the relationship between challenge and hindrance stressors and cognitive appraisals of those stressors; thus, due to similar linkages, engagement likely plays a role in the stress process as well.

STRESS AND HEALTH

There is substantial evidence of the links between distress and ill health (O'Connor et al., 2021; Quick et al., 1997). Conversely, research evidence concerning eustress suggests that the positive stress experience can have *beneficial* effects on health (Kupriyanov & Zhdanov, 2014). One review of the literature stated that "positive emotional states may promote healthy perceptions, beliefs, and physical well-being" (Salovey et al., 2000, p. 110). Likewise, after reviewing a variety of empirical findings, Edwards and Cooper (1988) found that the majority of evidence suggests a positive effect of eustress on health. The authors speculated that eustress may either improve health directly through physiological changes or indirectly by reducing existing distress. More recently, Parker and Ragsdale (2015) found that within persons, employees' experiences of distress predicted higher fatigue both in the morning and later in the workday, whereas two indicators of eustress—happiness and meaningfulness—predicted lower fatigue at both times of day. These results suggest differential effects of experiencing distress versus eustress: eustress may replenish energy (Zohar et al., 2003) and may directly improve self-efficacy, which in turn helps develop a range of positive resources and better health experiences (Gross et al., 2011).

Several empirical studies hypothesized that, in response to demands, hospital nurses would experience significant levels of both eustress and distress, and each stress response would have a separate effect on the nurses' perceptions of their health (Salovey et al., 2000). As hypothesized, even in the presence of a demanding work environment, nurses were actively engaged in their work and reported significant levels of eustress, and eustress in turn had a significant positive relationship with perceptions of their own health. Among all indicators of eustress, hope exhibited the strongest positive relationship with the nurses' perception of health. In addition to being healthy and productive themselves, eustressed nurses may have an increasingly positive effect on the health of patients by inspiring optimistic expectations and raising patients' levels of hope (Salovey et al., 2000).

Outside of the profession of nursing, it is likely that eustress has positive implications for the health of employees as well. Future research should continue to investigate the adaptive capacity of eustress for positive health outcomes and subjective well-being (Kupriyanov & Zhdanov, 2014). In doing so, organizations can not only learn about the positive implications of eustress in their employees but also engage in practices to promote and extend experiences of positive stress in the workplace.

MANAGING EUSTRESS AND DISTRESS

The research literature on work stress has focused strongly on pathology and on healing the wounded. The importance of this venture cannot be denied. Much has been learned about stressors, coping, and symptoms of distress, and great strides have been made in assisting both individuals and organizations in managing distress. These milestones, however, represent only half the battle. As a complement to healing the wounded, we must also find ways of building and capitalizing on strengths. Distress prevention and eustress generation together provide a more holistic framework for managing occupational health issues.

Distress Prevention

One framework that allows for a comprehensive gathering of distress-focused interventions is preventive stress management, as originally proposed by Quick and Quick (1984) and elaborated on by Quick et al. (1997). Central to this philosophy is the idea that stress is inevitable but distress is not. Rooted in a public health framework, the three levels of preventive stress management are primary prevention, secondary prevention, and tertiary prevention.

Primary prevention is intended to reduce, change, or eliminate stressors and often includes job redesign or time management efforts. Karasek's (1979) job strain model, for example, indicates that it is possible to increase the demand level of a job without making it distressful, so long as job discretion is also increased. Beyond job redesign, primary prevention strategies also involve efforts to change individual perceptions of stressors, such as cognitive restructuring and learned optimism that alter a person's internal self-talk.

When stressors cannot be eliminated through primary prevention, secondary prevention efforts are focused on modifying responses to stressors. For example, exercise, meditation, and other forms of relaxation and nutrition practices all focus on lowering the risk of disease following exposure to stressors. Notable among secondary prevention efforts is the work of Pennebaker and colleagues (e.g., Smyth & Pennebaker, 2001), which demonstrates the psychological and somatic health benefits of writing about traumatic events and stressors.

Finally, tertiary prevention is the most direct form of healing the wounds of distress once strains have developed over time. Specifically, tertiary prevention consists of professional help (e.g., counseling, physical therapy, medical treatment) for symptoms of distress. Organizational efforts of tertiary prevention are often facilitated by employee assistance programs.

Eustress Generation

Overall, we can tell individuals and organizations a great deal about how to prevent or resolve distress. While coping consists of voluntary self-regulation processes that individuals engage in as part of their reactions to distress, the positive counterpart to coping—*savoring*—involves enjoying the positive response to stress and dwelling on it with satisfaction or delight (Nelson & Simmons, 2004). As a complement to preventing and coping with distress, our next task, and a formidable one, is to learn how to help individuals and organizations generate eustress and reap the resulting benefits of increased health, well-being, and performance.

JD-R theory suggests that job conditions can be characterized as either job demands or resources, and each triggers a unique psychological process (Demerouti et al., 2001). Job demands impose energy costs or depletion and have been found to be the strongest predictors of distress. In contrast, job and personal resources are associated with motivational processes that promote engagement (an indicator of eustress) and well-being (Bakker & Demerouti, 2014), in addition to functioning as a buffer against the strain caused by demands. Said differently, high demands combined with low resources are a perfect recipe for distress, whereas high demands and high resources generate higher motivation (Demerouti & Bakker, 2011). Managers interested in eustress generation might start by identifying aspects of the work that help employees reserve and expand resources. Two popular concepts in positive psychology, job crafting and positive emotion regulation, may be effective self-regulatory strategies for countering distressful demands and developing job and personal resources.

Job Crafting

According to JD-R, employees do not simply react to their environment and play defense to cope with stressful situations. Instead, they can proactively make changes and alter various elements of work with an aim to increase the fit between work demands and their individual needs and capabilities (Berg et al., 2008). This bottom-up, individual job redesign strategy is referred to as *job crafting* (Wrzesniewski & Dutton, 2001).

Job crafting is resource expansion–oriented and can focus on either job demands or resources. Specifically, seeking resources (e.g., asking for feedback, increasing job autonomy, learning new skills, building social networks), seeking challenges (e.g., asking for extra responsibility, taking on challenging tasks), and optimizing demands (e.g., active improvement of work processes for better efficiency; planning and prioritization) are all forms of job crafting (Costantini et al., 2021; Demerouti & Peeters, 2018). These proactive efforts help employees build job and personal resources and optimize resource mobilization (Demerouti et al., 2015).

Job crafting leads to the accumulation of job and personal resources, which in turn helps enhance eustress in two ways. First, it serves an intrinsic motivational role and fulfills the basic human need for conserving and expanding valuable resources (Hobfoll, 2001). Second, this resource expansion plays an instrumental role in facilitating work task completion (Bakker & Demerouti, 2017). Proactive job crafters are found to be more confident and creative in finding innovative ways to solve problems (Petrou et al., 2012). A longitudinal study by Vogt and colleagues (2016) found that resource-expansion behaviors such as job crafting have direct positive effects on individuals' psychological capital (hope, resilience, self-efficacy, and optimism), which in turn improves work engagement (an indicator of eustress). As a whole, job crafting is a useful self-regulatory strategy for employees to proactively create resourceful work conditions to stay stimulated and thrive. Employees engaged in job crafting behaviors are likely to be more engaged, satisfied, resilient, and thriving at work (Berg et al., 2008).

Nonetheless, not all jobs provide opportunities to engage in job crafting. In jobs that do not have a high degree of autonomy or control, organizations can still help facilitate individuals savor the positive response to stress. Eustress recognition and interest in eustress generation will always be individualistic, but organizations can teach employees to recognize positive responses to stress and engage in practices to extend these experiences to capitalize on their potential health benefits.

Positive Emotion Regulation

Emotion plays an integral role in stress experiences. Stressful events elicit complex emotional responses that involve negative and positive emotions

(Folkman & Moskowitz, 2000) and both types of emotions play significant functional roles (Fredrickson, 1998). Negative emotions tend to trigger narrowly focused action, whereas positive emotions foster cognitive and psychological flexibility and facilitate generativity, higher level connectivity, and exploration (Fredrickson, 1998). These emotional effects have significant implications for personal resource development and eustress generation. Empirical findings show that there is a direct link between the effects of positive emotions that accumulate and compound over time and sustained psychological resilience (an enduring personal resource) and human flourishing (Fredrickson, 2004).

Depending on the emotion strategy employed in the stress response, there could be two resulting paths: negative emotional experiences, which represent an energy and resource depletion path of distress; or positive emotional experiences, which represent a resource development path of eustress (Quinones et al., 2017). Cultivating positive emotions through an emotion regulatory approach can be instrumental to effective stress management. Emotion regulatory behaviors have been known to help people sustain and maintain positive emotional experiences that are beneficial to well-being (Bryant, 2003), so emotion regulation can play an important role in *savoring*, or extending, eustress. Commonly recommended regulatory strategies include positive reappraisal (also known as deep acting) and infusing ordinary events with positive meaning (for a detailed review, see Folkman & Moskowitz, 2000). These cognitive and behavioral tools help maintain, prolong, and enhance positive emotion experiences, which in turn expand attention scopes, foster creative thinking, build enduring and vital psychological resources (e.g., efficacy, optimism, resilience), and ultimately promote eustress over time (Aspinwall, 1998, 2001).

THE MULTIFACETED ROLE OF PERSON–ENVIRONMENT FIT IN THE STRESS PROCESS

P-E fit describes the match between a person's attributes and those of an environment (Kristof-Brown et al., 2005). P-E fit can include many different individual attributes, including biological and psychological needs, personality traits, vocational interests, values, goals, and abilities (Cable & Edwards, 2004; Kristof, 1996). We posit that P-E fit plays a unique and multifaceted role in the holistic model of stress in that it may take on the role of a stressor, an individual difference, or a facilitator of coping and/or savoring.

First, P-E fit has typically been included in the stress literature as a potential stressor. Theories of fit describe an *adjustment process* in which individuals should increase their fit with their work environment over time (Dawis & Lofquist, 1984; French et al., 1974), and this process is often driven by negative stress experiences as a result of misfit (Caplan, 1987; Edwards et al., 1998). Specifically, when individuals are in environments that do not fit their values, interests, personality, abilities, or other needs, this misfit tends to produce stress. As a result, individuals will consciously or unconsciously undergo efforts to alleviate that stress (i.e., engage in coping) by changing their own attributes, changing their environment, or both (Caplan, 1987; French et al., 1974; Frese, 1982; Schneider, 1987).

Importantly, fit theories do not explicitly distinguish between distress and eustress, but misfit is often construed as undesirable, and adjustment processes typically refer to coping rather than savoring (Le Fevre et al., 2003). However, in light of the holistic model of stress (Figure 4.1), we propose that there are interesting opportunities to empirically examine misfit as a neutral stressor that may elicit distress, eustress, or both. For example, misfit may be in the form of either *excess* (i.e., the environment provides more of an attribute than the individual has or needs) or *deficiency* (i.e., the environment provides less of an attribute than the individual has or needs; Edwards & Parry, 1993; Wiegand et al., 2021). Previous research (e.g., Wiegand et al., 2021) has demonstrated that differential effects can result from different types of misfit: for example, outcomes like job satisfaction differ when people's interests are met and exceeded by their job, rather than under-supplied. These findings suggest that misfit may produce distress or eustress, depending on excess or deficiency. Likewise, when the demands of a job exceed a person's abilities, this may cause distress for the individual; on the other hand, when the person's abilities exceed the demands of their job, this may lead to eustress (Le Fevre et al., 2003).

Misfit may also simultaneously elicit distress and eustress. For instance, a person who values profits and success may experience misfit with an organization that donates a portion of their profits to environmental causes. That person may interpret this value misfit as both a hindrance (e.g., "My organization makes decisions that I do not agree with.") and a challenge (e.g., "I should be more sensitive to prosocial causes, such as saving the environment"). Based on each of these possibilities, researchers should empirically test both eustress and distress following experiences of misfit, rather than assuming that misfit will elicit negative responses.

In addition to P-E fit as a stressor, we propose that fit may also serve as an individual difference that predisposes a person to experience eustress or distress in the face of other stressors. Various types of P-E fit are important predictors of outcomes such as work attitudes (Hoff et al., 2020; Kristof-Brown et al., 2005), job performance (Nye et al., 2012, 2017), and turnover intentions (Kristof-Brown et al., 2005; Vancouver & Schmitt, 1991). As a result of these links, a person who "matches" their organization and job may be predisposed to view stressors as motivational challenges that elicit eustress responses, whereas a misfitting individual may be more likely to experience distress. For example, a person who works in a job that matches their interests may be more likely to be satisfied in that job and perform well (Hoff et al., 2020; Nye et al., 2012, 2017). If that person encounters stressors such as work overload or team pressures, they may view these stressors as opportunities to challenge themselves and perform at their best, whereas a person working in a job that does not match their interests may be more distressed as a result of those same demands. Despite its potential as a predisposition to stress responses, little empirical work has examined P-E fit as a moderator between exposure to stressors and experiences of distress and eustress. Similar to research on predispositions such as optimism (Peterson, 2000; Scheier & Carver, 1992) and hardiness (Florian et al., 1995; Kobasa et al., 1982), more research is needed to examine fit as a relevant individual difference characteristic following expo- sure to a stressor.

P-E fit may also facilitate coping and/or savoring, which can affect the link between stress and various work outcomes. One study that tested P-E fit as a moderator of the relationship between stress responses and work outcomes found that fit can serve as a buffer to reduce the negative effects of distress (Chu, 2014). Specifically, perceptions of distress in a sample of nurses were positively related to work–family conflict and negatively related to mental health, but these relationships were weaker for nurses who had better P-E fit with their jobs. In other words, for individuals with good fit, there was still some level of perceived distress, but this distress had fewer negative down- stream effects than it did for individuals with poor fit.

Aside from these findings, it is largely unknown how P-E fit can be used to strengthen coping and savoring processes. Because of adjustment processes in which individuals may strengthen their fit with their job and organization (Caplan, 1987; French et al., 1974; Frese, 1982; Schneider, 1987), there is certainly potential for these processes to involve coping and savoring in response to other stressors as well. As described earlier, one mechanism through which individuals may cope with misfit by changing their environment is job crafting (Tims et al., 2013). Given enough autonomy, individuals may actively work to change aspects of their job to help align their work environment with their own attributes (Li et al., 2022). In doing so, individuals may simulta- neously engage in active coping strategies that relieve or enhance other stressors. For instance, by changing how a workday is structured, an employee may both increase demands–abilities fit (i.e., the match between employees' abilities and the demands of their job; Kristof, 1996) and reduce role demands that were causing distress. Future research can further explore the possible role of P-E fit in facilitating such coping or savoring processes, as well as potential applications of fit in workshops designed to teach coping and savoring strategies.

METHODOLOGICAL CHALLENGES IN THE STUDY OF EUSTRESS

There are a number of methodological considerations in the stress literature, particularly when studying the positive experiences of eustress and savoring. First, an important consideration deals with the valence of psychological states and the need to conceptualize different valences on separate contin- uums, rather than bipolar ends of the same spectrum (e.g., positive affect vs. negative affect; Russell & Carroll, 1999). Likewise, one of the most promi- nent methodological challenges is that few measures are explicitly designed to capture the experience of eustress (Branson et al., 2019; Rodríguez et al., 2013). Because a person may experience a single stressor as both a positive challenge and a negative demand (Lazarus & Folkman, 1984; Van den Broeck et al., 2010), measures including items that address positive stress experiences are necessary. These measures allow for the evaluation of simultaneous experiences of distress and eustress following exposure to a neutral stressor, rather than treating eustress as the *opposite* of distress. Due to the lack of currently available measures, some researchers have undertaken efforts to develop their own measures with items designed for a particular study's goals (e.g., Cavanaugh et al., 2000; O'Sullivan, 2011). Nonetheless, more research on these measures is needed to advance the study of eustress and savoring, as well as more efforts to develop validated measures with high degrees of reliability.

Alternatively, factor analytic techniques may be used to conceptualize eustress as a higher order construct defined by other existing constructs such as hope, meaningfulness, vigor, and manageability (Simmons, 2000). This conceptualization via established, lower order constructs treats the higher order construct of eustress at a higher level of abstraction than the lower sub-dimension constructs (Credé & Harms, 2015; Sarstedt et al., 2019). This approach may complicate the construct validity regarding the definition of eustress and whether the measures truly reflect the construct as defined (Johnson et al., 2011). For example, whether eustress should be considered as more abstract than concepts like hope and vigor is a theoretical question. Higher order constructs are typically proposed because there is observed covariation among several existing constructs (Credé & Harms, 2015), rather than imposing a higher order factor analytic model to capture a construct that already exists on its own, such as eustress.

The use of higher order factor analysis also presents its own methodological challenges. Due to the complexity of such a model, researchers may experience convergence issues, and large samples are needed to test such models. As opposed to a direct measure of eustress, this method also requires empirical measurement of all indicator variables, which can induce survey fatigue due to the high number of items (Le et al., 2021).

Nonetheless, higher order factor analysis is a preferable method to conceptualize eustress compared with using a measure designed to assess distress, and this approach offers several advantages. For instance, building higher order, multidimensional constructs capitalizes on the bandwidth-fidelity argument that broader constructs are better predictors of other broad, multidimensional constructs (Jenkins & Griffith, 2004; Johnson et al., 2011). Additionally, when a set of variables all predict similar outcomes, it is more parsimonious to examine their common variance, which is captured by the higher order construct (Credé & Harms, 2015; Johnson et al., 2011).

Researchers choosing to conceptualize eustress as a higher order latent factor should follow recommendations to improve the construct validity and criterion-related validity of eustress, such as those outlined by Johnson and colleagues (2011): utilization of explicit inclusion criteria for the lower order factors (e.g., theoretical reasoning, a priori empirical factor loading cutoffs), a priori specification of the nature of the relations between the lower order constructs and the higher order eustress construct, ruling out potential alternative explanations for the emergence of eustress as the source of shared variance among the indicators (e.g., common method variance; Podsakoff et al., 2003), and demonstrating increased incremental prediction of outcomes from eustress compared with the lower order factors. Other such recommendations are presented by Credé and Harms (2015). Additionally, as more validated measures of eustress emerge, there will be interesting opportunities to explore competing models in which other psychological states are used as predictors of eustress, compared to indicators that define eustress.

Whether higher order factor analysis or an explicit, direct measure of eustress is used, it is important to conceptualize eustress as a psychological state that is experienced in a given moment as the result of a particular event. To capture in-the-moment psychological experiences, studies of eustress should ideally avoid cross-sectional designs. Experience sampling methodology, for example, provides an intriguing lens for studying stressors, eustress, and savoring as employees experience them at work (Rodell & Judge, 2009). Alternatively, field experiments could be used to study the causal mechanisms driving simultaneous experiences of distress and eustress, and longitudinal studies can track coping and savoring processes over time.

Along similar lines, interventions designed to promote primary eustress generation may also take the form of field experiments that include pre- and posttests with a control group to compare positive stress experiences before and after exposure to a stimulus. Otherwise, researchers may choose a longitudinal framework to understand how an intervention takes effect over time. These methods can help rule out threats to valid inferences, such as the Hawthorne effect (i.e., employees demonstrate positive psychological states simply because there are changes being made to their environment and work conditions, rather than states caused by the intervention). It is also possible that employees may experience something similar to a hedonic treadmill effect, in which there is an initial increase in eustress following an intervention, but over time employees return to their baseline psychological state and do not engage in savoring processes. For these reasons, longitudinal follow-ups are highly encouraged to understand the maintenance and longevity of effects from primary eustress generation efforts.

Finally, savoring, or the positive counterpart to coping, is a dynamic process that should unfold over time (see Figure 4.1). After an individual encounters a neutral stressor, that individual may experience eustress, distress, or both. Following an experience of eustress, the individual can savor and enjoy the positive experience of stress and may purposefully attempt to make that positive experience last longer (Nelson & Simmons, 2004; Peterson, 2006). Thus, savoring involves some level of self-awareness in order to understand that one is experiencing eustress. Individuals may lack this self-awareness or self-insight (Reilly & Doherty, 1989), in which case savoring will be difficult to measure, as well as difficult to train or enhance. This may be particularly true in cases when an individual simultaneously experiences eustress and distress, in which case the distress may be more salient due to its negative valence (Kanar et al., 2010). Researchers can develop interventions and training programs designed to teach employees how to recognize times in which they experience positive states of stress, the beneficial results that may arise from these experiences, and methods to savor those experiences to increase the likelihood of subsequent positive outcomes.

CONCLUSION

In conclusion, the holistic model of work stress presented here offers employees and organizations a framework to better understand how demands and stressors affect health and performance in the workplace. In line with the principles articulated by the JD-R model (Demerouti et al., 2001), distress and eustress capture the dual pathways of employees' stress experiences. Organizations can play a significant role in providing meaningful resources and helping employees build resilience in the face of challenges, particularly through facilitation of job crafting opportunities, providing training on emotion regulation and savoring, and promoting cultures of positive P-E fit through recruitment, hiring, and employee development initiatives (Hargrove et al., 2015).

As a result of these efforts, employees' stress response strategies of savoring eustress and coping with distress can manifest in employee outcomes that matter and result in sustained competitive advantage for organizations. Thus, a wide variety of outcomes may be further investigated in future work, including employees' positive and negative evaluations and feelings about their work (Warr, 2013), consistent and sustained levels of employee job performance following coping and savoring (Hargrove et al., 2015), reductions in employee withdrawal behaviors and eventual turnover, employees' organizational citizenship behaviors, and long-term experiences of subjective well-being and health implications following stress responses (Kupriyanov & Zhdanov, 2014).

REFERENCES

Aspinwall, L. G. (1998). Rethinking the role of positive affect in self-regulation. *Motivation and Emotion, 22*(1), 1–32. https://doi.org/10.1023/A:1023080224401

Aspinwall, L. G. (2001). Dealing with adversity: Self-regulation, coping, adaptation, and health. In A. Tesser & N. Schwarz (Eds.), *The Blackwell handbook of social psychology: Vol 1. Intra-individual processes* (pp. 591–614). Blackwell. https://doi.org/10.1002/9780470998519.ch27

Bakker, A. B., & Demerouti, E. (2014). Job demands–resources theory. In P. Y. Chen & C. L. Cooper (Eds.), *Wellbeing: A complete reference guide: Vol. 3. Work and Wellbeing* (pp. 37–64). Wiley-Blackwell. https://doi.org/10.1002/9781118539415.wbwell019

Bakker, A. B., & Demerouti, E. (2017). Job demands–resources theory: Taking stock and looking forward. *Journal of Occupational Health Psychology, 22*(3), 273–285. https://doi.org/10.1037/ocp0000056

Berg, J. M., Dutton, J. E., & Wrzesniewski, A. (2008). What is job crafting and why does it matter? *Center for Positive Organizational Scholarship, Ross School of Business, University of Michigan.* https://positiveorgs.bus.umich.edu/wp-content/uploads/What-is-Job-Crafting-and-Why-Does-it-Matter1.pdf

Branson, V., Dry, M., Palmer, E., & Turnbull, D. (2019). The Adolescent Distress-Eustress Scale: Development and validation. *SAGE Open, 9*(3). https://doi.org/10.1177/2158244019865802

Britt, T. W., Adler, A. B., & Bartone, P. T. (2001). Deriving benefits from stressful events: The role of engagement in meaningful work and hardiness. *Journal of Occupational Health Psychology, 6*(1), 53–63. https://doi.org/10.1037/1076-8998.6.1.53

Bryant, F. (2003). Savoring Beliefs Inventory (SBI): A scale for measuring beliefs about savoring. *Journal of Mental Health, 12*(2), 175–196. https://doi.org/10.1080/0963823031000103489

Cable, D. M., & Edwards, J. R. (2004). Complementary and supplementary fit: A theoretical and empirical integration. *Journal of Applied Psychology, 89*(5), 822–834. https://doi.org/10.1037/0021-9010.89.5.822

Caplan, R. D. (1987). Person–environment fit theory and organizations: Commensurate dimensions, time perspectives, and mechanisms. *Journal of Vocational Behavior, 31*(3), 248–267. https://doi.org/10.1016/0001-8791(87)90042-X

Cavanaugh, M. A., Boswell, W. R., Roehling, M. V., & Boudreau, J. W. (2000). An empirical examination of self-reported work stress among U.S. managers. *Journal of Applied Psychology, 85*(1), 65–74. https://doi.org/10.1037/0021-9010.85.1.65

Chu, L. C. (2014). The influence of perceived stress on work–family conflict and mental health: The moderating effect of person–environment fit. *Journal of Nursing Management, 22*(5), 613–620. https://doi.org/10.1111/jonm.12014

Costantini, A., Demerouti, E., Ceschi, A., & Sartori, R. (2021). Evidence on the hierarchical, multidimensional nature of behavioural job crafting. *Applied Psychology, 70*(1), 311–341. https://doi.org/10.1111/apps.12232

Credé, M., & Harms, P. D. (2015). 25 years of higher-order confirmatory factor analysis in the organizational sciences: A critical review and development of reporting recommendations. *Journal of Organizational Behavior, 36*(6), 845–872. https://doi.org/10.1002/job.2008

Dawis, R. V., & Lofquist, L. H. (1984). *A psychological theory of work adjustment: An individual-differences model and its applications.* University of Minnesota Press.

Demerouti, E., & Bakker, A. B. (2011). The job demands–resources model: Challenges for future research. *SA Journal of Industrial Psychology, 37*, 1–9. https://doi.org/10.4102/sajip.v37i2.974

Demerouti, E., Bakker, A. B., & Gevers, J. M. (2015). Job crafting and extra-role behavior: The role of work engagement and flourishing. *Journal of Vocational Behavior, 91*, 87–96. https://doi.org/10.1016/j.jvb.2015.09.001

Demerouti, E., Bakker, A. B., Nachreiner, F., & Schaufeli, W. B. (2001). The job demands–resources model of burnout. *Journal of Applied Psychology, 86*(3), 499–512. https://doi.org/10.1037/0021-9010.86.3.499

Demerouti, E., & Peeters, M. C. W. (2018). Transmission of reduction-oriented crafting among colleagues: A diary study on the moderating role of working conditions. *Journal of Occupational and Organizational Psychology, 91*(2), 209–234. https://doi.org/10.1111/joop.12196

Edwards, J. R., Caplan, R. D., & van Harrison, R. (1998). Person–environment fit. In C. Cooper (Ed.), *Theories of organizational stress* (pp. 28–67). Oxford University Press.

Edwards, J. R., & Cooper, C. L. (1988). The impacts of positive psychological states on physical health: A review and theoretical framework. *Social Science & Medicine, 27*(12), 1447–1459. https://doi.org/10.1016/0277-9536(88)90212-2

Edwards, J. R., & Parry, M. E. (1993). On the use of polynomial regression equations as an alternative to difference scores in organizational research. *Academy of Management Journal, 36*(6), 1577–1613. https://doi.org/10.5465/256822

Florian, V., Mikulincer, M., & Taubman, O. (1995). Does hardiness contribute to mental health during a stressful real-life situation? The roles of appraisal and coping. *Journal of Personality and Social Psychology, 68*(4), 687–695. https://doi.org/10.1037/0022-3514.68.4.687

Folkman, S., & Moskowitz, J. T. (2000). Positive affect and the other side of coping. *American Psychologist, 55*(6), 647–654. https://doi.org/10.1037/0003-066X.55.6.647

Fredrickson, B. L. (1998). What good are positive emotions? *Review of General Psychology, 2*(3), 300–319. https://doi.org/10.1037/1089-2680.2.3.300

Fredrickson, B. L. (2004). Gratitude, like other positive emotions, broadens and builds. In R. A. Emmons and M. E. McCullough (Eds.), *The psychology of gratitude* (pp. 145–166). Oxford University Press.

French, J. R., Rogers, W., & Cobb, S. (1974). A model of person–environment fit. In G. V. Coelho, D. A. Hamburgh, & J. E. Adams (Eds.), *Coping and adaptation* (pp. 316–333). Basic Books.

Frese, M. (1982). Occupational socialization and psychological development: An underemphasized research perspective in industrial psychology. *Journal of Occupational Psychology, 55*(3), 209–224. https://doi.org/10.1111/j.2044-8325.1982.tb00095.x

Gray-Toft, P., & Anderson, J. G. (1981). Stress among hospital nursing staff: Its causes and effects. *Social Science & Medicine. Part A, Medical Sociology, 15*(5), 639–647. https://doi.org/10.1016/0271-7123(81)90087-0

Gross, S., Semmer, N. K., Meier, L. L., Kälin, W., Jacobshagen, N., & Tschan, F. (2011). The effect of positive events at work on after-work fatigue: They matter most in face of adversity. *Journal of Applied Psychology, 96*(3), 654–664. https://doi.org/10.1037/a0022992

Hargrove, M. B., Becker, W. S., & Hargrove, D. F. (2015). The HRD eustress model: Generating positive stress with challenging work. *Human Resource Development Review, 14*(3), 279–298. https://doi.org/10.1177/1534484315598086

Hobfoll, S. E. (2001). The influence of culture, community, and the nested-self in the stress process: Advancing conservation of resources theory. *Applied Psychology, 50*(3), 337–421. https://doi.org/10.1111/1464-0597.00062

Hoff, K. A., Song, Q. C., Wee, C. J., Phan, W. M. J., & Rounds, J. (2020). Interest fit and job satisfaction: A systematic review and meta-analysis. *Journal of Vocational Behavior, 123*, 103503. https://doi.org/10.1016/j.jvb.2020.103503

Jenkins, M., & Griffith, R. (2004). Using personality constructs to predict performance: Narrow or broad bandwidth. *Journal of Business and Psychology, 19*(2), 255–269. https://doi.org/10.1007/s10869-004-0551-9

Johnson, R. E., Rosen, C. C., & Chang, C. H. (2011). To aggregate or not to aggregate: Steps for developing and validating higher-order multidimensional constructs. *Journal of Business and Psychology, 26*(3), 241–248. https://doi.org/10.1007/s10869-011-9238-1

Kahn, W. A. (1990). Psychological conditions of personal engagement and disengagement at work. *Academy of Management Journal, 33*(4), 692–724.

Kanar, A. M., Collins, C. J., & Bell, B. S. (2010). A comparison of the effects of positive and negative information on job seekers' organizational attraction and attribute recall. *Human Performance, 23*(3), 193–212. https://doi.org/10.1080/08959285.2010.487842

Karasek, R. A. (1979). Job demands, job decision latitude, and mental strain: Implications for job redesign. *Administrative Science Quarterly, 24*(2), 285–308. https://doi.org/10.2307/2392498

Kobasa, S. C., Maddi, S. R., & Kahn, S. (1982). Hardiness and health: A prospective study. *Journal of Personality and Social Psychology, 42*(1), 168–177. https://doi.org/10.1037/0022-3514.42.1.168

Kristof, A. L. (1996). Person-organization fit: An integrative review of its conceptualizations, measurement, and implications. *Personnel Psychology, 49*(1), 1–49. https://doi.org/10.1111/j.1744-6570.1996.tb01790.x

Kristof-Brown, A. L., Zimmerman, R. D., & Johnson, E. C. (2005). Consequences of individual's fit at work: A meta-analysis of person–job, person–organization, person–group, and person–supervisor fit. *Personnel Psychology, 58*(2), 281–342. https://doi.org/10.1111/j.1744-6570.2005.00672.x

Kupriyanov, R., & Zhdanov, R. (2014). The eustress concept: Problems and outlooks. *World Journal of Medical Sciences, 11*(2), 179–185. https://doi.org/10.5829/idosi.wjms.2014.11.2.8433

Lazarus, R. S., & Folkman, S. (1984). *Stress, appraisal and coping.* Springer.

Le, A., Han, B. H., & Palamar, J. J. (2021). When national drug surveys "take too long": An examination of who is at risk for survey fatigue. *Drug and Alcohol Dependence, 225*, 108769. https://doi.org/10.1016/j.drugalcdep.2021.108769

Le Fevre, M., Matheny, J., & Kolt, G. S. (2003). Eustress, distress, and interpretation in occupational stress. *Journal of Managerial Psychology, 18*(7), 726–744. https://doi.org/10.1108/02683940310502412

Li, J., Flores, L. Y., Yang, H., Weng, Q., & Zhu, L. (2022). The role of autonomy support and job crafting in interest incongruence: A mediated moderation model. *Journal of Career Development, 49*(5), 1181–1195. https://doi.org/10.1177/08948453211033903

Mittal, V., & Ross, W. T., Jr. (1998). The impact of positive and negative affect and issue framing on issue interpretation and risk taking. *Organizational Behavior and Human Decision Processes, 76*(3), 298–324. https://doi.org/10.1006/obhd.1998.2808

Nelson, D. L., & Simmons, B. L. (2003). Health psychology and work stress: A more positive approach. In J. C. Quick & L. E. Tetrick (Eds.), *Handbook of occupational health psychology* (pp. 97–119). American Psychological Association.

Nelson, D. L., & Simmons, B. L. (2004). Eustress: An elusive construct, an engaging pursuit. In P. L. Perrewe & D. C. Ganster (Eds.), *Research in occupational stress and well being: Vol. 3. Emotional and physiological processes and positive intervention strategies* (pp. 265–322). Elsevier. https://doi.org/10.1016/S1479-3555(03)03007-5

Nye, C. D., Su, R., Rounds, J., & Drasgow, F. (2012). Vocational interests and performance: A quantitative summary of over 60 years of research. *Perspectives on Psychological Science, 7*(4), 384–403. https://doi.org/10.1177/1745691612449021

Nye, C. D., Su, R., Rounds, J., & Drasgow, F. (2017). Interest congruence and performance: Revisiting recent meta-analytic findings. *Journal of Vocational Behavior, 98*, 138–151. https://doi.org/10.1016/j.jvb.2016.11.002

O'Connor, D. B., Thayer, J. F., & Vedhara, K. (2021). Stress and health: A review of psychobiological processes. *Annual Review of Psychology, 72*(1), 663–688. https://doi.org/10.1146/annurev-psych-062520-122331

O'Sullivan, G. (2011). The relationship between hope, eustress, self-efficacy, and life satisfaction among undergraduates. *Social Indicators Research, 101*(1), 155–172. https://doi.org/10.1007/s11205-010-9662-z

Parker, K. N., & Ragsdale, J. M. (2015). Effects of distress and eustress on changes in fatigue from waking to working. *Applied Psychology: Health and Well-Being, 7*(3), 293–315. https://doi.org/10.1111/aphw.12049

Peterson, C. (2000). The future of optimism. *American Psychologist, 55*(1), 44–55. https://doi.org/10.1037/0003-066X.55.1.44

Peterson, C. (2006). *A primer in positive psychology.* Oxford University Press.

Petrou, P., Demerouti, E., Peeters, M. C., Schaufeli, W. B., & Hetland, J. (2012). Crafting a job on a daily basis: Contextual correlates and the link to work engagement. *Journal of Organizational Behavior, 33*(8), 1120–1141. https://doi.org/10.1002/job.1783

Podsakoff, N. P., LePine, J. A., & LePine, M. A. (2007). Differential challenge stressor-hindrance stressor relationships with job attitudes, turnover intentions, turnover, and withdrawal behavior: A meta-analysis. *Journal of Applied Psychology, 92*(2), 438–454. https://doi.org/10.1037/0021-9010.92.2.438

Podsakoff, P. M., MacKenzie, S. B., Lee, J. Y., & Podsakoff, N. P. (2003). Common method biases in behavioral research: A critical review of the literature and recommended remedies. *Journal of Applied Psychology, 88*(5), 879–903. https://doi.org/10.1037/0021-9010.88.5.879

Quick, J. C., & Quick, J. D. (1984). *Organizational stress and preventive management.* McGraw-Hill.

Quick, J. C., Quick, J. D., Nelson, D. L., & Hurrell, J. J. (1997). *Preventive stress management in organizations.* American Psychological Association. https://doi.org/10.1037/10238-000

Quinones, C., Rodríguez-Carvajal, R., & Griffiths, M. D. (2017). Testing a eustress–distress emotion regulation model in British and Spanish front-line employees. *International Journal of Stress Management, 24*(Suppl. 1), 1–28. https://doi.org/10.1037/str0000021

Reilly, B. A., & Doherty, M. E. (1989). A note on the assessment of self-insight in judgment research. *Organizational Behavior and Human Decision Processes, 44*(1), 123–131. https://doi.org/10.1016/0749-5978(89)90038-1

Rich, B. L., LePine, J. A., & Crawford, E. R. (2010). Job engagement: Antecedents and effects on job performance. *Academy of Management Journal, 53*(3), 617–635. https://doi.org/10.5465/amj.2010.51468988

Rodell, J. B., & Judge, T. A. (2009). Can "good" stressors spark "bad" behaviors? The mediating role of emotions in links of challenge and hindrance stressors with citizenship and counterproductive behaviors. *Journal of Applied Psychology, 94*(6), 1438–1451.

Rodríguez, I., Kozusznik, M. W., & Peiró, J. M. (2013). Development and validation of the Valencia Eustress-Distress Appraisal Scale. *International Journal of Stress Management, 20*(4), 279–308. https://doi.org/10.1037/a0034330

Russell, J. A., & Carroll, J. M. (1999). On the bipolarity of positive and negative affect. *Psychological Bulletin, 125*(1), 3–30. https://doi.org/10.1037/0033-2909.125.1.3

Salovey, P., Rothman, A. J., Detweiler, J. B., & Steward, W. T. (2000). Emotional states and physical health. *American Psychologist, 55*(1), 110–121. https://doi.org/10.1037/0003-066X.55.1.110

Sarstedt, M., Hair, J. F., Jr., Cheah, J. H., Becker, J. M., & Ringle, C. M. (2019). How to specify, estimate, and validate higher-order constructs in PLS-SEM. *Australasian Marketing Journal, 27*(3), 197–211. https://doi.org/10.1016/j.ausmj.2019.05.003

Scheier, M. F., & Carver, C. S. (1992). Effects of optimism on psychological and physical well-being: Theoretical overview and empirical update. *Cognitive Therapy and Research, 16*(2), 201–228. https://doi.org/10.1007/BF01173489

Schneider, B. (1987). The people make the place. *Personnel Psychology, 40*(3), 437–453. https://doi.org/10.1111/j.1744-6570.1987.tb00609.x

Simmons, B. L. (2000). *Eustress at work: Accentuating the positive* [Unpublished doctoral dissertation]. Oklahoma State University.

Simmons, B. L., & Nelson, D. L. (2001). Eustress at work: The relationship between hope and health in hospital nurses. *Health Care Management Review, 26*(4), 7–18. https://doi.org/10.1097/00004010-200110000-00002

Simmons, B. L., & Nelson, D. L. (2007). Eustress at work: Extending the holistic stress model. In D. L. Nelson & C. L. Cooper (Eds.), *Positive organizational behavior* (pp. 40–54). Sage. https://doi.org/10.4135/9781446212752.n4

Simmons, B. L., Nelson, D. L., & Neal, L. J. (2001). A comparison of the positive and negative work attitudes of home health care and hospital nurses. *Health Care Management Review, 26*(3), 63–74. https://doi.org/10.1097/00004010-200107000-00007

Smyth, J. M., & Pennebaker, J. W. (2001). What are the health effects of disclosure? In A. Baum, T. A. Revenson, & J. E. Singer (Eds.), *Handbook of health psychology* (pp. 339–348). Erlbaum.

Tims, M., Bakker, A. B., & Derks, D. (2013). The impact of job crafting on job demands, job resources, and well-being. *Journal of Occupational Health Psychology, 18*(2), 230–240. https://doi.org/10.1037/a0032141

Van den Broeck, A., De Cuyper, N., De Witte, H., & Vansteenkiste, M. (2010). Not all job demands are equal: Differentiating job hindrances and job challenges in the Job Demands–Resources model. *European Journal of Work and Organizational Psychology, 19*(6), 735–759. https://doi.org/10.1080/13594320903223839

Vancouver, J. B., & Schmitt, N. W. (1991). An exploratory examination of person-organization fit: Organizational goal congruence. *Personnel Psychology, 44*(2), 333–352. https://doi.org/10.1111/j.1744-6570.1991.tb00962.x

Vogt, K., Hakanen, J. J., Brauchli, R., Jenny, G. J., & Bauer, G. F. (2016). The consequences of job crafting: A three-wave study. *European Journal of Work and Organizational Psychology, 25*(3), 353–362. https://doi.org/10.1080/1359432X.2015.1072170

Warr, P. (2013). How to think about and measure psychological well-being. In R. R. Sinclair, M. Wang, & L. E. Tetrick (Eds.), *Research methods in occupational health psychology: Measurement, design, and data analysis* (pp. 76–90). Routledge.

Watson, D., Clark, L. A., & Tellegen, A. (1988). Development and validation of brief measures of positive and negative affect: The PANAS scales. *Journal of Personality and Social Psychology, 54*(6), 1063–1070. https://doi.org/10.1037/0022-3514.54.6.1063

Wiegand, J. P., Drasgow, F., & Rounds, J. (2021). Misfit matters: A re-examination of interest fit and job satisfaction. *Journal of Vocational Behavior, 125*, 103524. https://doi.org/10.1016/j.jvb.2020.103524

Wrzesniewski, A., & Dutton, J. (2001). Crafting a job: Revisioning employees as active crafters of their work. *Academy of Management Review, 26*(2), 179–201. https://doi.org/10.2307/259118

Zohar, D., Tzischinski, O., & Epstein, R. (2003). Effects of energy availability on immediate and delayed emotional reactions to work events. *Journal of Applied Psychology, 88*(6), 1082–1093. https://doi.org/10.1037/0021-9010.88.6.1082

Controlling Occupational Safety and Health Hazards

Michael J. Smith, Pascale Carayon, and Peter Hoonakker

Certain events in history have had a major impact on the way work is organized and subsequently on the health and safety of workers. Think of the invention of the steam engine and electricity, which led to industrialization of society, which in turn had a major impact on work and how it was done. The COVID-19 pandemic had major effects on where people were working (or not working), how they carried out their jobs, and the kinds of hazards they encountered. The pandemic affected the nature and design of work organizations and supervision, how tasks were done, social and professional interactions with coworkers and customers, and resource availability for providing products and services, in addition to the rewards and satisfactions from doing work. The pandemic made us rethink workplace risks and safety in a broader context of "systems" that interact, as well as how external and internal risks relate to providing a "total" safety network to understand risks and hazards, how to apply controls, and how to redesign work systems.

This chapter examines occupational risks for injury and illness, in addition to some ways to reduce or control risks. It provides direction for establishing effective detection and control methods. First, we offer a simple model for examining safety and health risks. Then we examine different types of workplace hazards. Engineering and human factors approaches for eliminating or reducing hazards, injuries, and illnesses are presented. Then a systems-level model, model, Systems Engineering Initiative for Patient Safety (SEIPS), provides a total safety approach, followed by contemporary examples in the context of the COVID-19 pandemic.

https://doi.org/10.1037/0000331-005
Handbook of Occupational Health Psychology, Third Edition, L. E. Tetrick, G. G. Fisher, M. T. Ford, and J. C. Quick (Editors)

The building blocks of hazard identification and control are (a) hazard knowledge; (b) hazard identification and monitoring; (c) injury and illness surveillance; (d) interventions such as hazard removal, materials substitution, and/or changing the work processes; (e) interventions such as blocking access through guarding and/or barriers; (f) interventions that reduce exposures such as job rotation, time limits, and/or job redesign; (g) enhanced supervision and/or employee monitoring; (h) enhanced employee knowledge and skills through training; and (i) effective safety programs.

EXAMINING FACTORS THAT CAN LEAD TO EXPOSURES AND ACCIDENTS

Any strategy to control workplace exposures and accidents should consider the breadth of factors and their influences on each other (Carayon et al., 2012; Carayon & Smith, 2000, 2014; Smith & Carayon, 2011; Smith & Carayon-Sainfort, 1989). A *balance model*—with multiple components of the work system, including the person, task activities, the environment, technology, tools and machinery, the work organization, and supervision—is one way to organize safety efforts (Carayon, 2009; Smith & Carayon-Sainfort, 1989). For each component of the work system, there can be characteristics that cause hazardous exposures or provide controls for exposures. The components can interact to create a context for hazardous exposures. Understanding the contexts and interactions is essential for hazard identification and control.

The Person

A wide range of individual attributes can affect exposure and accident potential. Factors such as a person's intellectual capabilities and aptitudes, perceptual-motor abilities, physical capabilities, current health status, and personality can affect accident risk. For example, the ability for hazard recognition and the aptitude for training are important aspects of injury prevention. Employees must have the necessary physical resources, mental resources, knowledge, and skills to do the work safely. It is critical that a proper "fit" is achieved between an employee's capabilities and the demands of the job tasks. This can occur with appropriate selection, training, skill enhancement, hazard orientation, safety and ergonomic improvements, as well as proper engineering of the tasks, technology, and environment.

Machinery, Technology, and Materials

Machinery has moving parts that must be constructed to protect employees. Materials can be toxic, flammable, or combustible and must not contact employees. "Smart" technology is sometimes difficult to use and can develop "bugs" that lead to failure. General safety guidance is for moving parts to be guarded; less hazardous materials can be substituted for highly toxic materials; and backup for smart technology failure can be employed. When substitution is not possible for dangerous materials, "closed-system" production methods with extensive engineering controls can be used to contain the materials and to shield employees from exposures. Psychosocial stress from smart technology can be reduced by making it user friendly, as well as implementing the use of backup and recovery methods. Plans should be developed to deal with failures in the work processes that create production and safety risks. Resources for understanding and dealing with these hazards are provided at the end of this chapter.

Task Factors

The demands of work and the way it is conducted can influence the probability of exposures and accidents. These demands also influence employee attention, satisfaction, motivation, and behavior. Task considerations can be examined as the physical and mental requirements, as well as the psychological considerations. These affect the amount of energy expenditure, which affects physiological and mental load and fatigue, in addition to physical and psychological stress. Stress diminishes a worker's capabilities to recognize and respond to workplace hazards. Task considerations related to the physical work requirements include the workload, the pace or rate of work, the amount of repetition in task activities, and the extent of work pressure due to production demands. Psychosocial issues such as performance monitoring and social isolation can be stressors. These conditions may produce cumulative trauma disorders to the musculoskeletal system and cause mental distress. Sources for information on physical and psychological hazards are provided in the references.

The Physical Work Environment

The physical work environment exposes employees to materials, chemicals, physical agents, and climates that can cause harm or injury if the exposure exceeds safe limits. Such exposures vary widely from industry to industry, from job to job, and from task to task. The hazard potential of different environmental factors can be evaluated using various federal, state, and local codes and standards, as well as consensus standards for worker protection and exposure limits established by scientific and consensus groups. For access to standards and guidelines for particular chemicals, materials, technologies, processes, and industries, see the several sources listed at the end of the chapter. Environmental conditions may also hamper employees' ability to use their senses (poor lighting, excessive noise, overpowering smells, temperature) and thus reduce their capacity to respond or react to hazardous situations. The environment should be compatible with worker sensory capabilities, perceptual-motor skills, energy expenditure and endurance limits, and the motivational desire to do tasks in the proper and safe way. Air quality, lighting, and noise control can be designed to address these considerations.

Organizational Design and Management

Several aspects of organizational design and management can influence accident risk. These include management policies and procedures, the way in which work tasks are organized, supervision style, the motivational climate, the nature of the interaction among employees and organizational units, employee social support, as well as training and management attitude toward safety. Management attitude, involvement, and commitment are recognized as critical elements in successful safety programs. If managers have a disregard for safety, employees may not be motivated to work safely. If management considers safety to be important, managers, supervisors, and employees are motivated to work safely. An organizational climate that is conducive to cooperative efforts in hazard recognition and control, a management structure that provides for frequent employee interaction, a positive style of supervision, and social support all contribute to good safety performance.

WORKPLACE HAZARDS

The best sources for hazard information are the Occupational Safety and Health Administration (OSHA) standards, National Institute for Occupational Safety and Health (NIOSH) documents, and publications and resources from professional organizations and societies. Several are listed at the end of this chapter. There are also other international, federal, state, and local agencies that can provide information on occupational health and safety hazards and controls. The breadth and nature of occupational hazards is vast and can be classified into broad categories that help organize recognition and potential controls. These categories are (a) physical agents, such as noise, radiation, and heat; (b) powered mechanical agents, such as machinery and tools; (c) nonpowered mechanical agents, such as hammers, axes, and knives; (d) liquid chemical agents, such as benzene, toluene, and medications; (e) powdered materials, such as pesticides, asbestos, sand, and coal dust; (f) gaseous or vaporous chemical agents, such as nitrous oxide, carbon monoxide, and anhydrous ammonia; (g) heavy metals, such as lead, mercury, and chromium; (h) biological agents, such as bacteria, viruses and fungi; (i) genetically engineered agents; (j) nanotechnology; (k) medicines and drugs, such as pills, inhalants, and injections; (l) unsafe behaviors by self and others; (m) other hazards, such as wet working surfaces, working at height, and unguarded floor openings; (n) psychosocial job stressors; and (o) unknown and new and emerging hazards. These hazards affect the body through various routes, such as inhalation, absorption, ingestion, traumatic contact, and through cognitive mental processes. Many of these hazards, adverse exposure levels, and their health and injury effects are described in the sources identified at the end of this chapter.

The COVID-19 pandemic demonstrated the unpredictable and highly hazardous nature of biological agents. Traditional controls and disease treatments were only as good as the available knowledge, access to safety supplies, the ability to distribute and apply the controls, the availability of knowledgeable staff needed to apply the controls, the willingness of employees to accept new ways of doing work, and the capability to develop new controls and medical treatments. The COVID-19 pandemic increased physical and psychological work demands that led to physical stress and psychological stress problems. Insufficient staffing, longer work hours, shiftwork, fewer work breaks, and less time off all put heavier burdens on workers and their families. Such demands affect the quantity and quality of the products and services delivered.

Hopefully, one lesson learned was that efforts to decrease production and process costs by cutting staffing and making processes "lean" can backfire when emergencies occur. When the COVID-19 pandemic struck, there was a lack of necessary staff and critical supplies, and an inability to meet demand for products and services. Going "lean" and using a system of just-in-time delivery of supplies and parts meant there was no reserve to fall back on. People died as a result of the lack of facilities, services, supplies, and knowledge. Later in the chapter, we discuss a different approach, called the Systems Engineering Initiative for Patient Safety model, that we believe offers more possibilities for better outcomes.

MEASURING HAZARD POTENTIAL AND SAFETY PERFORMANCE

To successfully control occupational hazards as well as related illnesses and injuries, it is necessary to define their nature and predict when and where they will occur. This requires a process of hazard detection that defines their locations, nature, frequency seriousness, and amenability to control. Hazard identification can be examined by facility and work process through formal inspections, and by offline methods such as fault-free analysis, failure mode effects analysis, and employee hazard reporting programs. A parallel approach uses employee injury and company loss control information to define problem spots. In hazardous and complex work systems, incident reporting is often used before injuries or property damage occur.

Hazard Inspection Programs

Identifying hazards before an occupational injury occurs is a major goal of a hazard inspection program, which needs to be organized in a systematic way. Programs can be formalized using federal and state regulations that define potential health and safety hazards. Checklists can be used to document and organize hazard data, and employee interviews can elaborate on the hazards observed. Workers' compensation insurance carriers can also provide checklists and advice. Regular inspections are most effective in identifying permanent, fixed physical, biological, and environmental hazards that do not vary much over time. Inspections are not as effective in identifying transient hazards or unsafe workplace behaviors. To maintain a positive motivational influence, hazard inspections should not be a punitive process of placing blame, confrontation, or punishment. Highlighting the positive aspects of work areas is important for motivating safe behavior.

The frequency of inspections should be based on the frequency and injury or illness potential of the hazards being evaluated. Inspections should be conducted at least monthly and more frequently as needed. After a serious fixed physical hazard has been identified and controlled, periodic reinspection is required. Random spot-checking can be done. Hazards that are transient or intermittent will require more frequent inspection. In some cases of serious hazard potential, daily inspection is reasonable. Inspections should take place when and where the highest probability of a hazard exists, and reinspection can occur as needed. For infrequent intermittent hazards, employees are a good source of information and can be surveyed frequently.

Illness and Injury Statistics

There are four main uses of injury statistics: (a) to identify high-risk jobs or work areas, (b) to evaluate company health and safety performance, (c) to evaluate the effectiveness of hazard abatement approaches, and (d) to identify factors related to illness and injury causation. An illness and injury reporting and analysis system needs detailed information about the characteristics of illnesses and injuries as well as their frequency and severity. Information about the specific details of an exposure, accident, or incident should be collected. OSHA has illness and injury reporting and recording requirements that are mandatory for all employers, with certain exclusions. Regulations have been developed to define how employers are to adhere to these requirements (see https://www.osha.gov). Injury incidence and severity information provides the basis for directing a company's approach to health and safety. It can also serve as the basis of rewarding managers and workers for good performance.

CONTROLLING WORKPLACE HAZARDS

Having identified and defined workplace hazards, the next step is to eliminate them, where possible, or control them. There are six classes of interventions for achieving hazard control that are often used together to make a safety program. These include (a) identifying and eliminating the hazards; (b) blocking access to the hazards; (c) changing work practices and procedures to eliminate or reduce contact with the hazards; (d) warning about the hazards and how to avoid them; (e) educating and training about the hazards and how to avoid them; and (f) using personal protective equipment as a supplementary control.

Engineering Controls

The most effective way to deal with a hazard is to eliminate it. This is also called *primary prevention*. It can be accomplished by redesigning a product, tool, machine, process, or the environment, or through the substitution of a nonhazardous method, material, or technology. The second class of engineering controls is blocking employee access to the hazard. This can be achieved by putting up a barrier that prevents the employee from contacting the hazard or that keeps the employee from entering a hazardous area. Fences, guards, and shields over or around the hazard remove the potential for contact. With this type of intervention, the hazard remains but is controlled by restricting employees' access. It is sometimes the case that the hazard must be accessed for maintenance, repair, calibration, resetting, or other reasons. These situations require that the power to the hazard be shut down, locked out, and tagged. An important design feature is an interlock that keeps the hazard power off while employees are present in the danger zone. Containment is a special barrier guard or shield that is used for very dangerous chemicals and physical hazards, such as radiation or carcinogenic agents. It is a closed system with no access during operation, and extreme caution is maintained when the system is accessed for cleaning and repairs.

Another engineering control is the active removal of the hazard before it comes into contact with the employee. An example is a local scavenger ventilation system that sucks the fumes and mists produced by a process away from employees during operation. A related ventilation approach is to dilute exposure to airborne contaminants by bringing in more fresh air. This reduces the exposure concentrations below the danger threshold. When new materials or chemicals are introduced into the work process, or when additional airborne exposures are added into the environment, the adequacy of the ventilation dilution approach to provide safe levels for all exposure(s) must be verified. Combinations of multiple contaminant exposures add increased risks, as the science for defining safe limits for combinations of contaminants is incomplete.

Personal Protective Equipment

When engineering controls cannot provide complete protection or as a backup in case of an emergency, personal protective equipment must be worn by the employees. This is not a preferred method of control because there is a possibility that an employee may still be exposed to the hazard; therefore, it is a secondary prevention method. For example, a poorly fitted respirator mask will allow infiltration and unsafe exposure. This was demonstrated during the COVID-19 pandemic, when many employees lacked knowledge about the use and fit of face masks.

Keep in mind that it is an important rule of safety and health that the best method for controlling hazards is through engineering methods that eliminate or block access to them. Individual-focused controls are used when engineering controls are not feasible or not solely effective. Individual-focused controls are often necessary as supplements to engineering controls, but there are some instances where individual-focused controls are the only feasible and effective controls. These require close supervision.

Warnings and Instructions

Informing employees about workplace hazards has three aspects: (a) employees' right to know about potential hazard exposures, (b) warnings about the dangers of the hazards and how to avoid or control them, and (c) instructions on how to be protected from the hazards. Federal safety and health regulations, and many state and local regulations, specify that an employer has the obligation to inform employees of hazardous workplace exposures to chemicals, materials, and physical or biological agents that are known to cause harm. Employers must be aware of the requirements for specific hazards, as the requirements of informing may vary.

In general, an employer must provide information about the name of the material (hazard), its potential health effects, exposure levels that produce adverse health (safety), the typical kinds of exposures encountered in the facility, how to avoid exposures, and what to do if exposed. For each chemical, material, or agent classified as hazardous by OSHA and the Environmental Protection Agency (EPA), employers are required to maintain a safety document called a material safety data sheet that provides detailed information about the toxicity, potential injuries, control measures, and standard operating procedures for using the product. This document must be easily accessible to employees at or near the potential areas of exposure. A list of hazardous chemicals, materials, and physical agents can be obtained from OSHA (https://www.osha.gov) or the EPA (https://www.epa.gov).

Warnings are used to convey the message of extreme danger of serious injury or death. They are designed to catch the attention of the employee, to inform the employee about the hazard, and to instruct them how to avoid the hazard. The American National Standards Institute has developed standards for the design of visual warnings that provide guidelines as a starting point (https://www.ansi.org). Warnings are primarily visual and auditory but can also be olfactory (e.g., natural gas). The warning provides information about specific actions to take to avoid the hazard or to effectively deal with hazards. Warnings are the behavioral model that can be followed to increase the probability of safe behavior to eliminate or reduce the risk of exposure.

Promoting Safe Employee Behavior by Training

Training workers to improve their skills in recognizing hazardous conditions is a primary means for reducing hazard exposures and accidents. Safety and health training is effective in increasing employee knowledge about hazards and safe behavior as well as in reducing unsafe employee behavior. The training content should allow learners to achieve an effective level of health and safety knowledge and competence. The specifics of the content will meet the desired skills to be learned and the hazards to be recognized and controlled.

Hazard Reduction by Improved Work Practices

Many workplace hazards are produced by the interaction between employees, the technology and tools, and the environment. A human factors systems approach improves the interactions through technology redesign, enhanced environmental conditions, training, hazard monitoring, and improved work practices. Individual-focused approaches are often used when there are hazards that cannot be eliminated through engineering controls. This includes enhancing employee recognition of the hazards, following safe work procedures to ensure that hazards will not occur, using safe behaviors to eliminate contact with the hazards, and behavior-modification programs to instill the safe practices as habits.

SEIPS: A SYSTEMS APPROACH FOR SAFETY MANAGEMENT AND HAZARD CONTROL

The Systems Engineering Initiative for Patient Safety (SEIPS) model was developed to address patient safety and health care quality from a human factors and systems engineering perspective (Carayon et al., 2006). It builds on the balance model and the work system described previously (Smith & Carayon-Sainfort, 1989). According to the SEIPS model, the components and interactions of the work system (i.e., person, tasks, physical environment, tools and technologies, and organization) influence care processes, which in turn affect outcomes, particularly patient safety.

The SEIPS model has been used extensively to identify characteristics of the work system that affect health care workers' ability to do their job; obstacles and facilitators to work performance can be found in all components of the work system. For instance, in a study of 270 nurses in the intensive care units of seven hospitals, the most frequent performance obstacles were found in the physical work environment (e.g., noisy work environment, reported by 46% of nurses), the tasks (e.g., spending time dealing with family needs, reported by 35% of nurses), the organization (e.g., delay in getting medications from pharmacy, reported by 36% of nurses), and the tools and technologies (e.g., equipment not available, reported by 32% of nurses) (Gurses & Carayon, 2009, 2007). Performance obstacles and facilitators are anchored in the components of the work system and their interactions; they create hazards to health care workers performing their job safely and effectively.

Initially, the SEIPS model focused on safety in health care; however, it can be expanded to address safety in all industries and services. In the expanded version of the SEIPS model for occupational safety and health (the OSH-SEIPS model), the work system (i.e., its components and their interactions) influences production and service processes, which in turn impact occupational safety and health outcomes, such as injury and illnesses. Production and service processes represent how work is done and unfolds over time and are a direct output of the work system components and their interactions. See Figure 5.1 for a visual representation of the OSH-SEIPS model.

The OSH-SEIPS model includes feedback loops between the processes and the work system and between outcomes and the work system. These feedback loops are critical as they represent learning and improvement opportunities.

FIGURE 5.1.   OSH-SEIPS Model-Expanded SEIPS Model for Occupational Safety and Health

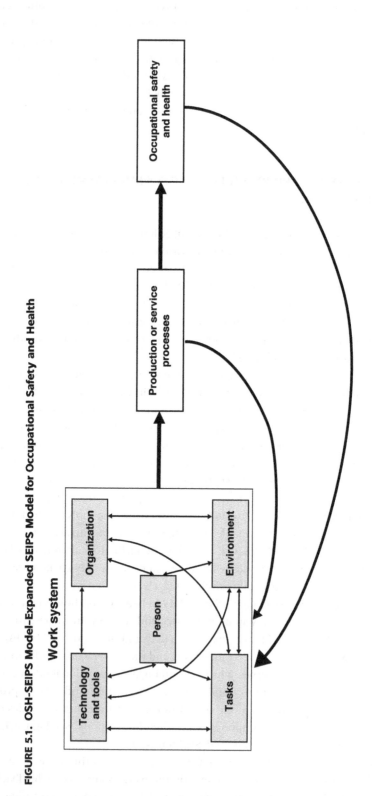

As described previously, effective controlling hazards should include methods and mechanisms for measuring hazard potential and safety performance. Hazard identification focuses on the production and service processes and produces information on the work system components and their interactions that have the potential to negatively affect safety and health (see the first feedback loop in Figure 5.1). Assessment of safety performance, for example, via illness and injury statistics, focuses on the right side of the OSH-SEIPS model, that is, the occupational safety and health outcomes (see the second feedback loop in Figure 5.1). Information from both assessments of hazard potential and safety performance feeds back to the work system and provides suggestions for implementation. This feedback is critical for continuous learning and improvement of work systems. The COVID-19 pandemic demonstrated that emergent changes can occur rapidly in how work is done and can thus affect the safety and health of workers. Therefore, organizations need to have structures, mechanisms, and methods in place to quickly identify hazards and address them in an efficient and effective manner; these are critical organizational learning processes for occupational safety and health.

EXAMPLES OF IMPROVING QUALITY MANAGEMENT STRATEGIES FOR OCCUPATIONAL SAFETY AND HEALTH

The following are examples that illustrate interventions where the OSH-SEIPS approach was used to improve safety and quality in a variety of industries with very different hazards and management issues. These illustrate the breadth of OSH-SEIPS capabilities for improving occupational safety and health while also improving productivity and quality of services and products.

Using OSH-SEIPS in Construction Operations

Some organizational strategies focus on improving production and service processes (e.g., lean management or total quality management), but they rarely integrate the human component in their approach. The result is increased efficiency but often at the cost of people and their health and safety. The OSH-SEIPS model integrates a focus on production and service processes with heightened attention to people and the rest of the work system in order to continually improve occupational safety and health.

Companies invest in various strategies aimed at improving the quality of their production, products, and services as well as for addressing occupational safety and management. A systematic review of the literature in the construction industry highlights the potential overlap between these two groups of organizational strategies (e.g., Loushine et al., 2006); however, very few studies have examined how quality management and safety management can be integrated within the construction industry. The authors of the systematic review highlighted the critical role of implementation factors as well as the need to develop a deep understanding of the nature of construction work; increased attention to these factors is critical to achieve production/ service improvements and optimal occupational safety and health.

In a mixed-methods study of construction contractors, Hoonakker and colleagues (2010) identified four main barriers to the implementation of quality management: (a) nature of construction projects that are often large, labor-intensive, and seldom situated in the same location; (b) large number of parties involved in the construction process that have their own interests and perspectives; (c) large variation within and across construction projects; and (d) organization of bidding process that often emphasizes efficiency and cost reduction at the expense of quality and occupational safety and health. The OSH-SEIPS model can be used to address these implementation barriers by focusing effort on the design of interconnected work systems and their interactions. This systems approach integrates the human component, as workers are at the center of the work systems and the objective is to improve their occupational safety and health.

As previously highlighted, another key characteristic of the OSH-SEIPS model is the feedback. The feedback loops are critical as they provide information on process and outcome measures, which can help identify areas of the work system in need of improvement. Improvement in the work systems can lead to improved safety performance; however, this often takes time. A longitudinal study of 912 contractors in the construction industry showed that safety efforts and initiatives produced benefits in safety performance, but only over time (Hoonakker et al., 2005). Therefore, the feedback loops of the OSH-SEIPS model are critical because they draw attention to organizational learning that occurs with information and over time.

Working From Home: Ergonomics and Job Design

The COVID-19 pandemic has introduced new psychosocial stressors and intensified traditional stressors. The world was not prepared to deal with this emergency. That signifies we need to implement resources for rapidly responding to unexpected and unplanned situations that can affect employee health and safety. In addition, these situations can cause psychosocial stressors, such as social isolation, reduced social support, or working at home with families, children, partners, and/or pets present, and can create more difficult environments with less job control, more demands, and fewer rest breaks. In addition, employers instituted more electronic job-performance monitoring of their employees. These job-design factors caused psychosocial stress levels to soar. In addition, a lack of access to acceptable computer/IT workstations and work areas while working at home led to increased ergonomic hazards and musculoskeletal discomfort and disorders.

For employees working from home, employers need to use ergonomic knowledge and principles to adapt technologies, activities, and environmental conditions to the physical, psychological, and social nature of these new working conditions. IT technology and workstation design must be more than just making the technology interfaces friendlier and having adjustable furniture. It must also integrate the design considerations with the work environment, the task requirements, the psychosocial aspects of work and job redesign. Critical considerations for good ergonomics practice include (a) reducing biomechanical loading on the back, neck, upper extremities, and legs to the lowest practical forces; (b) keeping repetition of body parts as low as practical; (c) keeping the back, neck, shoulders, and joints in good postures; (d) reducing the amount of time in static postures; (e) reducing the duration and extent of highly repetitive motions and/or high forces; (f) designing environmental conditions so that people can easily see, hear, and think; (g) providing frequent rest breaks from activities for resting, recovery and movement; and (h) providing healthy psychosocial working conditions. These conditions are not so easy to meet when an employee is working from home. Employer support with equipment, technology, and adjustments to job requirements can reduce the risk of injuries and stress.

There are many online and hardcopy resources that provide specific guidance for computer users in setting up and using fixed and portable computer/ IT workstations and work areas at home (Smith & Carayon, 2012; Smith et al., 2008). The primary working surface (e.g., those supporting the keyboard, the mouse, the monitor(s), and documents) should be sufficient to

- have the display screen at a comfortable viewing distance and height for comfortable head/neck and back postures and for easily reading the screen;

- have keyboard and mouse (or other pointing devices) at a height for comfortable head/neck, back, shoulder, arm, and wrist postures (wrist and arm supports have been shown to be effective);

- position documents for easy viewing and proper musculoskeletal alignment of the upper extremities, head, neck, and the back;

- provide easy access to materials and equipment, and comfortable postural shifts between the primary and secondary surfaces; and

- provide adequate knee and leg room for repositioning movements while working at primary and secondary surfaces.

In addition, ensure laptop or handheld devices (e.g., tablet, phone) are as thin and lightweight as possible; provide an adjustable table if possible as these are a better fit for users; and provide an adjustable height chair with swivel/tilt capabilities, adequate seat and back support, padding, and lumbar support. Other recommendations include setting up the workstation and area in a private location to reduce interruptions, distractions, and noise; getting away from the workstation and technology and move around after every hour of working; and designating set times each day to deal with personal and family matters.

Health Care Example: Systems Approach to Occupational Safety and Health

The COVID-19 pandemic has significantly affected the ways in which health care and patient care are organized and delivered. For instance, in a very short period of time, health care organizations have switched to telehealth with the use of audio and video remote technologies (Grossman et al., 2020). Health care organizations faced major challenges to protect their workers from physical and psychosocial hazards, such as lack of protective equipment, fear of exposure to virus, long work hours, as well as both overload and underload of critical information regarding protocols and organizational strategies (Carayon & Perry, 2020; Michaels & Wagner, 2020). Challenges of occupational safety and health in the health care industry were heightened by the COVID-19 pandemic, but many physical and psychosocial stressors and hazards were already present. Therefore, it is critical to reflect on and learn quickly from the effects of the COVID-19 pandemic so that health care organizations can engage in systems-based approaches for occupational safety and health.

Health care organizations should use the following principles in their continuous effort for improving occupational safety and health (Carayon & Perry, 2020): (a) Rely on local expertise to assess risks and hazards in the work system; (b) support resilience, adaptation, and creativity, particularly in case of a crisis such as the COVID-19 pandemic; (c) acknowledge that work systems are dynamic and influenced by both bottom-up and top-down interactions; (d) establish structures and processes for timely and accurate communication and coordination; and (e) institute short- and long-term learning at both individual and organizational levels. Genuine worker participation is key to developing an accurate assessment of what does and does not "work" in the work system; this can be done with multiple methods, such as survey, interview, focus group, and observation. Fostering worker participation is also important for creating an organizational climate and environment that helps develop creative and innovative solutions to complex problems of work organization. This will also help support opportunities for both individual and organizational learning. This systems approach to occupational safety and health in health care organizations is even more important as the COVID-19 pandemic extends and continues to challenge health care workers and affect their long-term health and safety.

Meat-Processing Plant

One of the authors of this chapter was consulted by a major grocery chain in the United States looking to reduce acute and cumulative trauma injuries in one of their large meat-processing facilities. The company management had been introduced to an early version of the SEIPS approach at a seminar. Plans were made for a hazard analysis to be conducted by ergonomic and safety professionals using a traditional inspection checklist. The company was comfortable using this approach because it fit with their own safety system. The professionals went into the food-processing production lines, warehouse, and shipping department. They found many safety and ergonomic hazards that fit the profile of potential causes for injuries in the facility. Having completed the evaluation and after examining the results, the management requested that the primary consultant and the ergonomic and safety professionals develop corrective measures. At this point in the process, it looked like a traditional approach would proceed.

The primary consultant reminded the management of the seminar they attended and reintroduced them to the SEIPS approach. There were management concerns about involving facility employees in the next steps. To allay the concerns, a training session was held with all employees in which the results of the evaluations were presented along with potential solutions. At the end of the training session, the primary consultant asked for questions and criticisms. The union steward immediately criticized the entire process for defining hazards as limited because the union and the employees were not involved. Other employees chimed in, expressing similar thoughts about the hazards and solutions, and a discussion ensued. Management became concerned about the dialogue and expressed the belief that it was management's responsibility to deal with safety issues related to OSHA.

After the meeting, the primary consultant suggested to management that committees of employees from each department be formed, including their direct supervisors. The purpose of the committees was to critique the work of the consultants and provide advice, from the employees' perspectives, on the hazards identified; to identify new hazards; and to propose solutions. Management agreed to have two high-risk departments carry this activity out for 1 month as a pilot test of efficacy.

The results from the two high-risk department committees were eye-opening to the consultants, management, and employees in other departments. The first critical outcome was improved communication between employees, their supervisors, and the union about safety. During the discussions, relations among employees, the union, and supervisors became more cooperative and less combative. They listened to each other, provided respectful critique, and reached a consensus. The second critical outcome was the identification of many hazards that were not observed by the ergonomic and safety consultants. This illustrated the limitation of walk-through inspections as the only means of defining hazards. Some hazards are cyclical, recurring, temporary, situational, unpredictable, and/or behavioral. Some of these would be missed by walk-through inspections. The employees knew about them, identified them, and provided potential solutions. Management was impressed and instituted committees in all departments.

As part of the initial evaluation of the facility, the primary consultant conducted work satisfaction and health symptom surveys of all employees and supervisors. The surveys were continued for each of the additional 4 years of the consultancy. In addition, an evaluation of the work injury records for the 5 years prior to the consultancy and going forward was conducted.

Over the first year of committee work, many additional hazards were defined beyond those found by the ergonomic and safety consultants. Solutions were proposed and evaluated. Some were implemented, and others were discarded for various reasons including feasibility, importance, impact, and cost. There was ongoing feedback between employees, the union, and management about potential new hazards and the effectiveness of solutions.

Some of the initial solutions were modified, others were dropped for ineffectiveness, and new solutions were proposed and implemented. The feedback process was a powerful tool to achieve success. The employees, the union, and management were in harmony dealing with the safety issues. The data on the injury experience showed marked reductions during the first year in terms of frequency, severity, and cost of injuries. The job satisfaction data showed that employees liked participating in defining hazards and potential solutions. The psychosocial stress levels of the employees decreased.

As the second year got underway, the union contract came up for negotiation. Tension occurred between the union and management, as well as among union employees in different job categories (skilled vs. unskilled, plant floor vs. warehouse). With the focus on pay increases and a potential strike, interest in safety waned. The union decided to use the SEIPS method of identifying the differences among various job categories on critical bargaining issues. The union assembled committees from each job category to develop the issues that were important to them. Then the committees were brought together to define and rank the bargaining issues.

At the same time, management determined that the cooperation developed with the union on the safety issues should be a way to work out differences in the contract negotiations. After a few months of management efforts to develop a cooperative discussion, management and the union came together and used feedback with their constituents. The cooperative discussion was a new context for management and labor that led to a new contract with which all sides (management, union, and employees) were satisfied.

Shortly after the contract was settled, renewed safety efforts started and carried on for the entire 5-year monitoring period by the primary consultant. Over those 5 years, the injury record for the facility continued to improve each year, and employee job satisfaction of the increased every year, except for the second year, when the new contract was being negotiated. The level of psychosocial stress of the employees was reduced each year except for the second year.

CONCLUSION

Reducing occupational injury and illness requires a multifaceted systems approach that can define hazards, evaluate and establish means to control risks, and actively include management, supervision, and employees in the process. It requires having an organization that has flexibility, resilience, and reserves to respond to current, emergent, and unexpected hazards and situations. Resilience requires adequate knowledge, skills, and resources to respond including staff, supplies and materials, expertise, a quick response management system, and flexibility to meet new challenges. The SEIPS approach provides this capability.

The following list includes some additional online resources:

- American Association of Occupational Health Nurses: https://www.aaohn.org
- American College of Occupational and Environmental Medicine: https://acoem.org/

- American Council of Government Industrial Hygienists: https://www.aiha.org/
- American Industrial Hygiene Association: https://www.aiha.org
- American National Standards Institute: https://www.ansi.org
- American Psychological Association: https://www.apa.org/
- American Society of Safety Professionals: https://www.assp.org
- ASTM International: https://www.astm.org/
- Centers for Disease Control and Prevention: https://www.cdc.gov/
- Environmental Health Sciences: https://www.niehs.nih.gov/
- Environmental Protection Agency: https://www.epa.gov/
- European Agency for Safety and Health at Work: https://osha.europa.eu/en
- Human Factors and Ergonomics Society: https://www.hfes.org/
- International Ergonomics Association: https://iea.cc/
- International Labor Office: https://www.ilo.org/global/lang--en/index.htm
- International Standards Organization: https://www.iso.org/home.html
- National Academy of Medicine: https://nam.edu/
- National Institute for Occupational Safety and Health: https://www.cdc.gov/niosh/index.htm
- National Safety Council: https://www.nsc.org/
- Occupational Safety and Health Administration: https://www.osha.gov/
- US Department of Labor: https://www.dol.gov/
- World Health Organization: https://www.who.int/

REFERENCES

Carayon, P. (2009). The balance theory and the work system model . . . Twenty years later. *International Journal of Human-Computer Interaction, 25*(5), 313–327. https://doi.org/10.1080/10447310902864928

Carayon, P., Hoonakker, P. L. T., & Smith, M. J. (2012). Human factors in organizational design and management. In G. Salvendy (Ed.), *Handbook of human factors and ergonomics* (4th ed., pp. 534–552). Wiley. https://doi.org/10.1002/9781118131350.ch18

Carayon, P., & Perry, S. (2020). Human factors and ergonomics systems approach to the COVID-19 healthcare crisis. *International Journal for Quality in Health Care, 33*(Suppl. 1), 1–3. https://doi.org/10.1093/intqhc/mzaa109

Carayon, P., Schoofs Hundt, A., Karsh, B.-T., Gurses, A. P., Alvarado, C. J., Smith, M., & Flatley Brennan, P. (2006). Work system design for patient safety: The SEIPS model. *Quality & Safety in Health Care, 15*(Suppl. 1), i50–i58. https://doi.org/10.1136/qshc.2005.015842

Carayon, P., & Smith, M. J. (2000). Work organization and ergonomics. *Applied Ergonomics, 31*(6), 649–662. https://doi.org/10.1016/S0003-6870(00)00040-5

Carayon, P., & Smith, M. J. (2014). The balance concept revisited: Finding balance to reduce stress in a frantic world of IT. In C. Korunka, & P. Hoonakker (Eds.), *The impact of ICT on quality of working life* (pp. 105–121). https://doi.org/10.1007/978-94-017-8854-0_7/

Grossman, S. N., Han, S. C., Balcer, L. J., Kurzweil, A., Weinberg, H., Galetta, S. L., & Busis, N. A. (2020). Rapid implementation of virtual neurology in response to the COVID-19 pandemic. *Neurology, 94*(24), 1077–1087. https://doi.org/10.1212/WNL.0000000000009677

Gurses, A. P., & Carayon, P. (2007). Performance obstacles of intensive care nurses. *Nursing Research, 56*(3), 185–194. https://doi.org/10.1097/01.NNR.0000270028.75112.00

Gurses, A. P., & Carayon, P. (2009). Exploring performance obstacles of intensive care nurses. *Applied Ergonomics, 40*(3), 509–518. https://doi.org/10.1016/j.apergo.2008.09.003

Hoonakker, P., Carayon, P., & Loushine, T. (2010). Barriers and benefits of quality management in the construction industry: An empirical study. *Total Quality Management & Business Excellence, 21*(9), 953–969. https://doi.org/10.1080/14783363.2010.487673

Hoonakker, P., Loushine, T., Carayon, P., Kallman, J., Kapp, A., & Smith, M. J. (2005). The effect of safety initiatives on safety performance: A longitudinal study. *Applied Ergonomics, 36*(4), 461–469. https://doi.org/10.1016/j.apergo.2004.07.006

Loushine, T. W., Hoonakker, P. L. T., Carayon, P., & Smith, M. J. (2006). Quality and safety management in construction. *Total Quality Management & Business Excellence, 17*(9), 1171–1212. https://doi.org/10.1080/14783360600750469

Michaels, D., & Wagner, G. R. (2020). Occupational Safety and Health Administration (OSHA) and worker safety during the COVID-19 pandemic. *JAMA, 324*(14), 1389–1390. Advance online publication. https://doi.org/10.1001/jama.2020.16343

Smith, M. J., & Carayon, P. (2011). Controlling occupational safety and health hazards. In J. C. Quick & L. E. Tetrick (Eds.), *Handbook of occupational health psychology* (2nd ed., pp. 75–93). American Psychological Association.

Smith, M. J., & Carayon, P. (2012). Design of fixed, portable and mobile information devices. In J. Jacko (Ed.), *The human–computer interaction handbook* (3rd ed., pp. 297–311). Lawrence Erlbaum Associates.

Smith, M. J., Carayon, P., & Cohen, W. J. (2008). Design of computer workstations. In A. Sears & J. A. Jacko (Eds.), *The human–computer interaction handbook* (2nd ed., pp. 313–236). Lawrence Erlbaum Associates.

Smith, M. J., & Carayon-Sainfort, P. (1989). A balance theory of job design for stress reduction. *International Journal of Industrial Ergonomics, 4*(1), 67–79. https://doi.org/10.1016/0169-8141(89)90051-6

An Integrated Framework for Organizational Well-Being

Updated Themes, Potential Competencies, and a Broader Horizon

Joel Bennett, Cristina Banks, and Aldrich Chan

I think we can finally figure this whole thing out together.

Workplaces are evolving to face complex pressures and new stressors. Four disruptive trends—volatility, uncertainty, complexity, and ambiguity (VUCA)—require employers to better engage employees and develop organizational agility (Baran & Woznyj, 2021). Worker mental health problems are also affecting businesses at an unprecedented rate, with fervent calls to action from corporate executives and occupational scientists. The recent publication *Dying for a Paycheck* (Pfeffer, 2018) and the research on which the publication is based (Goh et al., 2015) revealed what research has suggested for decades: Workplace stressors and managerial practices unnecessarily kill workers annually—120,000 workers—and cost businesses billions in health care.

There is a general lack of coordination among many professionals who, were they to work together, could potentially address this growing mass of stressors. We, along with positive organizational scholars (e.g., Cunha et al., 2020), believe the answer lies in having a holistic and human-centered vision of organizations composed of allies who work as a team and across multiple levels. Current solutions are limited partly due to overspecialization across disciplines, resulting in the proverbial blind men and the elephant. Occupational health practitioners, consultants, trainers, and vendors are focused suboptimally on one area—either the trunk, the tail, or a leg—without actively addressing the whole. Practitioners

https://doi.org/10.1037/0000331-006
Handbook of Occupational Health Psychology, Third Edition, L. E. Tetrick, G. G. Fisher, M. T. Ford, and J. C. Quick (Editors)

need a view of workplace health—and its contributors—that reaches beyond academic ideas and a myopic focus on specific topics.

As in the 2003 and 2013 versions of this chapter, we call for a transdisciplinary conception of healthy workplaces. This chapter further delineates core themes that exist in, and the occupational health psychology (OHP) competencies needed for, a healthy, human-centered workplace. Both the science and practice of a healthy workplace have advanced considerably. We offer an updated framework informed by these advances. We include studies that integrate health promotion and health protection to advance both worker and enterprise outcomes (e.g., Punnett et al., 2020); align prevention, the promotion of positive mental health, and treatment (LaMontagne et al., 2014); offer guidelines to promote positive mental health (Davenport et al., 2016); align job-related, employee, and interpersonal influences on thriving at work (Britt & Jex, 2015); and offer specific steps for facilitating and coordinating employer–employee alignment, organizational health, and the measurement of meaningful outcomes (Edington & Pitts, 2015).

We also include research reviews that have advanced the etiology and definition of organizational well-being, such as a meta-analysis ($k = 73$) of factors found to predict individual thriving at work (Kleine et al., 2019); a review of wellness culture studies ($k = 95$) that identified 24 distinct elements often relating to workplace social factors (e.g., peer support, employee involvement) (Flynn et al., 2018); syntheses of positive mental health interventions in the workplace (e.g., Carolan et al., 2017; Wagner et al., 2016); systematic reviews of positive organizational behavior (Cunha et al., 2020); and our own integral research (Bennett, 2018).

CHAPTER OVERVIEW

This chapter provides a synopsis of the considerable advances in the science and practice of workplace well-being since the first edition of this handbook. Our intent is to provide context for a transdisciplinary call to action and help readers recast other handbook chapters in this context. For example, while Chapter 3 discusses three major models of occupational stress, we ask readers to think about the application scenarios discussed within this chapter (e.g., techno-stress, job design, gig workers) and how OHP can engage other disciplines to practice these models in these scenarios. Alternatively, Chapter 5 provides a case study on occupational hazards. Readers can review this example (and others throughout this handbook) through the lens of our competency model, identifying and labeling specific competencies that consultants use in case studies.

First, we review then reframe and update our original model. We define *integral organizational wellness* (IOW) as the simultaneous, and mutually enhancing, promotion of individual, team, and organizational health by attending to reciprocal relationships across these levels and by equally addressing internal (psychological), social (relational), behavioral, environmental, and operational aspects of the business or agency. Specifically, a healthy organization (a) self-assesses its well-being and adapts accordingly, with awareness of (b) its level of internal and external fitness or congruence, (c) core tensions, and (d) cycles of growth and decay. Accordingly, it (e) makes efforts to promote well-being (f) across multiple dimensions (e.g., physical, emotional, spiritual) and (g) multiple levels (individual, team, organization). Previous versions of this chapter described these themes.

We add four new themes to address the increased importance of agility to business success. Healthy workplaces also possess (h) human-centered technologies, (i) healthy physical environments, and (j) organizational and job design features that prioritize human value. Our model also views (k) organizational culture as an attractive state supported by other themes.

This chapter is organized into sections as outlined in Figure 6.1 and includes (a) the 11 themes noted previously, (b) OHP competencies, (c) the competencies of well-being professionals and allies who work to promote health, (d) potential business partners and the ways they can influence organizational wellness, (e) the influence of all the aforementioned areas on business success, and (f) attentiveness to current trends. Figure 6.1 represents a working model. Each section of the figure is briefly described as follows, as a chapter overview. The chapter ends with a call to action.

1. **The key themes of organizational well-being** are practices that assess the state of well-being, maintain awareness of that state, and apply solutions.

2. **OHP competencies** occur in three areas related to the themes. This includes (3A) directly helping within the 11 theme areas—for example, assessing culture and consulting on health promotion efforts and job design. OHP practitioners can also (3B) translate themes and practices to help internal supporters in their own efforts: for example, helping them understand survey analyses and how to apply the latest research in any theme area. Such work is translational; it requires practitioners to be competent in translating ideas, information, and practices back and forth with internal collaborators. OHP practitioners can also (3C) work on cross-disciplinary teams with others who serve the organization. These collaborators include well-being allies (see 3) and other primary business roles (see 4).

3. **Internal well-being practitioners and allies** represent those who support healthy practices and the aptitudes they can develop through well-defined curricula, career application, and growth. Workplace wellness specialists, well-being champions, and mental health peer support coworkers each provide coworkers with tools that promote well-being. We compare the competencies of these roles, and those working in Total Worker Health®, with the OHP competencies.

4. **Other business functions and roles** include those working in safety, legal support, employee assistance, and other areas. These partners often have critical roles in protecting business success and information that practitioners can use.

FIGURE 6.1. Framework of Integral Organizational Wellness and Six Major Sections of Current Chapter

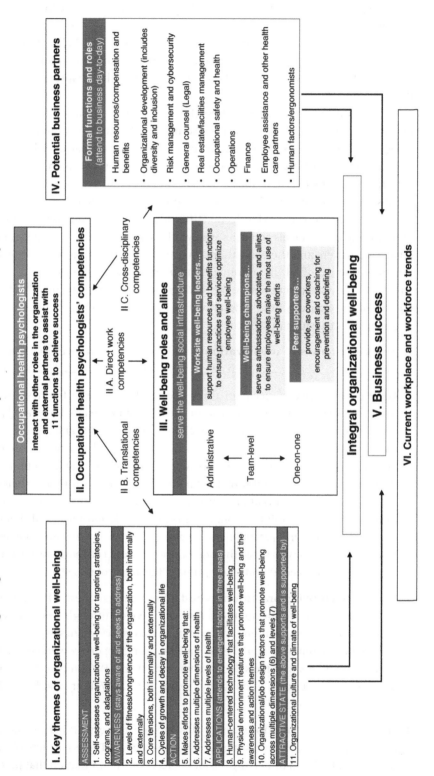

5. **Business success** is a significant consideration for worker health. It goes without saying that the themes—in addition to the practices and roles that sustain them—will not likely be seen as useful unless they promote business success.

6. **Current workplace and workforce trends** require ongoing attention. OHP professionals must stay attuned to changes in economy, the workforce, and technology. These changes include trends such as alternative or hybrid work arrangements, increased attention to mental health, and diversity. Practitioners can develop expertise to help employers adapt to these changes.

THE KEY THEMES OF ORGANIZATIONAL WELL-BEING

As noted, the current chapter reframes the first seven themes, described in previous editions, and outlines four new themes (Figure 6.1). We identify five theme categories: (a) assessment of organizational well-being; (b) awareness of factors that result from assessment; (c) actions that coordinate efforts toward well-being (particularly effective and supportive communications); (d) applications—from technology, organizational/job design, and environmental changes—that enhance well-being; and (e) attraction to a culture and climate of well-being. Applications and attraction are discussed in more depth in this section. Table 6.1 briefly defines all themes and lists OHP competencies related to each theme.

Attraction has a specific meaning in the revised framework and derives from the literature on organizational change and ambidexterity (Ford & Ford, 1994; Raisch & Birkinshaw, 2008). An agile organization adapts to change and stress. Instead of regressing, it resumes previous operations or moves to a new state of thriving. The attractive, telic, or purpose-oriented state is a healthy work culture (across the organization) or climate (locally, within departments or groups). Well-being is often defined by an ongoing attraction to enhancement, growth, and the ability to heal. The overall culture is the space wherein the eleven themes foster well-being.

Application: Human-Centered Technology

Workplace technology is ubiquitous and will become even more prevalent in the future (Oswald et al., 2019). Compared with technical-centered technology, human-centered technology focuses on (a) design led by humanistic values and devotion to human welfare, (b) enhancement of user skills and abilities, and (c) fit to human needs. Not all workplaces meet these expectations. Many cause harm physically and psychologically (e.g., keyboards, cell phones, office chairs, computer screens, surveillance cameras, and some social networking platforms; Salvendy, 2012). *Techno-stress* represents an opportunity to apply insights from psychology to inform information technology well-being design (e.g., La Torre et al., 2019). OHP practitioners can conduct techno-audits to identify risks and redesign technology to improve well-being.

TABLE 6.1. The 11 Themes: Five Areas, Activity of Occupational Health Psychologist, and Related Competencies

Area and theme	Activity of occupational health psychologist	Potential competencies
ASSESSMENT | A healthy organization . . .		
1. Self-assesses organizational well-being for targeting strategies, programs, and adaptations	Gathers reliable and valid information about areas below to continually maintain awareness of the organization's state of health and adapt to maintain optimal well-being across levels and dimensions.	• Applied psychometrics • Data analysis and synthesis • Data presentation
AWARENESS | A healthy organization stays aware of and seeks to address . . .		
2. Levels of fitness/congruence of the organization, both internally and externally	Consults on processes and strategies that improve fitness and congruence between: (a) the workplace and the external environment; and (b) functions within the organization.	• Environmental scan • Operations analysis • Leadership audit • Knowledge management • Multicultural competency
3. Core tensions, both internally and externally	Consults on processes and strategies that address various tensions involved in maintaining levels of optimal health and well-being.	• Humble inquiry • Organizational diagnosis • Continuous improvement tools
4. Cycles of growth and decay in organizational life	Maintains awareness of cycles of growth, regression, and deterioration in organizational vitality within areas that affect employee health and well-being.	
Awareness in these areas is used to make adjustments in strategies, approaches, and responses to resolve incongruities and tensions within and build the organization back toward growth and development.		
ACTION | A healthy organization . . .		
5. Makes efforts to promote well-being	OHP makes an ongoing effort to provide programs, policies, and practices that increase the health and well-being of employees.	• Curriculum design • Group facilitation • Coaching • Team building/team resilience • Leadership development
6. Addresses multiple dimensions of health	In these efforts, OHP considers multiple dimensions of well-being (spiritual, emotional, social), adopting a holistic view of employee health and well-being.	• Knowledge of mind–body, well-being, and resilience practices
7. Addresses multiple levels of health	In these efforts, OHP considers individuals, teams, and organizational level of well-being and the dynamic relationships across levels.	• Transfer of training tools

TABLE 6.1. The 11 Themes: Five Areas, Activity of Occupational Health Psychologist, and Related Competencies *(Continued)*

Area and theme	Activity of occupational health psychologist	Potential competencies
Actions in these areas are used to support and, whenever possible, coordinate with internal allies, external partners, and other stakeholders involved in the health and growth of the organization.		

APPLICATIONS | A healthy organization attends to emergent factors in three areas:

Area and theme	Activity of occupational health psychologist	Potential competencies
8. Human-centered technology that facilitates well-being, need fulfillment and productivity, and the reduction of unproductive or burdensome technology	Helps identify and implement technologies that promote employee health, well-being, and productivity through satisfaction of basic needs, making work efforts easier, simpler, user-friendly, and more efficacious, and lowers negative impacts to employee health and well-being.	• Macro-ergonomics • Health technologies • Communication technologies • AI-assisted work
9. Physical environment features that promote well-being and activities within the Awareness and Action themes	Is knowledgeable regarding physical environmental features that promote employee health and well-being, and implements strategies, programs, and practices that build in physical environmental features that support need fulfillment and productivity.	• IEQ standards and practices • Health and well-being environmental design • Postoccupancy evaluation
10. Organizational and job design factors that promote well-being across multiple dimensions (6) and levels (7)	Is knowledgeable regarding organizational and job design factors that promote employee health and well-being across dimensions and levels and make adjustments to designs that incorporate positive and remove negative factors to the greatest extent possible.	• Job and organization analysis • Employee surveys • Performance assessment • People analytics
Applications in these areas should remain sensitive to cross-disciplinary consultation with other allies and partners.		

ATTRACTIVE STATE | All of these areas and themes both support and are supported by:

Area and theme	Activity of occupational health psychologist	Potential competencies
11. Organizational culture and climate of well-being (the common or integrative goal of all preceding themes)	Helps cultivate an organizational culture and climate by engaging in compelling demonstrations of the organization's commitment to employee health and well-being. OHP takes actions to improve employee experience of the culture as well as support their well-being and growth.	• Collective leadership • Culture and climate assessments • Integrative scorecards • Metrics integration

To this end, we identify six categories needing attention, including (a) environment quality (EQ) controls: sensors/controls that measure/adjust temperature, humidity, air flow, noise, and lighting; (b) surveillance and occupancy: sensors that monitor occupancies, traffic flows through physical spaces, and employee behavior to adjust EQ and maximize use; (c) personal feedback: wearables/software that deliver coaching and personal health feedback such as time spent sitting, calories consumed, sleep quality, and heart rate; (d) communications: software delivered through devices that connect employees via social media, healthy behavior pop-up prompts, virtual meetings, podcasts, and more; (e) self-help: downloadable software and apps providing education, training, or just-in-time psychological support; and (f) productivity measurement: software and electronic monitoring devices that measure employee behavior such as time spent on a task, production per unit of time, website pages viewed, time spent on computer screen, clock-in and clock-out time, phone call duration, time at workstation, and time spent off the clock.

Nine criteria should be targeted by practitioner efforts in these areas. Technology should support (a) employees doing their work well, (b) opportunities for cognitive refreshment, (c) a comfortable degree of environmental control, (d) social connection, (e) employee safety and security, (f) worker choice in the location or timing of activities, (g) opportunities to bond with the organization, (h) actionable information to nudge healthy habits, and (i) positive nonverbal messages (Banks & Augustin, 2021). Sacasas (2021) also posed 41 questions, many related to well-being, for evaluating how technology is beneficial or detrimental to users. Practitioners can work toward shaping user experience to support rather than harm health and well-being. Regarding mental health, reviews of evidence-based apps may be especially useful to anyone working within OHP (Cunningham-Hill et al., 2020).

Application: The Physical Environment

Diverse professionals in human factors, industrial hygiene, and engineering have long sought to identify and remove or mitigate health risks—specifically, to remove negative factors from work environments and prevent illness, injury, and death. Recently, architects, designers, and psychologists have focused on positive factors that promote well-being. Architects, using design principles, can foster positive emotional and behavioral responses through physical place design. Interest in "well-being design" has forged partnerships between architects and psychologists to curate occupant experience via workplace features (e.g., Ayoko & Ashkanasy, 2019; Banks et al., 2019). OHP practitioners can collaborate with these designers. The following section explores some features related to health, job satisfaction, and productivity.

Indoor environmental quality (IEQ) includes fresh air treated with ultraviolet light to kill pathogens; temperature controls for comfort; noise reduction and noise masking (e.g., white noise); humidity controls to reduce molds; daylight and indoor lighting to mimic circadian rhythms; and scents and colors that stimulate productivity, creativity, and relaxation.

Floor plans include open and closed office design determined by the work performed; coworker proximity for safety and collaboration; placement of stairs to encourage physical movement; placement of walkways to increase privacy and noise reduction; safety barriers; and access to windows and outdoor spaces for cognitive refreshment.

Furnishings include ergonomic equipment and chairs for body support and postural variation; moderated visual complexity of the workspace; and biophilic materials, such as plants, natural materials such as wood, images of nature, and water features to promote restoration.

Nonverbal communications include workstation personalization to enhance a sense of belonging; posted messages of work values and meaningfulness; equitable access to resources; cultural symbols, such as flags, country, or group colors; and work areas to support inclusion.

Application: Organizational and Job Design

The trend toward reducing stressful work conditions has accelerated since 2000, and more so during the COVID-19 pandemic. Identifying risk factors dominated research and practice for much of this time. A positive turn toward well-being has led to new approaches (e.g., Chen & Cooper, 2014).

Healthy work design promotes (a) a life of purpose, (b) quality connections to others, and (c) positive self-regard and mastery (Quick & Macik-Frey, 2007). In the current IOW framework, organizational and job design should include (a) meaningful work; (b) helpful, respectful, and productive connections and communications with others; (c) sufficient support to meet work demands; (d) a safe environment; and (e) development of mastery and skill.

Several tested models of job design remain relevant for well-being: job characteristics model, job demand–control theory, job demand–resource theory, and self-determination theory. Research supports the following job characteristics: autonomy (choice), skill variety (job enrichment), task significance (importance), adequate resource support (time, technology, materials), and reductions to hindering job demands. Recently, need theory and person–job fit model have focused attention on the sufficiency of the job itself and organizational context for providing need satisfaction, which underlies well-being. Job crafting is also an emerging method that helps workers lower stress by managing job demands and acquiring resources to achieve more compatible work. A recent meta-analysis of job crafting found that it significantly improves job satisfaction, work engagement, work performance (Rudolph et al., 2017).

Looking to the future, artificial intelligence (AI)-assisted work (i.e., the symbiotic relationship between AI and humans in job performance) is expected to increase (Jarrahi, 2018). The combination of AI and human talent can help manage increasing work complexity and will be crucially important for jobs that require complex decision making. AI is likely to grow in importance in the development of exoskeletons to augment physical capabilities and stamina.

Application: Organizational Culture and Climate

The business literature is filled with articles about the importance of work culture or climate to employee well-being (e.g., Harvard Business Review, 2020). Few evidence-based practices (EBPs) specifically target culture. This section follows up on case studies of EBP interventions presented in the previous edition of this chapter (Bennett, Cook, & Pelletier, 2011). An example is culture-of-resilience programs implemented in a school district, a large manufacturing firm, a corporate wellness company, and an academic research group (Bennett, 2020).

In these and other implementations, we have applied the insights identified by Flynn and colleagues (2018) in their systematic review of evidence-based elements of healthy work cultures. While there is significant variation across workplaces regarding drivers of culture, certain factors appear to be more common: ongoing communication and feedback; training and learning; employee empowerment; authentic leadership; peer support; allocation of resources; and supportive policies and environments. OHP consultants cannot master the tools necessary to promote all of these drivers. However, they can become aware of the landscape and coordinate with other well-being advocates and business functions.

Accordingly, this theme of culture and climate integrates the four areas above. OHP consultants can assess culture and climate (area 1) using recently studied survey tools (e.g., Reynolds & Bennett, 2019). These assessments can be used to increase awareness—and readiness for culture change—among leaders and workers (area 2). Practitioners can use this awareness, along with research knowledge about what works to inform the selection, development, and design of actions and applications that have the greatest likelihood of succeeding (areas 3 and 4).

Specific competencies can enhance OHP professionals' contributions across these areas. Psychometric consultation on culture assessments can improve the utility of such instruments. This extends to understanding the limitations of wellness culture scorecards (e.g., Safeer & Allen, 2019). OHP scientists when working for a culture of health, can study shared leadership and its impact on employee health. Indeed, collective leadership may be the cardinal competency required to address the stressors discussed at the onset of this chapter (Contractor et al., 2012).

OHP COMPETENCIES

The good physician treats the disease; the great physician treats the patient who has the disease.

—attributed to SIR WILLIAM OSLER

We treat the whole patient, not just the hole in the patient.

—attributed to DR. CARRIE SUSSMAN

We view workplaces through the broad lens of positive psychology—human centered, growth oriented, and helping employees thrive. Integral OHP practice requires that organizations must, first and foremost, be approached as a living, whole entity with potential for health, growth, and healing. We need to know OHP-related research—such as that highlighted in this handbook, other key texts (e.g., Britt & Jex, 2015; Cunningham & Black, 2021; Schonfeld & Chang, 2017), and the *Journal of Occupational Health Psychology*. This knowledge is best used in the context of purpose-driven collaboration with others working across the 11 thematic areas.

These themes serve as a starting point for a competency-based approach to healthy organizations. The competencies (see Table 6.1, right column) help OHP professionals promote health in the organization as a whole. These professionals can apply competencies directly to benefit others working within or affected by the organization (e.g., employers, leaders, managers, employees, family members, customers, citizens); by translating them in dialogue with internal professionals and workers; and by collaborating with other business roles inside and outside the organization.

INTERNAL WELL-BEING ROLES AND ALLIES AND COMPETENCIES

OHP practitioners have many potential allies. We identify four here as well as the competencies they possess within their own domains of practice (see Figure 6.2). These allies include practitioners with training or certification: in *Total Worker Health®* (TWH), as a Workplace Wellness Specialist (or related title), as a Well-Being Champion or Ambassador, and as coworkers who have received some type of peer support training in mental health. OHP professionals can help these collaborators maximize their roles and also work together. As these professionals can foster IOW, we emphasize their unique involvement with allies because of training in personnel assessment, person–job fit, job design, job coaching, job crafting, and competency modeling. OHP professionals can contribute by helping to identify, develop, and support allies' competencies. Figure 6.2 is provided as an initial, synoptic guide to explore these possible competencies. The competencies for each ally are organized in the four areas of the IOW framework and should be viewed along with their related themes (see the final column in Table 6.1). Supportive communications to and for employees are a cardinal competency across all these allies. We also include communication as an additional subset of action.

Total Worker Health

Comparing the four allies, TWH professionals are the most likely to be academically certified through universities designated as TWH programs and the National Institute of Occupational Health and Safety (NIOSH). TWH takes a holistic approach to worker health, safety, and well-being by integrating protection from work-related safety and health hazards with promotion of injury

FIGURE 6.2. Competencies of *Total Worker Health* and Well-Being Allies: Definitions and Alignment With Integral Organizational Wellness

IOW Areas	*Total Worker Health®*	Workplace Wellness Specialist	Well-Being Champions	Mental Health Peer Support
Assessment	a) Evaluate intervention strategies		a) Evaluate progress	a) Has lived experiences b) Recognize crisis c) Recognize own biases d) Has emotional insight e) Is personable
Awareness	b) Understand prevention and health promotion disciplines	a) Evaluate data	b) Know infrastructure and resources	f) Engage in personal development g) Role model personal resilience (Contagion) h) Empower through communication
Action	c) Design, deliver, intervention strategies d) Understand and apply practices that affect the workers' well-being) e) Identify and disseminate evidence-based interventions	b) Drive employee engagement c) Implement best practices	c) Commitment to growth d) Plan well e) Gain support	i) Understand and collaborate with community support j) Maintain ethical responsibility
Communication	f) Communicate with multiple stakeholders	d) Communicate with workforce	f) Build partnerships g) Communicate well h) Grow ambassadors	
Application	g) Understand and/or develop policy h) Possess technical specializations	e) Know health-related regulations		
Attraction		f) Support organization culture	i) Scale the program j) Celebrate progress and wins k) Enhance wellness climate	

Definitions of Above

	Total Worker Health®	Workplace Wellness Specialist	Well-Being Champions	Mental Health Peer Support
a)	Can design, deliver, and evaluate TWH interventions	Understands and utilizes evaluation process to analyze wellness interventions and provide feedback to stakeholders	Evaluates outcomes and makes adjustment based on new information	Genuinely relates their own experiences to the experiences and challenges of their peers
b)	Understands how to apply prevention and health promotion disciplines to address workers' safety, health, and well-being	Drives engagement through multiple avenues (e.g., assessments, technologies, branding, process improvements)	Uses and maximizes worksite structure and health resources	Detects when a peer is in, or close to, a crisis and works with peer to deescalate with resources and services
c)	Assesses factors (e.g., noise, stress, addiction, health policies, health care) that influence a worker's well-being	Utilizes best practices to design and deliver holistic and evidence based practice	Engages and empowers employees to own the program for themselves	Has unconditional respect for the personal values, culture, and beliefs of the peer and their issues
d)	Identifies and adapts EBP to policies or programs to produce positive results (e.g., high productivity, health outcomes)	Communicate with the workforce during a wellness initiative to increase engagement, promote positive perceptions of the organization, support inclusiveness, and increase wellness	Has clear goals and milestones and tracks progress over time	Recognizes peer needs, and when one should broach difficult subjects to help the peer explore their options
e)	Articulates to multiple stakeholders (e.g., frontline workers, managers) how TWH aligns with the business strategy	Comprehends government policies (e.g., ACA, HIPAA, ADA) to help guide the formation of wellness programs	Builds buy-in from leaders, managers, and key allies	Has an outward demeanor (empathetic, nonjudgmental) and language (person centered and recovery oriented) to encourage open dialogue with the peer
f)	Understands how to apply prevention and health promotion disciplines to address workers' safety, health, and well-being	Has capacity to garner support for shifting an organization's culture into that of wellness	Collaborates with stakeholders	Seeks opportunities to develop peer-support skills
g)	Trained in areas (e.g., multilevel worker and workplace assessments, chronic disease management, persuasive speaking) that would assist in workplace health interventions		Effectively markets and builds campaigns	Role models' commitment to own self-care (e.g., stress management, resilience strategies, recovery, seeking help) approach evidence based intervention and describe to peers to initialize discovery
h)			Builds a team of other ambassadors who carry the message to others	Uses active listening and communication skills to fully understand the situation of the peer
i)			Has the ability to grow and replicate the program as needed	Communicates about community resources/services available; works with colleagues to meet needs
j)			Acknowledges, rewards, and celebrates others' progress with fun and play	Has knowledge of the laws and rules to ensure and protect the rights, privacy, and safety of the peers
k)			Monitors the local climate of receptivity and embracing of wellness	

Note. IOW = Integral organizational wellness; TWH = *Total Worker Health®*; EBP = evidence-based practice; ACA = Affordable Care Act; HIPAA = Health Insurance Portability and Accountability Act; ADA = Americans With Disabilities Act.

and illness prevention. NIOSH and the Centers for Disease Control and Prevention (CDC) wrote a workbook detailing the elements in a TWH approach while certificate programs for TWH developed additional competencies. These include knowledge of intervention strategy development, delivery, and evaluation; leadership communication and methods of influence; knowledge of scientific literature relevant to identifying health risks and safety hazards; technical knowledge in hazard prevention; and health promotion methodologies and subject matter (Lee et al., 2016).

There are similarities and differences between TWH and the IOW framework. For example, the physical environment and organizational/job design factors (in the IOW framework) overlap with TWH's competencies that serve to modify the workplace to promote wellness. Organizational culture and climate (in the IOW model) include competencies related to demonstrating leadership commitment to workers' safety and health as well as worker engagement. Both frameworks also emphasize the importance of making an effort to promote health. We also see important differences in emphasis between the two sets of competencies. IOW is less focused on the diverse antecedents to safety and health problems and more focused on keeping sight of the positive well-being potential and business success of the whole organization in addition to helping others from diverse areas to see where they fit in supporting the whole. Of course, these others include TWH practitioners but also all others described in this section (see Figure 6.2) and the next (Figure 6.3).

Workplace Wellness Specialists

Workplace wellness specialists (WWS) serve a different role than TWH practitioners because of a greater focus on workplace wellness programs, wellness vendor support, as well as strategies, programs, and incentives to engage workers in adapting a healthy lifestyle, often oriented toward physical health. There has been a growing interest among WWS to incorporate stress management, mindfulness, and resilience strategies as part of a mental well-being initiative within their workplaces. At least three programs train and certify WWS: the National Wellness Institute (https://www.nationalwellness.org), the Certified Corporate Wellness Specialist (https://www.corporatewellnesscertification.com), and Wellness Councils of America (https://www.welcoa.org). As shown in Figure 6.2, a key distinguishing competency among WWS is their attention to health-related policies and regulations as well as direct communications with employees. In-house WWS often work in human resources or risk management. Wellness vendors also assign external WWS as part of a comprehensive wellness program contract.

Well-Being Champions

Unlike WWS, champions are typically grown from within organizations through volunteering or nominations from supervisors and managers. Champions may also be called wellness ambassadors, advocates, or allies. They are typically at the "grassroots" (supervisory or employee) level. Their focus is to engage employees in local wellness-related activities (e.g., campaigns, fund-raising, sports), promote the wellness benefit, and encourage social ties among employees as part of the social dimension of wellness. In larger organizations, champions may be at the department, store, or location level and play a role in recruiting other ambassadors. The champion competencies listed in Figure 6.3 are derived from training the first author designed for diverse clients (see Bennett & Linde, 2016). The competencies behind a grassroots, voluntary, or peer-to-peer role is not as well documented or formalized as TWH or WWS. However, there is growing recognition that work peers can play a vital role in encouraging healthy behavior among their coworkers.

Mental Health Peer Support Workers

The growth in worker mental health and substance abuse concerns has led to the development of programs for training employees as peer supporters. In the United States, the Substance Abuse and Mental Health Services Administration (SAMHSA; 2015) has developed "Core Competencies for Peer Workers in Behavioral Health Services." The Mental Health Commission of Canada also published guidelines for peer support (Sunderland & Mishkin, 2013). Health and wellness coaching is a related and rapidly growing profession, although such coaches often do not address mental health issues and typically work outside the organization. Wellness coaches receive certification from a national agency that has identified competencies as well (Wolever et al., 2016). Overall, in the area of worker mental health, the employee assistance program can be a key ally that OHP practitioners should collaborate with too (Bennett et al., 2015; Herlihy et al., 2020)

POTENTIAL PARTNERS: BUSINESS FUNCTIONS AND ROLES

OHP practitioners, consultants, and scientists can also partner with traditional business functions that impact worker well-being. Ten business roles can assist in mitigating one or more of 11 work-related barriers to business success (see Figure 6.3). A barrier could be the result of one or several co-occurring factors. Accordingly, interrole collaboration, bilateral referral, and multipronged strategies could ensure a problem is (a) addressed in a holistic (vs. a short-term, expedient manner); and (b) does not reemerge in other areas where the problem is unaddressed.

Figure 6.3 views business functions in three categories (see rows): human resources (HR) and workplaces, risk and liability, and organizational and employee support. The figure also views barriers in two groups (see columns): organizational antecedents and psychosocial and organizational consequences. An *X* in a cell indicates domain responsibility. The figure is offered as a guide for collaboration across roles.

FIGURE 6.3. Work-Related Barriers to Business Success

Business functions and roles	Organizational antecedents					Psychosocial and organizational consequences					
	Job vacancies	Unskilled workers	Decision mistakes	Weak cultures	Management problems	Presenteeism	Sickness absence	Accidents/ injuries	Voluntary turnover	Illegal activity	Lawsuits
Human resources and workplaces											
Operations	X	X	X		X	X	X	X	X	X	X
Human resources/compensation and benefits	X	X			X	X	X		X	X	X
Real estate/facilities management	X		X	X		X	X	X	X		X
Risk and liability											
Risk management/cyber security	X	X	X	X			X	X	X	X	X
General counsel (Legal)	X	X	X	X	X				X	X	X
Finance	X	X	X	X	X	X	X	X	X	X	X
Organizational and employee supports											
Organizational development (D and I, DEI)		X	X	X	X	X	X		X	X	X
Occupational safety and health	X	X	X		X	X	X	X	X	X	X
Employee assistance/health care partners	X	X	X	X	X	X	X	X	X	X	X
Human factors/ergonomists	X	X	X	X	X	X	X	X	X	X	X

Work-related barriers to business success

Note. Cells marked with an "X" represent potential responsibilities for business functions and roles. Cells that are shaded may be especially relevant to particular roles. Relevance (represented by shading) may vary according to the project. D and I refers to diversity and inclusion; DEI refers diversity, equity, and inclusion. Adapted from *Blueprint for Building Business Success by Becoming a 'Healthcare Business'* [White paper] (p. 17), by C. G. Banks, 2023, Interdisciplinary Center for Healthy Workplaces, University of California, Berkeley (https://healthyworkplaces.berkeley.edu/sites/default/files/publications/blueprint_for_building_business_success_by_becoming_a_healthcare_business_jan_12_2023.pdf). Copyright 2023 by Cristina G. Banks. Adapted with permission.

We use the example of presenteeism to illustrate possible collaboration. *Presenteeism* is the practice of coming to work despite illness, injury, anxiety, and other personal issues. As presenteeism has a greater impact on productivity than absenteeism (Strömberg et al., 2017) and also increases safety risk (Widera et al., 2010), it concerns several business functions. Facilities management, HR, organizational development, and occupational medicine could co-investigate presenteeism's root causes (e.g., lack of paid sick leave, job insecurity, work overload, burnout, harmful physical conditions). Once potential problem sources are identified, collaborators could devise a holistic solution—if needed, across functions. Regardless of barrier type, external partners are essential to the success of many OHP efforts.

BUSINESS SUCCESS

For business leadership to support OHP practictioners' efforts, our themes have to be integral to business success. From an HR perspective, success translates into three outcomes: (a) All positions are filled by employees who have the knowledges, skills, and abilities to perform effectively and are motivated to do so; (b) all employees know what they are supposed to do and have the training and experience to execute; and (c) employees are committed to organizational priorities, are recognized for their contributions, and gain meaning from work.

Unfortunately, these outcomes face many threats: (a) vacant jobs; (b) management's poor decision making (e.g., flawed policies, processes, procedures, practices) resulting in confusion and lost productivity; (c) insufficient employee skills to perform effectively due to poor selection processes or failed training programs; (d) employee injuries due to accidents arising from ineffective safety controls and absence of a safety climate; (e) poorly managed employees causing frustration and lost productivity, often due to neglect, abusive management styles, poor accountability, or a lack of management training; (f) employee absences and presenteeism decreasing productivity; (g) voluntarily turnover; (h) weak culture and low morale undermining work motivation and productivity; and (i) complaints and lawsuits resulting from regulatory noncompliance. These outcomes create gaps between desired and actual business success.

The IOW themes and related OHP competencies directly impact business success. OHP practitioners minimize threats by moving the organization toward a positive cultural state in concert with key partners. Organizational well-being self-assessment bring potential threats to the surface for resolution. Awareness of the fitness and congruence of the organization, its core tensions, and the organization's position with respect to growth and decay in organizational life builds the organizational change agenda for better organizational functioning, and thus better employee health and well-being. Fruitful areas of change also include technology designed to meet user needs; a physical environment that removes harms and builds in features that enhance health and well-being; and organizational and job designs that lower job strain and promote thriving. Such changes result from programs designed to promote well-being and address multiple dimensions and levels of health.

Together, business partners and well-being allies (well-being specialists, champions, and peer supporters) can help OHP professionals fulfill their mission. Because the threats and opportunities described previously cut across multiple business functions, they reveal the critical role professionals can play by participating in and coordinating strategies and actions both hierarchically (with internal allies) and horizontally (with business partners) to support business success. Figure 6.3 indicates which partners can help OHP professionals avoid and eliminate threats by creating policies, practices, and programs that prevent negative and promote positive effects. The integral model illustrates how the execution of themes, supported by an expanded set of competencies, can be facilitated by genuine cross-functional teamwork and OHP leadership.

CURRENT WORKPLACE AND WORKFORCE TRENDS

For organizations to succeed, they have to respond to ongoing, emergent, and even disruptive trends and pressures. This is why, following assessment (theme 1), the awareness areas and themes of fitness (theme 2), tension (theme 3), and life cycle (theme 4) are essential. Current trends that impact well-being include the coronavirus pandemic, racial and social strife, political polarization, low-wage worker alienation, and cybersecurity breaches. We cannot cover all trends; we focus here on only three primary movers of daily life: (a) the pandemic, (b) growth in the gig economy, and (c) remote work. Readers are advised that multicultural wellness and guidance for addressing politics at work are also primary, but not pursued here (see Chow & Lees, 2021; Howard, 2019).

The Coronavirus Pandemic

Viruses are likely to pose continuous challenges to well-being and require new and creative solutions. COVID-19 emerged in January 2020 and changed the ways employees lived and worked, perhaps forever. After March 2020, lockdowns as a result of the pandemic meant that the vast majority of nonessential employees had no choice but to work remotely. Many modified their home into a workplace that may or may not have been conducive to performing work effectively. They experienced isolation, lack of connection to company culture, pressure to maintain pre-COVID productivity, and fuzzy boundaries between work and nonwork time. Essential workers experienced rapid acceleration of health and safety concerns, excessive workloads and fatigue, fear of exposing their family to COVID-19, physical separation from family members, and, for health care workers, exposure to severely ill and dying patients.

OHP scientists have outlined ways to address diverse COVID-19 stressors (Sinclair et al., 2020): mental health support for minority workers; ways employers can discourage workers caring for family members with COVID from excessive work; innovative work–family arrangements; ways to help locked-down workers stay socially active and to help essential workers manage death anxiety. This diversity of approaches testifies to the need for potential breadth of OHP competencies (see Table 6.1). At the same time, multiple challenges—across virtual and hybrid work environments—may lead to fragmentation in a work culture. Here, OHP professionals can strategically integrate approaches under the banner of an attractive cultural state and as a way to foster meaning and purpose.

The Growing Gig Economy

New work arrangements require innovation to promote well-being. *Gig workers* work without an employment contract (e.g., independent contractor, free-lancer). They decide when and where they work, and can work for a variety of organizations simultaneously. Although the numbers are difficult to track, the Bureau of Labor Statistics (Gallup, 2018) estimated that 36% of the U.S. workforce performed gig work in 2017. Gig work is predicted to constitute 52% of the workforce by 2023 (Karra, 2021). Gig work comes with considerable health, safety, and financial challenges, including loss of legal protections under occupational safety and health, civil rights, and wrongful termination laws, exposing gig workers to harm for which they have no redress. In response, gig workers have formed coalitions and worker groups (Johnston & Land-Kazlauskas, 2018) and have received psychosocial support through digital media (e.g., podcasts). The IOW framework offers new opportunities for addressing gig worker needs, such as safety training, consultation, work selection and job crafting, virtual culture development, human-centered technology, peer and app support, as well as online mental health resources.

Remote Work

OHP consultants can use the IOW framework to reimagine healthy work for remote and hybrid employees. As hybrid work arrangements become the norm, managers and employees will want to regain aspects of the attractive work culture they lost when working remotely (e.g., socializing, solving problems together), and also retain what they enjoyed from remote work (e.g., reduced commuting and nonessential meetings, greater discretion over time use). Research suggests it is possible to be productive and even thrive in either case (Burlacu & Monahan, 2021). OHP professionals can use this research to problem-solve with allies and partners, apply the IOW framework, and strategize on how to use the best of both work environments to promote well-being.

We suggest starting with an assessment of the desired culture (i.e., the attractive state) by asking, "What do you miss about not being at work?" Surveys suggest that it is often about the *experience* of social connection (e.g., GoBright, n.d.; Murray, 2021). Practitioners can also turn to the well-being allies who support the social infrastructure (e.g., wellness champions).

A review of their competencies (see Figure 6.2) shows that personable, engaging, and positive communication is essential. The newly added themes of physical environment and job design also suggest specific steps: cultural signs, symbols, folk objects, and other nonverbal communications can convey meaningfulness and belonging in the virtual space. Coaching workers on job crafting may also lead to innovation for remote and hybrid work (Ingusci et al., 2021).

CALL TO ACTION

This chapter asks readers to search the broader horizon. The preceding section on trends should make it clear that the field of OHP cannot evolve without innovation and adopting a larger futuristic view of well-being. Our call to action asks science practitioners to simultaneously promote business success, social well-being, and the overall health of the organization. Each of these corresponds to the three competency areas described previously. We need skills in order to work with business partners, well-being roles and allies, as well as with all employees themselves—from line-workers to the C-suite.

A great place to start is to illustrate how employer caring and human social connection promotes well-being (Eisenberger et al., 2020). OHP scientists can study how to build compassionate workplaces (Rynes et al., 2012), embrace virtue and spiritual values among workers and leaders (Neal, 2013), foster mindfulness in and through workplaces (Dhiman, 2020), and grow corporate social responsibility in ways that improve the health of both internal workers and the external community (Hiswåls et al., 2020; Zellner & Bowdish, 2017).

The IOW model also encourages collaboration between OHP practitioners, scientists, consultants with other professionals. Professional education programs should train on competencies that advance interdisciplinary health research (Gebbie et al., 2012) as well as interprofessional health practice (Schot et al., 2020). However, care should be taken to use collaboration judiciously to prevent "collaboration overload," which could hurt decision making and performance (Cross et al., 2018). More research is needed to identify the optimal circumstances for all competencies described in the IOW model: cross-disciplinary, translational, and direct.

We hope this chapter guides readers to help workers feel greater belonging, value, fairness, and respect regardless of business size, job level, or worker location. Those of us working in the field of OHP can cushion the harshness and trauma that comes with physical and psychological difficulty. When social connection is broken, so is loyalty, satisfaction, and productivity. To help recover from the coronavirus pandemic, future crises, and ongoing stressors, we must devote more effort to reestablish, strengthen, and enhance social bonds. When professionals work together, they both model social connection and also competently build a pathway back to well-being.

REFERENCES

Ayoko, O. B., & Ashkanasy, N. M. (Eds.). (2019). *Organizational behaviour and the physical environment*. Routledge.

Banks, C. G., & Augustin, S. (2021). Workplace technology that promotes health and well-being. *TMS Proceedings 2021*. https://doi.org/10.1037/tms0000155

Banks, C. G., DeClercq, C., & Thibau, I. J. C. (Eds.). (2019). *Built to thrive: How to build the best workplaces for health, well-being, and productivity*. Berkeley Interdisciplinary Center for Healthy Workplaces.

Banks, C. G. (2023, January 11). *Blueprint for building business success by becoming a 'healthcare business'* [White paper]. Interdisciplinary Center for Healthy Workplaces, University of California, Berkley. https://healthyworkplaces.berkeley.edu/sites/default/files/publications/blueprint_for_building_business_success_by_becoming_a_healthcare_business_jan_12_2023.pdf

Baran, B. E., & Woznyj, H. M. (2021). Managing VUCA: The human dynamics of agility. *Organizational Dynamics, 50*(2), Article 100787. https://doi.org/10.1016/j.orgdyn.2020.100787

Bennett, J. B. (2018). Integral Organizational Wellness™: An evidence-based model of socially inspired well-being. *Journal of Applied Biobehavioral Research, 23*(4), Article e12136. https://doi.org/10.1111/jabr.12136

Bennett, J. B. (2020, September). Toward evidence-based cultures of resilience: Authentic leadership, mental health and social connection. *Proceedings from HEROForum20: A Virtual Conference (September 2020)*. Health Enhancement Research Organization.

Bennett, J. B., Bray, J. W., Hughes, D., Hunter, J. F., Frey, J. J., Roman, P., & Sharar, D. (2015). *Bridging public health with workplace behavioral health services: A framework for future research and a stakeholder call to action* [White paper]. Interdisciplinary Center for Healthy Workplaces, University of California, Berkeley. https://www.eapassn.org/Portals/11/Docs/Newsbrief/PBRNwhitepaper.pdf

Bennett, J. B., Cook, R. F., & Pelletier, K. R. (2011). An integral framework for organizational wellness: Core technology, practice models, and case studies. In J. C. Quick & L. E. Tetrick (Eds.), *Handbook of occupational health psychology* (2nd ed., pp. 95–118). American Psychological Association.

Bennett, J. B., & Linde, B. D. (2016). *Well-being champions: A competency-based guidebook*. Organizational Wellness & Learning Systems.

Britt, T. W., & Jex, S. M. (2015). *Thriving under stress: Harnessing demands in the workplace*. Oxford University Press.

Burlacu, G., & Monahan, K. (2021, Autumn). Resources create a "productive anywhere" workforce: What we learned and confirmed about the job demands-resources model. *TIP, 59*(2), 22–23. https://www.siop.org/Portals/84/TIP/592/complete.pdf

Carolan, S., Harris, P. R., & Cavanagh, K. (2017). Improving employee well-being and effectiveness: Systematic review and meta-analysis of web-based psychological interventions delivered in the workplace. *Journal of Medical Internet Research, 19*(7), Article e271. https://doi.org/10.2196/jmir.7583

Chen, P. Y., & Cooper, C. L. (Eds.). (2014). *Work and wellbeing*. Wiley Blackwell.

Chow, D., & Lees, J. (2021, July 29). 3 strategies to address political polarization in the workplace. *Harvard Business Review*. https://hbr.org/2021/07/3-strategies-to-address-political-polarization-in-the-workplace

Contractor, N. S., DeChurch, L. A., Carson, J., Carter, D. R., & Keegan, B. (2012). The topology of collective leadership. *The Leadership Quarterly, 23*(6), 994–1011. https://doi.org/10.1016/j.leaqua.2012.10.010

Cross, R., Taylor, S., & Zehner, D. (2018). Collaboration without burnout. *Harvard Business Review, 96*(4), 134–137.

Cunha, M. P., Rego, A., Simpson, A. V., & Clegg, S. (2020). *Positive organizational behaviour: A reflective approach*. Routledge. https://doi.org/10.4324/9781315232249

Cunningham, C. J. L., & Black, K. J. (2021). *Essentials of occupational health psychology*. Routledge. https://doi.org/10.4324/9781351011938

Cunningham-Hill, M., Dodge-Rice, Z., Wilson-Myers, C., Sherman, C., Neary, M., & Schueller, S. M. (2020). *Digital tools and solutions for mental health: An employer's guide.* UMB Digital Archive. https://archive.hshsl.umaryland.edu/handle/10713/12802

Davenport, L. J., Allisey, A. F., Page, K. M., LaMontagne, A. D., & Reavley, N. J. (2016). How can organisations help employees thrive? The development of guidelines for promoting positive mental health at work. *International Journal of Workplace Health Management, 9*(4), 411–427. https://doi.org/10.1108/IJWHM-01-2016-0001

Dhiman, S. K. (Ed.). (2020). *The Routledge companion to mindfulness at work.* Routledge. https://doi.org/10.4324/9780429244667

Edington, D. W., & Pitts, J. S. (2015). *Shared values—shared results: Positive organizational health as a win–win philosophy.* Edington Associates.

Eisenberger, R., Shanock, L. R., & Wen, X. (2020). Perceived organizational support: Why caring about employees counts. *Annual Review of Organizational Psychology and Organizational Behavior, 7*(1), 101–124. https://doi.org/10.1146/annurev-orgpsych-012119-044917

Flynn, J. P., Gascon, G., Doyle, S., Koffman, D. M. M., Saringer, C., Grossmeier, J., Tivnan, V., & Terry, P. (2018). Supporting a culture of health in the workplace: A review of evidence-based elements. *American Journal of Health Promotion, 32*(8), 1755–1788. https://doi.org/10.1177/0890117118761887

Ford, J. D., & Ford, L. W. (1994). Logics of identity, contradiction, and attraction in change. *Academy of Management Review, 19*(4), 756–785. https://doi.org/10.2307/258744

Gallup. (2018). *Gallup's perspective on the gig economy and alternative work arrangements.* https://acrip.co/contenidos-acrip/gallup/2020/mayo/gallup-perspective-gig-economy-perspective-paper.pdf

Gebbie, K. M., Meier, B. M., Bakken, S., Carrasquillo, O., Formicola, A., Aboelela, S. W., Glied, S., & Larson, E. (2012). Training for interdisciplinary health research: Defining the required competencies. *Journal of Allied Health, 37*(2), 65–70.

GoBright. (n.d.). *What do you miss most about working at the office?* https://gobright.com/blogs/what-do-you-miss-most-about-working-at-the-office/

Goh, J., Pfeffer, J., & Zenios, S. A. (2015). The relationship between workplace stressors and mortality and health costs in the United States. *Management Science, 62*(2), 608–628. https://doi.org/10.1287/mnsc.2014.2115

Harvard Business Review. (2020). *Cultivating workforce well-being to drive business value: Research report.* https://hbr.org/resources/pdfs/comm/workplacewellbeing.pdf

Herlihy, P. A., Frey, J. J., Lin, N., & Kahn, A. (2020). International employee assistance digital archive: A new knowledge hub. *Journal of Workplace Behavioral Health, 35*(1), 6–13. https://doi.org/10.1080/15555240.2020.1724795

Hiswåls, A. S., Hamrin, C. W., Vidman, Å., & Macassa, G. (2020). Corporate social responsibility and external stakeholders' health and wellbeing: A viewpoint. *Journal of Public Health Research, 9*(1), Article 1742. https://doi.org/10.4081/jphr.2020.1742

Howard, L. (2019, June). Creating a multiculturally competent worksite wellness program: The why and the how. *Benefits Magazine, 56*(6), 14–21. https://withlindahoward.com/wp-content/uploads/2019/06/Howard-June-Ben-Mag-Reprint.pdf

Ingusci, E., Signore, F., Giancaspro, M. L., Manuti, A., Molino, M., Russo, V., Zito, M., & Cortese, C. G. (2021). Workload, techno overload, and behavioral stress during COVID-19 emergency: The role of job crafting in remote workers. *Frontiers in Psychology, 12*, Article 655148. https://doi.org/10.3389/fpsyg.2021.655148

Jarrahi, M. H. (2018). Artificial intelligence and the future of work: Human–AI symbiosis in organizational decision making. *Business Horizons, 61*(4), 577–586. https://doi.org/10.1016/j.bushor.2018.03.007

Johnston, H., & Land-Kazlauskas, C. (2018). *Organizing on-demand: Representation, voice, and collective bargaining in the gig economy.* International Labour Organization.

Karra, S. (2021, May 13). The gig or permanent worker: Who will dominate the post-pandemic workforce? *Forbes.* https://www.forbes.com/sites/forbeshumanresources

council/2021/05/13/the-gig-or-permanent-worker-who-will-dominate-the-post-pandemic-workforce/?sh=cecf7bc3cdc1

Kleine, A. K., Rudolph, C. W., & Zacher, H. (2019). Thriving at work: A meta-analysis. *Journal of Organizational Behavior, 40*(9–10), 973–999. https://doi.org/10.1002/job.2375

La Torre, G., Esposito, A., Sciarra, I., & Chiappetta, M. (2019). Definition, symptoms and risk of techno-stress: A systematic review. *International Archives of Occupational and Environmental Health, 92*(1), 13–35. https://doi.org/10.1007/s00420-018-1352-1

LaMontagne, A. D., Martin, A., Page, K. M., Reavley, N. J., Noblet, A. J., Milner, A. J., Keegel, T., & Smith, P. M. (2014). Workplace mental health: Developing an integrated intervention approach. *BMC Psychiatry, 14*(131). https://doi.org/10.1186/1471-244X-14-131

Lee, M. P., Hudson, H., Richards, R., Chang, C. C., Chosewood, L. C., & Schill, A. L. (2016). *Fundamentals of total worker health approaches: Essential elements for advancing worker safety, health, and well-being.* National Institute for Occupational Safety and Health.

Murray, J. K. (2021, March 29). *50% of remote employees miss their commute (and other surprising things people miss most about working in the office).* Indeed. https://www.indeed.com/career-advice/career-development/covid-19-what-people-miss-most-about-office-work/

Neal, J. (Ed.). (2013). *Handbook of faith and spirituality in the workplace: Emerging research and practice.* Springer. https://doi.org/10.1007/978-1-4614-5233-1

Oswald, F., Behrend, T. S., & Foster, L. (Eds.). (2019). *Workforce readiness and the future of work.* Routledge. https://doi.org/10.4324/9781351210485

Pfeffer, J. (2018). *Dying for a paycheck: How modern management harms employee health and company performance—and what we can do about it.* Harper Business.

Punnett, L., Cavallari, J. M., Henning, R. A., Nobrega, S., Dugan, A. G., & Cherniack, M. G. (2020). Defining "integration" for Total Worker Health®: A new proposal. *Annals of Work Exposures and Health, 64*(3), 223–235. https://doi.org/10.1093/annweh/wxaa003

Quick, J. C., & Macik-Frey, M. (2007). Healthy, productive work: Positive strength through communication competence and interpersonal interdependence. In D. L. Nelson & C. L. Cooper (Eds.), *Positive organizational behavior* (pp. 25–39). Sage Publications. https://doi.org/10.4135/9781446212752.n3

Raisch, S., & Birkinshaw, J. (2008). Organizational ambidexterity: Antecedents, outcomes, and moderators. *Journal of Management, 34*(3), 375–409. https://doi.org/10.1177/0149206308316058

Reynolds, G. S., & Bennett, J. B. (2019). A brief measure of organizational wellness climate: Initial validation and focus on small businesses and substance misuse. *Journal of Occupational and Environmental Medicine, 61*(12), 1052–1064. https://doi.org/10.1097/JOM.0000000000001739

Rudolph, C. W., Katz, I. M., Lavigne, K. N., & Zacher, H. (2017). Job crafting: A meta-analysis of relationships with individual differences, job characteristics, and work outcomes. *Journal of Vocational Behavior, 102*(1), 112–138. https://doi.org/10.1016/j.jvb.2017.05.008

Rynes, S. L., Bartunek, J. M., Dutton, J. E., & Margolis, J. D. (2012). Care and compassion through an organizational lens: Opening up new possibilities. *Academy of Management Review, 37*(4), 503–523. https://doi.org/10.5465/amr.2012.0124

Sacasas, L. M. (2021, June 4). *The questions concerning technology.* The Convivial Society. https://theconvivialsociety.substack.com/p/the-questions-concerning-technology

Safeer, R., & Allen, J. (2019). Defining a culture of health in the workplace. *Journal of Occupational and Environmental Medicine, 61*(11), 863–867. https://doi.org/10.1097/JOM.0000000000001684

Salvendy, G. (Ed.). (2012). *Handbook of human factors and ergonomics* (4th ed.). John Wiley & Sons. https://doi.org/10.1002/9781118131350

Schonfeld, I. S., & Chang, C. H. (2017). *Occupational health psychology.* Springer Publishing Company.

Schot, E., Tummers, L., & Noordegraaf, M. (2020). Working on working together. A systematic review on how healthcare professionals contribute to interprofessional collaboration. *Journal of Interprofessional Care, 34*(3), 332–342. https://doi.org/10.1080/13561820.2019.1636007

Sinclair, R. R., Allen, T., Barber, L., Bergman, M., Britt, T., Butler, A., Ford, M., Hammer, L., Kath, L., Probst, T., & Yuan, Z. (2020). Occupational health science in the time of COVID-19: Now more than ever. *Occupational Health Science, 4*(1–2), 1–22. https://doi.org/10.1007/s41542-020-00064-3

Strömberg, C., Aboagye, E., Hagberg, J., Bergström, G., & Lohela-Karlsson, M. (2017). Estimating the effect and economic impact of absenteeism, presenteeism, and work environment–related problems on reductions in productivity from a managerial perspective. *Value in Health, 20*(8), 1058–1064. https://doi.org/10.1016/j.jval.2017.05.008

Substance Abuse and Mental Health Services Administration. (2015). *Core competencies for peer workers in behavioral health services.* https://www.samhsa.gov/sites/default/files/programs_campaigns/brss_tacs/core-competencies_508_12_13_18.pdf

Sunderland, K., & Mishkin, W. (2013). *Guidelines for the practice and training of peer support.* Mental Health Commission of Canada. https://www.mentalhealthcommission.ca/English/document/18291/peer-support-guidelines

Wagner, S. L., Koehn, C., White, M. I., Harder, H. G., Schultz, I. Z., Williams-Whitt, K., Wärje, O., Dionne, C. E., Koehoorn, M., Pasca, R., Hsu, V., McGuire, L., Schulz, W., Kube, D., & Wright, M. D. (2016). Mental health interventions in the workplace and work outcomes: A best-evidence synthesis of systematic reviews. *The International Journal of Occupational and Environmental Medicine, 7*(1), 1–14. https://www.ncbi.nlm.nih.gov/pmc/articles/PMC6816521/

Widera, E., Chang, A., & Chen, H. L. (2010). Presenteeism: A public health hazard. *Journal of General Internal Medicine, 25*(11), 1244–1247. https://doi.org/10.1007/s11606-010-1422-x

Wolever, R. Q., Jordan, M., Lawson, K., & Moore, M. (2016). Advancing a new evidence-based professional in health care: Job task analysis for health and wellness coaches. *BMC Health Services Research, 16*(1), 1–11. https://doi.org/10.1186/s12913-016-1465-8

Zellner, S., & Bowdish, L. (2017). *The ROI of health and well-being: Business investment in healthier communities.* National Academy of Medicine. https://nam.edu/roi-health-well-business-investment-healthier-communities/

7

A Dual Process Model of Multidimensional Work–Nonwork Balance

Wendy J. Casper, Shelia A. Hyde, Hoda Vaziri, and Julie H. Wayne

Work–nonwork balance is a central concept in occupational health psychology, evidenced by the prominence of chapters in previous versions of the *Handbook of Occupational Health Psychology* (Frone, 2003; Greenhaus & Allen, 2011). Prior to the first handbook in 2003, there was discussion of balance in the literature but little consensus about how to define it. In this chapter, we review previous definitions of work–nonwork balance and then present our own dual process model.

PREVIOUS DEFINITIONS OF WORK–NONWORK BALANCE

Marks and MacDermid (1996) first defined *role balance* as "the tendency to become fully engaged in the performance of every role in one's total role system, to approach every typical role and role partner with an attitude of attentiveness and care" (p. 421). While this definition of balance impacted the academic literature, with 6,330 citations in Google Scholar (as of September 26, 2022), scholars continued to offer alternative conceptualizations of balance (Casper et al., 2018).

One reason Marks and MacDermid's (1996) definition failed to become the single accepted one in the literature may be that it was not well integrated with early theories of the work–family interface. For instance, the spillover model (Staines, 1980) suggested that positive or negative affective experiences in one

https://doi.org/10.1037/0000331-007
Handbook of Occupational Health Psychology, Third Edition, L. E. Tetrick, G. G. Fisher, M. T. Ford, and J. C. Quick (Editors)

domain (e.g., work) are carried into other domains (e.g., family): Negative affect from arguing with a spouse can bleed into work and damage work attitudes and behaviors, and/or positive mood from a fun night out with a spouse can also spill over into work as energy and joy during the workday.

The literature on negative spillover was a foundation for research on work–family conflict (Greenhaus & Beutell, 1985), which was the central construct in the work–family literature by the time Marks and MacDermid (1996) wrote about role balance. The construct of work–family conflict drew from the scarcity perspective, which viewed time and energy as finite and saw multiple role involvement as creating competition between roles (Goode, 1960). Greenhaus and Beutell (1985) defined *work–family conflict* as "a form of inter-role conflict that occurs when work and family are mutually incompatible in some respect" (p. 77). They suggested three types of work–family conflict. Time-based work–family conflict occurs when time demands of one role inhibit participation in another role. Strain-based conflict occurs when mental strain in one role interferes with engaging in another. Finally, behavior-based conflict occurs when behaviors that are adaptive in one domain are exhibited in a second domain where they are not adaptive. Research found that work–family conflict was bidirectional (work can interfere with family and vice versa) and linked to many deleterious outcomes (Eby et al., 2005).

Although early research mostly focused on conflict, some scholars documented positive spillover (Crouter, 1984; Grzywacz & Marks, 2000; Sieber, 1974; Wayne et al., 2004), which later was labeled *work–family enrichment*. Greenhaus and Powell (2006) defined *enrichment* as a bidirectional construct in which a skill, positive affect, or fulfillment in one domain (e.g., work) improves quality of life or performance in the other domain (e.g., family).

In the first edition of this handbook, Frone (2003) defined *work–family balance* as a function of conflict and enrichment, the focal constructs in the literature at the time. Frone presented a fourfold taxonomy in which both directions of conflict and both directions of enrichment created four possibilities for the level of balance. His taxonomy suggests that work–family balance is highest when there are low levels of both work-to-family and family-to-work conflict, in conjunction with high levels of work-to-family and family-to-work enrichment.

In the years that followed, various studies adopted Frone's (2003) definition and studied balance using measures of work–family conflict and enrichment (Aryee et al., 2005; Bulger et al., 2007; Gareis et al., 2009; Lu et al., 2009). Although some authors defined balance as a function of conflict and enrichment, an alternative literature continued to evolve depicting balance as a global, unidimensional construct distinct from conflict and enrichment, though there was little agreement about its definition (Casper et al., 2018).

In the second edition of the handbook, Greenhaus and Allen (2011) positioned conflict and enrichment as antecedents of balance rather than features of it, defining work–family balance as "an overall appraisal of the extent to which individuals' effectiveness and satisfaction in work and family roles are consistent with their life values at a given point in time" (p. 174). The authors theorized personal, work, and family characteristics as antecedents of bidirectional conflict and enrichment. In turn, they suggested that conflict damages while enrichment improves satisfaction and effectiveness in work and family roles—the proximal determinants of balance—which contribute to balance contingent on personal values. That is, satisfaction and effectiveness in more valued roles has a greater effect on balance than do experiences in less valued roles.

Around the same time, Maertz and Boyar (2011) argued that conflict and enrichment occur in "episodes" that accumulate and contribute to "levels" of balance. A few years later, Grawitch et al. (2013) found that conflict and enrichment predicted balance satisfaction, and studies began to coalesce around the idea of balance as distinct from conflict and enrichment. Wayne et al. (2017) compared four conceptualizations and operationalizations of balance and found important distinctions. Two operationalizations drew from Frone (2003)—an *additive* spillover approach (direct effects of bidirectional conflict and enrichment) and a *multiplicative* spillover approach (interactions between dimensions of conflict and enrichment). Wayne et al. suggested that the multiplicative spillover approach better reflected Frone's definition of a combination of low bidirectional conflict and high bidirectional enrichment.

Wayne et al. (2017) also found that two holistic operationalizations—*balance satisfaction* (Valcour, 2007), conceptualized as an attitude, and *balance effectiveness* (Carlson et al., 2009), defined as a self-evaluation of one's own cross-role performance—had vital theoretical differences and empirical implications. Balance effectiveness was related to family and job performance but not job or family satisfaction. Balance satisfaction predicted job satisfaction but not job or family performance. Wayne et al. (2017) also found that bidirectional conflict, enrichment, and their interactions were direct predictors of both balance effectiveness and balance satisfaction, supporting the idea of conflict and enrichment as predictors of balance. Yet, because they used a cross-sectional research design, there was no evidence of temporal precedence. Still, Wayne and colleagues (2017) concluded that the various operationalizations of balance are not interchangeable and that careful attention was needed to define and measure balance.

Rothbard et al. (2021) also proposed that depletion and enrichment ultimately result in work–life balance. For example, they suggested that the overall evaluation of balance may be determined by either the most recent role-experience evaluation or the extent of enrichment at its most meaningful point. This view reinforces the trend to conceptualize enrichment and conflict as antecedents of balance rather than core features of it, while also suggesting the importance of studying work–family experiences over time.

To continue to refine thinking on the conceptualization and measurement of balance, Casper et al. (2018) reviewed the definitions and measures of balance and concluded that balance is typically defined as a global nondirectional perception, distinct from conflict and enrichment, but that there are various meanings. The authors suggested that balance is a multidimensional construct that can be assessed as a global perception or via distinct facets. They defined *balance* as "employees' evaluation of the favorability of their combination of work and nonwork roles, arising from the degree to which their affective experiences and their perceived involvement and effectiveness in work and nonwork roles are commensurate with the value they attach to these roles" (p. 197). This suggests that balance has three facets: an affective facet (affective balance) and two cognitive facets (effectiveness balance and involvement balance).

Casper et al. (2018) proffered that each balance facet involves a self-evaluation of effectiveness, involvement, or affect in roles, while considering role centrality. *Affective balance* is defined as "the perception that one experiences sufficiently pleasant emotions in work and nonwork roles commensurate with the value attached to those roles" (Casper et al., 2018, p. 198). *Effectiveness balance* is "the perception that one's effectiveness in work and nonwork roles is commensurate with the value attached to the roles" (p. 198). *Involvement balance* is defined as "the perception that one's involvement in work and nonwork roles is commensurate with the value attached to the roles" (p. 198).

Most recently, Wayne et al. (2021) developed and validated a scale for global balance and its three facets (affective, involvement, effectiveness), based on Casper and colleagues' (2018) definition. Analyses suggested that balance is a hierarchical construct in which global balance functions at the apex of the balance hierarchy. While each facet shares variance with the second-order construct of balance, it also has unique variance not captured by global balance, with balance effectiveness having the largest unique variance. Their balance measure, particularly their global balance and affective balance facet, predicted outcomes such as organizational commitment, turnover intentions, emotional exhaustion, and self-reported health, above and beyond extant measures of balance satisfaction (Valcour, 2007) and balance effectiveness (Carlson et al., 2009).

Despite improved clarity in defining balance, studies of balance rarely reference theory; when they do, they use a wide range of theories often borrowed or adopted from other disciplines (Casper et al., 2018). In this chapter, we use theory blending to propose a model describing the process through which people come to experience work–nonwork balance.

A DUAL PROCESS MODEL OF MULTIDIMENSIONAL BALANCE

To advance theorizing about balance, we begin with the Greenhaus and Allen (2011) model and recent work on multidimensional balance (Casper et al., 2018) as the foundation of our dual process model of balance. We incorporate elements from two other balance models (Hirschi et al., 2019; Voydanoff, 2005), job demands–resources theory (JD-R; Demerouti et al., 2001), and the cross-domain thriving (CDT) model (Hyde et al., 2020; Hyde, 2021) to model how the experience of balance occurs (see Figure 7.1). A key element of our model is the adoption of Greenhaus and Allen's theorizing that personal characteristics, role demands, and role resources are distal antecedents that influence

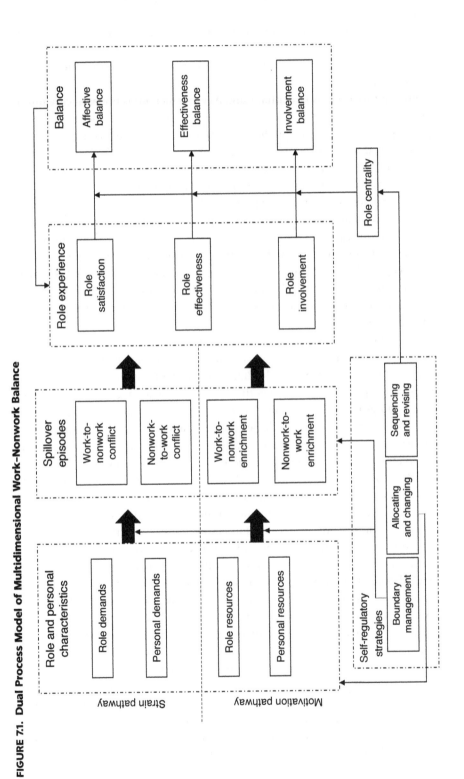

FIGURE 7.1. Dual Process Model of Multidimensional Work–Nonwork Balance

balance indirectly via bidirectional conflict and enrichment and in-role expe-riences (role satisfaction and effectiveness), sequentially.

Yet our model deviates from Greenhaus and Allen's (2011) model in three key ways. First, we conceptualize balance, consistent with Casper et al. (2018), as a holistic appraisal of how work and nonwork roles are combined, arising from affective, involvement, and effectiveness balance facets. This view differs from that proposed by Greenhaus and Allen, which (a) is not explicitly multi-dimensional and (b) excludes involvement from the definition of balance, positing involvement as a predictor of balance rather than a component of it. Casper et al.'s review found involvement was often invoked as a defining feature of balance, and they included it in their multidimensional definition. Second, we extend Greenhaus and Allen's model by proffering role involve-ment as an additional in-role experience that is an input to balance. Drawing from the compatibility principle in the attitude literature (Ajzen & Fishbein, 1977), we suggest that each in-role experience (e.g., role involvement) serves as an input into a conceptually matched facet of balance (e.g., involvement balance), as discussed later. Finally, Greenhaus and Allen posited that per-sonal characteristics, role demands, and role resources all relate to balance through both conflict and enrichment, whereas we suggest more specific mechanisms.

JD-R theory proposes that burnout and engagement occur through distinct processes (Demerouti et al., 2001). Burnout develops from excessive job demands that burden people, leading to exhaustion (strain process); engage-ment develops from job resources that enable people to meet demands, achieve goals, and grow (acting as a motivation process). JD-R theory also posits that dispositional traits can be both personal demands (e.g., neuroticism, perfec-tionism) and personal resources (e.g., optimism, self-efficacy) to directly affect strain and motivation pathways, respectively (Bakker & Demerouti, 2017).

We blend core elements of JD-R theory with Greenhaus and Allen's (2011) model to anchor our model of balance (Figure 7.1). Accordingly, we proffer that role demands and personal demands (sources of strain) inhibit, whereas role resources and personal resources (sources of motivation) enhance, goal focus, attention, and energy. Demands and resources, in turn, affect experiences of conflict and enrichment, respectively. Conflict and enrichment, in turn, impact one's degree of satisfaction, effectiveness, and involvement within valued roles, which predict one's experience of affective balance, effectiveness balance, and involvement balance, respectively, as well as global balance.

In the following section, we theorize about how distal antecedents relate to balance via two pathways. On the strain pathway, role and personal demands foster greater conflict. On the motivation pathway, role and personal resources lead to greater enrichment. As conflict and enrichment occur in episodes over time, people report their level of conflict or enrichment based on accumu-lated episodes of conflict and enrichment over time (Maertz & Boyar, 2011), which are proximal events that affect in-role experiences of role satisfaction, role effectiveness (Greenhaus & Allen, 2011), and role involvement, serving as inputs to balance.

Strain Pathway

Our model proposes that role and personal demands drain time, energy, and positive affect (Bakker & Demerouti, 2017), creating bidirectional work–nonwork conflict, which indirectly influence balance through diminished in-role experiences (Voydanoff, 2005).

Role and Personal Demands Foster Conflict

Both work and nonwork roles involve demands that are present in the role context. These *role demands* diminish time and energy for other roles and create work–nonwork conflict. *Personal demands,* which include self-imposed performance standards and dispositions that predispose people to negative affect and self-undermining behavior (Bakker & Demerouti, 2017), can also operate via the strain pathway to create conflict.

Conflict Leads to In-Role Experiences

As work–nonwork conflict is a stressor that creates strain, it harms in-role experiences, reducing satisfaction, performance, and involvement in a role. The *domain specificity hypothesis* (Frone et al., 1992) suggests that when people are overcome by demands in a domain (e.g., work), they struggle to meet obligations in another domain (e.g., family) and experience conflict (e.g., *work-to-family*) as well as diminishing quality of life and performance in the *receiving* (i.e., family) role. Ample evidence links work–family conflict to deleterious outcomes in the receiving role (Amstad et al., 2011; Frone et al., 1992). Though role involvement has not been widely theorized as an outcome of conflict, when one's time and energy in one role interferes with functioning in another, this should undermine involvement in the receiving role. However, the *source attribution perspective* suggests that conflict also has affective consequences for the source or originating domain (Shockley & Singla, 2011). As such, work-to-nonwork conflict may also be harmful to source role satisfaction as the source role is the basis for the conflict. In sum, our model posits that conflict impairs effectiveness and involvement in the receiving role and diminishes satisfaction in the source role.

Recursive Path Between In-Role Experiences and Balance

Greenhaus and Allen (2011) posited experiences in valued roles (i.e., role satisfaction and effectiveness) as inputs to balance. They suggested that self-evaluations of satisfaction and effectiveness in valued roles are cues individuals use to discern balance. We posit role involvement as another role experience that is a key input into self-evaluations of balance. As balance is an attitude in which the attitude object is one's evaluation of how work and nonwork roles fit together (Casper et al., 2018), we draw on *self-perception theory* (an attitude theory), which asserts that observations of our own behavior drive our attitudes (Bem, 1967), to suggest that role experiences and self-perceptions are inputs to balance facets that in turn relate to global balance.

Notably, this causal ordering is in direct opposition to role balance theory (Marks & MacDermid, 1996), which posits that balance contributes to better in-role experiences (e.g., satisfaction, performance). Drawing from Greenhaus and Allen (2011) and role balance theory, we posit in-role experiences as both predictors of and outcomes of balances (Marks & MacDermid, 1996), suggesting a bidirectional recursive process. That is, while balance develops as a function of in-role experiences, this initiates a positive feedback cycle in which work–nonwork balance and in-role experiences mutually reinforce one another. People judge how effective, satisfied, and involved they are in valued roles; these perceptions influence global balance indirectly via specific facets of balance. In turn, the harmony experienced as global balance fosters more positive in-role experiences in valued roles.

In contrast to Greenhaus and Allen's (2011) definition, we explicitly define balance as a multidimensional construct (Casper et al., 2018). Drawing from the compatibility principle in the attitude literature (Ajzen & Fishbein, 1977), we theorize that role satisfaction, role effectiveness, and role involvement serve as inputs into facets of balance. Specifically, role satisfaction is primarily an input to affective balance, role effectiveness to effectiveness balance, and role involvement to involvement balance. Our positioning of role experiences as proximal predictors of balance facets is consistent with Greenhaus and Allen's assertion that people

assess their effectiveness in each role against internal standards of performance, gauge the amount of satisfaction they derive from each role, and determine the degree to which their effectiveness and satisfaction are consistent with the value they attached to each role. (p. 174)

We also extend Greenhaus and Allen (2011) by proposing a recursive feedback loop such that in-role experiences drive balance, which leads to more positive in-role experiences, invoking a resource-gain spiral (Hobfoll, 2011). This approach blends elements of role balance theory (Marks & MacDermid, 1996) with Greenhaus and Allen's ideas to propose that positive in-role experiences and the experience of balance are mutually reinforcing.

The Impact of Role Centrality
Given an infinite number of roles, all roles are not equally important to one's sense of balance. Like Greenhaus and Allen (2011), we posit role centrality as a boundary condition that influences how much in-role experiences matter to balance, and position it as a moderator of the relationship between in-role experiences and balance facets. We suggest that the degree to which role experiences are important inputs to a conceptually matched facet of balance is dependent on the centrality of the role. Role experiences will be more pertinent to balance when roles are highly valued and core to one's self-concept and less pertinent if roles are less valued and central to the self (Greenhaus & Allen, 2011).

Summary of the Pathway
Integrating tenets from Greenhaus and Allen (2011) and JD-R theory (Demerouti et al., 2001), our model suggests a strain-based pathway that begins with role

and personal demands as the primary mechanism that impairs balance. These role and personal demands increase work–nonwork conflict, which negatively impacts role involvement, satisfaction, and effectiveness (Amstad et al., 2011; Shockley & Singla, 2011). These in-role experiences (i.e., role involvement, satisfaction, and effectiveness) serve as inputs to the appraisal of work and nonwork roles, which are combined (global balance) indirectly through self-assessments of the extent to which they are adequately involved, effective, and satisfied across valued work and nonwork roles (involvement, affective, and effectiveness balance, respectively). These relationships between role experiences and facets of balance (and, ultimately, global balance) are strengthened to the extent that people more strongly value a given role. Finally, balance feeds back to in-role experiences in a recursive process—a bidirectional positive feedback loop between balance and in-role experiences.

Examples of the Strain Pathway

Consider a job with difficult coworkers (work demand), which may foster work-to-nonwork conflict if an employee ruminates about work at home, interfering with being fully present for family life. Such distractions may impair effectiveness in the family role, undermining effectiveness balance to the extent that the family role is valued. This work-to-nonwork conflict also reduces job satisfaction when work is "blamed" for the deleterious effect on family (source attribution view), which impairs affective balance to the extent the work role is valued. Involvement, effectiveness, and affective balance, in turn, are the ultimate inputs into global balance. Finally, the sense of harmony that comes with global balance is a cue that initiates a reciprocal feedback process, reinforcing satisfaction, involvement, and effectiveness within roles.

Nonwork demands can also initiate the strain pathway. For instance, if a phone call comes from an employee's child's school while the employee is at work, and the employee learns that their teenage child faces suspension because alcohol was found in the child's locker, this produces negative affect (nonwork-to-work conflict) for the employee, promoting dissatisfaction in the family role (the source role) and impairing affective balance to the degree to which the nonwork (i.e., family) role is valued. If the employee must leave work midday to attend a meeting about their child at school, this reduces the employee's involvement in work meetings that day (low work involvement). Moreover, as they ruminate about the child's behavior and suspension, they may find it difficult to focus while at work and accomplish work tasks, reducing work effectiveness. To the degree that the work role is valued, low work involvement and effectiveness will have deleterious consequences for involvement and effectiveness balance, respectively. That reduced sense of balance reciprocally impairs role satisfaction, involvement, and effectiveness.

Finally, personal demands can also initiate the strain pathway. For example, perfectionism may cause an employee to spend extended time at work adjusting minor details, invoking work-to-nonwork conflict when family is neglected. The resulting low family role effectiveness is a negative input into effectiveness balance to the degree that the family role is valued, contributing to global balance. (Other examples are provided in Table 7.1.)

TABLE 7.1. Illustrations of Strain and Motivation Pathways to Balance

Source role and personal characteristics	Spillover episode	Role experience	Balance facet (role centrality moderator)
	Strain pathway		
Nonwork demand: Driving child to school at a specific time each workday	Arrival at work is delayed, invoking N-W conflict	Low work role effectiveness (Receiving role)	Low effectiveness balance (Work role)
Work demand: Long work hours	Reduced time for family invokes W-N conflict	Low nonwork role involvement (Receiving role)	Low involvement balance (Nonwork role)
Personal demand: Neurotic tendencies cause excessive rumination at home about work	Ruminating about work at home invokes W-N conflict	Low work role satisfaction (Source role)	Low affective balance (Work role)
	Motivation pathway		
Work resource: Flexibility to work at home	Accomplishing home tasks while working at home fosters W-N enrichment	High nonwork role effectiveness (Receiving role)	High effectiveness balance (Nonwork role)
Nonwork resource: Supportive spouse manages home responsibilities to facilitate late work hours	Assistance at home allows work responsibilities to be met (N-W enrichment)	High work role involvement (Receiving role)	High involvement balance (Work role)
Personal resource: Optimism results in appraisal of work reorganization as an exciting challenge rather than hindrance	Positive affect concerning work opportunity fosters W-N enrichment (i.e., good mood at home)	High work role satisfaction (Source role)	High affective balance (Work role)

Note. N–W = Nonwork-to-work; W–N = Work-to-nonwork.

Motivation Pathway

We propose that another pathway to balance begins with role and personal resources. Role resources are structural characteristics of roles (e.g., work support or spouse support) that enable improved functioning, whereas personal resources are individual differences in dispositions or beliefs that foster energy and positive emotions. Role resources and personal resources operate similarly as inputs to bidirectional work–nonwork enrichment (Demerouti et al., 2001; Voydanoff, 2005), which indirectly affects balance through diminished in-role experiences (Greenhaus & Allen, 2011). The motivation pathway is discussed further in the following section.

Role and Personal Resources Foster Enrichment

Resources are present in both work and nonwork roles (Voydanoff, 2005). As the JD-R theory suggests (Demerouti et al., 2001), role resources from a source role provide energy, skills, or positive emotions that foster engagement in the receiving role due to work–nonwork enrichment. Work role resources foster work-to-nonwork enrichment, whereas nonwork role resources influence nonwork-to-work enrichment. This theorizing is consistent with the CDT model (Hyde et al., 2020), which suggests that within-domain thriving produces role resources that promote work–nonwork enrichment (Hyde, 2021). Both work and nonwork roles provide access to enabling resources (e.g., autonomy) that foster effectiveness within and across domains, as well as psychological rewards (e.g., meaningful work) that promote positive affect within and across domains (Voydanoff, 2005). *Personal resources* include traits, mindsets, and beliefs that promote a sense of agency and control, positive affect, and effective coping, predisposing people to experience work–nonwork enrichment (Bakker & Demerouti, 2017). Meta-analytic evidence suggests that role resources relate to cross-domain enrichment (Lapierre et al., 2018).

Preliminary empirical tests of the CDT model support thriving as a resource-creation mechanism (Hyde, 2021). The CDT model posits cross-domain enrichment as a source of resource gain that occurs when thriving at work benefits nonwork to foster thriving in nonwork role(s). Resources are gained due to enrichment, and then such resources enhance enrichment across roles, spurring a virtuous process of resource-gain spirals (Hobfoll, 2011). Our dual process model depicts role and personal resources as distal antecedents that foster balance via resource gain spirals that play out as represented in Figure 7.1.

Enrichment Leads to In-Role Experiences
Enrichment involves resource transfer across the work–nonwork boundary. It can occur through an affective path, when positive affect from the source role is carried to the receiving role (Greenhaus & Powell, 2006). The source attribution view (Shockley & Singla, 2011) suggests that work–nonwork enrichment improves satisfaction in the source role due to appreciation of cross-role benefits. However, enrichment also results in tangible benefits to the receiving role, improving involvement and effectiveness in the receiving role as extra resources enter this role. Energy brought from the source role to the receiving role via enrichment can increase engagement in the receiving role, fostering receiving role involvement. Finally, when energy or skills developed in the source role benefit the receiving role, this can increase effectiveness in the receiving role.

Recursive Path Between In-Role Experiences and Balance
Though the motivational pathway differs from the strain pathway in antecedents (resources vs. demands) and intervening mechanisms (enrichment vs. conflict), once spillover processes affect in-role involvement, satisfaction, and effectiveness, the motivation pathway converges with the strain pathway. As described previously, we blend ideas from Greenhaus and Allen (2011) and role balance theory (Marks & MacDermid, 1996) to theorize a recursive feedback loop between in-role experiences and balance.

The Impact of Role Centrality

Likewise, as noted in the section on the strain pathway, role centrality strengthens the relationship of in-role experiences with balance facets. For instance, job satisfaction (an in-role experience) serves as an input to affective balance, and this relationship is strengthened when there is greater work role centrality.

Summary of the Pathway

The motivation pathway integrates ideas from models of balance (Greenhaus & Allen, 2011; Voydanoff, 2005) along with JD-R theory (Demerouti et al., 2001) and the CDT model (Hyde et al., 2020) to posit that role and personal resources exert their effects on balance via a series of indirect effects. The path begins with work, nonwork, and personal resources that foster work–nonwork enrichment in two ways. First, enrichment involves a transfer of resources from the source role to the receiving role, resulting in improved experiences (greater role effectiveness or involvement) in the receiving role. Second, enrichment positively affects source role satisfaction due to appreciation of the benefits provided by the source role. This process can also begin when personal resources predispose individuals to exhibiting more positive affect and energy, fostering cross-role enrichment and initiating positive experiences in the receiving role. Role experiences serve as inputs into aligned balance facets to the degree that the role is central to the self. Effectiveness balance, involvement balance, and affective balance ultimately determine global balance.

Examples of the Motivation Pathway

In this section and in Table 7.1, we provide examples of the motivation pathway. A work-role resource, such as feeling cared about at work (e.g., having a supportive employer), may increase positive affect, which is carried home to enrich nonwork domains, increasing work satisfaction due to gratitude for resources provided from work, which is an input to affective balance. Role experiences serve as inputs to facets of balance—in this case, work satisfaction to affective balance—to the degree that these roles are valued. The three facets of balance feed into global balance perceptions, which result in more positive in-role experiences.

Similarly, nonwork resources may foster nonwork–work enrichment and indirectly shape balance via in-role experiences. For instance, an employee who receives a phone call from a spouse to remind them they are loved gains positive affect, which influences their work (family-to-work enrichment). This fosters satisfaction with the family role (the source role), which will impact affective balance to the degree that the family role is valued.

Personal resources also influence balance through the motivation path. For example, high self-efficacy may allow an employee to confidently speak and share work-related expertise at their child's career night, supporting the Parent Teacher Association and fostering work-to-nonwork enrichment. Such involvement in the parent role should lead to high involvement balance if the parent role is valued. Finally, involvement balance is an input to global balance.

PURPOSEFUL ACTION REGULATION IN THE DUAL PROCESS MODEL OF MULTIDIMENSIONAL BALANCE

Often, scholarly and popular discussions imply that balance is largely determined by a person's situation (e.g., work hours, supervisor support, child's age). Yet people are not passive recipients of situational factors (e.g., role demands and resources); they can proactively influence them. In work–nonwork relationships, people are proactive agents that can craft boundaries between roles (de Bloom et al., 2020). Individuals may enhance their own balance by changing the demands imposed upon them, acquiring additional role resources, or adjusting life goals and values. Here, we draw from boundary theory (Ashforth et al., 2000; Nippert-Eng, 1996) and the action regulation view (Hirschi et al., 2019) to explore how employees' purposeful, self-regulatory actions impact their level of balance. In particular, we discuss three types of self-regulatory strategies—work–nonwork boundary management, engagement strategies, and disengagement strategies—as key moderating variables in our model (see Figure 7.1).

Boundary theory posits two ways that people enact boundaries, which are physical, temporal, emotional, cognitive, and relational restrictions around roles, to manage multiple roles (Ashforth et al., 2000). First, individuals adjust the extent to which interruptions from other roles are allowed (i.e., boundary permeability). Second, they control the extent to which they perform tasks related to a role in other settings or at other times (i.e., boundary flexibility). Boundary management behavior varies on a continuum from low flexibility and permeability, or segmentation, to high flexibility and permeability, or integration (Kreiner, 2006). Traditionally, research has conceptualized boundary management as a personal preference (Nippert-Eng, 1996), but these preferences may not match behavior, given that role demands may require the use of nonpreferred strategies (Ammons, 2013). For instance, an employee who prefers segmentation may feel the need to take phone calls from their boss at home. Scholars have theorized that employees may use a combination boundary management strategy known as cycling—at times using segmentation and at other times integration (Kossek, 2016), which may be the best strategy (Rothbard et al., 2021). For example, a cycler may allow integration of nonwork into work when work volume is low, taking calls from home and scheduling medical appointments as needed, but may enforce segmentation at work when work volume is high to foster concentration and productivity.

We posit that self-regulatory strategies such as boundary management moderate the degree to which role demands, role resources, and personal characteristics translate into conflict and enrichment—that is, whether work demands can intrude into nonwork when the work–nonwork boundary is permeable. Employees vary in the extent to which they read their work email during personal time. A segmentor may keep nonwork impermeable to work by refusing to read work-related email during nonwork hours. In contrast, an integrator may read email as soon as an email notification arrives, even during dinner with family. As such, boundary management behavior largely determines the degree to which role demands translate into work–nonwork conflict, which has downstream effects for balance.

Boundary management behavior also influences the degree to which role resources cross boundaries and foster enrichment. Integrators may develop personal friendships at work, such that work serves as a source of support during personal challenges. For example, after receiving a cancer diagnosis, a segmentor who prefers to keep personal life separate from work may keep this information private, disclosing only to a supervisor as absolutely needed for approval of medical leave. As such, the segmentor will have limited access to social support from work and experience minimal work-to-nonwork enrichment. In contrast, an integrator who discloses more widely at work may experience more work-to-nonwork enrichment due to receiving social support from colleagues.

The CDT model also posits employees as active agents who use self-regulatory boundary management (Hyde et al., 2020). Preliminary tests of the CDT model (Hyde, 2021) found that boundary management moderated the degree to which nonwork thriving, which produces role resources, crossed the nonwork-to-work boundary to foster enrichment, with the relationship stronger among integrators, as suggested in our model. In addition to its moderating role, Hyde (2021) found a direct effect of boundary management such that greater integration was associated with greater enrichment in both directions, whereas greater cycling was associated with greater nonwork-to-work enrichment but also greater nonwork-to-work conflict.

These results suggest potential benefits of both integration and cycling for enhancing enrichment. However, given that cycling was also associated with greater conflict, preliminary findings suggest integration may be the best approach to initiating the motivation pathway to balance without also initiating the strain pathway. As enrichment is theorized to influence affective, effectiveness, and involvement balance via role-specific experiences, empirical findings related to the CDT model (Hyde, 2021) support our dual process model in finding that boundary management has implications for balance via its impact on enrichment. Future research is needed to follow up on Hyde's (2021) preliminary results and determine whether boundary management can influence balance through its impact on conflict.

Another recent theoretical model discussed how people actively influence the resources available to them and the demands they face, in that they choose and change their priorities in an effort to gain balance (Hirschi et al., 2019). The action regulation perspective (Hirschi et al., 2019) suggests that individuals can use four action strategies (i.e., allocating resources, changing resources and barriers, sequencing goals, and revising goals) to attain work–family goals and thus experience greater balance. Allocating resources (i.e., "intentional activation and allocation of existing resources") as well as changing resources and barriers (i.e., "intentional increase of resources and/or reduction of barriers") are considered engagement strategies, whereas sequencing goals (i.e., "intentional prioritization of some work or family goals in the shorter term so that other goals can be attained in the longer term") and revising goals (i.e., "intentional revision of existing work or family goals and the selection of new goals") are considered disengagement strategies (Hirschi et al., 2019, p. 155). The action regulation model suggests that individuals prefer to use engagement strategies as they allow for more control and goal attainment; however, when engagement strategies are not viable, they may use disengagement strategies (i.e., change themselves) to assert control.

Accordingly, we argue that, in addition to boundary management, individuals' action regulation strategies to manage their work and nonwork roles are also important considerations in our dual process model of balance. We suggest that engagement strategies (allocating and changing) directly influence role demands and resources, which in turn lead to less conflict, more enrichment, and enhanced in-role experiences, fostering the experience of balance to the extent that the roles are valued. For example, a person with high work demands might have inadequate time for family (i.e., work-to-nonwork conflict), reducing family performance and balance effectiveness if the family role is valued. To improve balance, this person may proactively discuss these challenges with their supervisor and request additional resources (i.e., changing resources and barriers). These additional resources enable reduced work hours, freeing up time for family and improving balance. In another illustration of resource allocation, Calderwood and colleagues (2021) found that daily physical activity (i.e., steps taken) increased a person's bandwidth to achieve work (i.e., work recovery) and nonwork goals (i.e., family absorption) by enhancing boundary-spanning resources (i.e., vigor), ultimately enhancing satisfaction with work–life balance.

On the other hand, as disengagement strategies involve changes in the self (e.g., sequencing and revising goals and values), this may alter the centrality of roles. When a role becomes less central to the self via disengagement strategies, the influence of in-role experiences on the facets of balance is reduced. For instance, a person may feel ineffective in the friend role when they have no time to see friends due to excessive demands at work. If no engagement strategies is viable to free up time and energy to be more effective within the friend role, the person might revisit life priorities and assign a lower priority to their identity as a friend (i.e., revising goals) so that the friend role experiences (e.g., effectiveness) have a lower impact on felt balance. In sum, rather than being passive agents, people actively shape their demands and resources and make choices related to their role values, which ultimately influence their felt balance.

DIRECTIONS FOR FUTURE RESEARCH

The recent development of a scale to assess multidimensional balance (Wayne et al., 2021) enables exploration and comparison of people's experiences of balance. This can lead to recommendations for improving balance and for how organizations might support this effort. Research is needed to test aspects of our model that suggest actionable steps that individuals and organizations might take to enhance balance. There are also key questions about the multiple facets of balance. For instance, are the affective, effectiveness, and involvement facets of balance equally important to experiencing global balance? If one facet of balance (e.g., effectiveness) is more important to global balance than others, conceptually matched in-role experiences (e.g., role effectiveness) in highly valued roles may be a lever by which to improve this balance facet, and thereby global balance.

It is also important to consider how the relationships in our model unfold over time. As illustrated by the aforementioned study on physical activity and work–nonwork goals (Calderwood et al., 2021), daily experiences at work are linked to predictors that foster feelings of balance at the end of the workday. However, it is likely that the accumulation of role experiences over many days establishes a person's overall perception of balance. The episodic, configurational view (Rothbard et al., 2021) also provides an example of how cumulative experiences of enrichment and depletion may influence the perception of balance over time. Thus, while daily relationship studies provide critical insights into the short-term effects of demands and resources on balance outcomes, longitudinal studies would enable testing theorizing from the literature, such as the idea that conflict and enrichment are relatively dynamic and balance is more stable over time (Maertz & Boyar, 2011). Longitudinal studies with cross-lagged designs will also enable testing temporal ordering of variables proffered in our model. Such designs are critical to evaluate the relationship of in-role experiences with balance to determine whether in-role experiences precede balance (Greenhaus & Allen, 2011), whether balance precedes in-role experiences (Marks & MacDermid, 1996), or whether there is a bidirectional feedback loop between in-role experiences and balance (as suggested in our model). Cross-lagged designs would also enable the examination of relationships between the facets of balance. While preliminary evidence suggests the three facets of balance are correlated in a cross-sectional data collection (Wayne et al., 2021), the causal relationships between the facets of balance are not understood. Research with cross-lagged designs would allow exploration of temporal precedence of these facets. For instance, some degree of involvement balance may be necessary (but not sufficient) to experience effectiveness balance, as it is hard to imagine being effectively balanced across roles if you are uninvolved.

Research is also needed to explore self-regulatory strategies that hold promise for enhancing the experience of balance. Initially, survey research might measure the degree to which people engage in boundary management, engagement, and disengagement strategies to determine whether these self-regulatory behaviors operate as hypothesized in our model. If specific self-regulatory strategies are linked to greater balance, additional research could explore interventions that encourage the use of self-regulatory strategies to promote balance. If such interventions do, in fact, teach self-regulatory strategies that are associated with being more balanced, organizations might offer such interventions to help employees experience greater balance.

Another avenue for future research is to examine the factors that influence individuals' choice of self-regulatory strategies. For instance, role centrality may influence boundary management strategy, given evidence that distinct profiles of boundary management strategies relate to distinct role identities (Kossek et al., 2012). Engagement and disengagement strategies may also be related to role centrality. For instance, when a person decides to postpone pursuit of a personal goal until after an important career goal is achieved (e.g., postponing parenthood until after earning tenure), they are using a disengagement strategy to sequence goals, requiring them to make the postponed goal less central for the time being. Thus, additional research is needed to examine how the interplay of role centrality and self-regulatory strategies related to balance.

CONCLUSION

Our dual process model of multidimensional work–nonwork balance discusses how three facets of affective, involvement, and effectiveness balance develop to ultimately affect global balance. We incorporate theory and findings to describe two pathways—strain and motivation—that lead to in-role experiences and balance. In-role experiences are more significant to balance when they occur in roles that are highly valued and central to the self. Purposeful, self-regulation strategies, such as boundary management and (dis)engagement, also offer insight into differences in balance outcomes and are possible targets of interventions to foster balance.

REFERENCES

Ajzen, I., & Fishbein, M. (1977). Attitude-behavior relations: A theoretical analysis and review of empirical research. *Psychological Bulletin, 84*(5), 888–918. https://doi.org/10.1037/0033-2909.84.5.888

Allen, T. D., French, K. A., Dumani, S., & Shockley, K. M. (2020). A cross-national meta-analytic examination of predictors and outcomes associated with work–family conflict. *Journal of Applied Psychology, 105*(6), 539–576. https://doi.org/10.1037/apl0000442

Ammons, S. K. (2013). Work–family boundary strategies: Stability and alignment between preferred and enacted boundaries. *Journal of Vocational Behavior, 82*(1), 49–58. https://doi.org/10.1016/j.jvb.2012.11.002

Amstad, F. T., Meier, L. L., Fasel, U., Elfering, A., & Semmer, N. K. (2011). A meta-analysis of work–family conflict and various outcomes with a special emphasis on cross-domain versus matching-domain relations. *Journal of Occupational Health Psychology, 16*(2), 151–169. https://doi.org/10.1037/a0022170

Aryee, S., Srinivas, E. S., & Tan, H. H. (2005). Rhythms of life: Antecedents and outcomes of work–family balance in employed parents. *Journal of Applied Psychology, 90*(1), 132–146. https://doi.org/10.1037/0021-9010.90.1.132

Ashforth, B. E., Kreiner, G. E., & Fugate, M. (2000). All in a day's work: Boundaries and micro role transitions. *Academy of Management Review, 25*(3), 472–491. https://doi.org/10.2307/259305

Bakker, A. B., & Demerouti, E. (2017). Job demands–resources theory: Taking stock and looking forward. *Journal of Occupational Health Psychology, 22*(3), 273–285. https://doi.org/10.1037/ocp0000056

Bem, D. J. (1967). Self-perception: An alternative interpretation of cognitive dissonance phenomena. *Psychological Review, 74*(3), 183–200. https://doi.org/10.1037/h0024835

Bulger, C. A., Matthews, R. A., & Hoffman, M. E. (2007). Work and personal life boundary management: Boundary strength, work/personal life balance, and the segmentation-integration continuum. *Journal of Occupational Health Psychology, 12*(4), 365–375. https://doi.org/10.1037/1076-8998.12.4.365

Calderwood, C., Gabriel, A. S., Ten Brummelhuis, L. L., Rosen, C. C., & Rost, E. A. (2021). Understanding the relationship between prior to end-of-workday physical activity and work–life balance: A within-person approach. *Journal of Applied Psychology, 106*(8), 1239–1249. https://doi.org/10.1037/apl0000829

Carlson, D. S., Grzywacz, J. G., & Zivnuska, S. (2009). Is work–family balance more than conflict and enrichment? *Human Relations, 62*(10), 1459–1486. https://doi.org/10.1177/0018726709336500

Casper, W. J., Vaziri, H., Wayne, J. H., DeHauw, S., & Greenhaus, J. (2018). The jingle-jangle of work–nonwork balance: A comprehensive and meta-analytic review of its meaning and measurement. *Journal of Applied Psychology, 103*(2), 182–214. https://doi.org/10.1037/apl0000259

Crouter, A. (1984). Participative work as an influence on human development. *Journal of Applied Developmental Psychology, 5*(1), 71–90. https://doi.org/10.1016/0193-3973(84)90028-5

de Bloom, J., Vaziri, H., Tay, L., & Kujanpää, M. (2020). An identity-based integrative needs model of crafting: Crafting within and across life domains. *Journal of Applied Psychology, 105*(12), 1423–1446. https://doi.org/10.1037/apl0000495

Demerouti, E., Bakker, A. B., Nachreiner, F., & Schaufeli, W. B. (2001). The job demands-resources model of burnout. *Journal of Applied Psychology, 86*(3), 499–512. https://doi.org/10.1037/0021-9010.86.3.499

Eby, L. T., Casper, W. J., Lockwood, A., Bordeaux, C., & Brinley, A. (2005). A retrospective on work and family research in IO/OB: A content analysis and review of the literature (1980–2002) [Monograph]. *Journal of Vocational Behavior, 66*, 124–197. https://doi.org/10.1016/j.jvb.2003.11.003

Frone, M. R. (2003). Work–family balance. In J. C. Quick & L. E. Tetrick (Eds.), *Handbook of occupational health psychology* (pp. 143–162). American Psychological Association.

Frone, M. R., Russell, M., & Cooper, M. L. (1992). Antecedents and outcomes of work–family conflict: Testing a model of the work–family interface. *Journal of Applied Psychology, 77*(1), 65–78. https://doi.org/10.1037/0021-9010.77.1.65

Gareis, K. C., Barnett, R. C., Ertel, K. A., & Berkman, L. F. (2009). Work–family enrichment and conflict: Additive effects, buffering, or balance? *Journal of Marriage and Family, 71*(3), 696–707. https://doi.org/10.1111/j.1741-3737.2009.00627.x

Goode, W. (1960). A theory of strain. *American Sociological Review, 25*(4), 483–496. https://doi.org/10.2307/2092933

Grawitch, M. J., Maloney, P. W., Barber, L. K., & Mooshegian, S. E. (2013). Examining the nomological network of satisfaction with work–life balance. *Journal of Occupational Health Psychology, 18*(3), 276–284. https://doi.org/10.1037/a0032754

Greenhaus, J. H., & Allen, T. D. (2011). Work–family balance: A review and extension of the literature. In J. C. Quick & L. E. Tetrick (Eds.), *Handbook of occupational health psychology* (2nd ed., pp. 165–183). American Psychological Association.

Greenhaus, J. H., & Beutell, N. J. (1985). Sources of conflict between work and family roles. *Academy of Management Review, 10*(1), 76–88. https://doi.org/10.2307/258214

Greenhaus, J. H., & Powell, G. N. (2006). When work and family are allies: A theory of work–family enrichment. *Academy of Management Review, 31*(1), 72–92. https://doi.org/10.5465/amr.2006.19379625

Grzywacz, J. G., & Marks, N. F. (2000). Reconceptualizing the work–family interface: An ecological perspective on the correlates of positive and negative spillover between work and family. *Journal of Occupational Health Psychology, 5*(1), 111–126. https://doi.org/10.1037/1076-8998.5.1.111

Hirschi, A., Shockley, K. M., & Zacher, H. (2019). Achieving work–family balance: An action regulation model. *Academy of Management Review, 44*(1), 150–171. https://doi.org/10.5465/amr.2016.0409

Hobfoll, S. E. (2011). *Conservation of resources theory: Its implication for stress, health, and resilience.* Oxford University Press.

Hyde, S. (2021). *Self-regulation of boundaries for thriving, enrichment, and balance across the work-nonwork interface* [Unpublished doctoral dissertation]. University of Texas at Arlington.

Hyde, S., Casper, W. J., & Wayne, J. H. (2020). Putting role resources to work: The cross-domain thriving model. *Human Resource Management Review.* https://www.sciencedirect.com/science/article/abs/pii/S1053482220300929

Kossek, E. E. (2016). Managing work–life boundaries in the digital age. *Organizational Dynamics, 45*(3), 258–270. https://doi.org/10.1016/j.orgdyn.2016.07.010

Kossek, E. E., Ruderman, M. N., Braddy, P. W., & Hannum, K. M. (2012). Work–nonwork boundary management profiles: A person-centered approach. *Journal of Vocational Behavior, 81*(1), 112–128. https://doi.org/10.1016/j.jvb.2012.04.003

Kreiner, G. (2006). Consequences of work–home segmentation or integration: A person–environment fit perspective. *Journal of Organizational Behavior, 27*(4), 485–507. https://doi.org/10.1002/job.386

Lapierre, L. M., Li, Y., Kwan, H. K., Greenhaus, J. H., DiRenzo, M. S., & Shao, P. (2018). A meta-analysis of the antecedents of work–family enrichment. *Journal of Organizational Behavior, 39*(4), 385–401. https://doi.org/10.1002/job.2234

Lu, J. F., Siu, O. L., Spector, P. E., & Shi, K. (2009). Antecedents and outcomes of a fourfold taxonomy of work–family balance in Chinese employed parents. *Journal of Occupational Health Psychology, 14*(2), 182–192. https://doi.org/10.1037/a0014115

Maertz, C. P., Jr., & Boyar, S. L. (2011). Work–family conflict, enrichment, and balance under "levels" and "episodes" approaches. *Journal of Management, 37*(1), 68–98. https://doi.org/10.1177/0149206310382455

Marks, S. R., & MacDermid, S. M. (1996). Multiple roles and the self: A theory of role balance. *Journal of Marriage and Family, 58*(2), 417–432. https://doi.org/10.2307/353506

Nippert-Eng, C. (1996). *Home and work: Negotiating boundaries through everyday life.* University of Chicago Press. https://doi.org/10.7208/chicago/9780226581477.001.0001

Rothbard, N. P., Beetz, A. M., & Harari, D. (2021). Balancing the scales: A configurational approach to work-life balance. *Annual Review of Organizational Psychology and Organizational Behavior, 8*(1), 73–103. https://doi.org/10.1146/annurev-orgpsych-012420-061833

Shockley, K. M., & Singla, N. (2011). Reconsidering work–family interactions and satisfaction: A meta-analysis. *Journal of Management, 37*(3), 861–886. https://doi.org/10.1177/0149206310394864

Sieber, S. D. (1974). Toward a theory of role accumulation. *American Sociological Review, 39*(4), 567–578. https://doi.org/10.2307/2094422

Staines, G. L. (1980). Spillover versus compensation: A review of the literature on the relationship between work and nonwork. *Human Relations, 33*(2), 111–129. https://doi.org/10.1177/001872678003300203

Valcour, M. (2007). Work-based resources as moderators of the relationship between work hours and satisfaction with work–family balance. *Journal of Applied Psychology, 92*(6), 1512–1523. https://doi.org/10.1037/0021-9010.92.6.1512

Voydanoff, P. (2005). Toward a conceptualization of perceived work–family fit and balance: A demands and resources approach. *Journal of Marriage and Family, 67*(4), 822–836. https://doi.org/10.1111/j.1741-3737.2005.00178.x

Wayne, J. H., Butts, M., Casper, W. J., & Allen, T. D. (2017). In search of balance: A conceptual and empirical integration of multiple meanings of work–family balance. *Personnel Psychology, 70*(1), 167–210. https://doi.org/10.1111/peps.12132

Wayne, J. H., Musisca, N., & Fleeson, W. (2004). Considering the role of personality in the work–family experience: Relationships of the Big Five to work–family conflict and facilitation. *Journal of Vocational Behavior, 64,* 108–130. https://doi.org/10.1016/S0001-8791(03)00035-6

Wayne, J. H., Vaziri, H., & Casper, W. J. (2021). Work–nonwork balance: Development and validation of a global and multidimensional measure. *Journal of Vocational Behavior, 127*(103565). https://doi.org/10.1016/j.jvb.2021.103565

Cross-Cultural Occupational Health Psychology

An Updated Review

William Scott, Chu-Hsiang Chang, and Paul E. Spector

The roots of occupational health psychology (OHP) can be traced to early work by Nordic scholars (Barling & Griffiths, 2003), making it international from the beginning. Cultural factors can affect psychological processes that contribute to employee health, well-being, and safety. Indeed, at the societal level, cultural factors are connected to the sociopolitical environment in which organizations operate (Levi, 1990), thereby affecting employees' organizational experiences. Cultural characteristics also have implications for individual employees' own values, which can shape how they perceive, regard, and respond to their work context (Das & Kumar, 2010). Cross-cultural considerations of OHP aim to address the challenges associated with understanding the diverse psychological mechanisms underlying the employee health and well-being across the national boundaries, which serves as the topic of this chapter.

CULTURAL CONTEXT AND VALUES

Cross-cultural research has largely focused on values. The Global Leadership and Organizational Behavior Effectiveness (GLOBE) project (House et al., 2004), for example, collected data from 62 countries measuring values in addition to leadership attributes. The GLOBE project expanded upon the five culture dimensions developed by Hofstede (2001) to include nine dimensions,

https://doi.org/10.1037/0000331-008
Handbook of Occupational Health Psychology, Third Edition, L. E. Tetrick, G. G. Fisher, M. T. Ford, and J. C. Quick (Editors)

listed in Table 8.1, along with how they map onto Hofstede's culture value taxonomy.

In addition to the dimensional differences highlighted in Table 8.1, the GLOBE study measured the cultural dimensions across both actual societal practices ("As Is") and values ("Should Be"), whereas the Hofstede (2001) dimensions were focused purely on the practices. Despite the differences between the two, both the Hofstede and GLOBE studies have provided scholars with significant insights into the structure of national culture values.

Another recent addition to cross-cultural research dimensions that go beyond values is the cultural tightness and looseness dimensions proposed by Gelfand et al. (2006). Gelfand and colleagues noted that societal tightness-looseness has two key components: "the strength of social norms, or how clear and pervasive norms are within societies, and the strength of sanctioning, or how much tolerance there is for deviance from norms within societies" (p. 7). A culturally tight society tends to have strong and clear social norms that are pervasive, as well as having little tolerance for deviance from these norms.

TABLE 8.1. Cultural Value Taxonomies and Definitions

GLOBE culture values	Hofstede culture values	GLOBE value definition
Uncertainty avoidance	Uncertainty avoidance	The extent to which members of an organization or society strive to avoid uncertainty by reliance on social norms, rituals, and bureaucratic practices to alleviate the unpredictability of future events
Power distance	Power distance	The degree to which members of an organization or society expect and agree that power should be unequally shared
Institutional collectivism	Individualism-collectivism	The degree to which organizational and societal institutional practices encourage and reward collective distribution of resources and collective action
Ingroup collectivism		The degree to which individuals express pride, loyalty, and cohesiveness in their organizations or families
Gender egalitarianism	Masculinity	The extent to which an organization or a society minimizes gender role differences
Assertiveness		The degree to which individuals in organizations or societies are assertive, confrontational, and aggressive in social relationships
Future orientation	Long-term orientation	The degree to which individuals in organizations or societies engage in future-oriented behaviors such as planning, investing in the future, and delaying gratification
Performance orientation		The extent to which an organization or society encourages and rewards group members for performance improvement and excellence
Humane orientation		The degree to which individuals in organizations or societies encourage and reward individuals for being fair, altruistic, friendly, generous, caring, and kind to others

OHP TOPICS FROM A CROSS-CULTURAL PERSPECTIVE

It is important to distinguish between cross-cultural versus cross-national research. *Cross-national* (CN) research compares participants from different countries, with the assumption that differences in the national cultures explain the observed differences in the focal phenomenon (Tsui et al., 2007). *Cross-cultural* (CC) research directly incorporates assessment of the cultural variables such as values into an investigation (Tsui et al., 2007). Whereas CN studies require sampling across national boundaries, CC research can be conducted within a single country by isolating cultural factors that vary across people.

Job Stress

Most theories of job stress adopt either explicitly or implicitly the environment-response or stressor-strain framework (Spector, 1992), best reflected in the transactional approach (Lazarus, 1991) in which the work environment (stressor) is assumed to cause responses in the person (strain). *Stressors* are conditions in the environment that require an adaptive response (Jex, 1998). Numerous stressor types are inherent in the nature of the job (e.g., uncertainty over required job tasks), whereas other types are more social by nature (e.g., being bullied). *Strains* are reactions to stressors that can be classified as physical (e.g., increased blood pressure), psychological (anger), or behavioral (alcohol consumption).

International Replications
The most common international studies are international replications in a single country. Such studies generally make no explicit attempt to compare results quantitatively to another country, and most make no claim at being cross-cultural. For example, Bishop et al. (2003) found support for the demand-control model in the context of analyzing the responses of a sample of Singaporean police officers. Lu and colleagues (2005) noted that extending Western findings to China was the purpose of their study about the role of self-efficacy in the job stress process. Similarly, Chen et al. (2003) were interested in exploring sources of stress specifically among Chinese citizens, and how these sources might vary as a function of personality. This literature is fragmented and provides limited insights concerning generalizability because there are too few studies in too few countries using too many diverse measures and samples from which to draw definitive conclusions.

Transporting Assessments
Conducting CC and CN research often requires the translation of assessments from the source language in which they were developed to the target language in the countries being studied. To maintain meaning, an assessment is translated from the source to the target language and vice versa (Brislin, 1986). It is also important to establish measurement equivalence and invariance (ME/I) using complex statistical methods to demonstrate that the factorial structure of the instrument has been maintained (Spector et al., 2015).

An examination of the CC and CN literature will reveal many examples of ME/I tests, but there have been few systematic attempts to explore how culture and language might affect transportability. Perhaps the most comprehensive is a series of studies by Puig and colleagues that compared the psychometric properties of burnout for counselors across several Asian countries (e.g., Carrola et al., 2012; S. M. Lee et al., 2007; Puig et al., 2014; Shin et al., 2013).

Cross-National Job Stress

CN studies comparing stress variables reveal inconsistencies across countries (Spector, in press). For example, Glazer and Amren (2018) looked at the buffering effect on job satisfaction on the stressor–job attitude relationship. The effect on the relationship was expected to be lessened when the level of social support was high compared with when it was low. They surveyed employees in 25 countries from nine world regions and found that the buffering effect occurred in only one third of the regions, and the reverse buffering effect was found in two. Like other CN studies, these surveys were unable to provide much insight into why the differences occurred and the extent to which they might be attributable to some aspect of culture.

Another question is whether the nature of stressors might differ across national boundaries. For example, Liu and colleagues (2007) used a mixed-methods approach with their comparative study of job stress in China and the United States. Their results showed that interpersonal conflict differed in nature across cultures. Chinese conflict was mainly indirect, involving bad-mouthing and undermining colleagues, whereas American conflict mainly involved direct confrontation.

Cross-Cultural Job Stress

CC studies include cultural variables to investigate how culture itself is a factor in job stress. When multiple countries are examined, multilevel modeling is useful; country-level cultural variables can serve as moderators of relationships among stressors, strains, and other stress-relevant variables at the individual employee level. Examples of this multilevel approach include Fisher (2014), who studied role overload across 18 countries, and Yang et al. (2012), who studied workload across 24 countries. Both studies used Hofstede's (2001) values as the cultural variables of interest. Although it is assumed that culture is an important factor in individuals' responses to job conditions, the role of culture is not clear. Only a handful of studies have investigated cultural variables, leaving little upon which one can base conclusions and theories about how culture affects the experience of work.

Work–Family Issues

The interplay between work and family domains has implications for employee health and well-being. Of particular concern is the interrole conflict of work–family conflict (WFC), which is the incompatibility of demands between the work and family domains (Greenhaus & Allen, 2011). WFC has been categorized into two forms: *work–family conflict*, in which the general demands of time devoted to, and strain created by, the job interfere with performing family-related responsibilities; and *family–work conflict*, in which the general demands of, time devoted to, and strain created by the family interfere with performing work-related responsibilities (Greenhaus & Allen, 2011). In the work–family research area is the concept of *work–family enrichment* (WFE), which refers to the positive process at the work–life interface, whereby experience or participation in one role increases the quality or performance in the other role (Greenhaus & Allen, 2011).

Recent CC and CN research in WFC has revealed similar and different antecedents and outcomes of WFC across different countries and cultures. Ollo-López and Goñi-Legaz (2017) found that participants from countries higher in uncertainty avoidance had lower WFC. Ollo-López and Goñi-Legaz also found that humane orientation was negatively related to WFC, while ingroup collectivism and power distance were not significantly related to WFC. Billing and colleagues (2014) found that employees in predominantly individualistic countries (e.g., the United States and Canada) were better able to deal with WFC and did not experience as much psychological strain when they had sufficient decision latitude in performing the duties and responsibilities associated with their work roles. However, decision latitude did not moderate the relationship between WFC and psychological strain in collectivistic contexts (e.g., India, Indonesia, South Korea). Billing et al. noted that this may be because the degree of emotional interconnectedness among the members of the family is stronger in collectivistic countries, and it may not be necessary for a collectivistic working member of the family to either seek or have decision latitude to mitigate the effects of WFC (Sanchez-Burks & Lee, 2007).

The distinction between work–family and family–work conflict is especially important when it comes to CN comparisons. Galovan et al. (2010) found that in the United States, work–family conflict was more strongly associated with depression than was family–work conflict. Conversely, in Singapore, family–work conflict was more strongly associated with depression than was work–family conflict. Moreover, work–family conflict was significantly and negatively related to job satisfaction in the United States but not in Singapore. Galovan et al. argued that work may bring honor to the families in collectivist cultures, and that when family demands interfere with work, employees may be more likely to develop depression because they are unable to enhance their family reputation (Redding, 1993).

Another area to explore is the effects of formal support programs on WFC in different contexts. Stock et al. (2016) found that formal work–family programs, such as offering child care and flexible work time options (Batt & Valcour, 2003), were positively related to job satisfaction and subsequent performance in the United States and India but had no significant effect on employee satisfaction or performance in China. Stock and colleagues proposed that this may be because employees in more collectivistic cultures may rely on help from family members instead of using formal support programs. Although India may also be more of a collectivistic culture than the United

States, economic developments in India continue to encourage the transmission of Western cultural values (Kulkarni et al., 2010), thus causing the adoption of more individualistic values.

In addition to individualism–collectivism, Beham et al. (2013) found that in countries with extensive governmental support and high gender-equality values (e.g., Sweden, the Netherlands, Germany), organizations provided more resources to support employees in meeting their nonwork responsibilities, thus leading to lower WFC. In less gender-egalitarian countries (e.g., the United Kingdom, Portugal) with less state support, the organizational provision of work–family support also tended to be low, and employees experienced higher WFC. These results suggest that gender egalitarianism may be a predictor of WFC, especially for women in less gender-egalitarian countries.

O'Brien and colleagues (2014) found that although there was no difference in WFC, American and Israeli mothers had higher levels of WFE than Korean mothers. Meanwhile, Korean mothers reported the lowest levels of spousal support and employer support, as well as the highest levels of depression relative to their American and Israeli counterparts. This may be due to the low gender-egalitarianism practice score in South Korea (House et al., 2004; Sohn, 2005).

One CN study by Ollier-Malaterre et al. (2020) examined the interplay between Family-Supportive Organizational Perception (FSOP), which helped enhance employees' experience of WFE, and the humane orientation cultural value in predicting employees' job burnout (e.g., emotional exhaustion, cynicism) across five countries. They found that FSOP was related to reduced emotional exhaustion and cynicism in cultures that were higher in humane orientation, whereas FSOP was unrelated to emotional exhaustion or cynicism in cultures that were lower in humane orientation. Specifically, employees in countries with higher humane orientation value (e.g., New Zealand, Malaysia) experienced a greater beneficial effect of FSOP. Since higher humane orientation countries encourage and reward the demonstration of kindness and compassion toward others (House et al., 2004), witnessing kind behaviors in one's context may help bolster the effects of FSOP on reducing burnout symptoms (Ollier-Malaterre et al., 2020).

Accidents, Injuries, and Work-Related Musculoskeletal Disorders

Workplace accidents refer to "discrete occurrence in the course of work leading to physical or mental occupational injury" (European Commission, 2001, p. 12). In the United States, private industry employers reported 2.8 million non-fatal workplace injuries and illnesses in 2019, with almost one third of these injuries resulting in a worker missing at least 1 day of work (Bureau of Labor Statistics, 2020).

GLOBE cultural values have been found to impact safety and accident outcomes. Mohamed et al. (2009) found that workers' attitudes regarding safety and accidents were influenced by the cultural values of their work environment, as workers in a more collectivist, feminist, and higher uncertainty avoidance environment had greater safety awareness and beliefs. García-Arroyo and Segovia (2020) found in Spain that immigrant workers' native language and cultural distance from Spanish culture were associated with number of accidents. Specifically, immigrant workers from non-Spanish-speaking countries had fewer accidents compared with Spanish-speaking immigrant workers. Moreover, immigrants whose home cultures were more distant from the host (i.e., Spanish) culture and shared fewer norms and values (Hofstede, 2001) experienced fewer accidents. García-Arroyo and Segovia suggested that there is more direct and close supervision of immigrant workers who tend to have more difficulties at work because of cultural and language differences. Additionally, certain groups of immigrant workers (e.g., workers from China or Bangladesh) were also likely to have higher long-term orientation and uncertainty avoidance values compared with Spanish-speaking immigrants, which is a factor that may also contribute to having fewer accidents.

Another CN study found that accident rates were higher in Spain versus Sweden (Morillas et al., 2013). This difference may be due to the strong emphasis and consistent practice of safety and health training both in the school curriculum and the organizational policy in Sweden. Taking a broader view of Europe, Reniers and Gidron (2013) examined the relationship between Hofstede's (2001) cultural values and fatal work injuries (FWIs) of European countries. FWIs had a positive relationship with power distance and a negative relationship with individualism, after controlling for the countries' income and alcohol consumption levels. Reniers and Gidron (2013) suggested that employees in countries with high individualism and low power distance may be more likely to be proactive and contribute to safety-related practices at work, which may help prevent errors and FWIs.

There may also be cultural differences regarding how employees think about and communicate safety-related thoughts and concerns. *Error orientation* is the extent to which employees perceive errors as learning opportunities, appraise errors in a favorable light, and constructively cope with errors (Rybowiak et al., 1999). Zotzmann et al. (2019) found among eight diverse countries that the United States had the highest error orientation and Japan the lowest, and that power distance and masculinity were negatively related to error orientation, which may explain the CN differences in error orientation.

Another study examining the safety perceptions of employees found that Western pilots were more willing than Chinese pilots to share information and knowledge that would help improve safety for the organization with other pilots (Liao, 2015). Chinese pilots, particularly if the pilot was junior in rank, felt that sharing information and knowledge was an indication of showing off. Chinese pilots may be worried about the negative consequences related to submitting safety-related reports or reporting their higher ranking crewmembers' rule violations due to the power distance. Thus, creating a psychologically safe environment in which error reporting is not perceived as relationship-damaging or status quo–challenging may be critical for improving safety in the Chinese context (Liao, 2015).

It is important to recognize that certain occupations have a higher risk of accidents and injuries, such as manual labor (especially laborers from immigrant groups), firefighters, police officers, and construction workers (Schonfeld & Chang, 2017). One study focusing on firefighters found differences in post-traumatic stress disorder (PTSD) prevalence rates among the firefighters from eight European countries (Kehl et al., 2015). In particular, 19.4% of Polish firefighters were at risk of PTSD, followed by 9.4% of U.K. firefighters and 9% of Turkish firefighters. On the other hand, firefighters in the Czech Republic and Spain both had lower than a 3% PTSD prevalence rate, and 0% of the Swedish firefighters were at risk for PTSD. Kehl and colleagues (2015) suggested that some cultures may be higher in masculinity value and encourage the adoption of a "macho" image or "stiff-upper lip," thereby causing distress to be bottled up and postevent growth to be stifled. Indeed, masculinity was higher in Poland and the United Kingdom compared with Spain and Sweden (Hofstede, 2001). Additionally, organizational difficulties, such as poor communication and an administrative burden, may also directly affect postevent distress (Kehl et al., 2015).

One prominent type of occupational injury is work-related musculo-skeletal disorders (WRMSDs). WRMSDs are disorders of the nerves, tendons, muscles, and supporting tissues that result from overexertion or repetitive strain (Cohen et al., 1997). Physical load, which is defined as biomechanical forces occurring in the body resulting from individuals' job tasks, is a primary predictor of WRMSDs (Eatough et al., 2012). Additionally, research has found that work-related psychosocial factors (high psychological job demands, low decision latitude, low social support, and job insecurity) were associated with psychological strain (Karasek, 1979), putting employees at increased risk of stress-related health problems, including WRMSDs (Eatough et al., 2012; Golubovich et al., 2014). Therefore, WRMSDs may come from a combination of physical load and psychosocial stressors, and research has begun to explore whether there are cultural or national differences relating to WRMSDs.

Focusing specifically on migrant workers, H. Lee and colleagues (2011) found that the WRMSD prevalence rates differed among workers from different countries, as Vietnamese female workers reported more WRMSDs than did Thai or Filipino female workers. Interestingly, H. Lee et al. also found that the acculturation strategy of migrant workers, which is defined as how an individual goes about their life during cultural and psychological change (Berry, 2006), was partially associated with increased risk of WRMSDs. Migrant workers with a separation strategy that leans toward maintaining the original culture and rejecting relationships with the host group reported an increased risk of WRMSDs. H. Lee et al. suggested the use of interventions that will encourage migrant workers to interact with host country populations and to participate in joint activities to help curtail WRMSDs among female migrant workers.

A CN study found differences in the prevalence rate of self-reported WRMSD symptoms between Malaysia and Australia (Maakip et al., 2017). Significantly more Malaysian respondents (92.8%) reported MSD discomfort than

Australian respondents (71.2%). Maakip et al. (2017) suggested that one possible reason for this result is that in Australia, significant efforts have been undertaken to mitigate hazards and risks associated with MSDs (Ireland, 1995). Malaysia differs in this regard, as MSDs have only recently been recognized as a work-related problem (L. T. Lee, 2007). Another CN study by Carugno et al. (2012) evaluated the WRMSDs for Brazilian and Italian nurses and found similar prevalence rates. The one exception was that Brazilian nurses reported more shoulder problems, with significant differences for shoulder pain in the past month and shoulder pain causing absence from work in the past year. Carugno et al. found that for both countries, somatizing tendencies appeared to be a relevant risk factor for the WRMSD-related outcomes, particularly multisite pain—pain that occurred in three or more sites within the past month—and sickness absence—when the worker is absent due to pain. *Somatization* refers to the tendency to experience and communicate somatic distress in response to psychosocial stress and to seek medical help for the discomfort (Lipowski, 1988). It may occur when psychological concerns about health are converted into physical symptoms, as it is a defense against the awareness or expression of psychological distress (Katon et al., 1982). Carugno et al. suggested that regardless of country, nurses with a higher tendency to engage in somatization were more likely to experience WRMSDs and sickness absence.

Taken together, accidents, injuries, and WRMSDs appear to be influenced by a combination of cultural values and national differences in public policy. Values such as collectivism, feminism, uncertainty avoidance, and long-term orientation are associated with greater safety and lower accidents or injuries, while values such as masculinity and power distance are associated with lower degrees of safety. However, there are conflicting results regarding the effect of individualism–collectivism on safety. More research is needed on the relationship between the cultural value of individualism–collectivism and occupational safety across industries.

Workplace Mistreatment

Workplace mistreatment is another important occupational health concern to evaluate, as it is a broader construct than stress/WRMSDs. Workplace mistreatment comes in several forms, including physical assault, homicide, verbal abuse, bullying or mobbing, and sexual, racial, and psychological harassment (Chappell & Di Martino, 2006). Lanctôt and Guay (2014) noted that mistreatment directed at employees by customers, clients, patients, students, or others for whom an organization provides services, and mistreatment against coworkers, supervisors, or managers by a present or former employee, are the most common types of workplace violence. Lanctôt and Guay's review also identified seven categories of consequences of workplace mistreatment: (a) physical, (b) psychological, (c) emotional, (d) work functioning, (e) relationship with patients/quality of care, (f) social/general, and (g) financial. Workplace violence rates may also depend on the type of industry, as Piquero and colleagues (2013) found that workers within the health care, education, public safety, retail, and justice industries are more prone to experiencing workplace mistreatment.

Research has suggested CN and CC differences in different forms of workplace mistreatment. For example, Jacobson et al. (2014) focused on assertiveness, ingroup collectivism, and power distance to help explain differences in workplace bullying. *Workplace bullying* is a form of workplace mistreatment characterized by repeated, regular, aggressive, and negative treatment directed at an employee (or several employees) by one or more coworkers and/or superiors in a situation where the target finds it difficult to defend him/herself (Einarsen et al., 2011). Jacobson and colleagues argued that while assertiveness and bullying are not precisely the same, it does follow that more assertive cultures will have more aggression and therefore more bullying. Similarly, organizations located within cultures with higher assertive values are likely to have more aggression and bullying. For example, Sweden had the lowest score of assertiveness (House et al., 2004), and it also had the lower rate of workplace bullying (3.5%) compared with 10% in the United States and 15% in the United Kingdom (Keashly & Jagatic, 2003). However, Jacobson et al. also noted that lower levels of assertiveness may not lead to an absence of bullying, as bullying may manifest in a more covert manner in low-assertiveness cultures (Morita et al., 1999).

There may be differences in workplace violence across individuals from the same country who have different ethnic backgrounds. For example, Sabri and colleagues (2015) found in a U.S. sample that while there were no significant differences between the racial/ethnic groups in frequency of abuse, Black and Asian employees were less likely to be knowledgeable about resources and were more likely to express uncertainty regarding organizational policies and procedures on workplace violence. In addition, among victims of workplace violence, Black and Asian people were almost 51% less likely than White people to use formal resources to address the mistreatment. Workplace violence resource utilization includes the use of formal (e.g., counseling services) and informal resources (e.g., family and friends). Previous research has shown that ethnic minorities and immigrant workers tend to underutilize formal services offered by their work organizations (Sabri et al., 2015). One solution for closing this gap is to establish training programs to develop awareness about violence prevention resources for workers in high-risk occupations.

Bergbom et al. (2015) found that cultural distance from the host country affected the risk of being bullied among immigrant workers in Finland. Immigrants whose culture is the least distant from the Finnish culture, for instance, Estonians and Swedes, were at the lowest risk of being bullied. Compared with native citizens, the risk of being bullied was nearly 3 times higher in the intermediate-distance group of immigrants (i.e., western and southern Europeans), and nearly 8 times higher in the most culturally distant group (i.e., sub-Saharan and northern Africans). The negative act immigrants were primarily subjected to was social exclusion. Bergbom et al. suggested that higher cultural distance between employees may increase the likelihood of communication misunderstandings and conflict, which over time may escalate into bullying.

It is important to note that there may be different reasons for bullying across countries. D'Cruz et al. (2016) found that employees from Australia, Turkey, and India reported that gender-based harassment and racial discrimination were common reasons for workplace bullying. However, religious and regional harassment was noted as a reason for workplace bullying by only Indian employees. D'Cruz et al. suggested that this may be because Indian social identities are hierarchically rather than democratically organized, with strong ingroup and outgroup alignments, thereby restricting tolerance and inclusion. Another key difference between the countries was the prevalence of formal and institutionalized avenues of support in addition to interventions to address workplace bullying. Professional psychological and psychiatric help, grievance mechanisms, and union actions were available in Australia but less so in India and Turkey (D'Cruz et al., 2016). These results indicate that employees in India and Turkey may have to rely more on informal support when facing workplace bullying.

The CN differences in workplace bullying may also be partially due to differences in willingness to report when workplace bullying had actually occurred. For example, Lopes and colleagues (2020) found that U.K. teachers reported significantly more work-related bullying than French teachers. Research supported that in contrast to U.K. teachers, French teachers tend to underreport mental health symptoms (e.g., burnout) and deviant or unethical personal behaviors (Vercambre et al., 2009). These differences may be because there is a social stigma in France concerning the report of personal health problems or issues in the workplace (Angermeyer et al., 2013). Lopes et al. suggested that French teachers may have felt ashamed or uncomfortable to report negative experiences in the workplace, which may result in the underreporting of workplace bullying in France.

The CC/CN differences in prevalence rates of bullying may also be due to the different definitions of workplace bullying. In a sample of employees from 13 counties, Salin et al. (2019) found that participants agreed that physical violence or intimidation and personal harassment in the form of insults, verbal abuse, and jokes constituted workplace bullying. However, participants from different countries differed on how they categorized social exclusion. *Workplace social exclusion* is defined as the perception of an individual that they are being excluded, rejected, or ignored by another individual within the workplace, such that their ability to establish or maintain positive interpersonal relationships is hindered (Pereira et al., 2013). European interviewees considered social exclusion to be a core part of bullying, whereas Asian, African, and U.S. participants were less likely to view exclusion as part of bullying. Additionally, Salin et al. found that participants from countries with lower ingroup collectivism were particularly sensitive to negative behavior toward minority group employees and considered exclusion to be an important issue in workplace bullying. In contrast, participants from Middle Eastern countries saw differences in terms of gender, religion, or country of origin as factors that could make social exclusion acceptable or even desirable. Salin and colleagues argued that high ingroup collectivism may lead to a bigger distinction between ingroups and outgroups (Jacobson et al., 2014), thereby justifying the different treatment or exclusion of outgroup members as part of the cultural norm, rather than workplace bullying.

Last, Power et al. (2013) examined the effects of GLOBE cultural values on the acceptability of workplace bullying among employees from 14 countries. Participants from cultures with a higher performance orientation (e.g., Confucian Asia) reported a greater tolerance for workplace bullying compared with those from cultures with a lower performance orientation (e.g., Latin America, sub-Saharan Africa). In contrast, cultures with higher humane orientation were associated with a greater disapproval of workplace bullying. Likewise, future orientation was related to lower acceptance of workplace bullying. Power et al. suggested that cultures of a higher future orientation may view workplace bullying as a risk to the future success of the organization, as it may potentially result in the turnover of valuable employees. Additionally, regardless of cultural values, physical violence was considered less acceptable than verbal aggression by employees across all countries.

Abusive supervision—the extent to which supervisors engage in the sustained display of hostile verbal and nonverbal behaviors (Tepper, 2000)—is another type of workplace mistreatment. Recent research has suggested CC/CN differences in how subordinates perceive and respond to abusive supervision. For example, Vogel and colleagues (2015) found that compared with the subordinate employees from Western cultures, those from the Confucian Asian culture were more likely to view abusive supervision as acceptable and interpersonally just, and were more likely to trust their supervisor and engage in constructive efforts at work. Vogel et al. suggested that the high power distance[1] orientation in Confucian Asian cultures may legitimize the use of hostility as a form of social control for subordinates. Lian et al. (2012) found similar results that subordinates in higher power distance cultures viewed abusive supervision as more interpersonally fair. However, they also noted that these subordinates were more likely to engage in interpersonal deviance when experiencing highly abusive supervision compared with those in lower power distance cultures. These results may be in part because individuals with a high power distance orientation are more likely to mimic the abusive behaviors displayed by their supervisors, perceiving that they may be rewarded for doing so (Lian et al., 2012).

Outside of workplace bullying and abusive supervision, a few studies have compared CC/CN differences in other forms of workplace mistreatment. For example, Shao and Skarlicki (2014) found differences in how employees

---

[1]High power distance refers to supervisors having a high level of power compared with subordinate employees. Low power distance cultures distribute power more evenly among supervisors and subordinates.

responded to perceived customer aggression and mistreatment. Employees from Canada were more likely to engage in sabotage toward the aggressive customers compared with employees from China. Shao and Skarlicki noted that employees from individualistic and collectivistic countries may use different coping strategies to deal with the workplace stress stemming from mistreatment. Employees from an individualistic culture may prioritize personal interests over group interests and are likely to cope with workplace stress with direct and active strategies, such as sabotaging customers, to express their self-interests. On the other hand, collectivistic employees may be more likely to use indirect and passive coping strategies, such as reduced helping behaviors toward customers, to cope with customer mistreatment. Last, Welbourne et al. (2015) found differences across cultures when reporting workplace incivility, defined as "low-intensity deviant behavior with ambiguous intent to harm the target, in violation of workplace norms for mutual respect" (Andersson & Pearson, 1999, p. 457). Welbourne and colleagues found that although there was no difference between Hispanic and non-Hispanic employees in terms of experienced incivility, the relationships between workplace incivility and job satisfaction and burnout were weaker for Hispanic employees. Welbourne et al. suggested that because Hispanic employees were found to be less individualistic than non-Hispanic employees, they may have greater social resources and support to cope with stress such as workplace incivility, thus mitigating the impact of incivility on work outcomes (Chun et al., 2006).

Taken together, there appear to be CC/CN differences in the prevalence, responses, and perceptions of workplace mistreatment. In general, employees in cultures of higher assertiveness, power distance, individualism, cultural distance, and performance orientation are more likely to experience workplace bullying. In contrast, employees in cultures of higher ingroup collectivism, humane orientation, and future orientation are less likely to experience bullying. Results from multiple studies find that immigrants and individuals from minority groups (e.g., ethnic, religious) may be more likely to experience specific forms of workplace bullying compared with the native or majority population (Bergbom et al., 2015; D'Cruz et al., 2016; Salin et al., 2019). Finally, differences in power distance and individualism–collectivism may explain how employees respond differently to different forms of workplace violence.

CONCLUSION

Perhaps the most reasonable conclusion to be drawn about CC/CN OHP is that differences occur across culture and national boundaries, but these differences have been inconsistent across studies and across the OHP topics. Due to the paucity of systematic comparative research, firm conclusions about why differences occur cannot be drawn. Additionally, although CC research can allow us to make inferences about how cultural values explain the between-group differences observed in various OHP phenomena, most research reviewed in the current chapter adopted the CN design. Thus, we recommend that future researchers incorporate the assessment of cultural values in CN research to provide more insights on how values may explain CC/CN differences in OHP topics. Specifically, a research design that measures individual participants' cultural values (or other cultural variables) in a CN study can offer unique insights about how values and cultures may affect the processes underlying different OHP topics. For example, value assessments may be considered as individual differences unique to the individual participants. It is also possible to aggregate them to the country level to evaluate how CN differences in values, on average, may affect OHP phenomena. Additionally, country-level variations in cultural values may also be estimated to examine their effects. Finally, a limited number of countries have been investigated, as well as a limited number of cultural variables. More systematic studies are needed so we can begin to draw firm conclusions and develop theories to explain the differences in occupational health and safety among people from different cultures and places.

REFERENCES

Andersson, L. M., & Pearson, C. M. (1999). Tit for tat? The spiraling effect of incivility in the workplace. *Academy of Management Review, 24*(3), 452–471. https://doi.org/10.2307/259136

Angermeyer, M. C., Millier, A., Rémuzat, C., Refaï, T., & Toumi, M. (2013). Attitudes and beliefs of the French public about schizophrenia and major depression: Results from a vignette-based population survey. *BMC Psychiatry, 13*(1), 1–12. https://doi.org/10.1186/1471-244X-13-313

Barling, J., & Griffiths, A. (2003). A history of occupational health psychology. In J. C. Quick & L. E. Tetrick (Eds.), *Handbook of occupational health psychology* (pp. 19–31). American Psychological Association.

Batt, R., & Valcour, P. M. (2003). Human resources practices as predictors of work–family outcomes and employee turnover. *Industrial Relations, 42*(2), 189–220. https://doi.org/10.1111/1468-232X.00287

Beham, B., Drobnič, S., & Präg, P. (2013). The work–family interface of service sector workers: A comparison of work resources and professional status across five European countries. *Applied Psychology, 63*(1), 29–61. https://doi.org/10.1111/apps.12012

Bergbom, B., Vartia-Vaananen, M., & Kinnunen, U. (2015). Immigrants and natives at work: Exposure to workplace bullying. *Employee Relations, 37*(2), 158–175. https://doi.org/10.1108/ER-09-2014-0101

Berry, J. W. (2006). Acculturation: A conceptual overview. In M. H. Bornstein & L. R. Cote (Eds.), *Acculturation and parent–child relationships: Measurement and development* (pp. 13–32). Lawrence Erlbaum Associates Publishers. https://psycnet.apa.org/record/2006-02515-002

Billing., T. K., Bhagat, R. S., Babakus, E., Krishnan, B., Ford Jr., D. L., Srivastava, B. N., Rajadhyaksha, U., Shin, M., Kuo, B., Kwantes, C., Setiadi, B., & Nasurdin, A. M. (2014). Work–family conflict and organisationally valued outcomes: The moderating role of decision latitude in five national contexts. *Applied Psychology, 63*(1), 62–95. https://psycnet.apa.org/record/2006-02515-002

Bishop, G. D., Enkelmann, H. C., Tong, E. M., Why, Y. P., Diong, S. M., Ang, J., & Khader, M. (2003). Job demands, decisional control, and cardiovascular responses. *Journal of Occupational Health Psychology, 8*(2), 146–156. https://doi.org/10.1037/1076-8998.8.2.146

Brislin, R. W. (1986). The wording and translation of research instruments. In W. J. Lonner & J. W. Berry (Eds.), *Field methods in cross-cultural research* (pp. 137–164). Sage.

Bureau of Labor Statistics. (2020). *Employer reported workplace injuries and illnesses—2020* [News release]. U.S. Department of Labor. https://www.bls.gov/news.release/pdf/osh.pdf.

Carrola, P. A., Yu, K., Sass, D. A., & Lee, S. M. (2012). Measurement invariance of the Counselor Burnout Inventory across cultures: A comparison of U.S. and Korean counselors. *Measurement & Evaluation in Counseling & Development, 45*(4), 227–244. https://doi.org/10.1177/0748175612447630

Carugno, M., Pesatori, A. C., Ferrario, M. M., Ferrari, A. L., Silva, F. J., Martins, A. C., Felli, V. E., Coggon, D., & Bonzini, M. (2012). Physical and psychosocial risk factors for musculoskeletal disorders in Brazilian and Italian nurses. *Cadernos de Saude Publica, 28*(9), 1632–1642. https://doi.org/10.1590/S0102-311X2012000900003

Chappell, D., & Di Martino, V. (2006). *Violence at work.* International Labour Organization.

Chen, W.-Q., Wong, T.-W., Yu, T.-S., Lin, Y.-Z., & Cooper, C. L. (2003). Determinants of perceived occupational stress among Chinese offshore oil workers. *Work and Stress, 17*(4), 287–305. https://doi.org/10.1080/02678370310001647302

Chun, C., Moos, R. H., & Cronkite, R. C. (2006). Culture: A fundamental context for the stress and coping paradigm. In P. T. P. Wong & L. C. J. Wong (Eds.), *Handbook of multicultural perspectives on stress and coping* (pp. 29–53). Spring Publications. https://doi.org/10.1007/0-387-26238-5_2

Cohen, A. L., Gjessing, C. C., Fine, L. J., Bernard, B. P., & McGlothin, J. D. (1997). *Elements of ergonomics programs: A primer based on workplace evaluations of musculoskeletal disorders* (Publication No. 97–117). US Department of Health and Human Services, Public Health Service, Centers for Disease Control and Prevention, National Institute for Occupational Safety and Health, DHHS (NIOSH).

D'Cruz, P., Paull, M., Omari, M., & Guneri-Cangarli, B. (2016). Target experiences of workplace bullying: Insights from Australia, India and Turkey. *Employee Relations, 38*(5), 805–823. https://doi.org/10.1108/ER-06-2015-0116

Das, T. K., & Kumar, R. (2010). Interpartner sensemaking in strategic alliances: Managing cultural differences and internal tensions. *Management Decision, 48*(1), 17–36. https://doi.org/10.1108/00251741011014436

Eatough, E. M., Way, J. D., & Chang, C.-H. (2012). Understanding the link between psychosocial work stressors and work-related musculoskeletal complaints. *Applied Ergonomics, 43*(3), 554–563. https://doi.org/10.1016/j.apergo.2011.08.009

Einarsen, S., Hoel, H., Zapf, D., & Cooper, C. L. (2011). The concept of bullying and harassment at work: The european tradition. In S. Einarsen, H. Hoel, D. Zapf, & C. L. Cooper (Eds.), *Bullying and harassment in the workplace: Developments in theory, research, and practice* (2nd Ed., pp. 3–39). CRC Press.

European Commission, Directorate-General for Employment & Social Affairs, Unit EMPL/D. (2001). *European Statistics on Accidents at Work (ESAW): Methodology.* Office for Official Publications of the European Communities.

Fisher, D. M. (2014). A multilevel cross-cultural examination of role overload and organizational commitment: Investigating the interactive effects of context. *Journal of Applied Psychology, 99*(4), 723–736. https://doi.org/10.1037/a0035861

Galovan, A. M., Fackrell, T., Buswell, L., Jones, B. L., Hill, E. J., & Carroll, S. J. (2010). The work–family interface in the United States and Singapore: Conflict across cultures. *Journal of Family Psychology, 24*(5), 646–656. https://doi.org/10.1037/a0020832

García-Arroyo, J. A., & Segovia, A. O. (2020). Occupational accidents in immigrant workers in Spain: The complex role of culture. *Safety Science, 121*, 507–515. https://doi.org/10.1016/j.ssci.2019.09.027

Gelfand, M. J., Nishii, L. H., & Raver, J. L. (2006). On the nature and importance of cultural tightness-looseness. *Journal of Applied Psychology, 91*(6), 1225–1244. https://doi.org/10.1037/0021-9010.91.6.1225

Glazer, S., & Amren, M. (2018). Culture's implications on support as a moderator of the job stressor–outcome relationship. *International Journal of Stress Management, 25*, 7–25. https://doi.org/10.1037/str0000087

Golubovich, J., Chang, C. H., & Eatough, E. M. (2014). Safety climate, hardiness, and musculoskeletal complaints: A mediated moderation model. *Applied Ergonomics, 45*(3), 757–766. https://doi.org/10.1016/j.apergo.2013.10.008

Greenhaus, J. H., & Allen, T. D. (2011). Work–family balance: A review and extension of the literature. In J. C. Quick & L. E. Tetrick (Eds.), *Handbook of occupational health psychology* (2nd ed., pp. 165–183). American Psychological Association.

Hofstede, G. (2001). *Culture's consequences: Comparing values, behaviors, institutions and organizations across nations.* Sage Publications.

House, R. J., Hanges, P. J., Javidan, M., Dorfman, P. W., & Gupta, V. (Eds.). (2004). *Culture, leadership, and organizations: The GLOBE study of 62 societies.* Sage.

Ireland, D. C. (1995). Repetition strain injury: The Australian experience—1992 update. *The Journal of Hand Surgery, 20*(3), S53–S56. https://doi.org/10.1016/S0363-5023(95)80170-7

Jacobson, K. J., Hood, J. N., & Van Buren, H. J., III. (2014). Workplace bullying across cultures: A research agenda. *International Journal of Cross Cultural Management, 14*(1), 47–65. https://doi.org/10.1177/1470595813494192

Jex, S. M. (1998). *Stress and job performance: Theory, research, and implications for managerial practice.* Sage.

Karasek, R. (1979). Job demands, job decision latitude and mental strain: Implication for job redesign. *Administrative Science Quarterly, 24*(2), 285–308. https://doi.org/10.2307/2392498

Katon, W., Kleinman, A., & Rosen, G. (1982). Depression and somatization: A review. Part I. *The American Journal of Medicine, 72*(1), 127–135. https://doi.org/10.1016/0002-9343(82)90599-X

Keashly, L., & Jagatic, K. (2003). By any other name: American perspectives on workplace bullying. In S. Einarsen, H. Hoel, D. Zapf, & C. Cooper (Eds.), *Bullying and emotional abuse in the workplace: International perspectives in research and practice* (pp. 31–61). Taylor & Francis.

Kehl, D., Knuth, D., Hulse, L., Schmidt, S., & the BeSeCu-Group. (2015). Predictors of postevent distress and growth among firefighters after work-related emergencies—A cross-national study. *Psychological trauma: Theory, research, practice, and policy, 7*(3), 203–211. https://doi.org/10.1037/a0037954

Kulkarni, S. P., Hudson, T., Ramamoorthy, N., Marchev, A., Georgieva-Kondakova, P., & Gorskov, V. (2010). Dimensions of individualism-collectivism: A comparative study of five cultures. *Current Issues of Business and Law, 5*, 93–109. https://citeseerx.ist.psu.edu/viewdoc/download?doi=10.1.1.613.4362&rep=rep1&type=pdf

Lanctôt, N., & Guay, S. (2014). The aftermath of workplace violence among healthcare workers: A systematic literature review of the consequences. *Aggression and Violent Behavior, 19*(5), 492–501. https://doi.org/10.1016/j.avb.2014.07.010

Lazarus, R. S. (1991). Psychological stress in the workplace. *Journal of Social Behavior and Personality, 6*, 1–13.

Lee, H., Ahn, H., Park, C. G., Kim, S. J., & Moon, S. H. (2011). Psychosocial factors and work-related musculoskeletal disorders among Southeastern Asian female workers living in Korea. *Safety and Health at Work, 2*(2), 183–193. https://doi.org/10.5491/SHAW.2011.2.2.183

Lee, L. T. (2007, 1 Nov.). *Opening address of chairman, NIOSH* [Conference proceedings]. Agriculture Ergonomics Development Conference. Kuala Lumpur, Malaysia.

Lee, S. M., Baker, C. R., Cho, S. H., Heckathorn, D. E., Holland, M. W., Newgent, R. A., Ogle, N. T., Powell, M. L., Quinn, J. J., Wallace, S. L., & Yu, K. (2007). Development and initial psychometrics of the Counselor Burnout Inventory. *Measurement and Evaluation in Counseling and Development, 40*(3), 142–154. https://doi.org/10.1080/0 7481756.2007.11909811

Levi, L. (1990). Occupational stress. Spice of life or kiss of death? *American Psychologist, 45*(10), 1142–1145. https://doi.org/10.1037/0003-066X.45.10.1142

Lian, H., Ferris, D. L., & Brown, D. J. (2012). Does power distance exacerbate or mitigate the effects of abusive supervision? It depends on the outcome. *Journal of Applied Psychology, 97*(1), 107–123. https://doi.org/10.1037/a0024610

Liao, M. (2015). Safety culture in commercial aviation: Differences in perspective between Chinese and Western pilots. *Safety Science, 79*, 193–205. https://doi.org/ 10.1016/j.ssci.2015.05.011

Lipowski, Z. J. (1988). Somatization: The concept and its clinical application. *The American Journal of Psychiatry, 145*(11), 1358–1368. https://doi.org/10.1176/ajp.145.11.1358

Liu, C., Spector, P. E., & Shi, L. (2007). Cross-national job stress: A quantitative and qualitative study. *Journal of Organizational Behavior, 28*(2), 209–239. https://doi.org/ 10.1002/job.435

Lopes, B. C. D. S., Bortolon, C., Macioce, V., & Raffard, S. (2020). The positive relationships between paranoia, perceptions of workplace bullying, and intentions of workplace deviance in United Kingdom and French teachers: Cross-cultural aspects. *Frontiers in Psychiatry, 11*, 14–27. https://doi.org/10.3389/fpsyt.2020.00203

Lu, C., Siu, O., & Cooper, C. L. (2005). Managers' occupational stress in China: The role of self-efficacy. *Personality and Individual Differences, 38*(3), 569–578. https://doi.org/ 10.1016/j.paid.2004.05.012

Maakip, I., Keegel, T., & Oakman, J. (2017). Predictors of musculoskeletal discomfort: A cross-cultural comparison between Malaysian and Australian office workers. *Applied Ergonomics, 60*, 52–57. https://doi.org/10.1016/j.apergo.2016.11.004

Mohamed, S., Ali, T. H., & Tam, W. Y. V. (2009). National culture and safe work behaviour of construction workers in Pakistan. *Safety Science, 47*(1), 29–35. https:// doi.org/10.1016/j.ssci.2008.01.003

Morillas, R. M., Rubio-Romero, J. C., & Fuertes, A. (2013). A comparative analysis of occupational health and safety risk prevention practices in Sweden and Spain. *Journal of Safety Research, 47*, 57–65. https://doi.org/10.1016/j.jsr.2013.08.005

Morita, Y., Soeda, H., Soeda, K., & Taki, M. (1999). Japan. In P. K. Smith, Y. Morita, J. Junger-Tas, D. Olweus, R. Catalano, & P. Slee (Eds.), *The nature of school bullying: A cross-national perspective* (pp. 309–323). Routledge.

O'Brien, K. M., Ganginis Del Pino, H. V., Yoo, S. K., Cinamon, R. G., & Han, Y. J. (2014). Work, family, support, and depression: Employed mothers in Israel, Korea, and the United States. *Journal of Counseling Psychology, 61*(3), 461–472. https://doi.org/ 10.1037/a0036339

Ollier-Malaterre, A., Haar, J. M., Sunyer, A., & Russo, M. (2020). Supportive organizations, work–family enrichment, and job burnout in low and high humane orientation cultures. *Applied Psychology, 69*(4), 1215–1247. https://doi.org/10.1111/apps.12217

Ollo-López, A., & Goñi-Legaz, S. (2017). Differences in work–family conflict: Which individual and national factors explain them? *The International Journal of Human Resource Management, 28*(3), 499–525. https://doi.org/10.1080/09585192.2015.1118141

Pereira, D., Meier, L. L., & Elfering, A. (2013). Short-term effects of social exclusion at work and worries on sleep. *Stress and Health, 29*(3), 240–252. https://doi.org/10.1002/ smi.2461

Piquero, N. L., Piquero, A. R., Craig, J. M., & Clipper, S. J. (2013). Assessing research on workplace violence, 2000–2012. *Aggression and Violent Behavior, 18*(3), 383–394. https://doi.org/10.1016/j.avb.2013.03.001

Power, J. L., Brotheridge, C. M., Blenkinsopp, J., Bowes-Sperry, L., Bozionelos, N., Buzády, Z., Chuang, A., Drenvich, D., Garzon-Vico, A., Leighton, C., Madero, S. M., Mak, W., Matthew, R., Monserrat, S. I., Mujtaba, B. G., Olivas-Lujan, M. R., Polycroniou, P., Sprigg, C. A., Axtell, C. . . . Nnedumm, A. U. O. (2013). Acceptability of workplace bullying: A comparative study on six continents. *Journal of Business Research, 66*(3), 374–380. https://doi.org/10.1016/j.jbusres.2011.08.018

Puig, A., Yoon, E., Callueng, C., An, S., & Lee, S. M. (2014). Burnout syndrome in psychotherapists: A comparative analysis of five nations. *Psychological Services, 11*(1), 87–96. https://doi.org/10.1037/a0035285

Redding, S. G. (1993). *The spirit of Chinese capitalism.* De Gruyter.

Reniers, G., & Gidron, Y. (2013). Do cultural dimensions predict prevalence of fatal work injuries in Europe? *Safety Science, 58,* 76–80. https://doi.org/10.1016/j.ssci.2013.03.015

Rybowiak, V., Garst, H., Frese, M., & Batinic, B. (1999). Error orientation questionnaire (EOQ): Reliability, validity, and different language equivalence. *Journal of Organizational Behavior, 20*(4), 527–547. https://doi.org/10.1002/(SICI)1099-1379 (199907)20:4<527::AID-JOB886>3.0.CO;2-G

Sabri, B., St. Vil, N. M., Campbell, J. C., Fitzgerald, S., Kub, J., & Agnew, J. (2015). Racial and ethnic differences in factors related to workplace violence victimization. *Western Journal of Nursing Research, 37*(2), 180–196. https://doi.org/10.1177/0193945914527177

Salin, D., Cowan, R., Adewumi, O., Apospori, E., Bochantin, J., D'Cruz, P., Djurkovic, N., Durniat, K., Escartín, J., Guo, J., Išik, I., Koeszegi, S. T., McCormack, D., Monserrat, S. I., & Zedlacher, E. (2019). Workplace bullying across the globe: A cross-cultural comparison. *Personnel Review, 48*(1), 204–219. https://doi.org/10.1108/PR-03-2017-0092

Sanchez-Burks, J., & Lee, F. (2007). Cultural psychology of workways. In S. Kitayama & D. Cohen (Eds.), *Handbook of cultural psychology* (pp. 346–369). Guilford Press.

Schonfeld, I. S., & Chang, C.-H. (2017). *Occupational health psychology: Work, stress, and health.* Springer Publishing Company.

Shao, R., & Skarlicki, D. P. (2014). Service employees' reactions to mistreatment by customers: A comparison between North America and East Asia. *Personnel Psychology, 67*(1), 23–59. https://doi.org/10.1111/peps.12021

Shin, H., Yuen, M., Lee, J., & Lee, S. M. (2013). Cross-cultural validation of the Counselor Burnout Inventory in Hong Kong. *Journal of Employment Counseling, 50*(1), 14–25. https://doi.org/10.1002/j.2161-1920.2013.00021.x

Sohn, S. Y. (2005). Labor experiences and dilemma of highly-educated professional women in Korea. *Korean Journal of Women's Studies, 21*(3), 67–97.

Spector, P. E. (1992). A consideration of the validity and meaning of self-report measures of job conditions. In C. L. Cooper & I. T. Robertson (eds.) *International Review of Industrial and Organizational Psychology: 1992* (pp. 123–151). John Wiley.

Spector, P. E. (in press). Occupational stress in the global world. In M. J. Gelfand & M. Erez (Eds.), *The Oxford handbook of culture and organizations.* Oxford University Press.

Spector, P. E., Liu, C., & Sanchez, J. I. (2015). Methodological and substantive issues in conducting multinational and cross-cultural research. *Annual Review of Organizational Psychology and Organizational Behavior, 2*(1), 101–131. https://doi.org/10.1146/annurev-orgpsych-032414-111310

Stock, R. M., Strecker, M. M., & Bieling, G. I. (2016). Organizational work–family support as universal remedy? A cross-cultural comparison of China, India and the USA. *International Journal of Human Resource Management, 27*(11), 1192–1216. https://doi.org/10.1080/09585192.2015.1062039

Tepper, B. J. (2000). Consequences of abusive supervision. *Academy of Management Journal, 43* (2), 178–190. https://www.researchgate.net/publication/228079372_Consequences_of_Abusive_Supervision

Tsui, A. S., Nifadkar, S. S., Ou, A. Y., & the Amy Yi Ou. (2007). Cross-national, cross-cultural organizational behavior research: Advances, gaps, and recommendations. *Journal of Management, 33*(3), 426–478. https://doi.org/10.1177/0149206307300818

Vercambre, M. N., Brosselin, P., Gilbert, F., Nerrière, E., & Kovess-Masféty, V. (2009). Individual and contextual covariates of burnout: A cross-sectional nationwide study of French teachers. *BMC Public Health, 9*(1), 1–12. https://doi.org/10.1186/1471-2458-9-333

Vogel, R. M., Mitchell, M. S., Tepper, B. J., Restubog, S. L., Hu, C., Hua, W., & Huang, J. C. (2015). A cross-cultural examination of subordinates' perceptions of and reactions to abusive supervision. *Journal of Organizational Behavior, 36*(5), 720–745. https://doi.org/10.1002/job.1984

Welbourne, J. L., Gangadharan, A., & Sariol, A. M. (2015). Ethnicity and cultural values as predictors of the occurrence and impact of experienced workplace incivility. *Journal of Occupational Health Psychology, 20*(2), 205–217. https://doi.org/10.1037/a0038277

Yang, L.-Q., Spector, P. E., Sanchez, J. I., Allen, T. D., Poelmans, S., Coopers, C. L., Lapierre, L. M., O'Driscoll, M. P., Abarca, N., Alexandrova, M., Antoniou, A.-S., Beham, B., Brough, P., Çarikçi, I., Ferreiro, P., Fraile, G., Geurts, S., Kinnunen, U., Lu, C., & Lu, L. (2012). Individualism–collectivism as a moderator of the work demands–strains relationship: A cross-level and cross-national examination. *Journal of International Business Studies, 43*(4), 424–443. https://doi.org/10.1057/jibs.2011.58

Zotzmann, Y., van der Linden, D., & Wyrwa, K. (2019). The relation between country differences, cultural values, personality dimensions, and error orientation: An approach across three continents—Asia, Europe, and North America. *Safety Science, 120*, 185–193. https://doi.org/10.1016/j.ssci.2019.06.013

CAUSES AND RISKS

INTRODUCTION: CAUSES AND RISKS

From a public health protection and prevention perspective, causes and health risks are the primary agents of concern. These health risk factors cause diseases and disorders, and manifest symptoms. Part III of this handbook contains a set of six chapters that focus on a range of health risk factors that cause ill health, injury, and in the worst case, premature death. Public health's preferred point of intervention is always primary prevention, which aims to identify, isolate, remove, and/or ameliorate these causes and health risks to preclude symptomatic responses, diseases, and disorders. Although not an exhaustive coverage of occupational health risks, these six chapters provide significant coverage of structural causes and risk factors.

Chapter 9 examines the linkages between organizational climate and occupational health. The authors note that past emphasis has been on identifying toxic and noxious dimensions of an organization's environment, whereas recent consideration has been given to positive characteristics of safe and healthy work environments. They explore best practices for examining an organization's work environment and climate. Chapter 10 covers non-standard work schedules with a comprehensive examination of the impact of shift work on occupational health. In addition to shift work, the chapter includes consideration of flextime and teleworking, each of which may be considered nonstandard work arrangements. Chapter 11, which describes nonstandard work arrangements, can be considered a companion to Chapter 10. This chapter examines the implications of gig work arrangements on the occupational health of the workers and the organizations they inhabit. Chapter 12 focuses on a vitally important emergent issue in occupational health psychology: sleep and fatigue. The primary consideration in the chapter is how employee sleep behavior at home impacts occupational health and performance in the work environment. Although there are work and non-work boundaries at play here, what happens in the work environment is of legitimate concern to the organization. Chapter 13 takes a broad and robust view of justice, beyond organizational justice, as a component of occupational health. Examining both evolutionary and philosophical background issues, Chapter 13 discusses how individuals' health and well-being improves with fair and just treatment for all concerned. Chapter 14 addresses the important issue of mistreatment in organizations. In this chapter the principal goals are, first, to assess the current state of evidence on the impact of mistreatment on occupational health, and, second, to chart out the direction of OHP in this important interpersonal domain.

Organizational Climate and Occupational Health

Mark G. Ehrhart and Maribeth Kuenzi

To best understand key individual-level outcomes in occupational health psychology (OHP), such as health, safety, well-being, and stress, it is critical to address the organizational environment in which those individuals work. Traditionally, OHP has focused on the elimination of risks to employees' health and safety (Di Fabio, 2017). However, more recently, researchers have started looking at how to promote positive experiences in the workplace through the development of safe and healthy work environments (Tamers et al., 2019). Indeed, researchers suggest that a healthy organization cannot focus only on profits but also must promote a healthy environment for the well-being of its workers (Grawitch & Ballard, 2016). One of the most common ways that the organizational environment has been conceptualized and studied is in terms of *organizational climate*, or the "shared meaning organizational members attach to the events, policies, practices, and procedures they experience and the behaviors they see being rewarded, supported, and expected" (Ehrhart et al., 2014, p. 69). Organizational climate has over a 40-year history in OHP, going back to Zohar's (1980) introduction of the concept of safety climate. Recent years have seen an application to a broader array of OHP topics, including sexual harassment, mistreatment, stress, and health.

This chapter has four major goals. The first is to provide some brief history and background on the concept of organizational climate. The second is to provide a focused review of how organizational climate has been studied within the field of OHP. The third goal is to give an overview of best practices in research on

https://doi.org/10.1037/0000331-009
Handbook of Occupational Health Psychology, Third Edition, L. E. Tetrick, G. G. Fisher, M. T. Ford, and J. C. Quick (Editors)

climate as a resource for OHP scholars. Finally, the fourth goal is to identify ideas for future research on OHP that integrates organizational climate.

ORGANIZATIONAL CLIMATE: A BRIEF OVERVIEW

A full history of the concept of organizational climate can be found in Ehrhart et al. (2014); for the purposes of this chapter, we provide a brief overview to help frame the development of the construct and explain why it is approached the way it is today. Research on organizational climate began in earnest in the late 1960s. Psychologists who had tended to focus on individual-level phenomena were gaining interest in the influence of the work environment, which raised the question of how to define and measure that environment. In response, research on organizational climate was born. The following decade could be characterized by a burst of research on the topic followed by a series of criticisms (e.g., Guion, 1973) and subsequent clarifications about what climate was and how it should best be studied (e.g., Schneider, 1975). Some core questions were whether climate should be studied at the individual or unit level, whether it was different from job attitudes, and whether climate should capture the entirety of the work environment versus those elements most relevant to a particular outcome of interest. Many researchers (most notably, Schneider, 1975) advocated that climate should capture employees' descriptions of their work environment (vs. their attitudes or evaluations), should be focused on those elements most relevant for a particular outcome (vs. a more general or molar approach), and should be defined as a unit-level concept (rather than an individual-level one). However, there has not been uniformity within research on climate (e.g., Jones & James, 1979), such as studies that approach climate more from an individual approach (i.e., psychological climate) or attempt to capture the overall work environment (i.e., molar climate).

After a relatively stagnant period from the mid-1980s through the mid-1990s, climate research saw a rise in interest starting in the late 1990s that continues to this day. The focused or facet-specific approach to climate has proliferated, with a wide variety of climates being studied throughout the organizational research literature. The most commonly studied are safety climate and service climate, which have the deepest roots going back to the research by Zohar (1980) on safety climate and Schneider and colleagues (1980) on service climate. Also commonly studied are climates for justice (Colquitt et al., 2002), diversity (Holmes et al., 2021), ethics (Kuenzi et al., 2020), and innovation (Anderson & West, 1998). Early climate research tended to focus on the relationship between climate and organizational outcomes, such as customer perceptions of service quality for service climate or injury rates for safety climate. Over time, climate has been studied in a wider variety of ways, such as the extent to which climate mediates the effects of other organizational variables, like leadership, on outcomes, or what other variables mediate climate's effects (e.g., Barling et al., 2002; Schneider et al., 2005). Climate has been examined as a moderator of both individual-level and unit-level relationships, demonstrating how the predictors of work outcomes vary depending on the unit climate (e.g., McKay et al., 2008). Moderators of climate have been another focus, demonstrating the boundary conditions for when climate is likely to have more or less of an influence on outcomes (Dietz et al., 2004; Hofmann & Mark, 2006). One such moderator has been climate strength, or the extent to which there is agreement among unit members about the climate. Although such research has tended to focus on climate strength's moderating influence (e.g., Schneider et al., 2002), it has also been studied as a variable of interest in its own right (e.g., Colquitt et al., 2002). As more and more focused climates have been studied, researchers have begun to examine how multiple climates operate and interact with each other (e.g., McKay et al., 2011; Williams et al., 2018) and how they operate simultaneously across organizational levels (Zohar & Luria, 2005). Finally, researchers have developed and tested interventions to improve climate and its outcomes, especially within the realm of safety climate (e.g., Zohar & Polachek, 2014).

ORGANIZATIONAL CLIMATE IN OCCUPATIONAL HEALTH PSYCHOLOGY

To better understand how organizational climate has been studied in the domain of occupational health psychology, we conducted a focused review of research published in the *Journal of Occupational Health Psychology (JOHP)* over the past 20 years. Our goal was not to provide an exhaustive review of the study of climate in OHP, but rather to sample from that literature to provide a flavor of what has been done up to this point. The result of this process was 34 articles (including 30 empirical articles and four reviews or meta-analyses) that directly addressed climate in *JOHP* between the years of 2001 and 2020. Of the 34 studies within the 30 primary research articles (because some articles included multiple studies), most studies ($n = 25$) measured climate at the individual level (i.e., psychological climate). The majority of the articles we reviewed (32 out of 34) fell into the focused climate category. Of those, we identified three general categories for the types of climates covered: safety climates, mistreatment climates, and health-related climates. In the following sections, we highlight some of the representative articles from our review from each of these three categories, in addition to providing a brief overview of the larger literature on these climates to give a sense of the overall state of research in these areas. We follow with a description of the research on molar climates and some general conclusions that can be drawn from our review.

Safety Climate

Not surprisingly, one of the most widely studied focused climates in our review of *JOHP* was safety climate, with nine total articles. These articles include a review of safety climate and culture published in the *JOHP* 20th anniversary issue (Casey et al., 2017), a systematic review of the safety climate intervention literature (Lee et al., 2019), and an early meta-analysis on safety climate and safety performance by Clarke (2006). All six of the empirical articles examined safety climate at the individual level of analysis; one highly cited representative article was by Kelloway et al. (2006), who showed that individual-level safety climate perceptions mediated the relationship between the effects of leadership perceptions on safety events and outcomes.

There is an over 40-year history of research on safety climate, starting with the original work by Zohar (1980), that has made it a central topic in the field of OHP. Space does not allow for a detailed review of the safety climate literature, although a number of reviews have been published, including in past editions of this handbook (e.g., Zohar, 2011) and elsewhere (Griffin & Curcuruto, 2016; Zohar 2010, 2014). Examples of highly cited safety climate research include articles by Zohar (2000) showing the relationship between group-level safety climate and microaccidents; by Zohar (2002) demonstrating the mediating role of safety climate between leadership and injury rate; by Hofmann et al. (2003) featuring safety climate as a cross-level moderator of the relationship between leader-member exchange and safety citizenship role definitions; by Griffin and Neal (2000) highlighting manager values, safety communication, safety practices, safety training, and safety equipment as dimensions of safety climate as well as outlining safety knowledge, safety motivation, and two forms of safety behavior, safety compliance and safety participation, as intermediary outcomes of safety climate; and by Zohar and Luria (2005) highlighting the multilevel effects of climate, including the role of climate strength or variability. These articles only scratch the surface of safety climate research, and as a result, numerous meta-analyses have been published that address the antecedents and outcomes of safety climate (e.g., Beus et al., 2010; Christian et al., 2009; Clarke, 2006, 2010; He et al., 2019; Jiang et al., 2019). Overall, these meta-analyses show that safety climate is consistently one of the strongest predictors of safety behavior and injuries in organizations.

Mistreatment Climates

Mistreatment climates were also a frequent topic in *JOHP*, with nine total articles. We included a few focused climates under this general category, including climates related to sexual harassment (four articles), incivility and mistreatment (two articles), racial/ethnic harassment (one article), violence prevention (one article), and discrimination across a variety of domains (one article). Examining the literature on mistreatment climates outside of our review of the last 20 years of *JOHP*, it is clear that although the history of research in this area is not as extensive as research on safety or service climate, the field of OHP has propelled research on mistreatment climates forward over the past 15 to 20 years. Perhaps the most research related to mistreatment climate has been conducted on climate for sexual harassment, sometimes discussed in terms of organizational tolerance for sexual harassment (e.g., Fitzgerald et al., 1997). Early work on the organizational antecedents of sexual harassment focused on the role of climate (e.g., Hulin et al., 1996), and meta-analytic work has identified climate as an important antecedent of sexual harassment experiences (Willness et al., 2007). There has been less research on an organization's tolerance of racial discrimination and harassment (Bergman et al., 2012) because this literature tends to focus on the role of the climate for diversity or inclusion (see the recent meta-analysis by Holmes et al., 2021). The literature on violence prevention climate has grown over the last decade (e.g., C. H. Chang et al., 2012; Yang & Caughlin. 2017), especially within the nursing literature (e.g., Y. P. Chang et al., 2018). Interest in incivility has grown dramatically in recent years, with over 89 empirical articles included in a recent meta-analysis on the topic (Yao et al., 2022). The role of organizational antecedents has been a major part of that growing literature, and a distinction has been made between a climate for incivility that addresses management policies and procedures related to incivility (e.g., Gallus et al., 2014) and a norm for incivility that addresses coworker views and performance of incivility within the work unit (e.g., Walsh et al., 2012), although these are sometimes merged together (e.g., Yao et al., 2022). Overall, there is a clear, growing trend of interest within OHP and related fields in the influence of organizational climate for a variety of types of worker mistreatment.

Health-Related Climates

Seven studies in our review were related to the health of employees and the organizations, almost all of which were published since 2013, reflecting the relatively recent growth in applying the climate construct to the topic of health. Four of the seven articles focused specifically on *psychosocial safety climate* (PSC), which Dollard and Baker (2010) defined as "policies, practices, and procedures for the protection of worker psychological health and safety" (p. 580). Although the definition mentions both health and safety, only three of the items on the scale most commonly used to measure PSC (the PSC-12; Hall et al., 2010) mention safety, with the rest focusing on psychological health. Research on PSC has shown that in a 3-month lag study, emotional demands mediated the relationship between unit-level PSC and emotional exhaustion, but not depression (Idris et al., 2014), and although PSC level was a better predictor than PSC strength on a variety of OHP-related outcomes, PSC level and strength interacted to predict employee engagement (Afsharian et al., 2018).

Outside of research on PSC, researchers have investigated a wide variety of health-related organizational climates, going back to early research by Ribisl and Reischl (1993) and including research on the general health climates in organizations (Zweber et al., 2016) and much more specific health-related climates, such as the climate for healthy weight maintenance (Sliter, 2013). A recent systematic review of research on climate and health outcomes showed that a variety of climates have been tied to health, including safety climate, service climate, team climate, and molar climate (Loh et al., 2019). As we highlight later in this chapter, more research is needed to understand how these other climates relate to health-specific climates in predicting employees' health outcomes.

Molar Climates

Two papers in our review examined climate as a broader or more generic concept than the other more focused climates. As an example, in their study of nurses, von Treuer et al. (2014) used a work environment measure capturing 10 molar climate dimensions, such as cohesion, supervisor support, autonomy, work pressure, and role clarity. Although studying focused climates is the more dominant approach in contemporary organizational research, some of the earliest research on climate took a molar climate approach (e.g., Litwin & Stringer, 1968), and molar climate research has continued (e.g., Patterson et al., 2005). The challenge with molar climate is that it is very broad and tends to subsume a wide variety of discrete organizational constructs that have their own literatures and unique effects (e.g., cohesion, participation in decision-making, role clarity, stress). As a result, theorizing about molar climate is difficult, as there are likely specific reasons for the individual molar climate dimensions to be linked to health, safety, and well-being outcomes. One approach is to consider organizational profiles of the molar climate dimensions to better distinguish how organizations differ in their pattern of scores across the molar climate dimensions (Schulte et al., 2009). Another option is to consider how molar climate may form a foundation for focused climates (see examples for service climate by Schneider et al., 1998, or for implementation climate by Williams et al., 2018).

Summary and Key Takeaways

Several insights can be gathered from our review. The focus on climates related to safety, mistreatment, and health is not surprising, as these broadly capture the organizational environment issues most closely linked to the health and well-being outcomes that are important to the OHP literature. That being said, we also found a variety of other climates that have been shown to be relevant for OHP-related outcomes, even if the content of the climate was not as directly related to those outcomes (e.g., research on service climate and employee well-being by Drach-Zahavy, 2010, or research on job insecurity climate and safety outcomes by Jiang & Probst, 2016). This research parallels the rise of interest in focused climates in the general organizational research literature (Ehrhart et al., 2014; Kuenzi & Schminke, 2009). We also saw a wide variety of approaches to studying climate; although initial research on individual focused climates has tended to address their relationship with outcomes, the expansion of research to consider more complex mediating, moderating, and cross-level or multilevel relationships has tended to occur as research areas have matured, such as with safety and service climate. We also saw a wide variety of approaches to measuring climate, potential overlap with other unit-level constructs (e.g., norms), and a relative shortage of research on climate at the group or organizational level. We return to these issues shortly as we consider best practices and future directions for climate research in OHP.

BEST PRACTICES FOR STUDYING ORGANIZATIONAL CLIMATE

Numerous reviews of the climate literature provide a great starting point for researchers who are new to studying climate, as these reviews cover many of the debates and best practices in the climate literature (Ehrhart et al., 2014; Kuenzi & Schminke, 2009; Ostroff et al., 2012; Schneider et al., 2013; Zohar & Hofmann, 2012). However, because much of the climate literature is housed in the specific research domain where it is studied (e.g., safety, service, justice, innovation, diversity), there can be some inconsistencies in the conceptualization and measurement of climate. As a resource for OHP researchers considering climate research, we summarize some of the most important best practices for conducting research in this area.

One critical issue when conducting climate research is to align the level of theory with the level of analysis. Too often, researchers theorize about organizational climate but then measure psychological climate and test models at the individual level. Doing so is an example of the atomistic fallacy (Diez-Roux, 1998), which occurs when researchers use the results from individual-level studies to reach conclusions about higher level units of analysis, such as groups or organizations. Using the safety climate literature as an example, meta-analyses reveal that research on safety climate at the unit level is outnumbered by safety climate at the individual level by roughly a 3-to-1 margin or more (see Beus et al., 2010; Christian et al., 2009; Clarke, 2006). Given that climate is usually conceptualized as a unit-level construct (Ehrhart et al., 2014), the potential prevalence of the atomistic fallacy is concerning. However, even when researchers are careful to ensure their conclusions are focused on the individual level, research on psychological climate can still be subject to another fallacy, what has sometimes been referred to as the psychologistic fallacy (Diez-Roux, 1998). This fallacy occurs when relevant unit-level factors are ignored in favor of individual-level factors when predicting individual outcomes. In most cases, studies of psychological climate do not also include climate at the unit level, and thus it is unclear whether the results for psychological climate actually reflect cross-level effects of unit-level climate. These issues are not just statistical; they have critical implications for the practical application of the research. For instance, if the effects of climate are largely due to unit-level climate, then the focus of any change efforts will likely be on leaders and the policies, practices, and procedures they put into place. However, if the effects are due to psychological climate, independent from unit-level climate, then that is essentially a within-group effect, meaning that individuals are experiencing the policies, practices, and procedures within the group differently, and thus the focus would shift to why that is the case. In summary, these levels of analysis issues are critical, and researchers should address them starting with theoretical development, throughout the design and analysis stages, and finally in the conclusions reached based on the research (see Klein & Kozlowski, 2000, for a thorough discussion of these issues). Ideally, we would see more OHP research conducted on climate at the unit level, and research on individual-level outcomes would include climate at both the individual and unit levels to best understand the unique effects of climate at different levels.

This brings us to a second issue: consensus surrounding climate perceptions. When studying unit-level climate, it is important to demonstrate that perceptions are shared among unit or organizational members before data are aggregated. Typically, researchers justify aggregation using indicators of interrater agreement and interrater reliability. Interrater agreement examines the extent to which raters provide the same value for each item being rated (LeBreton & Senter, 2008). Interrater agreement can be measured in a variety of ways, with the most common likely being $r_{WG(j)}$ (James et al., 1984). Although most researchers have used .70 or higher as the accepted standard, this cutoff is arbitrary, resulting in some researchers recommending a continuum of levels of agreement (LeBreton & Senter, 2008). Interrater reliability examines the extent to which the rank ordering of the ratings is consistent across the people in the unit. Typically, intraclass correlations (ICCs) have been used to evaluate interrater reliability, although technically these indicators capture information about both interrater agreement and reliability (LeBreton & Senter, 2008). ICC(1) is the ratio of between unit variance to total variance (Bliese, 2000). There is no specific cutoff used for ICC(1); LeBreton and Senter (2008) suggested values of .01 as a small effect, .10 as a medium effect, and .25 as a large effect. A second intraclass correlation, ICC(2) or ICC(K), is an index of reliability of group means (Bliese, 2000; LeBreton & Senter, 2008). ICC(2) values are evaluated similarly to traditional reliability ratings, with values of .70 or higher viewed as acceptable. ICC(2) values are heavily influenced by group size, and thus smaller values are typical when studying small groups. Researchers should report a variety of aggregation statistics to provide a clear picture of the nature of their multilevel data, considering the context of the research when interpreting the values.

However, just because a construct shows good agreement among unit members, it does not necessarily mean that the organizational climate is being measured. Thus, a third issue in climate research is the appropriateness of the climate label. One of the early challenges in climate research was clarifying its distinctiveness relative to other constructs, such as job satisfaction, which led climate researchers to clarify that climate is a description of the work environment as opposed to an affect-laden evaluation of it (Schneider, 1975). In line with this perspective, we recommend the use of definitions of climate that emphasize perceptions of the organization's policies, practices, procedures, and events (Ehrhart et al., 2014) as opposed to feelings, emotions, or attitudes. Furthermore, there is a tendency for researchers to apply the climate label anytime survey data are aggregated, whether or not the aggregate construct is measured in line with the definition of climate. However, there are other shared unit-level constructs such as norms or culture that are not climate. An example related to OHP comes from the literature on sexual harassment. Researchers studying general levels of sexual harassment in a work group have used the term "ambient sexual harassment" (Glomb et al., 1997). This is distinct from the research on sexual harassment climate described previously, which addresses the extent to which policies and practices in the organization tolerate the occurrence of sexual harassment (Fitzgerald et al., 1997). Another example mentioned earlier is the distinction between a climate for incivility that addresses management policies and procedures related to incivility (e.g., Gallus et al., 2014) and a norm for incivility that addresses the level of incivility within the work unit (e.g., Walsh et al., 2012). Such a distinction is particularly helpful because behavioral norms are considered a proximal outcome of climate (Ehrhart & Raver, 2014). The point is that there are many options for labeling aggregate constructs, and researchers need to be clear and thoughtful as to what they are actually measuring and not just use the climate label for any aggregated measure.

A fourth issue to consider when conducting climate research is how climate items should be written. The items should focus on policies, practices, and procedures, and researchers should also consider the referent of the items (e.g., team, department, organization). Although climate stems from individual perceptions, it is typically considered a property of the unit (Ehrhart et al., 2014). As a result, the best way to phrase items related to organizational climate is with unit-level referent, such that the items refer to the attributes of the unit or organization rather than an individual's own perspective (Chan, 1998). Klein et al. (2001) found that using a unit referent for the climate items rather than an individual-level referent resulted in greater within-group agreement and more between-group variability. In addition, Wallace et al. (2016) found stronger relationships with performance outcomes when items had a unit-level referent versus an individual-level referent (noting that relationships were stronger for attitudes when an individual-level referent was used). In general, the use of a unit referent is a best practice in climate research to ensure the focus is on what is happening in the unit as a whole and to best differentiate from individual-level, evaluative constructs such as job attitudes. Which referent level (e.g., team, department, organization) is used should match the theory and the research question being asked.

Fifth, researchers should consider what related climate constructs have been addressed in the literature before proposing a new type of climate and/or developing a new climate measure. In our review, we found that multiple measures are often used to study the same type of climate, which can be limiting when comparing findings across studies. Researchers should review the literature to see whether there is already a validated scale that is usable before creating a new measure. If a new measure is warranted, then justification for the new scale is needed and the measure should be validated. Good examples of climate measure development include Tracey and Tews (2005) and Kuenzi et al. (2020). Researchers also need to consider the width of the climate's focus. Although a narrower focus may make sense from the perspective of aligning the bandwidth of the scale with the outcome of interest, it can also raise questions about whether such a narrow climate exists in organizations. If a new climate measure is warranted, it should be based on strong theory and follow best practices in measure development (e.g., Hinkin, 1998).

Finally, transparency is needed in organizational climate research in the reporting of the data. Researchers need to provide adequate information on the design of the study and the multilevel nature of the data so the research can be properly understood and interpreted. For instance, the referent for the items assessing climate (e.g., group, organization, individual) should be clear. Researchers should provide the sample size at the individual and unit levels, including the average and range of individuals per unit and the response rates for both the overall study and the average within-unit response rate across units. The criteria for inclusion should also be clear, for example, whether units were dropped because the within-unit response rate was too low or the number of respondents for the unit was too low. Such information is critical for understanding and evaluating the research as well as for future meta-analyses to compare sample and design-related issues across studies.

FUTURE DIRECTIONS FOR STUDYING CLIMATE IN OHP

Our consideration of the study of climate in the OHP literature leads to a number of possible directions for future research, particularly when comparing research on climate in the OHP literature with the developments in climate research in the broader organizational research literature, as reviewed earlier in this chapter. One such direction is the consideration of the climates that have not typically been studied in the OHP literature. For instance, service climate was one of the earliest focused climates to be studied in the climate literature, yet its connection to the OHP literature has been limited. However, there is evidence that service climate influences the emotional labor (Katz-Navon et al., 2020) and burnout that service workers experience (Drach-Zahavy, 2010); additional research could clarify our understanding of these relationships. Other climates that have received ample attention outside of OHP could have implications for OHP-related outcomes, such as climates for ethics (Kuenzi et al., 2020) or innovation (Anderson & West, 1998). For instance, an ethical climate could contribute to decreased employee mistreatment or impact how employees conceptualize employee safety. A climate for innovation or creativity that welcomes employees' ideas and input could have implications for employee well-being; however, it could also be experienced as pressure to come up with new ideas that could have negative implications for employee health and well-being. Relatedly, climates could be studied in combination with one another. Zohar's work on safety climate has typically emphasized the competing demands of the workplace, and other climates could be studied with safety climate to better understand these competing demands. Alternatively, ethical climate or innovation climate could be viewed as enhancing the effectiveness of a safety climate, as they may tie safety to moral reasoning or allow for innovations to enhance safety, respectively.

Along similar lines, more developed climate literatures can provide a road map for research on other climates in terms of the types of questions and complexity of models that could be considered in future research. For instance, research on safety climate and service climate have begun to disentangle the leader behaviors that help create a climate from perceptions of the policies, procedures, and systems that are the focus of climate, which has led to research on safety-specific (Barling et al., 2002) and service-specific (Schneider et al., 2005) leadership as antecedents of safety and service climate, respectively. In terms of outcomes, these literatures have also identified mediating mechanisms between climate and outcomes, such as employee knowledge, motivation, and behavior or behavioral norms (e.g., Griffin & Neal, 2000). Researchers can investigate the moderating role of climate (e.g., Burke et al., 2008) and moderators of climate's effects (e.g., Dietz et al., 2004), as well as the role of climate strength (e.g., Schneider et al., 2002). The multilevel effects of climate are also an important possibility for future research; research by Zohar and Luria (2005) provides an excellent example of the role of climate at different levels and the importance of alignment across levels. Again, although the literatures on safety and service climate have addressed many of these issues, such models provide a template for newer climate literatures, such as mistreatment and health climates.

One topic that often arises in the climate literature is its relationship with organizational culture. Culture and climate have been described as "sibling" constructs (Schneider et al., 2011), and although both address the work environment, they have unique qualities. Ehrhart et al. (2014) provided an in-depth discussion of the similarities and differences between the literatures on these topics, and Zohar and Hofmann (2012) discussed how focused climates, which represent shared perceptions of the enacted values and priorities of management, can be compared to espoused values to give insights into the deeper layers of culture. From a methodological perspective, qualitative methodologies tend to be used more in research on organizational culture, whereas quantitative methodologies tend to be used more in research on organizational climate. An integration of concepts and methodologies from the culture and climate literatures would deepen our understanding of the work environment and its implications for OHP-related outcomes.

Finally, future research should consider interventions specifically targeted at organizational climate. There have been numerous efforts in this regard in the literature on safety climate; Lee et al. (2019) identified 19 articles testing safety climate interventions. However, such interventions are less commonly found for other focused climates. Thus, the literature on safety climate interventions can spur future research on other climates to better understand how organizational climate can be developed and changed. Such research also provides a foundation for the practical implications of climate, as interventions provide a clear road map for organizations to utilize the climate literature to improve organizational effectiveness and employee well-being.

CONCLUSION

The organizational environment plays a critical role in influencing employee health, safety, and well-being. The organizational climate literature has provided useful insights into the implications of the organizational environment for OHP, especially on the topics of safety, mistreatment, and health. Continued research on these topics and other related climates, including the study of multiple climates and competing priorities, can build on the foundation of climate research to date and provide a deeper understanding of how organizational leaders can build climates in their organizations to support employees and OHP-related efforts.

REFERENCES

Afsharian, A., Zadow, A., Dollard, M. F., Dormann, C., & Ziaian, T. (2018). Should psychosocial safety climate theory be extended to include climate strength? *Journal of Occupational Health Psychology, 23*(4), 496–507. https://doi.org/10.1037/ocp0000101

Anderson, N. R., & West, M. A. (1998). Measuring climate for work group innovation: Development and validation of the team climate inventory. *Journal of Organizational Behavior, 19*(3), 235–258. https://doi.org/10.1002/(SICI)1099-1379(199805)19:3<235::AID-JOB837>3.0.CO;2-C

Barling, J., Loughlin, C., & Kelloway, E. K. (2002). Development and test of a model linking safety-specific transformational leadership and occupational safety. *Journal of Applied Psychology, 87*(3), 488–496. https://doi.org/10.1037/0021-9010.87.3.488

Bergman, M. E., Palmieri, P. A., Drasgow, F., & Ormerod, A. J. (2012). Racial/ethnic harassment and discrimination, its antecedents, and its effect on job-related outcomes. *Journal of Occupational Health Psychology, 17*(1), 65–78. https://doi.org/10.1037/a0026430

Beus, J. M., Payne, S. C., Bergman, M. E., & Arthur, W., Jr. (2010). Safety climate and injuries: An examination of theoretical and empirical relationships. *Journal of Applied Psychology, 95*(4), 713–727. https://doi.org/10.1037/a0019164

Bliese, P. (2000). Within-group agreement, non-independence, and reliability: Implications for data aggregation and analysis. In K. J. Klein & S. W. J. Kozlowski (Eds.), *Multilevel theory, research and methods in organizations* (pp. 512–556). Jossey-Bass.

Burke, M. J., Chan-Serafin, S., Salvador, R., Smith, A., & Sarpy, S. A. (2008). The role of national culture and organizational climate in safety training effectiveness. *European Journal of Work and Organizational Psychology, 17*(1), 133–152. https://doi.org/10.1080/13594320701307503

Casey, T., Griffin, M. A., Flatau Harrison, H., & Neal, A. (2017). Safety climate and culture: Integrating psychological and systems perspectives. *Journal of Occupational Health Psychology, 22*(3), 341–353. https://doi.org/10.1037/ocp0000072

Chan, D. (1998). Functional relations among constructs in the same content domain at different levels of analysis: A typology of composition models. *Journal of Applied Psychology, 83*(2), 234–246. https://doi.org/10.1037/0021-9010.83.2.234

Chang, C. H., Eatough, E. M., Spector, P. E., & Kessler, S. R. (2012). Violence-prevention climate, exposure to violence and aggression, and prevention behavior: A mediation model. *Journal of Organizational Behavior, 33*(5), 657–677. https://doi.org/10.1002/job.776

Chang, Y. P., Lee, D. C., & Wang, H. H. (2018). Violence-prevention climate in the turnover intention of nurses experiencing workplace violence and work frustration. *Journal of Nursing Management, 26*(8), 961–971. https://doi.org/10.1111/jonm.12621

Christian, M. S., Bradley, J. C., Wallace, J. C., & Burke, M. J. (2009). Workplace safety: A meta-analysis of the roles of person and situation factors. *Journal of Applied Psychology, 94*(5), 1103–1127. https://doi.org/10.1037/a0016172

Clarke, S. (2006). The relationship between safety climate and safety performance: A meta-analytic review. *Journal of Occupational Health Psychology, 11*(4), 315–327. https://doi.org/10.1037/1076-8998.11.4.315

Clarke, S. (2010). An integrative model of safety climate: Linking psychological climate and work attitudes to individual safety outcomes using meta-analysis. *Journal of Occupational and Organizational Psychology, 83*(3), 553–578. https://doi.org/10.1348/096317909X452122

Colquitt, J., Noe, R., & Jackson, C. (2002). Justice in teams: Antecedents and consequences of procedural justice climate. *Personnel Psychology, 55*(1), 83–109. https://doi.org/10.1111/j.1744-6570.2002.tb00104.x

Di Fabio, A. (2017). Positive healthy organizations: Promoting well-being, meaningfulness, and sustainability in organizations. *Frontiers in Psychology, 8,* 1938. https://doi.org/10.3389/fpsyg.2017.01938

Dietz, J., Pugh, S. D., & Wiley, J. (2004). Service climate effects on customer attitudes: An examination of boundary conditions. *Academy of Management Journal, 47*(1), 81–92. https://doi.org/10.2307/20159561

Diez-Roux, A. V. (1998). Bringing context back into epidemiology: Variables and fallacies in multilevel analysis. *American Journal of Public Health, 88*(2), 216–222. https://doi.org/10.2105/AJPH.88.2.216

Dollard, M. F., & Bakker, A. B. (2010). Psychosocial safety climate as a precursor to conducive work environments, psychological health problems, and employee engagement. *Journal of Occupational and Organizational Psychology, 83*(3), 579–599. https://doi.org/10.1348/096317909X470690

Drach-Zahavy, A. (2010). How does service workers' behavior affect their health? Service climate as a moderator in the service behavior–health relationships. *Journal of Occupational Health Psychology, 15*(2), 105–119. https://doi.org/10.1037/a0018573

Ehrhart, M. G., & Raver, J. L. (2014). The effects of organizational climate and culture on productive and counterproductive behavior. In B. Schneider & K. Barbera (Eds.), *The Oxford handbook of organizational climate and culture* (pp. 153–176). Oxford University Press.

Ehrhart, M. G., Schneider, B., & Macey, W. H. (2014). *Organizational climate and culture: An introduction to theory, research, and practice.* Routledge.

Fitzgerald, L. F., Drasgow, F., Hulin, C. L., Gelfand, M. J., & Magley, V. J. (1997). Antecedents and consequences of sexual harassment in organizations: A test of an integrated model. *Journal of Applied Psychology, 82*(4), 578–589. https://doi.org/10.1037/0021-9010.82.4.578

Gallus, J. A., Bunk, J. A., Matthews, R. A., Barnes-Farrell, J. L., & Magley, V. J. (2014). An eye for an eye? Exploring the relationship between workplace incivility experiences and perpetration. *Journal of Occupational Health Psychology, 19*(2), 143–154. https://doi.org/10.1037/a0035931

Glomb, T. M., Richman, W. L., Hulin, C. L., Drasgow, F., Schneider, K. T., & Fitzgerald, L. F. (1997). Ambient sexual harassment: An integrated model of antecedents and consequences. *Organizational Behavior and Human Decision Processes, 71*(3), 309–328. https://doi.org/10.1006/obhd.1997.2728

Grawitch, M. J., & Ballard, D. W. (Eds.). (2016). *The psychologically healthy workplace: Building a win–win environment for organizations and employees.* American Psychological Association. https://doi.org/10.1037/14731-000

Griffin, M. A., & Curcuruto, M. (2016). Safety climate in organizations. *Annual Review of Organizational Psychology and Organizational Behavior, 3*(1), 191–212. https://doi.org/10.1146/annurev-orgpsych-041015-062414

Griffin, M. A., & Neal, A. (2000). Perceptions of safety at work: A framework for linking safety climate to safety performance, knowledge, and motivation. *Journal of Occupational Health Psychology, 5*(3), 347–358. https://doi.org/10.1037/1076-8998.5.3.347

Guion, R. (1973). A note on organizational climate. *Organizational Behavior and Human Performance, 9*(1), 120–125. https://doi.org/10.1016/0030-5073(73)90041-X

Hall, G. B., Dollard, M. F., & Coward, J. (2010). Psychosocial safety climate: Development of the PSC-12. *International Journal of Stress Management*, 17(4), 353–383. https://doi.org/10.1037/a0021320

He, Y., Wang, Y., & Payne, S. C. (2019). How is safety climate formed? A meta-analysis of the antecedents of safety climate. *Organizational Psychology Review*, 9(2–3), 124–156. https://doi.org/10.1177/2041386619874870

Hinkin, T. R. (1998). A brief tutorial on the development of measures for use in survey questionnaires. *Organizational Research Methods*, 1(1), 104–121. https://doi.org/10.1177/109442819800100106

Hofmann, D., & Mark, D. (2006). An investigation of the relationship between safety climate and medication errors as well as other nurse patient outcomes. *Personnel Psychology*, 59(4), 847–869. https://doi.org/10.1111/j.1744-6570.2006.00056.x

Hofmann, D. A., Morgeson, F. P., & Gerras, S. J. (2003). Climate as a moderator of the relationship between leader-member exchange and content specific citizenship: Safety climate as an exemplar. *Journal of Applied Psychology*, 88(1), 170–178. https://doi.org/10.1037/0021-9010.88.1.170

Holmes, I. V. O., IV, Jiang, K., Avery, D. R., McKay, P. F., Oh, I.-S., & Tillman, C. J. (2021). A meta-analysis integrating 25 years of diversity climate research. *Journal of Management*, 47(6), 1357–1382. https://doi.org/10.1177/0149206320934547

Hulin, C. L., Fitzgerald, L. F., & Drasgow, F. (1996). Organizational influences on sexual harassment. In M. S. Stockdale (Ed.), *Sexual harassment in the workplace: Perspectives, frontiers, and response strategies* (pp. 127–150). Sage Publications. https://doi.org/10.4135/9781483327280.n7

Idris, M. A., Dollard, M. F., & Yulita. (2014). Psychosocial safety climate, emotional demands, burnout, and depression: A longitudinal multilevel study in the Malaysian private sector. *Journal of Occupational Health Psychology*, 19(3), 291–302. https://doi.org/10.1037/a0036599

James, L. R., Demaree, R. G., & Wolf, G. (1984). Estimating within-group interrater reliability with and without response bias. *Journal of Applied Psychology*, 69(1), 85–98. https://doi.org/10.1037/0021-9010.69.1.85

Jiang, L., Lavaysse, L. M., & Probst, T. M. (2019). Safety climate and safety outcomes: A meta-analytic comparison of universal vs. industry-specific safety climate predictive validity. *Work and Stress*, 33(1), 41–57. https://doi.org/10.1080/02678373.2018.1457737

Jiang, L., & Probst, T. M. (2016). A multilevel examination of affective job insecurity climate on safety outcomes. *Journal of Occupational Health Psychology*, 21(3), 366–377. https://doi.org/10.1037/ocp0000014

Jones, A. P., & James, L. R. (1979). Psychological climate: Dimensions and relationships of individual and aggregated work environment perception. *Organizational Behavior and Human Performance*, 23(2), 201–250. https://doi.org/10.1016/0030-5073(79)90056-4

Katz-Navon, T., Vashdi, D. R., & Naveh, E. (2020). The toll of service climate on employees: An emotional labor perspective. *Journal of Service Theory and Practice*, 30(2), 105–121. https://doi.org/10.1108/JSTP-12-2018-0291

Kelloway, E. K., Mullen, J., & Francis, L. (2006). Divergent effects of transformational and passive leadership on employee safety. *Journal of Occupational Health Psychology*, 11(1), 76–86. https://doi.org/10.1037/1076-8998.11.1.76

Klein, K. J., Conn, A. B., Smith, D. B., & Sorra, J. S. (2001). Is everyone in agreement? An exploration of within-group agreement in employee perceptions of the work environment. *Journal of Applied Psychology*, 86(1), 3–16. https://doi.org/10.1037/0021-9010.86.1.3

Klein, K. J., & Kozlowski, S. W. J. (Eds.). (2000). *Multilevel theory, research and methods in organizations: Foundations, extensions, and new directions*. Jossey-Bass.

Kuenzi, M., Mayer, D. M., & Greenbaum, R. L. (2020). Creating an ethical organizational environment: The relationship between ethical leadership, ethical organizational climate, and unethical behavior. *Personnel Psychology, 73*(1), 43–71. https://doi.org/10.1111/peps.12356

Kuenzi, M., & Schminke, M. (2009). Assembling fragments into a lens: A review, critique, and proposed research agenda for the organizational work climate literature. *Journal of Management, 35*(3), 634–717. https://doi.org/10.1177/0149206308330559

LeBreton, J. M., & Senter, J. L. (2008). Answers to 20 questions about interrater reliability and interrater agreement. *Organizational Research Methods, 11*(4), 815–852. https://doi.org/10.1177/1094428106296642

Lee, J., Huang, Y. H., Cheung, J. H., Chen, Z., & Shaw, W. S. (2019). A systematic review of the safety climate intervention literature: Past trends and future directions. *Journal of Occupational Health Psychology, 24*(1), 66–91. https://doi.org/10.1037/ocp0000113

Litwin, G. H., & Stringer, R. A. (1968). *Motivation and organizational climate.* Harvard Business School.

Loh, M. Y., Idris, M. A., Dormann, C., & Muhamad, H. (2019). Organisational climate and employee health outcomes: A systematic review. *Safety Science, 118*, 442–452. https://doi.org/10.1016/j.ssci.2019.05.052

McKay, P. F., Avery, D., Lioa, H., & Morris, M. (2011). Does diversity climate lead to customer satisfaction? It depends on the service climate and business unit demography. *Organization Science, 22*(3), 788–803. https://doi.org/10.1287/orsc.1100.0550

McKay, P. F., Avery, D. R., & Morris, M. A. (2008). Mean racial-ethnic differences in employee sales performance: The moderating role of diversity climate. *Personnel Psychology, 61*(2), 349–374. https://doi.org/10.1111/j.1744-6570.2008.00116.x

Ostroff, C., Kinicki, A. J., & Muhammad, R. S. (2012). Organizational culture and climate. In N. W. Schmitt & S. Highhouse (Eds.), *Handbook of psychology: Vol. 12. Industrial and organizational psychology* (2nd ed., pp. 643–676). Wiley.

Patterson, M., West, M., Shackleton, V., Dawson, J., Lawthom, R., Matlis, S., Robinson, D. L., & Wallace, A.M. (2005). Validating the organizational climate measure: Links to managerial practices, productivity and innovation. *Journal of Organizational Behavior, 26*(4), 379–408. https://doi.org/10.1002/job.312

Ribisl, K. M., & Reischl, T. M. (1993). Measuring the climate for health at organizations. Development of the worksite health climate scales. *Journal of Occupational Medicine, 35*(8), 812–824. https://doi.org/10.1097/00043764-199308000-00019

Schneider, B. (1975). Organizational climates: An essay. *Personnel Psychology, 28*(4), 447–479. https://doi.org/10.1111/j.1744-6570.1975.tb01386.x

Schneider, B., Ehrhart, M. G., & Macey, W. H. (2011). Perspectives on organizational climate and culture. In S. Zedeck (Ed.), *APA handbook of industrial and organizational psychology: Vol. 1. Building and developing the organization* (pp. 373–414). American Psychological Association. https://doi.org/10.1037/12169-012

Schneider, B., Ehrhart, M. G., & Macey, W. H. (2013). Organizational climate and culture. *Annual Review of Psychology, 64*(1), 361–388. https://doi.org/10.1146/annurev-psych-113011-143809

Schneider, B., Ehrhart, M. J., Mayer, D. M., Saltz, J. L., & Niles-Jolly, K. (2005). Understanding organizational links in service settings. *Academy of Management Journal, 48*(6), 1017–1032. https://doi.org/10.5465/amj.2005.19573107

Schneider, B., Parkington, J. J., & Buxton, V. M. (1980). Employee and customer perceptions of service in banks. *Administrative Science Quarterly, 25*(2), 252–267. https://doi.org/10.2307/2392454

Schneider, B., Salvaggio, A. N., & Subirats, M. (2002). Climate strength: A new direction for climate research. *Journal of Applied Psychology, 87*(2), 220–229. https://doi.org/10.1037/0021-9010.87.2.220

Schneider, B., White, S. S., & Paul, M. C. (1998). Linking service climate and customer perceptions of service quality: Test of a causal model. *Journal of Applied Psychology*, *83*(2), 150–163. https://doi.org/10.1037/0021-9010.83.2.150

Schulte, M., Ostroff, C., Shmulyian, S., & Kinicki, A. (2009). Organizational climate configurations: Relationships to collective attitudes, customer satisfaction, and financial performance. *Journal of Applied Psychology*, *94*(3), 618–634. https://doi.org/10.1037/a0014365

Sliter, K. A. (2013). Development and validation of a measure of workplace climate for healthy weight maintenance. *Journal of Occupational Health Psychology*, *18*(3), 350–362. https://doi.org/10.1037/a0033132

Tamers, S. L., Chosewood, L. C., Childress, A., Hudson, H., Nigam, J., & Chang, C.-C. (2019). Total Worker Health® 2014–2018: The novel approach to worker safety, health, and well-being evolves. *International Journal of Environmental Research and Public Health*, *16*(3), 321. https://doi.org/10.3390/ijerph16030321

Tracey, J. B., & Tews, M. (2005). Construct validity of a general training climate scale. *Organizational Research Methods*, *8*(4), 353–374. https://doi.org/10.1177/1094428105280055

von Treuer, K., Fuller-Tyszkiewicz, M., & Little, G. (2014). The impact of shift work and organizational work climate on health outcomes in nurses. *Journal of Occupational Health Psychology*, *19*(4), 453–461. https://doi.org/10.1037/a0037680

Wallace, J. C., Edwards, B. D., Paul, J., Burke, M., Christian, M., & Eissa, G. (2016). Change the referent? A meta-analytic investigation of direct and referent-shift consensus models for organizational climate. *Journal of Management*, *42*(4), 838–861. https://doi.org/10.1177/0149206313484520

Walsh, B. M., Magley, V. J., Reeves, D. W., Davies-Schrils, K. A., Marmet, M. D., & Gallus, J. A. (2012). Assessing workgroup norms for civility: The development of the Civility Norms Questionnaire-Brief. *Journal of Business and Psychology*, *27*(4), 407–420. https://doi.org/10.1007/s10869-011-9251-4

Williams, N. J., Ehrhart, M. G., Aarons, G. A., Marcus, S. C., & Beidas, R. S. (2018). Linking molar organizational climate and strategic implementation climate to clinicians' use of evidence-based psychotherapy techniques: Cross-sectional and lagged analyses from a 2-year observational study. *Implementation Science*, *13*, 85. https://doi.org/10.1186/s13012-018-0781-2

Willness, C., Steel, P., & Lee, K. (2007). A meta-analysis of the antecedents and consequences of workplace sexual harassment. *Personnel Psychology*, *60*(1), 127–162. https://doi.org/10.1111/j.1744-6570.2007.00067.x

Yang, L. Q., & Caughlin, D. E. (2017). Aggression-preventive supervisor behavior: Implications for workplace climate and employee outcomes. *Journal of Occupational Health Psychology*, *22*(1), 1–18. https://doi.org/10.1037/a0040148

Yao, J., Lim, S., Guo, C. Y., Ou, A. Y., & Ng, J. W. X. (2022). Experienced incivility in the workplace: A meta-analytical review of its construct validity and nomological network. *Journal of Applied Psychology*, *107*(2), 193–220.https://doi.org/10.1037/apl0000870

Zohar, D. (1980). Safety climate in industrial organizations: Theoretical and applied implications. *Journal of Applied Psychology*, *65*(1), 96–102. https://doi.org/10.1037/0021-9010.65.1.96

Zohar, D. (2000). A group-level model of safety climate: Testing the effect of group climate on microaccidents in manufacturing jobs. *Journal of Applied Psychology*, *85*(4), 587–596. https://doi.org/10.1037/0021-9010.85.4.587

Zohar, D. (2002). The effects of leadership dimensions, safety climate, and assigned priorities on minor injuries in work groups. *Journal of Organizational Behavior*, *23*(1), 75–92. https://doi.org/10.1002/job.130

Zohar, D. (2010). Thirty years of safety climate research: Reflections and future directions. *Accident Analysis and Prevention*, *42*(5), 1517–1522. https://doi.org/10.1016/j.aap.2009.12.019

Zohar, D. (2011). Safety climate: Conceptual and measurement issues. In J. C. Quick & L. E. Tetrick (Eds.), *Handbook of occupational health psychology* (2nd ed., pp. 141–164). American Psychological Association.

Zohar, D. (2014). Safety climate: Conceptualization, measurement, and improvement. In B. Schneider & K. M. Barbera (Eds.), *The Oxford handbook of organizational climate and culture* (pp. 317–334). Oxford University Press.,

Zohar, D., & Hofmann, D. H. (2012). Organizational culture and climate. In S. W. J. Kozlowski (Ed.), *The Oxford handbook of industrial and organizational psychology* (pp. 643–666). Oxford University Press.

Zohar, D., & Luria, G. (2005). A multilevel model of safety climate: Cross-level relationships between organization and group-level climates. *Journal of Applied Psychology, 90*(4), 616–628. https://doi.org/10.1037/0021-9010.90.4.616

Zohar, D., & Polachek, T. (2014). Discourse-based intervention for modifying supervisory communication as leverage for safety climate and performance improvement: A randomized field study. *Journal of Applied Psychology, 99*(1), 113–124. https://doi.org/10.1037/a0034096

Zweber, Z. M., Henning, R. A., & Magley, V. J. (2016). A practical scale for Multi-Faceted Organizational Health Climate Assessment. *Journal of Occupational Health Psychology, 21*(2), 250–259. https://doi.org/10.1037/a0039895

10

Nonstandard Work Schedules

Philip Tucker and Göran Kecklund

An increasing proportion of the global workforce have some form of "nonstandard" schedule—a pattern of work hours that differs markedly from what society considers to be "normal" (where a normal schedule might be, for example, 9 a.m. to 5 p.m., Monday through Friday). A nonstandard schedule might involve working outside these normal daily hours and outside the normal workweek and might also involve variations from day-to-day in which hours are worked and from week-to-week in which days are worked. Such nonstandard work schedules may be a necessity of the job, or they may be an option available to the employee for their own convenience, or it may be a combination of the two.

An employee's work schedule is key to their effectiveness at work and to the effect that their job has on their own health, well-being, and safety. For example, work-related fatigue can be exacerbated by schedules that restrict opportunities for sleep and recovery, or it can be mitigated by working time arrangements that allow the employee to rest when they need to (Kecklund & Axelsson, 2016). Similarly, schedules that restrict opportunities for socializing with family and friends can be a source of psychological strain, whereas flexible working can help optimize the fit between work and nonwork life, thereby potentially improving the employee's quality of life and their job satisfaction (Nijp et al., 2012).

This chapter examines the employee health and safety implications of two of the main forms of nonstandard work schedules: shift work and flexible working. In the case of flexible working, while the focus is on flexible work

https://doi.org/10.1037/0000331-010
Handbook of Occupational Health Psychology, Third Edition, L. E. Tetrick, G. G. Fisher, M. T. Ford, and J. C. Quick (Editors)

hours, the discussion also encompasses the closely related phenomenon of flexible workplace location (i.e., remote working and teleworking).

SHIFT WORK

When one thinks of shift work, one most commonly thinks of employees divided into teams who take turns to work duty periods (or "shifts") that cover the operating hours of the organization. The term *shift work* is also used to encompass night working—indeed, the two terms are often used interchangeably. However, shift working does not necessarily have to involve night work, and night work does not necessarily have to involve handing operations over to a team of day workers, for example, if the organization only operates at night. Shift workers may alternate which shifts they work— so-called rotating shifts, whereby their daily work hours (start and finish times) change in a more or less regular sequence over the shift cycle (e.g., a combination of morning, afternoon/evening, and night shifts). Or they may only ever work one type of shift—so-called permanent or fixed shifts (e.g., permanent night shifts).

The proportion of workers involved In some kind of shift work is between 10% and 20% in most of the countries for which recent data are available (Eurofound & ILO, 2019). However, in the United States the figure is higher at 38%, with 30% carrying out night work. In Europe, the corresponding proportions are 21% and 19%; in Turkey, 11% and 16%; in the Republic of Korea, 9% and 13%; and in Argentina, 12% and 11%.

Shift working is commonly associated with the disturbance of sleep and other biological functions as well as the disruption of social and family life. These disturbances are thought to underlie many of the psychological and physical health problems that tend to be more prevalent among shift workers than among typical day workers. Sleep disturbances and consequent fatigue are also likely to be responsible for the greater risk of accidents and injuries that tends to be associated with shift working. Moreover, workers who are at greater risk of fatigue and ill health may be less productive, more likely to be absent from work, and more inclined to quit their job altogether.

Mechanisms Underlying the Impact of Shift Work on Health and Performance

Human beings have evolved as diurnal creatures; they are naturally active during the day and inclined toward rest, recovery, and sleep at night. These tendencies are reflected in human circadian rhythms, the regular oscillations of physiological and psychological functions that cycle with a 24-hour period (e.g., the sleep-wake cycle). This circadian rhythmicity is primarily controlled by an internal mechanism ("the body clock"), located in the suprachiasmatic nuclei area of the brain, in the hypothalamus (see also Chapter 12, this volume).

Under normal circumstances, the cycle of our body clock is synchronized with our daily routine. During the daytime, when our daily routine is focused on activity (e.g., working, socializing), the body clock is promoting wakefulness and mobilizing bodily resources for energy expenditure, as well as the ingestion and absorption of food. Conversely, at nighttime when our daily routine is focused on rest and recovery, the body clock is promoting sleep, bodily restitution, and repair. However, under some circumstances the body clock can become desynchronized from the daily routine. When we make long-distance journeys by airplane between time zones, or when we change between working day shifts and night shifts, we may find ourselves needing to be active when the body clock is promoting sleep, and trying to sleep when the body clock is promoting wakefulness. The body clock rhythm is inherently stable, and so, depending on the degree of desynchrony (e.g., how many time zones we have crossed or how great the change in our shift start time is), it can take days for the body clock and our circadian rhythms to fully realign themselves with our new daily routine (i.e., the timing of the new activity-rest cycle), if it happens at all.

The mechanism that promotes the body clock's realignment to a new time zone or work shift is known as *entrainment*. This is the influence on the timing of the body clock of environmental factors (or *zeitgebers*) such as work, activity, sleep, meals, and, in particular, light exposure. Exposure to bright light (and most especially light in the blue part of the spectrum) suppresses the secretion of melatonin—a hormone that is central in the regulation of the body clock. Hence melatonin levels are normally low during daylight hours and increased during nighttime. When we travel between time zones, exposure to the new day–night cycle at our destination helps our body clock adjust. Shift workers swapping from day shifts to night shifts have no such advantage. For them, the timing of most zeitgebers, including the exposure to daylight, does not change, and so their adjustment tends to be much slower.

Effects of Shift Work on Workers

The impacts that shift work have upon workers range from acute effects (e.g., the disturbed sleep and excess fatigue that may occur when working certain shifts) to chronic effects on psychological well-being and physical health.

Sleep, Fatigue, and Accident Risk

While the evidence is fairly clear that shift workers experience *acute* sleep problems when working certain shifts (i.e., night shifts and early morning shifts; Kecklund & Axelsson, 2016), the evidence is equivocal that shift workers are at greater risk of developing *chronic* sleep problems, such as symptoms of insomnia, to a degree that is clinically significant. A systematic review reported only a trend toward increased risk for shift workers (Linton et al., 2015). Caution is required when interpreting this finding as suggesting that shift workers are not at risk of developing serious sleep problems. Method-ological issues such as loose definitions of shift-work exposure, inaccurate measurement of outcomes (e.g., self-reported symptoms), and biased sam-pling may have led to an underestimation of effects.

Shift working is also associated with increased fatigue-related errors, acci-dents, and injury risk. A meta-analysis determined that accident risk is higher on night shifts as compared with daytime shifts and on shifts longer than 9 hours in duration, that the trend for risk to increase over the course of a shift is offset by scheduling of intrashift rest breaks, and that risk accumulates over consecutive morning or night (but not afternoon/evening) shifts (Fischer et al., 2017).

Psychological–Emotional Disorders

Shift workers may experience additional psychosocial strain and emotional dis-tress compared with day workers, not least because of the impact that the anti-social work hours of shift work have on their personal lives, with the effect being greater among women than men (Torquati et al., 2019). However, studies that have used objective indices of clinically diagnosed mental health disorders (e.g., recorded prescription of psychotropic medication, hospital medical records, records of sickness absence related to mental health) have produced mixed results (Jørgensen et al., 2021). Methodological issues are likely to underlie this diversity of findings. A commonly discussed problem is one of selection—the so-called healthy shift worker effect (Knutsson & Åkerstedt, 1992). Shift workers who develop health problems as a result of their exposure are more likely to leave their position and transfer into day work, leaving a "survivor population" of exceptionally robust, healthy shift workers. This survivor population is then compared with a sample of day workers, which includes those individuals who left shift work and who may still be suffering ill health as a result of their pre-vious exposure. Hence the effect of shift work on the health outcome being studied is underestimated.

Chronic Cognitive and Neurological Impairment

While several studies have observed acute fatigue-related cognitive impair-ment on certain shifts, most commonly night shifts (de Cordova et al., 2016), the picture regarding longer term effects of shift work on cognition is less clear. A study of employees in a range of occupations found that participants with more than 10 years of exposure to shift work were cognitively impaired by the equivalent of 6.5 years of normal cognitive aging, when compared with unexposed workers (Marquié et al., 2015). However, these findings con-trast with two other prospective cohort studies that found no evidence of greater within-subject cognitive decline due to shift work, either in a large sample of older nurses (Devore et al., 2013) or a smaller population-based sample of older adults (Bokenberger et al., 2017). Prolonged exposure to shift work may also increase the risk of developing dementia, with some evidence that risk is greatest among shift workers with a genetic predisposition (Leso et al., 2021).

The mechanisms underlying the possible chronic cognitive and neurological impairment of shift workers have yet to be ascertained. Impaired cognitive performance may be the result of chronic exposure to circadian disruption and consequent physiological stress, which has been shown to have an impact on cerebral structures involved in cognition and mental health over the lifespan (Marquié et al., 2015). The link between shift work and dementia may be mediated by chronic sleep disturbance or restriction. Chronic sleep impairment impacts the clearance of metabolites that are a hallmark protein in Alzheimer's disease (Spira et al., 2013), and it is also associated with cortical thinning, a clinical marker found in certain dementia patients (Wennberg et al., 2017). Alternatively, the link with dementia may be mediated through shift workers' increased susceptibility to cardiometabolic diseases, which are strong risk factors for dementia (Fillit et al., 2008).

Physical Health Complaints With a Psychosocial Etiology
Sleep disruption is thought to underlie many of the physical health complaints that are more prevalent among shift workers compared with day workers. However, evidence of a clear causal pathway between shift work, insufficient sleep, and ill health remains to be established (Kecklund & Axelsson, 2016). Circadian disruption is also likely to play a crucial role in shift workers' health problems, as a cause of the sleep problems and by way of disrupting other physiological functions. Another potential health issue for shift workers is that they are more likely to be overweight and to engage in risk behaviors, such as leading a sedentary lifestyle.

Shift work has been linked to the development of cardiovascular disease (CVD; Torquati et al., 2018). Multiple potential pathways link shift work with increased risk of CVD (Puttonen et al., 2010). These include the psychosocial strain of working antisocial hours and of restricted recovery opportunities; behavioral factors such as smoking and weight gain, which tend to be more prevalent among shift workers; and physiological mechanisms such as activation of the autonomic nervous system, inflammation, and alteration of lipid and glucose metabolism.

Shift work alters workers' eating habits. This altered pattern is potentially problematic in terms of the digestion of the food itself and the metabolism of energy and nutrients it contains. Digestive processes (e.g., gastric pH) vary as a function of time of day, with the absorptive system being less prepared for handling food at nighttime. This is thought to be one of the main reasons that night workers report greater incidence of gastrointestinal problems (e.g., irritable bowel syndrome, upper gastrointestinal dyspepsia, peptic ulcer; Lowden et al., 2010).

The processes of metabolism (i.e., the extraction of energy from food and its subsequent utilization) are also normally synchronized to the day–night and rest–activity cycle. When we eat at night, our capacity for metabolizing both glucose and fats is reduced. Eating during the "circadian night" also reduces levels of leptin (an appetite-suppressing hormone that is normally present at night). These affects are thought to be linked to shift workers' greater susceptibility to developing metabolic syndrome (i.e., the association of even moderate degrees of visceral obesity, dyslipidemia, abnormal blood pressure, and serum glucose levels in the same individual), when compared with day workers (Wang et al., 2014). The circadian disruption of the metabolic system, including altered eating habits, may well underlie the higher prevalence of other health complaints among shift workers, such as CVD, Type 2 diabetes, and obesity. The likely importance of eating habits to shift workers' health has prompted the development of dietary recommendations for managing the nutrition of shift workers (see Lowden et al., 2010).

Individual Differences

The impact of shift work on health and well-being varies substantially between individuals, due to differences in the working conditions (e.g., psychosocial and physical demands), individual circumstances (e.g., domestic situation), and psychobiological differences between individuals. There are differences in human circadian rhythms that can affect how well workers cope with shift work. The mostly widely discussed parameter of individual difference in circadian rhythms is chronotype (see Chapter 12, this volume). Typically, early chronotypes (or "morning types") spontaneously wake early in the morning, prefer undertaking activities (e.g., involving physical or mental effort, eating meals) earlier in the day, and prefer to retire to bed relatively early. Conversely, late chronotypes ("evening types") prefer later rising and bedtimes and prefer undertaking activities later in the day. Early chronotypes tend to have more difficulties adjusting to night work, particularly with respect to sleep and alertness (Booker et al., 2018). A mismatch between chronotype and shift timing (e.g., early chronotypes working late shifts and vice versa) may predict increased risk of diseases such as cancer and metabolic disorders (Hittle & Gillespie, 2018). Matching workers' schedules to their chronotype (i.e., abolishing morning shifts for extreme late chronotypes and night shifts for extreme early ones) can improve individuals' sleep and well-being (Vetter et al., 2015).

Shift working exacerbates the normal age-related decline in sleep quality and the increasing instability of our circadian rhythms (Costa & Di Milia, 2008). Consequently, shift workers become more vulnerable to the negative effects of shift work on sleep and health when they enter middle age (40–50 years old), although the evidence is mixed (Saksvik et al., 2011). Some studies have reported that while sleep problems increase with age, they appear to plateau at around 45 years (e.g., Tucker et al., 2011), with the suggestion being that many of those who experience sustained sleep disruption have left shift work by middle age (see the discussion of selection effects). Other possible explanations for the plateau are that (a) people's expectations of what constitutes a "good sleep" may lessen in older age and (b) older workers' actual need for sleep may reduce (Härmä, 1996). Older workers benefit from a change to a so-called very rapidly forward-rotating shift schedule (Viitasalo et al., 2015). Very rapid rotation involves working only very few (e.g., one or two) consecutive shifts of one sort (e.g., morning shifts) before either changing to the next type of shift (e.g., afternoon/evening shifts) or having a rest day. Forward rotation is when the change between the type of shift involves a delay of the circadian rhythm (e.g., changing from morning to afternoon/evening shifts, or from afternoon/evening to night shifts). Besides the sequencing of shifts, other factors that are likely to be helpful for older shift workers are allowing flexibility in work hours—that is, employee-oriented work time control (Loudoun et al., 2014)—and a general reduction in the number of night shifts.

Gender differences in the effects of shift work vary by outcome. Earlier studies found that female shift workers tend to be at greater risk of sleep problems, fatigue, and sleepiness compared with male shift workers (Saksvik et al., 2011). However, a more recent systematic review found that the majority of selected studies of health care workers found no gender differences in the association between shift work and sleep (Booker et al., 2018). Moreover, another review noted some evidence of higher rates of shift-work disorder (a circadian rhythm sleep disorder characterized by excessive sleepiness and complaints of insomnia related to the work schedule) in males than in females (Kervezee et al., 2018). Female shift workers are at greater risk of disability pension, mortality, factors relating to obesity (Saksvik et al., 2011), metabolic syndrome (Wang et al., 2014), Type 2 diabetes (Gao et al., 2020), and mental health disorders (Torquati et al., 2019).

Several factors contribute to the greater impact of shift work on certain aspects of women's sleep and health, compared with men's. Biological differences, including in the circadian system (e.g., women are more likely to be early chronotypes), may make women more vulnerable to the effects of night work (e.g., on sleep and alertness; Boivin et al., 2016). In many societies, working women still undertake the majority of unpaid domestic chores, including child care, which can be especially burdensome when their paid job involves a demanding work schedule. Shift-working women and shift-working men tend to work in different occupational sectors, and so there may be differences in their working conditions or in their shift patterns that could result in apparent gender differences in the effects of shift work.

Countermeasures

Light treatment can be used to help shift workers adapt to a nocturnal routine, with blue-green light being the most effective. Exposing shift workers to blue light in the evening, while also reducing their exposure to outdoor morning light after the end of the shift (using sunglasses or goggles), improves their alertness and performance at night, and their ability to sleep during the day. However, the long-term health effects of repeated readjustment of circadian rhythms using light treatment are unknown (Lowden et al., 2019).

There is only very limited evidence that hypnotics improve daytime sleep in night workers, and they do not improve nighttime alertness. Clinical trials have shown that the wakefulness-promoting agents modafinil and armodafinil reduce nighttime sleepiness and improve performance without causing any objectively measurable impairments of daytime sleep (Liira et al., 2014).

Taking a nap during the night shift reduces sleepiness, improves performance on the shift, and is unlikely to affect daytime sleep during the following day (Ruggiero & Redeker, 2014). However, naps are often followed by sleep inertia, a brief period (20–30 minutes) of decreased cognitive function and performance immediately after a period of sleep, and so it is desirable to allow time for recuperation after a nap. Naps taken prior to the night shift were found to reduce accident rates by 48% in a study of police drivers (Garbarino et al., 2004).

A work schedule that minimizes circadian disruption and accumulated sleep loss, and that permits sufficient recovery during days off, should be beneficial for alertness, sleep, and health. Forward-rotating shift schedules have most consistently been identified as being beneficial with respect to chronic disease and sleep, while changing from slow to rapid rotation has also been linked to slight improvements in subjectively reported health (Kecklund & Axelsson, 2016). The avoidance of short intershift intervals (i.e., ≤ 11 hours) has also been identified as being beneficial to sleep, sleepiness, and fatigue (Vedaa et al., 2016). A review focusing on the scheduling of night shifts concluded that the risk of injuries and possibly breast cancer could be reduced by implementing schedules that have (a) ≤ 3 consecutive nights, (b) shift intervals of ≥ 11 hours, and (c) night shifts of ≤ 9 hours in duration (Garde et al., 2020).

Few who work permanent (i.e., nonrotating) night shifts show complete circadian adaption to nights (Folkard, 2008). However, such schedules may be appropriate for those with extreme evening-orientation, those who can remain on a nocturnal rhythm on rest days and in circumstances where exposure to daylight is limited (e.g., oil rigs; Bjorvatn et al., 2006). There is mixed evidence regarding the effects of compressing the working week into fewer longer shifts (e.g., 12 hours), with successful implementation possibly depending upon how the shifts are arranged (e.g., in terms of start and finish times, distribution of rest within and between shifts; Ferguson & Dawson, 2012). Allowing the individual some control over their hours of work can produce improvements in the health and organizational effectiveness of shift workers (Bambra et al., 2008). Chapter 12 in this book discusses additional approaches to tackling employees' sleep problems.

FLEXIBLE WORKING

Flexible working arrangements (FWAs) are when the possibility exists for an employee's work hours (e.g., their start and finish times, when they take breaks, which days or shifts they work) and workplace location (e.g., the employer's premises or the employee's home) to change from day to day, from week to week, or over longer periods. Crucially, the timing and place of work may vary at the discretion of the employee, to suit their individual needs and wishes (employee-oriented flexibility); at the discretion of the employer, to suit the business need (employer-oriented flexibility); or a combination of the two.

In the United States in the period 2013 to 2017, 28% of employees worked outside their place of work on at least some days (Krantz-Kent, 2019), while in Europe in 2019, 9% of employees worked from home at least sometimes, up from 5% in 2009 (Milasi et al., 2020). The prevalence of flexible work hours also varies widely between countries. In 2019, it was estimated that 40% of workers in the United States were able to adjust their own work hours, while elsewhere the proportions ranged from 19% in the EU, down to 6% in Korea and 4% in Turkey (Eurofound & ILO, 2019). The proportions of workers with FWA increased substantially during the COVID-19 pandemic (Brynjolfsson et al., 2020), but at the time of writing it remains to be seen whether the figures will return closer to prepandemic levels at some point in the future.

Mechanisms Underlying the Impact of Flexible Working Arrangements on Health and Performance

Employee-oriented flexibility is generally associated with positive or protective effects on an employee's well-being, whereas employer-oriented flexibility is more likely to be associated with negative effects. The mechanisms underlying these associations are not fully understood. Regarding flexible work hours, two potential mediators have been identified, namely, *work–life balance* (WLB, a term that also encompasses the more specific term *work–family balance*) and the process of recovery from the strain and effort associated with work. By having influence over their work hours, employees are better able to align their work commitments with their private life. This reduces the strain associated with conflicts between work and nonwork life, promoting more positive health outcomes. Having influence over work hours also allows employees to optimize their recovery from the stresses and strains of work, both while at work and outside of work—for example, by taking rest breaks when highly fatigued, or by matching one's start and finish times to one's diurnal preference (see the discussion of chronotype in the Shift Work section).

WLB also plays a role in the effects of workplace flexibility, and in particular, *teleworking* (i.e., working away from the central workplace, typically from home, using technology to interact with others as needed to conduct work tasks; Allen et al., 2015), on health and performance. In accordance with the theory of boundary management, employees with access to flexible working arrangements sit on a continuum between integration and segmentation (Kossek et al., 2006). Employees who prefer to integrate work and nonwork life have permeable borders between the two domains, mixing work and nonwork activities. They may take private calls while at work, and work remotely at home while remaining accessible to members of their family and friends. Employees preferring segmentation seek to maintain boundaries between the two domains, keeping personal calls to a minimum during work hours, avoiding working from home, having separate email accounts for work and personal use, and not checking work emails outside normal work hours. Integration may be preferred by teleworkers as a way of enhancing WLB. However, too much integration may have the opposite effect if it leads to extended work hours (e.g., checking work emails in the evening).

Work-Hours Flexibility: Effects and Moderators

Flexibility can have very different impacts on the worker, depending upon whether the timing and place of work varies at the discretion of the employee or at the discretion of the employer.

Employee-Oriented Work-Hours Flexibility—Work-Time Control

Work-time control (WTC) refers to an individual's autonomy over the duration and distribution of their working time. It is usually measured through self-reports, either as a single-item global measure or, preferably, as a multidimensional index score. Enhanced WTC helps employees manage their workload and recovery by giving them influence over their daily work hours (e.g., being able to determine the length of the workday, start and finish times) and by having control over their time off (e.g., deciding when to take breaks, being able to run personal errands during work time, choosing when to take paid leave; Albrecht et al., 2016). Some of the clearest evidence of the beneficial effects of WTC is seen with regard to its impact on WLB (Nijp et al., 2012). There is also a growing body of evidence that WTC protects against mental ill-health, musculoskeletal disorders (Albrecht, Kecklund, & Leineweber, 2020), sleep disturbance (Salo et al., 2014), and accident risk (Tucker et al., 2016). WTC is also associated with reduced sickness absence (Albrecht, Leineweber, et al., 2020) and the voluntary postponement of retirement (Virtanen et al., 2014).

Enhanced WTC may be especially beneficial for some groups of workers; conversely, some workers may experience negative side effects. Women have been found to benefit from WTC more than men with respect to WLB and health, reflecting the greater level of family and household responsibilities undertaken by women in many societies (Nijp et al., 2012). However, there is also a risk that when women use WTC to take on more of these nonwork responsibilities, rather than using it to enhance recovery from strain, it may be harmful to their well-being. This is one example of a more general concern with enhanced WTC and other forms of flexible working: given the freedom to choose their own working arrangements, employees may make "unhealthy" choices that, for example, limit their opportunities for recovery. Such potentially unhealthy choices might include self-imposed long weekly work hours, or choosing to compress the working week into fewer longer shifts with limited breaks between shifts to facilitate longer periods of time off.

Employer-Oriented Work-Hours Flexibility and Work-Time Variability

The primary purpose of employer-oriented flexible work hours, or work-time variability (WTV), is to promote an organization's efficiency, performance, and accessibility to clients. It can place heavy demands on employees, such as requiring them to work long weekly hours, on weekends, and on call. This can result in the employee experiencing impaired recovery and sleep, disruption of WLB, and difficulties planning. This negative impact is likely to be exacerbated if the imposed work hours are often changing in a largely unpredictable manner. Hence WTV is associated with negative effects on subjective health, psychological well-being, sleep quality, and the experience of leisure time (Bohle et al., 2004, 2011; Janssen & Nachreiner, 2004; Martens et al., 1999).

WTV has become increasingly prevalent as a result of the increase in precarious work and associated working time arrangements such as zero-hour contracts, casual work, and on-call work. In these situations, WTV may coexist alongside some form of WTC. Where this is the case, the hours worked by the employee could reflect a negotiated process of meeting the requirements of the employee and the employer. However, in practice, variable work hours that are irregular and unpredictable are usually associated with poorer WLB and health (e.g., CVD, fatigue, and mental ill-health; Arlinghaus et al., 2019). Nevertheless, in situations where WTV and WTC do coexist, the negative effects of WTV on WLB and mental health can be offset by greater WTC (Bohle et al., 2011).

Teleworking: Effects and Moderators

Like WTC, allowing employees the possibility to work remotely (i.e., working elsewhere than the main workplace, such as at home) is generally associated with positive health outcomes, reduced absenteeism, and greater job satisfaction (Charalampous et al., 2019; Shifrin & Michel, 2021). Indeed, some of the observed positive effects of remote working may be due to the flexible work hours that are often (although not necessarily) synonymous with teleworking. The possibility to work from home is often regarded as a job perk, with employees expressing willingness to take a pay cut in order to be able to work remotely (Mas & Pallais, 2017). However, during the COVID-19 pandemic, large numbers of employees had remote working at home imposed upon them for the first time. This seismic shift from voluntary working at home, perhaps just for a few days a week, to mandatory full-time working from home highlighted some of the potential risks of remote working.

Teleworking is associated with longer work hours (Noonan & Glass, 2012) and the intensification of work activity (Kelliher & Anderson, 2010). Though potentially beneficial for productivity in the short term, this may have negative consequences for recovery and health. Teleworking employees may choose to work longer hours and more intensively (a) because they have opportunity to do so (e.g., choosing to work during the time that would otherwise have been spent commuting; being able to work without interruptions from colleagues), (b) as an act of reciprocation for being allowed to work flexibly, or (c) because they feel compelled to do so (Kelliher & Anderson, 2010). The latter motivation reflects the "always on" culture that is associated with the use of mobile information and communication technology for work. Especially when workloads are high and there are ambiguous expectations about work hours and goals, teleworkers may feel obliged to be available outside normal work hours (e.g., checking messages and taking phone calls), resulting in overwork (see also Chapter 12). Working after hours in this way may make it difficult for employees to psychologically detach from thoughts of work, such that work never stops. This prevents the employee from unwinding in the evenings, leading to increased stress, and the impairment of sleep and recovery. Moreover, working outside normal hours may lead to conflict between work and nonwork life, which could explain why teleworking is only relatively weakly associated with lower work–nonwork conflict, despite the possibilities it offers for managing WLB (Demerouti et al., 2014).

Teleworking often involves working physically apart from one's colleagues and clients, which can leave employees feeling isolated and lacking social support at work, with potentially negative consequences for their well-being and job engagement. While remote working has the potential to reduce distractions from coworkers in the workplace, it also reduces spontaneous interactions as well as the informal exchange of ideas and information with colleagues and clients (Charalampous et al., 2019).

One of the major ongoing debates about remote working that was reignited in the wake of the COVID-19 pandemic concerns the impact of remote working on productivity. Findings on the impact of flexible working on organizational outcomes have been mixed. One meta-analysis identified small positive associations between flexible working arrangements and self-reported productivity, performance, organizational commitment, and retention (Martin & MacDonell, 2012). However, a systematic review conducted around the same time concluded that the mixed evidence failed to demonstrate a business case for the use of FWAs (de Menezes & Kelliher, 2011). Several obstacles confront those attempting aggregate findings from this vast literature, including the wide and varied forms that FWAs take, as well as the influence of a range of moderating factors at the both the individual and organizational level (Allen et al., 2015).

Frequency of Teleworking

Prior to the COVID-19 pandemic, teleworking was rarely an all-or-nothing activity, with most teleworkers dividing their time between home working and days spent at their employer's premises. The extent to which an employee works away from the office moderates the impact of FWAs on a range of job-related outcomes (e.g., job satisfaction; Golden & Veiga, 2005). Many studies of teleworking have ignored this moderating factor, treating teleworking as a dichotomous variable, which has likely contributed to the diversity of findings in the field and some inappropriate conclusions being drawn (Allen et al., 2015). Few studies have focused on full-time teleworking, which calls into question the applicability of much of the current literature to the situation of employees who became teleworkers as a result of the COVID-19 pandemic.

Employees who engage in teleworking to a moderate degree report higher satisfaction, compared with those teleworking more or less frequently, suggesting a threshold in the extent of teleworking, beyond which there are diminishing returns, at least with respect to organizational outcomes (Golden & Veiga, 2005). This may reflect the social and professional isolation that teleworkers experience when spending much of their working lives away from the office (Allen et al., 2015). It remains to be established empirically whether a balance between teleworking and face-to-face working is also optimal with respect to health outcomes. A meta-analysis found that while quality of coworker relationships diminished above 2.5 days per week working away from the office, a higher frequency of teleworking was associated with improved work–family conflict (Gajendran & Harrison, 2007).

Individual Differences

We have already noted in the discussion of WTC that while FWAs can be particularly beneficial for women's health, there is a potential conflict if the flexibility is used to take on more nonwork responsibilities, thereby restricting opportunities for recovery. Accordingly, a small number of studies have found FWAs to be less beneficial, or more negative, for women than for men (Hall et al., 2019; Oakman et al., 2020). Personality, domestic circumstances, job competencies, and job characteristics are potential moderators of employees' experience of, and satisfaction with, teleworking (Allen et al., 2015; Charalampous et al., 2019). For example, teleworking has been found to be less suited to jobs with a high degree of interdependency among workers, where the need to rely on electronic communication may frustrate the rapid and efficient exchange of information (Golden & Veiga, 2005). Whether such barriers can be overcome with the development of richer and more immersive forms of communication technology (e.g., virtual reality) remains to be seen.

Availability and Use of Flexible Working Arrangements

There is an important distinction to be drawn between the *availability* of FWAs and the extent to which the flexibility is actually *used* by employees to vary the timing or location of their work. Two meta-analyses focusing on this distinction found that the availability of FWAs can be a stronger predictor of WLB (Allen et al., 2013) and physical health (Shifrin & Michel, 2021) than their actual use. This was interpreted as the availability of flexibility providing employees with a greater sense of autonomy, to the benefit of both WLB and stress-related health outcomes. Use of FWAs, on the other hand, may not always be beneficial if, for example, the organizational climate (e.g., attitude of coworkers and supervisors) is not supportive of the practice. When employees are given the opportunity to work flexibly, it is important that they are not inadvertently punished for doing so (e.g., by being regarded as insufficiently committed to the job and are hence overlooked for promotion). Supervisors may not always be predisposed to an FWA as it can present them with managerial challenges. For example, flexibility can impede communication and coordination with and between employees, which may thus require additional planning and implementation costs (Baltes et al., 1999). Another suggested explanation for the lack of positive effects of FWA usage is whether the flexibility is imposed (Allen et al., 2013), such as when many workers were compelled to work at home during the COVID-19 pandemic. This latter explanation highlights the importance of distinguishing between employee- and employer-oriented flexibility.

Implementation of Flexible Working Arrangements

Organizational and supervisory support for workers who choose to use FWAs is critical to its successful implementation. The lack of an employee's physical presence at the employer's premises should not mean that the employee is overlooked, or that they are expected to assume full responsibility for their own work-related health and safety. In addition, managers should take steps to avoid the "always on" culture associated with teleworking by promoting an appropriate balance between the use of communication technology that allows employees to be contactable 24/7 and employees' nonwork lives. Furthermore, given the risks of employees with FWAs choosing "unhealthy" FWAs (e.g., extending the workday into the evening), organizations could consider offering training on the importance of recovery, and teaching techniques to promote unwinding and psychologically detaching from thoughts about work in the evenings. Teleworkers may also benefit from skills training (e.g., in planning and self-regulatory behaviors) so that they can function effectively in an environment that provides them with a great deal of control (e.g., by helping employees focus on work tasks and ignore conflicting demands and cues; Allen et al., 2015).

The beneficial effects of a change to FWAs may take time to manifest themselves, as employees will need a period to adjust and acquire the appropriate skills and strategies to handle this new way of working. This was demonstrated by a meta-analysis which found that beneficial effects of teleworking on WLB and on role stress were only present among employees with more than 1 year's experience with teleworking (Gajendran & Harrison, 2007).

CONCLUSION

Shift work is necessary: Society depends on shift workers for the provision of essential (and nonessential) services outside "normal" working hours, and for its economic sustainability. This dependence on shift working entails health and safety risks—for the shift workers and for the wider public they serve. These risks can be mitigated by measures that seek to minimize the impact of disruption to shift workers' sleep and their circadian rhythms. FWAs that give workers discretion over when and where they work offer many potential benefits, but they also come with their own set of possible risks. However, if implemented and managed in the right way, FWAs have the potential to make working life more sustainable for many workers.

REFERENCES

Albrecht, S. C., Kecklund, G., & Leineweber, C. (2020). The mediating effect of work-life interference on the relationship between work-time control and depressive and musculoskeletal symptoms. *Scandinavian Journal of Work, Environment & Health, 46*(5), 469–479. https://doi.org/10.5271/sjweh.3887

Albrecht, S. C., Kecklund, G., Tucker, P., & Leineweber, C. (2016). Investigating the factorial structure and availability of work time control in a representative sample of the Swedish working population. *Scandinavian Journal of Public Health, 44*(3), 320–328. https://doi.org/10.1177/1403494815618854

Albrecht, S. C., Leineweber, C., Ojajärvi, A., Oksanen, T., Kecklund, G., & Härmä, M. (2020). Association of work-time control with sickness absence due to musculo-skeletal and mental disorders: An occupational cohort study. *Journal of Occupational Health, 62*(1), e12181. https://doi.org/10.1002/1348-9585.12181

Allen, T. D., Golden, T. D., & Shockley, K. M. (2015). How effective is telecommuting? Assessing the status of our scientific findings. *Psychological Science in the Public Interest, 16*(2), 40–68. https://doi.org/10.1177/1529100615593273

Allen, T. D., Johnson, R. C., Kiburz, K. M., & Shockley, K. M. (2013). Work–family conflict and flexible work arrangements: Deconstructing flexibility. *Personnel Psychology, 66*(2), 345–376. https://doi.org/10.1111/peps.12012

Arlinghaus, A., Bohle, P., Iskra-Golec, I., Jansen, N., Jay, S., & Rotenberg, L. (2019). Working Time Society consensus statements: Evidence-based effects of shift work and non-standard working hours on workers, family and community. *Industrial Health, 57*(2), 184–200. https://doi.org/10.2486/indhealth.SW-4

Baltes, B. B., Briggs, T. E., Huff, J. W., Wright, J. A., & Neuman, G. A. (1999). Flexible and compressed workweek schedules: A meta-analysis of their effects on work-related criteria. *Journal of Applied Psychology, 84*(4), 496–513. https://doi.org/10.1037/0021-9010.84.4.496

Bambra, C. L., Whitehead, M. M., Sowden, A. J., Akers, J., & Petticrew, M. P. (2008). Shifting schedules: The health effects of reorganizing shift work. *American Journal of Preventive Medicine, 34*(5), 427–434.e30. https://doi.org/10.1016/j.amepre.2007.12.023

Bjorvatn, B., Stangenes, K., Oyane, N., Forberg, K., Lowden, A., Holsten, F., & Åkerstedt, T. (2006). Subjective and objective measures of adaptation and readaptation to night work on an oil rig in the North Sea. *Sleep, 29*(6), 821–829. https://doi.org/10.1093/sleep/29.6.821

Bohle, P., Quinlan, M., Kennedy, D., & Williamson, A. (2004). Working hours, work-life conflict and health in precarious and "permanent" employment. *Revista de Saude Publica, 38*(Suppl.), 19–25. https://doi.org/10.1590/S0034-89102004000700004

Bohle, P., Willaby, H., Quinlan, M., & McNamara, M. (2011). Flexible work in call centres: Working hours, work-life conflict & health. *Applied Ergonomics, 42*(2), 219–224. https://doi.org/10.1016/j.apergo.2010.06.007

Boivin, D. B., Shechter, A., Boudreau, P., Begum, E. A., & Ng Ying-Kin, N. M. (2016). Diurnal and circadian variation of sleep and alertness in men vs. naturally cycling women. *Proceedings of the National Academy of Sciences of the United States of America, 113*(39), 10980–10985. https://doi.org/10.1073/pnas.1524484113

Bokenberger, K., Ström, P., Dahl Aslan, A. K., Åkerstedt, T., & Pedersen, N. L. (2017). Shift work and cognitive aging: A longitudinal study. *Scandinavian Journal of Work, Environment & Health, 43*(5), 485–493. https://doi.org/10.5271/sjweh.3638

Booker, L. A., Magee, M., Rajaratnam, S. M. W., Sletten, T. L., & Howard, M. E. (2018). Individual vulnerability to insomnia, excessive sleepiness and shift work disorder amongst healthcare shift workers: A systematic review. *Sleep Medicine Reviews, 41*, 220–233. https://doi.org/10.1016/j.smrv.2018.03.005

Brynjolfsson, E., Horton, J. J., Ozimek, A., Rock, D., Sharma, G., & TuYe, H. Y. (2020). *COVID-19 and remote work: An early look at US data* (No. w27344). National Bureau of Economic Research. https://doi.org/10.3386/w27344

Charalampous, M., Grant, C. A., Tramontano, C., & Michailidis, E. (2019). Systematically reviewing remote e-workers' well-being at work: A multidimensional approach. *European Journal of Work and Organizational Psychology, 28*(1), 51–73. https://doi.org/10.1080/1359432X.2018.1541886

Costa, G., & Di Milia, L. (2008). Aging and shift work: A complex problem to face. *Chronobiology International, 25*(2), 165–181. https://doi.org/10.1080/07420520802103410

de Cordova, P. B., Bradford, M. A., & Stone, P. W. (2016). Increased errors and decreased performance at night: A systematic review of the evidence concerning shift work and quality. *Work, 53*(4), 825–834. https://doi.org/10.3233/WOR-162250

de Menezes, L. M., & Kelliher, C. (2011). Flexible working and performance: A systematic review of the evidence for a business case. *International Journal of Management Reviews, 13*(4), 452–474. https://doi.org/10.1111/j.1468-2370.2011.00301.x

Demerouti, E., Derks, D., ten Brummelhuis, L. L., & Bakker, A. B. (2014). New ways of working: Impact on working conditions, work–family balance, and well-being. In C. Korunka & P. Hooakker (Eds.), *The impact of ICT on quality of working life* (pp. 123–141). Springer Science+Business Media. https://doi.org/10.1007/978-94-017-8854-0_8

Devore, E. E., Grodstein, F., & Schernhammer, E. S. (2013). Shift work and cognition in the Nurses' Health Study. *American Journal of Epidemiology, 178*(8), 1296–1300. https://doi.org/10.1093/aje/kwt214

Eurofound, & ILO. (2019). *Working conditions in a global perspective.* Publications Office of the European Union and International Labour Organization.

Ferguson, S. A., & Dawson, D. (2012). 12-h or 8-h shifts? It depends. *Sleep Medicine Reviews, 16*(6), 519–528. https://doi.org/10.1016/j.smrv.2011.11.001

Fillit, H., Nash, D. T., Rundek, T., & Zuckerman, A. (2008). Cardiovascular risk factors and dementia. *The American Journal of Geriatric Pharmacotherapy, 6*(2), 100–118. https://doi.org/10.1016/j.amjopharm.2008.06.004

Fischer, D., Lombardi, D. A., Folkard, S., Willetts, J., & Christiani, D. C. (2017). Updating the "Risk Index": A systematic review and meta-analysis of occupational injuries and work schedule characteristics. *Chronobiology International, 34*(10), 1423–1438. https://doi.org/10.1080/07420528.2017.1367305

Folkard, S. (2008). Do permanent night workers show circadian adjustment? A review based on the endogenous melatonin rhythm. *Chronobiology International, 25*(2), 215–224. https://doi.org/10.1080/07420520802106835

Gajendran, R. S., & Harrison, D. A. (2007). The good, the bad, and the unknown about telecommuting: Meta-analysis of psychological mediators and individual consequences. *Journal of Applied Psychology, 92*(6), 1524–1541. https://doi.org/10.1037/0021-9010.92.6.1524

Gao, Y., Gan, T., Jiang, L., Yu, L., Tang, D., Wang, Y., Li, X., & Ding, G. (2020). Association between shift work and risk of Type 2 diabetes mellitus: A systematic review and dose-response meta-analysis of observational studies. *Chronobiology International, 37*(1), 29–46. https://doi.org/10.1080/07420528.2019.1683570

Garbarino, S., Mascialino, B., Penco, M. A., Squarcia, S., De Carli, F., Nobili, L., Beelke, M., Cuomo, G., & Ferrillo, F. (2004). Professional shift-work drivers who adopt prophylactic naps can reduce the risk of car accidents during night work. *Sleep, 27*(7), 1295–1302. https://doi.org/10.1093/sleep/27.7.1295

Garde, A. H., Begtrup, L., Bjorvatn, B., Bonde, J. P., Hansen, J., Hansen, A. M., Härmä, M., Jensen, M. A., Kecklund, G., Kolstad, H. A., Larsen, A. D., Lie, J. A., Moreno, C. R., Nabe-Nielsen, K., & Sallinen, M. (2020). How to schedule night shift work in order to reduce health and safety risks. *Scandinavian Journal of Work, Environment & Health, 46*(6), 557–569. https://doi.org/10.5271/sjweh.3920

Golden, T. D., & Veiga, J. F. (2005). The impact of extent of telecommuting on job satisfaction: Resolving inconsistent findings. *Journal of Management, 31*(2), 301–318. https://doi.org/10.1177/0149206304271768

Hall, A. L., Kecklund, G., Leineweber, C., & Tucker, P. (2019). Effect of work schedule on prospective antidepressant prescriptions in Sweden: A 2-year sex-stratified analysis using national drug registry data. *BMJ Open, 9*(1), e023247. https://doi.org/10.1136/bmjopen-2018-023247

Härmä, M. (1996). Ageing, physical fitness and shiftwork tolerance. *Applied Ergonomics, 27*(1), 25–29. https://doi.org/10.1016/0003-6870(95)00046-1

Hittle, B. M., & Gillespie, G. L. (2018). Identifying shift worker chronotype: Implications for health. *Industrial Health, 56*(6), 512–523. https://doi.org/10.2486/indhealth.2018-0018

Janssen, D., & Nachreiner, F. (2004). Health and psychosocial effects of flexible working hours. *Revista de Saúde Pública, 38*(Suppl. 1), 11–18. https://doi.org/10.1590/S0034-89102004000700003

Jørgensen, J. T., Rozing, M. P., Westendorp, R. G. J., Hansen, J., Stayner, L. T., Simonsen, M. K., & Andersen, Z. J. (2021). Shift work and incidence of psychiatric disorders: The Danish Nurse Cohort study. *Journal of Psychiatric Research, 139*, 132–138. https://doi.org/10.1016/j.jpsychires.2021.05.045

Kecklund, G., & Axelsson, J. (2016). Health consequences of shift work and insufficient sleep. *BMJ, 355*, i5210. https://doi.org/10.1136/bmj.i5210

Kelliher, C., & Anderson, D. (2010). Doing more with less? Flexible working practices and the intensification of work. *Human Relations, 63*(1), 83–106. https://doi.org/10.1177/0018726709349199

Kervezee, L., Shechter, A., & Boivin, D. B. (2018). Impact of shift work on the circadian timing system and health in women. *Sleep Medicine Clinics, 13*(3), 295–306. https://doi.org/10.1016/j.jsmc.2018.04.003

Knutsson, A., & Åkerstedt, T. (1992). The healthy-worker effect: Self-selection among Swedish shift workers. *Work and Stress, 6*(2), 163–167. https://doi.org/10.1080/02678379208260350

Kossek, E. E., Lautsch, B. A., & Eaton, S. C. (2006). Telecommuting, control, and boundary management: Correlates of policy use and practice, job control, and work–family effectiveness. *Journal of Vocational Behavior, 68*(2), 347–367. https://doi.org/10.1016/j.jvb.2005.07.002

Krantz-Kent, R. (2019). *Where did workers perform their jobs in the early 21st century?* U.S. Bureau of Labor Statistics. https://www.bls.gov/opub/mlr/2019/article/where-did-workers-perform-their-jobs.htm

Leso, V., Caturano, A., Vetrani, I., & Iavicoli, I. (2021). Shift or night shift work and dementia risk: A systematic review. *European Review for Medical and Pharmacological Sciences, 25*(1), 222–232. https://doi.org/10.26355/eurrev_202101_24388

Liira, J., Verbeek, J. H., Costa, G., Driscoll, T. R., Sallinen, M., Isotalo, L. K., & Ruotsalainen, J. H. (2014). Pharmacological interventions for sleepiness and sleep disturbances caused by shift work. *Cochrane Database of Systematic Reviews, 8*, CD009776. Advance online publication. https://doi.org/10.1002/14651858.CD009776.pub2

Linton, S. J., Kecklund, G., Franklin, K. A., Leissner, L. C., Sivertsen, B., Lindberg, E., Svensson, A. C., Hansson, S. O., Sundin, Ö., Hetta, J., Björkelund, C., & Hall, C. (2015). The effect of the work environment on future sleep disturbances: A systematic review. *Sleep Medicine Reviews, 23*, 10–19. https://doi.org/10.1016/j.smrv.2014.10.010

Loudoun, R. J., Muurlink, O., Peetz, D., & Murray, G. (2014). Does age affect the relationship between control at work and sleep disturbance for shift workers? *Chronobiology International, 31*(10), 1190–1200. https://doi.org/10.3109/07420528.2014.957307

Lowden, A., Moreno, C., Holmbäck, U., Lennernäs, M., & Tucker, P. (2010). Eating and shift work–effects on habits, metabolism and performance. *Scandinavian Journal of Work, Environment & Health, 36*(2), 150–162. https://doi.org/10.5271/sjweh.2898

Lowden, A., Öztürk, G., Reynolds, A., & Bjorvatn, B. (2019). Working Time Society consensus statements: Evidence based interventions using light to improve circadian adaptation to working hours. *Industrial Health, 57*(2), 213–227. https://doi.org/10.2486/indhealth.SW-9

Marquié, J. C., Tucker, P., Folkard, S., Gentil, C., & Ansiau, D. (2015). Chronic effects of shift work on cognition: Findings from the VISAT longitudinal study. *Occupational and Environmental Medicine, 72*(4), 258–264. https://doi.org/10.1136/oemed-2013-101993

Martens, M. F. J., Nijhuis, F. J. N., Van Boxtel, M. P. J., & Knottnerus, J. A. (1999). Flexible work schedules and mental and physical health. A study of a working population with non-traditional working hours. *Journal of Organizational Behavior, 20*(1), 35–46. https://doi.org/10.1002/(SICI)1099-1379(199901)20:1<35::AID-JOB879>3.0.CO;2-Z

Martin, B. H., & MacDonell, R. (2012). Is telework effective for organizations? A meta-analysis of empirical research on perceptions of telework and organizational outcomes. *Management Research Review, 35*(7), 602–616. https://doi.org/10.1108/01409171211238820

Mas, A., & Pallais, A. (2017). Valuing alternative work arrangements. *The American Economic Review, 107*(12), 3722–3759. https://doi.org/10.1257/aer.20161500

Milasi, S., Gonzalez-Vazquez, I., & Fernandes-Macias, E. (2020). *Telework in the EU before and after the COVID-19: Where we were, where we head to.* European Commission. https://ec.europa.eu/jrc/sites/default/files/jrc120945_policy_brief_-_covid_and_telework_final.pdf

Nijp, H. H., Beckers, D. G., Geurts, S. A., Tucker, P., & Kompier, M. A. (2012). Systematic review on the association between employee worktime control and work–non-work balance, health and well-being, and job-related outcomes. *Scandinavian Journal of Work, Environment & Health, 38*(4), 299–313. https://doi.org/10.5271/sjweh.3307

Noonan, M. C., & Glass, J. L. (2012). The hard truth about telecommuting. *Monthly Labor Review, 135*(6), 38–45.

Oakman, J., Kinsman, N., Stuckey, R., Graham, M., & Weale, V. (2020). A rapid review of mental and physical health effects of working at home: How do we optimise health? *BMC Public Health, 20*(1), 1825. https://doi.org/10.1186/s12889-020-09875-z

Puttonen, S., Härmä, M., & Hublin, C. (2010). Shift work and cardiovascular disease–pathways from circadian stress to morbidity. *Scandinavian Journal of Work, Environment & Health, 36*(2), 96–108. https://doi.org/10.5271/sjweh.2894

Ruggiero, J. S., & Redeker, N. S. (2014). Effects of napping on sleepiness and sleep-related performance deficits in night-shift workers: A systematic review. *Biological Research for Nursing, 16*(2), 134–142. https://doi.org/10.1177/1099800413476571

Saksvik, I. B., Bjorvatn, B., Hetland, H., Sandal, G. M., & Pallesen, S. (2011). Individual differences in tolerance to shift work—A systematic review. *Sleep Medicine Reviews, 15*(4), 221–235. https://doi.org/10.1016/j.smrv.2010.07.002

Salo, P., Ala-Mursula, L., Rod, N. H., Tucker, P., Pentti, J., Kivimäki, M., & Vahtera, J. (2014). Work time control and sleep disturbances: Prospective cohort study of Finnish public sector employees. *Sleep, 37*(7), 1217–1225. https://doi.org/10.5665/sleep.3842

Shifrin, N. V., & Michel, J. S. (2021). Flexible work arrangements and employee health: A meta-analytic review. *Work and Stress, 35*(1), 60–85. https://doi.org/10.1080/02678373.2021.1936287

Spira, A. P., Gamaldo, A. A., An, Y., Wu, M. N., Simonsick, E. M., Bilgel, M., Zhou, Y., Wong, D. F., Ferrucci, L., & Resnick, S. M. (2013). Self-reported sleep and β-amyloid deposition in community-dwelling older adults. *JAMA Neurology, 70*(12), 1537–1543. https://doi.org/10.1001/jamaneurol.2013.4258

Torquati, L., Mielke, G. I., Brown, W. J., Burton, N. W., & Kolbe-Alexander, T. L. (2019). Shift work and poor mental health: A meta-analysis of longitudinal studies. *American Journal of Public Health, 109*(11), e13–e20. https://doi.org/10.2105/AJPH.2019.305278

Torquati, L., Mielke, G. I., Brown, W. J., & Kolbe-Alexander, T. (2018). Shift work and the risk of cardiovascular disease. A systematic review and meta-analysis including dose–response relationship. *Scandinavian Journal of Work, Environment & Health, 44*(3), 229–238. https://doi.org/10.5271/sjweh.3700

Tucker, P., Albrecht, S., Kecklund, G., Beckers, D. G., & Leineweber, C. (2016). Work time control, sleep & accident risk: A prospective cohort study. *Chronobiology International*, 33(6), 619–629. https://doi.org/10.3109/07420528.2016.1167723

Tucker, P., Folkard, S., Ansiau, D., & Marquié, J. C. (2011). The effects of age and shift-work on perceived sleep problems: Results from the VISAT combined longitudinal and cross-sectional study. *Journal of Occupational and Environmental Medicine*, 53(7), 794–798. https://doi.org/10.1097/JOM.0b013e318221c64c

Vedaa, Ø., Harris, A., Bjorvatn, B., Waage, S., Sivertsen, B., Tucker, P., & Pallesen, S. (2016). Systematic review of the relationship between quick returns in rotating shift work and health-related outcomes. *Ergonomics*, 59(1), 1–14. https://doi.org/10.1080/00140139.2015.1052020

Vetter, C., Fischer, D., Matera, J. L., & Roenneberg, T. (2015). Aligning work and circadian time in shift workers improves sleep and reduces circadian disruption. *Current Biology*, 25(7), 907–911. https://doi.org/10.1016/j.cub.2015.01.064

Viitasalo, K., Puttonen, S., Kuosma, E., Lindström, J., & Härmä, M. (2015). Shift rotation and age–interactions with sleep–wakefulness and inflammation. *Ergonomics*, 58(1), 65–74. https://doi.org/10.1080/00140139.2014.958573

Virtanen, M., Oksanen, T., Batty, G. D., Ala-Mursula, L., Salo, P., Elovainio, M., Pentti, J., Lybäck, K., Vahtera, J., & Kivimäki, M. (2014). Extending employment beyond the pensionable age: A cohort study of the influence of chronic diseases, health risk factors, and working conditions. *PLOS ONE*, 9(2), e88695. https://doi.org/10.1371/journal.pone.0088695

Wang, F., Zhang, L., Zhang, Y., Zhang, B., He, Y., Xie, S., Li, M., Miao, X., Chan, E. Y., Tang, J. L., Wong, M. C., Li, Z., Yu, I. T., & Tse, L. A. (2014). Meta-analysis on night shift work and risk of metabolic syndrome. *Obesity Reviews*, 15(9), 709–720. https://doi.org/10.1111/obr.12194

Wennberg, A. M. V., Wu, M. N., Rosenberg, P. B., & Spira, A. P. (2017). Sleep disturbance, cognitive decline, and dementia: A review. *Seminars in Neurology*, 37(4), 395–406. https://doi.org/10.1055/s-0037-1604351

11

Nonstandard Work Arrangements

Regina Pana-Cryan, John Howard, and Tim Bushnell

There are several types of work arrangements between those who perform work and those who provide jobs. Standard arrangements continue to be the most prevalent, but the prevalence of some types of nonstandard arrangements seem to be increasing. While there are no commonly accepted definitions for all types of work arrangements, and they are typically understudied in the occupational health psychology literature, evidence continues to build on the different ways they affect the safety, health, and well-being of workers. This chapter reviews the definitions, classification, and prevalence of nonstandard work arrangements and related concepts. It also provides a curated literature review on their impact on healthy work design and worker well-being, in addition to their role in the future of work.

DEFINITIONS AND CLASSIFICATION OF WORK ARRANGEMENTS

The lack of commonly accepted definitions of work arrangements affects the ability to accurately assess prevalence estimates of work arrangement types and, in turn, work design and worker well-being research findings based on these estimates. To help clarify this issue, we provide an overview of a two-tiered approach to classify work arrangements. The first tier is a legal approach to classifying employed, coemployed, and nonemployee workers (e.g., independent

This chapter was coauthored by employees of the United States (U.S.) government as part of official duty and is considered to be in the public domain. Any views expressed herein do not necessarily represent the views of the U.S. government, and the authors' participation in the work is not meant to serve as an official endorsement.

https://doi.org/10.1037/0000331-011

Handbook of Occupational Health Psychology, Third Edition, L. E. Tetrick, G. G. Fisher, M. T. Ford, and J. C. Quick (Editors)
In the public domain.

contractors or businesspersons). The second-tier approach is based on important characteristics of all work arrangements that vary by arrangement (e.g., earnings security). Unless otherwise mentioned, we discuss workers' main job, on which most data sources collect information.

First, we discuss the legal first-tier approach used to establish employment, described in detail by Howard (2017) and summarized here. In the standard (industrial model) work arrangement type, the employer controls the manner and means by which the worker provides services; this legally establishes the employment relationship (Estreicher et al., 2015, Chapter 1, Section 1.01). The employer is legally responsible for protecting the safety and health of employees. The main types of nonstandard arrangements in this first-tier approach include agency, contract, and gig arrangements. In an agency arrangement, employees are hired by an agency labor supplier for time-limited work assignments at the premises of another employer. The staffing agency-based temporary help services arrangement is a type of coemployment or joint employment arrangement (Cappelli & Keller, 2013), with the two employers sharing legal responsibility for protecting the safety and health of employees (Occupational Safety and Health Administration & National Institute for Occupational Safety and Health [NIOSH], 2015). Workers in contract work arrangements are independent contractors or businesspersons rather than employees and are excluded from federal labor law protections (Muhl, 2002). In this arrangement, the payer controls or directs only the result of the work and not what will be done and how it will be done (Internal Revenue Service, 2016) and the worker provides services to a firm through a business rather than an employment relationship (Estreicher et al., 2015, Chapter 1, Section 1.01). Advances in digital technology gave rise to work intermediated by digital online platforms. Workers in this type of arrangement are often referred to as app-based, platform, or gig workers. Here and unless otherwise noted, we define gig workers as those who provide work intermediated by digital platforms. These workers are typically classified as independent contractors, but many of them may be misclassified employees. Note that there is no commonly accepted definition of "gig worker." For example, the U.S. Bureau of Labor Statistics (BLS) has no official definition of gig workers and acknowledges that "researchers use many different definitions, many of which are likely to include electronically mediated workers" (BLS, 2018d). While jobs obtained through an online platform may be the most commonly cited example of gig work, the term *gig work* is often used more broadly to refer to jobs that are of relatively short duration, often limited to a specific project or task.

Several household surveys use a similar first-tier approach to broadly classify workers as employed, coemployed, or nonemployees when considering their main job. An important example is the Contingent Worker Supplement (CWS) of the Current Population Survey (CPS), administered by the BLS. CWS uses several questions to classify an individual's type of work arrangement and defines the following nonstandard (or alternative) arrangements (see https://www.bls.gov/cps/contingent-and-alternative-arrangements-faqs.htm#alternative):

- *Temporary help agency workers*—Workers who were paid by a temporary help agency, whether or not their job was temporary

- *Workers provided by contract firms*—Workers who are employed by a company that provides them or their services to others under contract and who are usually assigned to only one customer and usually work at the customer's worksite

- *Independent contractors*—Workers who were identified as independent contractors, independent consultants, or freelance workers, whether they were self-employed or wage and salary workers

- *On-call workers*—Workers who are called to work only as needed, although they can be scheduled to work for several days or weeks in a row

A recent National Academies of Sciences, Engineering, and Medicine (NASEM) report provided recommendations for improving the CWS measurement of nonstandard work arrangements (NASEM, 2020). The report mentioned that, to reduce misclassification and distinguish independent contractors from business operators, CWS asks self-employed workers: "Are you self-employed as an independent contractor, independent consultant, freelance worker, or something else (such as a shop or restaurant owner)?" In addition, CWS asks wage and salary workers: "Last week, were you working as an independent contractor, an independent consultant, or a freelance worker? That is, someone who obtains customers on their own to provide a product or service" (BLS, 2018c). Accordingly, the types of arrangements used by CWS identify whether a worker is an employee of the organization for whom he or she is performing work and allow the classification of a respondent's main job into one of several mutually exclusive categories:

- employees, not in a nonstandard work arrangement

- workers in intermediated arrangements, including
  - temporary agency workers
  - contract firm workers, other than agency workers

- those who are not employees or are self-employed
  - independent contractors
  - self-employed, not independent contractors

The NASEM report also claimed that while the CWS question that asks wage and salary workers whether they work on an on-call or day laborer basis (i.e., only when needed) addresses the temporariness of the relationship between employer and employee, it also addresses the degree of earnings security. The report concluded that the degree of earnings security is a characteristic of all work arrangements. This is consistent with our including it in the second-tier classification approach.

Finally, the NASEM report stated that on-demand platform (gig) work, captured only in the 2017 CWS (BLS, 2018b), was a hybrid of contract firm and independent contractor arrangements, and that there was policy and research interest in distinguishing between gig workers who were W-2 employees and gig workers who were in self-employment or nonemployee arrangements.

Beyond the CWS, other surveys, such as the General Social Survey (GSS) and its Quality of Worklife Supplement (QWL), as well as the National Health Interview Survey (NHIS) and its Occupational Health Supplement (OHS; data are currently available from 2010 and 2015), use similar but not identical first-tier definitions of work arrangement types (see https://gss.norc.org/Pages/quality-of-worklife.aspx and https://www.cdc.gov/niosh/topics/nhis/questions.html). For example, the QWL module of GSS, started in 2002 and conducted every 4 years since, has been assessing work arrangement type in the main job using the following responses to a single question: I work as an independent contractor, independent consultant, or freelance worker; I am on call and work only when called to work; I am paid by a temporary agency; I work for a contractor who provides workers and services to others under contract; and I am a regular permanent employee (in a standard work arrangement). NHIS[BT(4]-OHS also has only used a similar, single question to determine work arrangement types. However, GSS-QWL and NHIS-OHS also collect additional data that relate to characteristics of work that may be considered defining aspects of work arrangements within our second-tier approach, including the safety, health, and well-being of workers.

The second tier of our approach to classify work arrangements uses basic characteristics of both standard and nonstandard arrangements that are recognized as important determinants of worker well-being, including by NASEM (2020) and NIOSH (https://www.cdc.gov/niosh/about/strategicplan/; Bushnell et al., 2017). These characteristics include job security, work schedule, compensation type, earnings level and security, and benefits. Nonstandard work arrangements are a priority focus area for NIOSH, the only federal agency whose mission focuses on worker safety and health research, through its Healthy Work Design and Well-Being Program (https://www.cdc.gov/niosh/programs/hwd/default.html).

To better understand work arrangements, it is important to understand related concepts including contingent work and work precariousness. CWS uses three definitions to construct estimates of the number of contingent workers, listed as follows in order from narrowest to broadest (https://www.bls.gov/cps/contingent-and-alternative-arrangements-faqs.htm):

- wage and salary workers who expect their jobs will last for an additional year or less and who had worked at their jobs for 1 year or less

- workers, including the self-employed and independent contractors, who expect their employment to last for an additional year or less and who had worked at their jobs (or been self-employed) for 1 year or less

- workers who do not expect their jobs to last

While there is no standardized definition of *work precariousness*, its characteristics include insecurity; temporariness; vulnerability to unfair treatment; lack of ability to negotiate pay, benefits, and work schedule; lack of ability to take leave; and lack of a social safety net including unemployment and workers' compensation insurance (Bhattacharya & Ray, 2021; Bushnell et al., 2017; Vives et al., 2010).

Information on jobs other than the worker's main one (second and third jobs) is also important to collect in order to understand work arrangements and worker well-being. Definitions of multiple jobholders may vary among sources. For example, the U.S. Census Bureau's Longitudinal Employer-Household Dynamics (LEHD), a longitudinally linked employer–employee administrative data set created by the U.S. Census Bureau, defines a multiple jobholder as anyone who holds two or more jobs in a quarter and at least one of these jobs "is a long-lasting, stable job," that is, "held in the previous, current, and following quarters" (Bailey & Spletzer, 2020). In addition to understanding all the jobs held by a worker, it is also important to understand all the jobs held within a household (NASEM, 2020). For example, access to benefits by one household member might also enable access to benefits by another household member. Note that unless otherwise mentioned, we do not consider the unemployed and we use the term *agency workers* in lieu of *temporary help agency workers*.

PREVALENCE OF NONSTANDARD WORK ARRANGEMENTS

As discussed in the previous section, estimates of the size of the nonstandard workforce are based on data collected in different years and using different definitions and methods, making occupational safety and health surveillance and research challenging (Government Accountability Office [GAO], 2015; Howard, 2017). NASEM (2020) provided specific recommendations for improving CWS estimates that may also apply to other surveys, including the length of reference periods and the related underreporting of some types of arrangements (e.g., gig). In this section, we provide prevalence estimates of workers in different work arrangements, contingent workers, workers experiencing work precariousness, and multiple jobholders. We also provide selected work arrangement prevalence estimates by worker demographics.

Table 11.1 presents the prevalence of nonstandard work arrangements using CWS data from multiple years during 1995–2017 and the 2015 RAND–Princeton

TABLE 11.1. Workers in Nonstandard Work Arrangements as a Percentage of Workers in all Arrangements, CWS, 1995-2017, and RPCWS, 2015

Work arrangement type	CWS						RPCWS, 2015	
	1995	1997	1999	2001	2005	2017	Initial estimate	Revised estimate, 2019
Agency workers	1.0	1.0	0.9	0.9	0.9	0.9	1.6	1.7
Contract firm workers	0.5	0.6	0.6	0.5	0.6	0.6	3.1	2.5
Independent contractors	6.7	6.7	6.3	6.4	7.4	6.9	8.4	7.2
On-call workers	1.7	1.6	1.5	1.6	1.8	1.7	2.6	2.4
Total	9.9	9.9	9.3	9.4	10.7	10.1	15.8	13.7

Note. CWS = Contingent Worker Supplement; RPCWS = RAND–Princeton Contingent Work Survey. Data from Bureau of Labor Statistics (BLS; 2001a): CWS (1995, 1997, 1999); BLS (2001b): CWS (2001); BLS (2005): CWS (2005); Katz and Krueger (2016, 2019): RPCWS (2015); BLS (2018a): CWS (2017).

Contingent Work Survey (RPCWS; Katz & Krueger, 2016). According to CWS, the overall prevalence of nonstandard work arrangements increased from 9.9% in 1995 to 10.7% in 2005, decreasing to 10.1% in 2017. Even though RPCWS was based on CWS, the definitions of work arrangements by these two surveys were slightly different. RPCWS-based estimates showed that 15.8% of workers were in nonstandard work arrangements in 2015, up from the 10.7% 2005 CWS-based estimate (Katz & Krueger, 2016). However, CWS-based estimates in 2017 (BLS, 2018a) were lower than those from 2005, suggesting no increase in the prevalence of nonstandard arrangements. Subsequently, Katz and Krueger (2019) examined potential causes of this discrepancy, revised their overall prevalence estimate downward to 13.7% (shown in the last column of Table 11.1), and adjusted BLS estimates upward (not included in Table 11.1) to make them more comparable to their revision, and concluded that there likely had been a modest upward trend in the share of the U.S. workforce in nonstandard work arrangements during 2000–2017.

Findings based on 2002–2018 GSS-QWL data (presented in Table 11.2) show a higher percentage of workers in nonstandard arrangements than CWS but corroborate CWS-based findings in that the total percentage of workers in nonstandard work arrangements has not significantly changed in recent years. Alterman et al. (2013) used similar survey items and data from the 2010 NHIS-OHS survey, estimating that 18.7% of U.S. workers were in nonstandard arrangements, compared with the 21.1% estimated by Ray et al. (2017), based on 2010 GSS-QWL data. Considering the CWS, RPCWS, GSS-QWL, and NHIS-OHS estimates discussed here, and the difficulty of deriving work arrangement prevalence estimates from surveys, the prevalence of nonstandard work arrangements likely ranged from 9.3% (1999 CWS) to 21.1% (2010 GSS-QWL) during 1995–2018.

RPCWS also included questions on gig work obtained through online intermediaries. Based on responses to these questions, 0.5% of workers were working through online intermediaries in 2015 (Katz & Krueger, 2016). Smith (2016) used 2016 Pew Research Center data and estimated that 8% of Americans earned money from online gig platforms in the previous year; of that 8%, 29%, or 2% of all workers, said that income from their gig work

TABLE 11.2. Workers in Nonstandard Work Arrangements as a Percentage of Workers in all Arrangements, GSS-QWL, 2002–2018

Work arrangement type	Year				
	2002	2006	2010	2014	2018
Agency workers	0.8	1.2	1.4	0.6	1.6
Contract firm workers	2.4	3.5	2.7	3.1	3.5
Independent contractors	14.0	13.9	13.4	14.2	12.2
On-call workers	2.3	2.5	3.6	2.9	2.9
Total	19.5	21.1	21.1	20.8	20.1

Note. GSS-QWL = General Social Survey-Quality of Worklife Supplement. Data from Ray et al. (2017): GSS-QWL (2002, 2006, 2010, 2014); Ray and Pana-Cryan (2021): GSS-QWL (2018).

was essential to meeting their basic needs. Data from the 2017 CWS indicated that electronically mediated workers accounted for 1% of all workers (BLS, 2018a). However, BLS noted that these questions did not capture information as intended, and consequently NASEM (2020) provided BLS recommendations for improved measurement. Based on the RPCWS, Pew Research Center, and CWS estimates we discussed and considering the difficulty of deriving work arrangement prevalence estimates from surveys, the prevalence of electronically mediated work likely ranged from 0.5% to 8% during 2015–2017.

CWS data indicated a downward trend in the prevalence of contingent workers between 1995 and 2017, regardless of which of the three alternative definitions of *contingent worker* was used (estimate 1 from 2.2% to 1.3%, estimate 2 from 2.8% to 1.6%, and estimate 3 from 4.9% to 3.8%; BLS, 2001b, 2001c, 2005, 2018a). Using the 2017 CWS data and the broadest contingent worker estimate 3, the percentage of workers in nonstandard arrangements who also were classified as contingent workers ranged from 3.2% for independent contractors to 42% for agency workers. In addition, 1.0% to 1.3% of workers in standard arrangements reported being contingent in 2017 (BLS, 2018a).

To generate a scale to measure work precariousness, Bhattacharya and Ray (2021) used GSS-QWL 2002–2014 data. The scale, inspired by the Employment Precariousness Scale (Vives et al., 2010), included four precariousness components: (a) temporariness, (b) disempowerment, (c) vulnerability, and (d) wages.[1] Agency workers reported the highest percentage of high work precariousness (62.6%), while independent contractors reported high work precariousness least frequently (22.5%) and less often than did workers in standard arrangements (33.5%).

In addition to understanding the prevalence of work arrangement types, it is important to assess the distribution of work arrangements by gender, age, race and ethnicity, and education. According to CWS, in 2017, the population of agency workers had the highest percentages of 16- to 24-year-old men (8.9% and 8.5%, respectively) and women (7.4% and 5.8%, respectively) followed by on-call workers. Independent contractors had the highest percentage of White workers (84.6%) and agency workers the highest percentage of Hispanic workers (25.4%). Agency workers reported the lowest percentage of having a bachelor's degree or above (26.3%; BLS, 2018a).

---

[1]Temporariness included job security, salaried or wage earner status, and job tenure. Disempowerment included ability to make decisions, ability to change job schedule, union membership, relationship between management and workers, having enough help and equipment to get the job done, mandatory overtime, and opportunity to develop one's own special abilities. Vulnerability included respect at the workplace, trust toward management, job conditions that allow worker to be productive, age discrimination, race discrimination, and workers and management working together to ensure safe working conditions. Wages included satisfaction with family financial situation, personal income level, satisfaction with family income, fringe benefits, and chances for promotion.

To measure multiple jobholding, Bailey and Spletzer (2020) used LEHD data and found that the percentage of workers with more than one job increased from the second quarter of 1996 to the first quarter of 2018. During this period, the seasonally adjusted quarterly time series of the multiple job-holding rate (i.e., the number of multiple jobholders in a quarter divided by the total number of workers) increased from 6.8% to 7.8%. The authors pointed out that their findings differed from those derived from other data sources, such as, for example, CPS that uses household survey data and showed that the rate has been declining. They mentioned that the rate rose during economic expansions and fell during recessions, and that women held multiple jobs at a higher rate than men. For men the rate did not change much over the last 20 years, increasing from 6.3% to 6.6%, but for women the rate increased from 7.5% to 9.1%. The authors concluded that holding multiple jobs was more important in the U.S. economy than the CPS data had showed.

WORK DESIGN AND WORKER WELL-BEING

In this section, we focus on organizational characteristics, psychosocial working conditions, work–life balance, earnings and benefits, flexibility, and prefer-ence for types of work arrangement by workers in different arrangements (including gig workers and multiple jobholders). While findings depend on the data sources used, considering these findings together provides some gen-eral understanding of potential trends and opportunities for improvements in work design that, in turn, could improve worker well-being. We then discuss selected recent findings on worker well-being.

Work Design

Using 2002–2014 GSS-QWL data, Ray et al. (2017) examined the association of work arrangement with a variety of organizational and other work charac-teristics. They concluded that occupation, industry, hours of work and shift type, and part-time or full-time status were significantly associated with work arrangement. Thirty-nine percent of independent contractors and 36% of workers in standard arrangements were in management occupations. The highest percentages of contract firm workers worked in the construction (34%) and services (31%) industry sectors. Over half of on-call workers worked in services (52%), while the highest percentages of agency workers worked in services (35%) and manufacturing (32%). Compared with other arrange-ment groups, a higher percentage of independent contractors (33%) worked more than 49 hours per week. Independent contractors also reported the highest percentage of irregular schedules (30%). Of all on-call workers, 44.7% reported working full-time on average from 2002–2014, compared with 85% of workers in standard arrangements and lower than in other non-standard arrangements. According to 2017 CWS data, the percentage of on-call workers working full-time was somewhat higher, at 55.4%, and a lower per-centage of on-call workers worked full-time compared with workers in other arrangements (BLS, 2018a).

Some of the psychosocial working conditions and work–life balance indi-cators assessed by Ray et al. (2017) were significantly associated with work arrangement. Agency workers reported the highest percentages of being overworked and working very fast, and the lowest percentages of having lots of say about what happens on the job, freedom to decide how they do their work, job security, good benefits, as well as safe and healthy workplace con-ditions. However, agency workers also reported the lowest percentage of family matters interfering with work. Independent contractors reported the lowest percentage of working very fast and the highest percentages of having control over what happens on the job, freedom to decide how they do their work, as well as safe and healthy workplace conditions. On-call workers also reported the lowest percentage of working very fast—the same percentage reported by independent contractors—and the highest percentage of family matters interfering with work. Workers in standard arrangements reported the highest percentages of having job security and good benefits.

Next, we assess earnings levels and access to specific benefits. CWS data from 2017 demonstrated that among full-time workers, agency workers reported the lowest median usual weekly earnings ($521). Agency workers also reported the lowest percentage of having health insurance coverage (67.35%), followed by independent contractors (75.4%), and eligibility for an employer-provided pension or retirement plan (12.7%), followed by on-call workers (35.4%; BLS, 2018a).

Tsai et al. (2019) used 2015 NHIS-OHS data and examined how the avail-ability of and participation in workplace health promotion programs (WHPPs) varied by work arrangement. WHPP availability was highest for workers in stan-dard arrangements (49.2%), followed by agency and contract firm workers com-bined (26.9%), independent contractors (22.2%), and other workers (21.5%). Of those who reported WHPP availability, workers in standard arrangements reported the highest participation (57.4%), followed by independent contractors (49.4%), other (47.9%), and agency and contract firm workers combined (38.7%). Findings pointed to opportunities for improving participation that could potentially improve worker physical and mental health.

Based on 2017 CWS data, worker preferences for type of work arrange-ment demonstrated that 79.1% of independent contractors preferred their arrangement, while 43.8% of on-call workers and 38.5% of agency workers preferred their arrangements over a standard arrangement (BLS, 2018a).

In terms of multiple jobholding, Bailey and Spletzer (2020) used LEHD data and reported that during the period from the second quarter of 1996 to the first quarter of 2018, most multiple jobs were found in a few industries, with the percentage of second jobs being 16.8% in health care and social assistance, 16.7% in accommodation and food services, 14.5% in retail trade, and 10.8% in administrative and support and waste management and remediation services. Workers who were not multiple jobholders earned, on average, $15,750 from their full-quarter job in the first quarter of 2018. Workers who were multiple jobholders and had full-quarter jobs earned an average $9,770 from their primary job in the first quarter of 2018 and an average $3,780 from all secondary jobs during that same quarter, for a total of $13,550 from all jobs. This means that, on average, earnings from secondary jobs accounted for 28% of a multiple jobholder's total earnings. The authors mentioned that this earnings differential was due to age, gender, and the industries that employ multiple jobholders. Using different data from a special module of the 2016 and 2017 Survey of Household Economics and Decisionmaking, Abraham and Houseman (2019) found that over the course of a month, more than one-quarter of adults engaged in some "informal" work outside of a main job, including as independent contractors. The authors concluded that informal work was an important source of household income, including for independent contractors, but could not compensate for the lack of benefits typical of independent contractor work.

Work flexibility is yet another term with no standardized definition, but common work-flexibility types include being able to work at home, take time off when needed, and change one's work schedule. Given the ongoing changes in and increasing importance of work flexibility, Ray and Pana-Cryan (2021) used 2002–2018 GSS-QWL data and found that when compared with those in other nonstandard work arrangements, independent contractors reported the highest percentage of access to all three types of flexibility (13.7%). Considering each type of flexibility for all arrangements, a higher percentage of on-call workers reported being able to change their schedule, but a lower percentage of those workers reported being able to work at home than those in standard arrangements. Agency workers reported the lowest percentages of access to each of the three flexibility types.

Next, we compare flexibility statistics from two different BLS sources, the American Time Use Survey (ATUS; BLS, 2023) and CPS (BLS, 2022), before and during the ongoing COVID-19 pandemic. According to ATUS, changes in the percentages of workers working at home between the period of May–December 2019 and the period of May–December 2020 varied by gender: women reported an increase from 25.9% to 49.3% and men reported an increase from 19.7% to 35.5%. Comparing May 2020, July 2021, and August 2021 data from CPS showed that in each of the selected months, women teleworked or worked at home more than men, but the percentages of both men and women with this type of flexibility decreased from May 2020 to July 2021 and remained relatively stable in August 2021.

The ability to work at home has been especially important for workers during the ongoing pandemic. According to April and May 2020 data from the COVID Impact Survey (Wozniak et al., 2020), of those who continued to work during the pandemic, many were unable to work remotely. In addition to being less exposed to infection, those working remotely were better able to preserve their economic security. In the period examined, 57% of those in households earning more than $125,000 per year reported working remotely, but only 19% of those in households earning less than

$60,000 per year reported having this ability (Pana-Cryan et al., 2020). This points to the need to understand the interrelated elements of work design and their implications, including overlapping vulnerabilities experienced by some workers and their families.

To better understand work design aspects of platform-based gig workers, we looked for potential evidence of a pay gap between men and women as well as workers' characteristics and preferences for portable benefits that move with them as they change jobs. Using January 2016–June 2017 data from CloudResearch, an online microtask platform connecting employers to workers who perform research-related tasks, Litman et al. (2020) found that, on average, women's hourly earnings were 10.5% lower than men's and highlighted the need to identify possible causes of this gap. Using proprietary data on Canadian gig economy workers (who included both workers who provide work interme- diated by digital online platforms and other gig workers) from a 2021 survey, Advanis (2021) clarified the characteristics and needs of freelance and gig workers roles. In this survey, freelance workers doing higher-paid professional work were distinguished from gig workers doing lower-paid relatively low- skilled work. Compared with gig workers, more freelancers were men with a college degree, higher income, and living in urban areas versus gig workers who connected with clients via an internet platform but performed more manual tasks. The percentage of freelancers and gig workers who desired, but did not have, a consistent income, health insurance coverage, or employer- funded retirement plans ranged from 40% to 64% (e.g., 64% of gig workers desired consistent income). In addition, 77% of freelancers and 68% of gig workers reported desiring some form of portable benefits.

Worker Well-Being

Howard (2017) provided references and summarized findings published in the previous 20 years about the health and safety risks for workers in non- standard work arrangements, contingent workers, and workers in arrange- ments with work precariousness characteristics. Here we build on these findings by highlighting several studies that have been published since 2017.

A comparative analysis of injury risks among agency workers and workers in standard arrangements used Ohio workers' compensation data on claims of injury during 2001–2013 and concluded that agency workers had higher injury rates in addition to lower lost-time and medical costs. Differences were pronounced for certain industries and injury events. These findings along with mostly similar findings from other studies using workers' compensation data from the states of Washington and Illinois point to opportunities for prevention (Al-Tarawneh et al., 2020).

Ray et al. (2017) assessed the association between job stress and well-being by work arrangement, using 2002–2014 GSS-QWL data. Descriptive analyses demonstrated that contract firm workers reported the highest percentage of pre- viously injured workers (14%) and agency workers the lowest (3%). On-call workers reported the highest percentage in general good health in the last year

(80%), followed by independent contractors (74%), agency workers (67%), and contract firm workers (66%). On-call workers were the least frequently stressed (20%) and contract firm workers were the most frequently stressed (34%). Independent contractors reported job satisfaction most frequently (94%) and agency workers least frequently (73%). Regression analyses demonstrated that work arrangement was an important risk factor for perceived job stress. Independent contractors (odds ratio [OR] = 0.71) and on-call workers (OR = 0.71) had significantly lower odds of reporting job stress compared with workers in standard arrangements. Stressed workers were at higher risk of experiencing unhealthy days (defined as the number of days in poor physical and mental health within the last 30 days), and the strength of association between job stress and unhealthy days varied by work arrangement. The relative risk of experiencing unhealthy days (incidence) among workers in standard arrangements and independent contractors was almost twice as high for those with job stress compared with those without job stress. In standard arrangements, stressed workers had almost double the risk of experiencing days with activity limitations due to health problems compared with nonstressed workers. Among agency workers, those who were stressed were 5 times more likely to experience days with activity limitations compared with nonstressed workers.

Kang et al. (2019) investigated work-related factors that contribute to early retirement due to ill health (ERIH) among middle-aged and elderly individuals using a sample from a Korean longitudinal survey conducted biennially from 2006 to 2014. Work-related factors included work arrangements, physical working conditions, and job satisfaction. The authors found no significant associations among women. However, the risk for ERIH in men was significantly higher among those with high physical demands, awkward posture, dissatisfaction with the working environment, and no industrial compensation insurance or retirement benefits.

The level, time trend, and variability of earnings are all important for worker well-being. Access to benefits is also important for the well-being of workers and their families. Both access to paid sick leave and the ability to take time off for doctor visits affect the health care of children (Asfaw and Colopy, 2017). Access to paid sick leave also is positively associated with a lower probability of spread of infectious disease at work (Asfaw et al., 2017) and suffering an occupational injury (Asfaw et al., 2012).

Bhattacharya and Ray (2021) assessed work precariousness, job stress, and well-being using 2002–2014 GSS-QWL data. As mentioned previously, the study generated a work precariousness scale and examined the associations among work precariousness scores derived by this scale and job stress, unhealthy days, and days with activity limitations due to health problems. The authors found a significant positive association between job stress and work precariousness. Workers reporting work precariousness were likely to experience more unhealthy days and more days with activity limitations due to health problems.

Two recent studies used European Working Conditions Survey (EWCS) data to assess associations between work arrangements and well-being.

Julià et al. (2019) used 2010 data to estimate the contribution of different contract arrangements (i.e., permanent, temporary, and informal) and working and employment precariousness variables on health outcomes, including psychosocial well-being and self-rated health. Findings included that the prevalence of informal employment among salaried employees was 4% among men and 5% among women; poor working conditions and employment precariousness varied by type of contract arrangement, with the best conditions observed among permanent employees and the worst among informal employees; and there was no evidence that health outcomes varied by type of contract arrangement. The authors noted that theirs was the first study to characterize working and employment conditions of informal employees, their precariousness, and the relationship with health outcomes in the context of high-income countries, and to compare them to other arrangements.

The second study (Reuter at al., 2020) used 2010 and 2015 EWCS data to assess the associations between precarious employment and unwanted sexual attention (UWSA) and precarious employment and sexual harassment (SH), which are prevalent experiences for working women and often accompanied by poor health. The authors assessed precarious employment using seven indicators and an index they derived from them: (a) temporary employment, (b) contractual duration of less than 1 year, (c) schedule unpredictability, (d) involuntary part-time work, (e) low information on occupational safety and health (OSH) risks, (f) low pay, and (g) holding multiple jobs. UWSA was reported in the previous month by 0.8% of men and 2.6% of women. SH in the previous year was reported by 0.4% of the men and 1.3% of the women in the study. For both men and women, precariousness was significantly associated with elevated prevalence of UWSA and SH, especially when reporting schedule unpredictability, low information on OSH risks, and holding multiple jobs.

Ray and Pana-Cryan (2021) assessed the association of well-being and flexibility indicators measured as workers' ability to work at home, take time off when needed, or change one's schedule, using 2002–2018 GSS-QWL data. The authors measured well-being using job stress, job satisfaction, healthy days (measured as unhealthy days subtracted from the previous 30 days), and days with activity limitations. The ability to work at home increased the likelihood of job stress by 22% and job satisfaction by 65%. The ability to take time off when needed decreased the likelihood of job stress by 56% and days with activity limitations by 24%, and more than doubled the likelihood of job satisfaction. The ability to change one's schedule decreased the likelihood of job stress by 20% and increased the likelihood of job satisfaction by 62%.

Two recent European studies reported on flexibility and worker well-being. The first, by Rodríguez-Modroño and López-Igual (2021), assessed the effect of telework on different dimensions of job quality using 2015 EWCS data. Findings showed that occasional teleworkers reported the best job quality, while highly mobile teleworkers reported the worst job quality and work–life balance. Compared with highly mobile workers, home-based teleworkers, especially women, reported better working-time quality and intensity but also lower skills and discretion, income, and career prospects. The second study (Vanajan et al., 2020) used data on older workers (60–65 years) in the Netherlands to assess the effect of flexibility (i.e., working-time flexibility, workplace flexibility, phased retirement) and organizational climate (i.e., healthy aging climate, psychologically safe climate) on health-related work limitations among workers experiencing chronic health conditions. These findings demonstrated that access to flexible working hours and a psychologically safe organizational climate was associated with fewer health-related work limitations among older workers with chronic health conditions. This implies that offering flexible working hours and ensuring a psychologically safe climate in which older workers with health issues are inclined to share their work needs and preferences are likely to contribute to healthy aging in the workplace.

WORK ARRANGEMENTS AND THE FUTURE OF WORK

In this section, we summarize the main points from the previous sections, identify research, policy, and practice gaps, and discuss the role of work arrangements in the future of work. We have addressed the need for standardized definitions and classification of work arrangements. We described a two-tiered approach to define and classify work arrangements and discussed related concepts that included contingent work and work precariousness. Using findings from different surveys, we concluded that the overall prevalence of nonstandard work arrangements did not increase, and the prevalence of contingent workers decreased, over the past 20 years. We discussed findings from selected studies examining specific aspects of work arrangements, work precariousness, multiple jobholding, and flexibility, as well as their association with specific indicators of work design and well-being. Job stress was an important determinant of other well-being outcomes (e.g., days with activity limitations due to health problems) for workers in all work arrangements, with stressed workers faring worse than non-stressed workers across arrangements.

Overall, workers in standard arrangements did not consistently fare better than others, except with regard to access to benefits. Agency workers fared worse than others in many aspects of work design and well-being, while independent contractors fared better than others, including those in standard arrangements, and most often reported a preference for their arrangement. Those working at home had access to an important type of flexibility and positive well-being outcomes but also reported more frequent work–life imbalance. While not all gig economy workers are similar in terms of demographics, work design, and well-being, one survey indicated that 40% or more of them reported not having but desiring a consistent income and access to health and retirement benefits (Advanis, 2021).

While there is a wealth of challenges to resolve and specific findings to explore further, we have mentioned the relatively new findings on the importance of secondary jobs for the overall earnings of multiple jobholders along with evidence of increasing multiple jobholding rates for women and a gender pay gap among gig workers. These findings support the need to further explore and address disparities in earnings and benefits, which are important determinants of worker and family well-being.

Highlighting the importance of access to benefits, there are several proposals for benefits that move with workers as they change jobs. We summarize some aspects of the proposals by Lehrer (2016) and the Aspen Institute (Reder et al., 2019) as examples of plans that place different emphases on private and public sector roles. Lehrer proposed enabling a gig economy (which would include both workers who provide work intermediated by digital online platforms and other gig workers) that allows more opportunities for part-time work for those who cannot or will not work full-time. He suggested four main policy changes: (a) reducing professional-licensing mandates, (b) creating a new employment status called the "flexible worker," (c) recognizing a new type of employer called a "job platform," and (d) developing a mostly private social safety-net system made up of worker-controlled benefits exchanges (WCBEs) to provide a minimum level of social protection to these flexible workers. Flexible workers would have civil-rights protections, access to state and federal worker protections to ensure that platforms pay them as promised for work, and control over their own hours and conditions of work. While flexible workers would not receive most of the fringe benefits of standard employers or collect unemployment insurance, a safety net would consist of the new WCBEs. The new product provided through WCBEs would provide a replacement-income stream, a type of insurance that would replace unemployment insurance, sick leave, and some aspects of workers' compensation for platforms that remain outside the workers' compensation system. Similar to unemployment and private disability insurance, the amount of replacement income would be pegged to a percentage of earnings but would be portable, individualized, and privately funded but regulated like other insurance products.

Reder et al. (2019) advocated for a new system of effective benefits that are portable (connected to the worker not the employer), prorated (provided according to the work performed), and universal (accessible to workers regardless of their work arrangement). These benefits would aim to improve worker and household financial security, create more equity among workers in standard and nonstandard arrangements, and result in a more dynamic labor market. Examples of programs that provide portable, prorated, and increasingly universal benefits are the Social Security program and the Affordable Care Act. Reder et al. (2019) provided specific examples of proposed new state-based systems or expanding existing and emerging government programs to allow participation by all workers. Social insurance programs, like paid family and medical leave or unemployment insurance, and savings programs, like state-facilitated retirement accounts, can be expanded to serve more workers.

Additional challenges include the need to

- improve surveillance methods to include emerging determinants of well-being such as increased flexibility for workers and organizations;

- assess the effects of evolving advanced technologies and worker demographics on work arrangements;

- assess the effects of work arrangement types and characteristics over the span of a working life, considering all jobs held simultaneously, the sequence of jobs, and periods of unemployment, in addition to the work arrangements of other household members;

- determine barriers and aids to implementing cost-effective safety and health programs for workers in nonstandard work arrangements;

- conduct intervention studies to assess the cost- and comparative-effectiveness of programs and trainings to improve the well-being of workers in non-standard arrangements;

- assess potential work arrangement-related and additional overlapping vulnerabilities experienced by workers in specific demographic groups; and

- conduct systems research on how macro-level external factors such as economic conditions or climate change may affect all types of work arrangements.

NIOSH efforts to advance research on work arrangements include plans currently being implemented to address research gaps identified by the Healthy Work Design and Well-Being Cross-Sector Council (https://www.cdc.gov/nora/councils/hwd/), ongoing research aiming to address related strategic goals (https://www.cdc.gov/niosh/about/strategicplan/), and the development of a strategic plan for the Future of Work Initiative (https://www.cdc.gov/niosh/topics/future-of-work/default.html) that includes an emphasis on work arrangements. Efforts to improve surveillance on work arrangements include data currently being collected by the NHIS-OHS with support from NIOSH. The 2021 NHIS-OHS questions (National Center for Health Statistics, 2022) ask about whether employers deduct or withhold taxes from pay (to ascertain employee versus independent contractor status), the magnitude of month-to-month changes in earnings, usual shift (e.g., day, evening, night), ability to change work schedule, frequency of changes in work schedule on the part of supervisors, advance knowledge of work schedule, and the likelihood of losing one's job in the next year. Information from this data collection can guide data collection by other surveys such as GSS-QWL and can be analyzed in combination with well-being indicators (NASEM, 2020). Given the findings and ongoing and emerging challenges discussed, additional research on the issues presented in this chapter could aim to improve work design and arrangements that will in turn improve the well-being of workers in all work arrangements.

REFERENCES

Abraham, K. G., & Houseman, S. N. (2019). Making ends meet: The role of informal work in supplementing Americans' income. *The Russell Sage Foundation Journal of the Social Sciences: RSF, 5*(5), 110–131. https://doi.org/10.7758/rsf.2019.5.5.06

Advanis. (2021). *Searching for well-being and financial stability in the Canadian gig economy* [Infographic]. https://f.hubspotusercontent40.net/hubfs/19523297/Gig%20Economy%20Canada%20Infographic.pdf

Al-Tarawneh, I. S., Wurzelbacher, S. J., & Bertke, S. J. (2020). Comparative analyses of workers' compensation claims of injury among temporary and permanent employed workers in Ohio. *American Journal of Industrial Medicine, 63*(1), 3–22. https://doi.org/10.1002/ajim.23049

Alterman, T., Luckhaupt, S. E., Dahlhamer, J. M., Ward, B. W., & Calvert, G. M. (2013). Prevalence rates of work organization characteristics among workers in the U.S.: Data from the 2010 National Health Interview Survey. *American Journal of Industrial Medicine, 56*(6), 647–659. https://doi.org/10.1002/ajim.22108

Asfaw, A., & Colopy, M. (2017). Association between parental access to paid sick leave and children's access to and use of healthcare services. *American Journal of Industrial Medicine, 60*(3), 276–284. https://doi.org/10.1002/ajim.22692

Asfaw, A., Pana-Cryan, R., & Rosa, R. (2012). Paid sick leave and nonfatal occupational injuries. *American Journal of Public Health, 102*(9), e59–e64. https://doi.org/10.2105/AJPH.2011.300482

Asfaw, A., Rosa, R., & Pana-Cryan, R. (2017). Potential economic benefits of paid sick leave in reducing absenteeism related to the spread of influenza-like illness. *Journal of Occupational and Environmental Medicine, 59*(9), 822–829. https://doi.org/10.1097/JOM.0000000000001076

Bailey, K. A., & Spletzer, J. R. (2020). *A new measure of multiple jobholding in the U.S. economy* (Discussion Paper CES 20–26). U.S. Census Bureau, Center for Economic Studies. https://www2.census.gov/ces/wp/2020/CES-WP-20-26.pdf

Bhattacharya, A., & Ray, T. (2021). Precarious work, job stress, and health-related quality of life. *American Journal of Industrial Medicine, 64*(4), 310–319. https://doi.org/10.1002/ajim.23223

Bureau of Labor Statistics. (2001a). *Characteristics of and preference for alternative work arrangements, 1999.* https://www.bls.gov/opub/mlr/2001/03/art2full.pdf

Bureau of Labor Statistics. (2001b). *Contingent and alternative employment arrangements, February 2001.* https://www.bls.gov/news.release/history/conemp_05242001.txt

Bureau of Labor Statistics. (2001c). *Contingent work in the late-1990s.* https://www.bls.gov/opub/mlr/2001/03/art1full.pdf

Bureau of Labor Statistics. (2005). *Contingent and alternative employment arrangements, February 2005.* https://www.bls.gov/news.release/archives/conemp_07272005.pdf

Bureau of Labor Statistics. (2018a). *Contingent and alternative employment arrangements—May 2017* [Press release]. https://www.bls.gov/news.release/pdf/conemp.pdf

Bureau of Labor Statistics. (2018b). *Electronically mediated work: New questions in the Contingent Worker Supplement.* https://www.bls.gov/opub/mlr/2018/article/electronically-mediated-work-new-questions-in-the-contingent-worker-supplement.htm

Bureau of Labor Statistics. (2018c). *Labor Force Statistics from the Current Population Survey – Frequently asked questions about data on contingent and alternative employment arrangements.* https://www.bls.gov/cps/contingent-and-alternative-arrangements-faqs.htm#alternative

Bureau of Labor Statistics. (2018d). *Labor Force Statistics from the Current Population Survey – Frequently asked questions about data on electronically mediated employment.* https://www.bls.gov/cps/electronically-mediated-employment-faqs.htm#gig

Bureau of Labor Statistics. (2022, November 2). *Labor force statistics from the Current Population Survey: Effects of the coronavirus COVID-19 pandemic (CPS).* https://www.bls.gov/cps/effects-of-the-coronavirus-covid-19-pandemic.htm

Bureau of Labor Statistics. (2023, June 22). *American Time Use Survey—2022 results* [Press release]. https://www.bls.gov/news.release/pdf/atus.pdf

Bushnell, T., Scharf, T., Alterman, T., Cummings, K. J., Luckhaupt, S. E., Ray, T. K., Rosa, R. R., & Su, C. P. (2017, June 8). *Developing a taxonomy of work arrangements to examine relationships with worker safety, health, and well-being* [Poster presentation]. Work, Stress, and Health Conference, Minneapolis, MN, United States. https://www.bls.gov/news.release/pdf/conemp.pdf

Cappelli, P., & Keller, J. R. (2013). Classifying work in the new economy. *Academy of Management Review, 38*(4), 575–596. https://doi.org/10.5465/amr.2011.0302

Estreicher, S., Bodie, M. T., Harper, M. C., & Schwab, S. J. (2015). *Restatement of the Law: Employment Law.* American Law Institute. https://www.ali.org/publications/show/employment-law/#_tab-volumes

Howard, J. (2017). Nonstandard work arrangements and worker health and safety. *American Journal of Industrial Medicine, 60*(1), 1–10. https://doi.org/10.1002/ajim.22669

Internal Revenue Service. (2016). Independent contractor defined. https://www.irs.gov/businesses/small-businesses-self-employed/independent-contractor-defined

Julià, M., Belvis, F., Vives, A., Tarafa, G., & Benach, J. (2019). Informal employees in the European Union: Working conditions, employment precariousness and health. *Journal of Public Health, 41*(2), e141–e151. https://doi.org/10.1093/pubmed/fdy111

Kang, M. Y., Myong, J. P., & Kim, H. R. (2019). Job characteristics as risk factors for early retirement due to ill health: The Korean Longitudinal Study of Aging (2006–2014). *Journal of Occupational Health, 61*(1), 63–72. https://doi.org/10.1002/1348-9585.12014

Katz, L. F., & Krueger, A. B. (2016). The rise and nature of alternative work arrangements in the United States, 1995–2015. *National Bureau of Economic Research.* https://scholar.harvard.edu/files/lkatz/files/katz_krueger_cws_v3.pdf?m=1459369766

Katz, L. F., & Krueger, A. B. (2019). Understanding trends in alternative work arrangements in the United States. *National Bureau of Economic Research.* https://www.nber.org/papers/w25425.pdf

Lehrer, E. (2016). The future of work. *National Affairs.* https://www.nationalaffairs.com/publications/detail/the-future-of-work

Litman, L., Robinson, J., Rosen, Z., Rosenzweig, C., Waxman, J., & Bates, L. M. (2020). The persistence of pay inequality: The gender pay gap in an anonymous online labor market. *PLOS ONE, 15*(2), e0229383. https://doi.org/10.1371/journal.pone.0229383

Muhl, C. J. (2002). What is an employee? The answer depends on federal law. *Monthly Labor Review,* 3–11. https://www.bls.gov/opub/mlr/2002/01/art1full.pdf

National Academies of Sciences, Engineering, and Medicine (NASEM). (2020). *Measuring alternative work arrangements for research and policy.* The National Academies Press. https://doi.org/10.17226/25822

National Center for Health Statistics. (2022, August 8). *National Health Interview Survey: 2021 NHIS.* Centers for Disease Control and Prevention.

Pana-Cryan R., Ray T. K., Bushnell T., & Quay, B. (2020). Economic security during the COVID-19 pandemic: A healthy work design and well-being perspective. *NIOSH Science Blog.* https://blogs.cdc.gov/niosh-science-blog/2020/06/22/economic-security-covid-19/

Occupational Safety and Health Administration, & National Institute for Occupational Safety and Health. (2015). *Protecting temporary workers.* https://www.cdc.gov/niosh/docs/2014-139/pdfs/2014-139.pdf

Ray, T. K., Kenigsberg, T. A., & Pana-Cryan, R. (2017). Employment arrangement, job stress, and health-related quality of life. *Safety Science 100*(Pt. A), 46–56. https://doi.org/10.1016/j.ssci.2017.05.003

Ray, T. K., & Pana-Cryan, R. (2021). Work flexibility and work-related well-being. *International Journal of Environmental Research and Public Health, 18*(6), 3254. https://doi.org/10.3390/ijerph18063254

Reder, L., Steward, S., & Foster, N. (2019). *Designing portable benefits: A resource guide for policymakers*. The Aspen Institute Future of Work Initiative. https://www.aspeninstitute. org/publications/designing-portable-benefits/

Reuter, M., Wahrendorf, M., Di Tecco, C., Probst, T. M., Chirumbolo, A., Ritz-Timme, S., Barbaranelli, C., Iavicoli, S., & Dragano, N. (2020). Precarious employment and self-reported experiences of unwanted sexual attention and sexual harassment at work. An analysis of the European Working Conditions Survey. *PLOS ONE, 15*(5), e0233683. https://doi.org/10.1371/journal.pone.0233683

Rodríguez-Modroño, P., & López-Igual, P. (2021). Job quality and work–life balance of teleworkers. *International Journal of Environmental Research and Public Health, 18*(6), 3239. https://doi.org/10.3390/ijerph18063239

Smith, A. (2016). *Gig work, online selling and home sharing*. Pew Research Center. https:// www.pewinternet.org/2016/11/17/gig-work-online-selling-and-home-sharing/

Tsai, R., Alterman, T., Grosch, J. W., & Luckhaupt, S. E. (2019). Availability of and participation in workplace health promotion programs by sociodemographic, occupation, and work organization characteristics in US workers. *American Journal of Health Promotion, 33*(7), 1028–1038. https://doi.org/10.1177/0890117119844478

U.S. Government Accountability Office. (2015). *Contingent workforce: Size, characteristics, earnings, and benefits* (GAO Publication No. GAO-15-168R). https://gao.gov/assets/ 670/669899.pdf

Vanajan, A., Bültmann, U., & Henkens, K. (2020). Health-related work limitations among older workers—the role of flexible work arrangements and organizational climate. *The Gerontologist, 60*(3), 450–459. https://doi.org/10.1093/geront/gnz073

Vives, A., Amable, M., Ferrer, M., Moncada, S., Llorens, C., Muntaner, C., Benavides, F. G., & Benach, J. (2010). The Employment Precariousness Scale (EPRES): Psychometric properties of a new tool for epidemiological studies among waged and salaried workers. *Occupational and Environmental Medicine, 67*(8), 548–555. https://doi.org/ 10.1136/oem.2009.048967

Wozniak, A., Willey, J., Benz, J., & Hart, N. (2020). *COVID Impact Survey* (Version 1) [Data set]. National Opinion Research Center, University of Chicago. https://www. covid-impact.org/results

12

Sleep and Fatigue in Occupational Health Psychology Research

Larissa K. Barber and Christopher J. Budnick

Sleep is an important activity that affects how people function in their day-to-day lives. Without good sleep, at work we can be emotionally reactive, unfocused, and unable to perform well (Banks & Dinges, 2007; Zohar et al., 2005). For this reason, researchers have been building a case for why companies should be interested in how employee sleep impacts job behaviors due to fatigue (Barnes & Watson, 2019; Mullins et al., 2014). Sleep issues are the most influential cause of work fatigue, especially 24 to 48 hours before employee work shifts (Dawson & McCulloch, 2005; Techera et al., 2016). Poor sleep is implicated in a diverse set of work problems, such as poorer work performance, unsafe work behaviors, lower work engagement, and more intentions to leave the organization (Henderson & Horan, 2021; Litwiller et al., 2017)

In this chapter, we cover sleep and fatigue from an occupational health psychology (OHP) perspective with an emphasis on psychological processes among employees in field research (for reviews on physiological sleep processes, see Carskadon & Dement, 2005; Techera et al., 2016). We first provide an overview of common applied assessments of work fatigue and sleep concepts in organizational research. We then examine organizational strategies for addressing employee sleep and work fatigue issues, including organizational risk factors detrimental to sleep managing work fatigue arising from poor sleep during nonwork hours. We also discuss considerations for future research in each area.

https://doi.org/10.1037/0000331-012

Handbook of Occupational Health Psychology, Third Edition, L. E. Tetrick, G. G. Fisher, M. T. Ford, and J. C. Quick (Editors)

UNDERSTANDING SLEEP AND WORK FATIGUE IN ORGANIZATIONAL RESEARCH

Applied research in organizations often emphasizes psychological processes when studying work fatigue and sleep from an OHP perspective. This section covers common conceptualizations and assessments of work fatigue and sleep, as well as the link between them.

Conceptualizing and Assessing Work Fatigue

Work fatigue is important to organizations, as it is one of the top three drivers of health care and productivity costs, right behind back/neck pain and depression (Loeppke et al., 2007). Meta-analysis research also shows higher work fatigue is associated with lower job performance in terms of in-role tasks, helping others at work, and customer satisfaction (Taris, 2006). It is therefore of no surprise that fatigue is a key concept in many occupational stress theories linking work demands to performance and long-term well-being.

The concept of work fatigue represents a low-energy state of exhaustion or tiredness that reduces one's capacity to function well on the job (Frone & Tidwell, 2015). As a psychophysiological state, it contains a mix of low physiological energy but also includes a lack of motivational effort (Meijman & Mulder, 1998; Zijlstra et al., 2014). In other words, fatigue cannot be solely understood as a lack of physical energy or ability to exert effort; it is essentially an emotionally driven psychological state that results in reduced motivation to allocate remaining energy to work goals and tasks (see Hockey, 2013). This framing is important for applied researchers in OHP because it is often practically difficult to disentangle physiological ability for workers to exert effort (i.e., what an employee can do) from motivational preferences to conserve their energy (i.e., what an employee is willing to do) when observing behavioral work outcomes associated with fatigue.

Many researchers conceptualize work fatigue as a short-term stress response (i.e., acute strain) arising from work demands, an expected part of the stress process that rest and recovery can overcome. However, long-term or chronic work fatigue that occurs with prolonged exposure to work demands without sufficient recovery is often of concern for long-term employee health and well-being (Meijman & Mulder, 1998; Van Dijk & Swaen, 2003). For example, meta-analysis research shows that work fatigue is associated with more errors, injuries, and physical illness (Techera et al., 2016). A longitudinal research review suggests that work fatigue increases sickness absences over time (Sagherian et al., 2019) and is central to many poor well-being outcomes associated with stress, such as work burnout and depression (Van Dijk & Swaen, 2003).

Work fatigue is assessed with self-report measures that range from general experiences of fatigue adapted from state mood or affective well-being measures (e.g., Michielsen et al., 2003; van Hooff et al., 2007) to multidimensional approaches assessing typical fatigue experiences at the end of the workday (see Table 12.1). For example, one measure distinguishes between acute and chronic

TABLE 12.1. Work Fatigue Measurement Examples in Occupational Health Psychology

General fatigue	Multidimensional fatigue
The Fatigue Assessment Scale	Three-dimensional work fatigue inventory
(Michielsen et al., 2003)	(Frone & Tidwell, 2015)
• Mentally, I feel exhausted. • I am bothered by fatigue.	• Physical—I feel physically exhausted at the end of the workday. • Mental—I feel mentally worn out at the end of the workday. • Emotional—I want to emotionally shut down at the end of the workday.
Single-Item Fatigue Measure	The occupational fatigue exhaustion/recovery scale
(Van Hooff et al., 2007)	(Winwood et al., 2005)
• How fatigued do you currently feel?	• Chronic work fatigue—I often feel at the end of my rope with work. • Acute work fatigue—I have plenty of reserve energy when I need it. • Recovery between work periods—I don't get enough time between work shifts to recover my energy fully.

Note. Examples are not intended to be comprehensive.

fatigue (Windwood et al., 2005). Another multidimensional approach distinguishes between physical, mental, and emotional aspects of extreme tiredness and low functional capacity at the end of the workday (Frone & Tidwell, 2015). Specifically, work fatigue can manifest as difficulties engaging in physical work tasks, problems concentrating on mental tasks, and challenges with managing emotions arising from interacting with others at work.

Approaches to conceptualizing and measuring work fatigue often overlap with other commonly studied strain concepts in occupational health research. One similar concept is the work exhaustion or emotional exhaustion components of work burnout. Chronic fatigue or exhaustion is a critical component of work burnout, with other work attitudes or beliefs such as low professional efficacy and cynicism (Maslach et al., 1996) or disengagement (Demerouti et al., 2003) included as a holistic assessment of the work burnout syndrome. Yet other burnout measures focus only on general work exhaustion (e.g., Kristensen et al., 2005) and multidimensional aspects of exhaustion (physical, cognitive, and emotional; e.g., Shirom & Melamed, 2006) have stronger similarities to work fatigue.

Conceptualizing and Assessing Employee Sleep in Organizational Research

Sleep is a complex and dynamic process during which individuals display a reversible state of disengagement from their surroundings (Carskadon & Dement, 2005). Sleep seems critical for replenishing physiological and cognitive functions needed to regulate how we think, feel, and behave (Barnes,

2012; Gordon et al., 2017). Ultimately a physiological process, much basic sleep research explores sleep "cycles." These include different sleep stages (e.g., rapid eye movement) within nightly sleep experiences and aspects of the daily sleep/wake cycle (circadian rhythms) that explain alertness variations over a 24-hour period (Carskadon & Dement, 2005).

Applied occupational health research, however, often focuses on three key sleep proxies used to infer whether individuals experienced a productive or replenishing sleep process (see Table 12.2). These include sleep duration (sleep quantity), the number of disturbances during sleep (sleep quality), and the desire to fall asleep (sleepiness). Popular self-report questionnaires that include both sleep-quality (often one item) and sleep-quantity assessments (one item and multi-item) are the Karolinska Sleep Diary and the Pittsburgh Sleep Quality Index. Sleepiness can be measured with multiple items using the Epworth Sleepiness Scale or one item using the Stanford Sleepiness Scale (for a review of these and other measures, see Pilcher et al., 2012).

For sleep quality and quantity during nonwork hours, wrist-worn actigraphy devices that measure movements are used to assess sleep objectively (Sadeh, 2011). Applied researchers have widely adopted actigraphy, as these wearable devices can be implemented in field research (see Eatough et al., 2016) and appear to approximate sleep patterns well compared with the gold standard of polysomnography assessment. Polysomnography requires a sleep lab to assess multiple physiological sleep indicators such as electrical brain wave activity, oxygen levels and breathing, blood pressure, and physical movements (for an overview, see Van de Water et al., 2011). The Multiple

TABLE 12.2. Sleep Measurement Examples in Occupational Health Psychology

	Sleep quantity	Sleep quality	Sleepiness
Definition	Amount of sleep	Disturbances to sleep	Desire to sleep
Objective assessment example	Actigraphy Data (Sadeh, 2011) Total sleep duration	Actigraphy Data (Sadeh, 2011) Sleep efficiency (ratio of time asleep compared to time in bed), number and length of sleep awakenings	Multiple Sleep Latency Test (Carskadon et al., 1986) Sleep laboratory assessment using polysomnography that assesses time to fall asleep
Subjective assessment example	Pittsburgh Sleep Quality Index (Buysse et al., 1989) How many hours of actual sleep do you get at night?	Karolinka Sleep Diary (Åkerstedt et al., 1994) How well did you sleep?	Epworth Sleepiness Scale (Johns, 1991) How likely are you to nod off or fall asleep in the following situations, in contrast to feeling just tired?

Note. Examples are not intended to be comprehensive (for more information, see Pilcher et al., 2012).

Sleep Latency Test is also an objective measure of sleepiness conducted in a sleep laboratory using polysomnography (Carskadon et al., 1986).

Meta-analyses of employee samples show that overall (i.e., combining objective and subjective assessments) these sleep aspects' different operationalizations are rather distinct with low intercorrelations. Sleep quality and quantity only have a small but significant relationship ($r = .16$), and sleepiness has similar correlations in the negative direction with both sleep quantity and quality (Litwiller et al., 2017). Objective and subjective sleep-quantity measures are also more strongly associated with each other than sleep-quality measures (Litwiller et al., 2017).

Of special note, sleepiness is often confused with fatigue given both overlap with the colloquial use of the term "tired" (Shen et al., 2006). Yet sleepiness captures the subjective experience of drowsiness whereas fatigue represents a diminished capacity to exert effort. Although both can certainly co-occur, fatigued individuals can recover with periods of rest or relaxation while staying awake whereas those who are sleepy need to fulfill a drive to fall asleep. Therefore, applied researchers must determine whether they are more interested in indicators of sleep quantity or quality during workers' previous sleep period(s) or their subjective feelings of sleepiness during their waking hours either before or during work. The former approach asks about past sleep behaviors whereas the latter assesses the current desire to fall asleep.

The Link Between Sleep and Work Fatigue

In occupational health research, sleep is considered a key recovery process (Åkerstedt et al., 2009; Sonnentag, 2018). The concept of work recovery is important for understanding how employees can manage ongoing work demands that require sustained effort or exertion. Prolonged exertion on physical, mental, and emotional tasks lead to temporary states of fatigue that can be reversed with periods of rest. Although many different nonwork activities can contribute to work recovery (e.g., psychological detachment, physical relaxation, leisure activities), sleep is the most critical given it is a basic, physiological drive critical for brain functioning (Sonnentag, 2018). Therefore, better sleep can reduce work fatigue through both physiological processes related to neurological processing and felt energy needed for motivation.

The sleep–work fatigue link appears consistent across applied sleep measurement strategies, although the relationship's exact strength may somewhat vary (Litwiller et al., 2017). Fatigue is more strongly associated with sleep quality than sleep quantity, especially when using multi-item rather than single-item measures. This may be due to individual sleep need differences that make it difficult to use overall sleep duration as a useful proxy for sufficient sleep in some research designs. The "8 hours of sleep a day" recommendation is often seen as misguided given that there is considerable variation in sleep need that can range from 6 to more than 9 hours (Ferrara & De Gennaro, 2001). Daily diary method approaches can somewhat circumvent this issue, as deviations in sleep duration can be compared to average levels within each person.

Additionally, subjective sleep-quality measures more strongly relate to fatigue than objective ones; the reverse is true for sleep quantity (Litwiller et al., 2017). However, relatively few studies have objectively measured sleep quality and quantity. In fact, most organizational research examining sleep and fatigue focuses on self-report sleep-quality measures.

Future Considerations for Studying the Sleep and Fatigue Link in Organizations

Current approaches in applied research may benefit from further exploration of nuances involved in sleep and fatigue measurement. A few example considerations are noted in this section.

Other Fatigue Conceptualizations

A newer fatigue-related concept in OHP studies, adopted from social psychology research, is *ego depletion* (or self-control depletion; e.g., Baumeister, 2002). This idea describes reduced efforts to engage in acts of self-control (i.e., resisting impulses, making decisions, regulating thoughts/emotions/behaviors) following initial exertion. Some consider the term *depletion* a slight misnomer because rest or incentives can reverse this temporary state (Masicampo et al., 2014). Researchers have thus argued for the term *self-regulatory fatigue* (Evans et al., 2016), a specific short-term mental fatigue that occurs after exerting self-control (Inzlicht et al., 2014). Indeed, self-regulatory fatigue self-report measures include items approximating mental, physical, and emotional fatigue in addition to motivation deficits concerning upcoming effortful tasks (also in the general fatigue concept, see Meijman & Mulder, 1998). Fatigue and self-regulatory fatigue measures are rarely included in the same study to evaluate their distinctions. One exception found that state self-regulatory fatigue was strongly associated with general state fatigue ($r = .70$) and similarly related to state sleepiness and sleep loss (Barber & Budnick, 2015).

Self-regulatory fatigue is still a compelling area of study; it is strongly related to poor sleep among employees and is an explanatory mechanism between sleep and work behaviors (Barnes et al., 2015; Christian & Ellis, 2011). However, future work would benefit from distinguishing between work fatigue and self-regulatory fatigue at work given that the latter is typically contrasted only with negative affect. Negative affect measures lump together low activated states with fatigue (e.g., sadness) and even highly activated emotions (e.g., hostility, anger). Further differentiating among affective reactions and assessing multidimensional work fatigue aspects (physical, cognitive, and emotional components; Frone & Tidwell, 2015) would help establish if self-regulatory fatigue is a unique concept and measurement approach in the work fatigue literature.

Other Sleep Conceptualizations

The dual process model of sleep suggests two primary physiological influences on sleep behavior and sleepiness (Borbély et al., 2016). Usually, organizational sleep researchers draw from the homeostatic process perspective of sleep, which assumes sleep pressure (Process S), or the drive to fall asleep, increases linearly during the day accompanied by declining energy and functioning. Sleep periods are then a restorative process related to this sleep drive, with better sleep leading to improved work outcomes due to less fatigue. From this perspective, sleep quantity and quality are behavioral proxies for assessing this nightly restorative process, and sleepiness most directly measures the drive to fall asleep. However, there is a second circadian process of alertness that fluctuates over the course of the day (Process C). This perspective suggests that our energy and functioning may depend on our position in this cycle. Therefore, sleep's impact on fatigue and performance may also depend on a circadian mismatch based on the time of day and an individual's sleep/wake cycle.

One approach to examining circadian mismatches is assessing *chronotype*, or individual differences in worker sleep/wake cycle preferences that may conflict with the timing of work demands. Early chronotypes (morning types) sleep/awaken early and are most alert in the morning, whereas late chrono-types (evening types) sleep/awaken late and are most alert in the afternoon or evening (Kim & Kim, 2020). Most researchers rely on self-report instruments to assess chronotypes in field research, as objective approaches involve invasive physiological measures of core body temperature or melatonin levels (Baron & Reid, 2014). Fortunately, validated self-report questionnaires are also available, such as the Morningness-Eveningness Questionnaire and its reduced version (the five-item rMEQ amenable to field research), Composite Scale of Morning-ness, Preference Scale, Munich Chronotype Questionnaire, and the Morningness-Eveningness-Stability-Scale (for a review, see Kim & Kim, 2020).

Other Objective Measurement Strategies for Field Research
Objective measures are often prized in organizational and occupational health research given the documented limitations of self-report data (Eatough & Spector, 2013). However, objective measures are not without disadvantages; they can also produce biased information due to issues with training on pro-cedures, measurement calibration, participant compliance, and participants' reactivity to being monitored with devices (Eatough et al., 2016; Ganster et al., 2018). Strategies incorporating wrist-worn actigraphy measures are often useful for field research given they can be worn for many days and capture evening sleep parameters as well as other movements throughout the day (Eatough et al., 2016; Sadeh, 2011). Medical-grade devices validated against polysomnography in laboratory studies are particularly important, as com-mercially available options on smartphones or other wearable devices may not produce reliable data. It is critical that inferences we make in research regarding the distinctions between subjective versus objective measures of sleep are not driven by methodological artifacts.

Yet some newer technologies targeting fitness crowds may be promising. Recent work compared a commercial smartwatch (Samsung) and a smartring (Oura) to a medical-grade actigraphy device (Asgari Mehrabadi, 2020). Although the commercial devices performed adequately compared with actigraphy, actigraphy was still more accurate (followed by the ring, with the smartwatch being lowest). Other work suggests a commercial wrist-worn activity tracker (i.e., Fitbit) estimates sleep parameters well compared with polysomnography (de Zambotti et al., 2018). Future validation studies comparing commercial to medical-grade devices like the actigraph could provide valuable information about more commonly available real-time data sources.

PRIMARY AND SECONDARY INTERVENTION STRATEGIES FOR SLEEP AND WORK FATIGUE

This section reviews key intervention strategies for addressing sleep and work fatigue issues in organizations. These strategies may include improving sleep by altering aspects of the work environment or mitigating work fatigue after sleep problem have already occurred.

Addressing Sleep-Related Organizational Risk Factors

Various aspects of the work environment have a powerful influence on employee sleep. Therefore, identifying, targeting, and reducing organizational risk factors that affect employee sleep can be a critical primary intervention approach to combating sleep-related work fatigue (see Figure 12.1). First, organizations can consider reducing work demands—aspects of the work environment that require sustained effort in terms of physical, mental, or emotional tasks (Bakker & Demerouti, 2017). In addition to leading to work fatigue and long-term health and well-being outcomes, many work demands are anticipated to also affect sleep through emotional, cognitive, and behavioral processes. For example, work demands can interfere with sleep through negative emotional activation (tension, anxiety) and work-related cognitions (rumination) in the evening that make it difficult to fall asleep at bedtime

FIGURE 12.1. Sleep and Work Fatigue Intervention Approaches

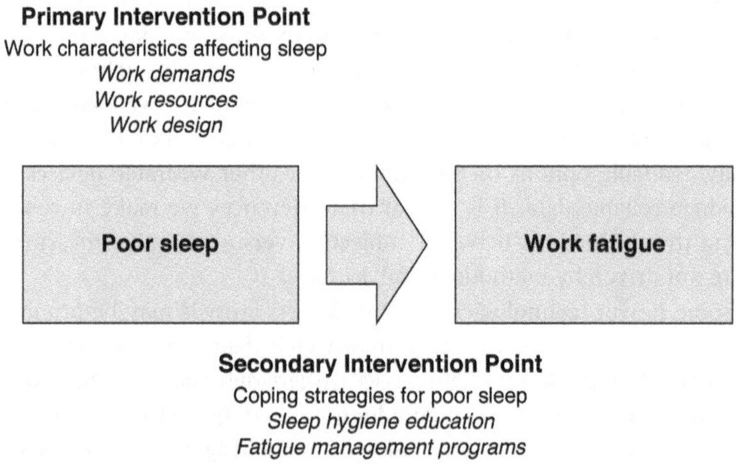

Primary Intervention Point
Work characteristics affecting sleep
Work demands
Work resources
Work design

Poor sleep   **Work fatigue**

Secondary Intervention Point
Coping strategies for poor sleep
Sleep hygiene education
Fatigue management programs

(Sonnentag, 2018). Additionally, some research has implicated behavioral processes related to managing time. Workers may "borrow" from sleep time during periods of longer work hours given that time is a limited resource (Barnes et al., 2012).

Surprisingly, meta-analytic work in organizational studies indicates that workload is only modestly, but consistently, associated with poorer sleep-quality (including sleep disturbances) and sleep-quantity measures (Litwiller et al., 2017; Nixon et al., 2011). Focusing on hours worked, however, appears to produce different results depending on the sleep measurement approach. There is a fairly weak relationship between hours worked and sleep quality, but more hours worked does have a moderate relationship with lower sleep quantity. However, intervention work in this area does show improvement on both sleep indicators using employees from a variety of worksites and sectors (i.e., social services, technical services, care and welfare, and call center managers/administrators). When reducing work time by 25% while keeping pay steady, sleep quality and duration improved 18 months later (Schiller et al., 2017). Employees also reported reduced sleepiness, stress, and worries or stress at bedtime on workdays.

Work resources may be another critical intervention point for sleep. Work resources are generally considered to be motivational aspects of the work environment that help people manage work demands. In occupational health theories, resources typically include psychosocial factors such as perceived control over work time or job autonomy, supervisor support, and fair work environments (Bakker & Demerouti, 2017). The mechanisms by which work resources might affect sleep would likely differ based on the type of resource offered. For example, job autonomy could help employees coordinate work around their preferred schedules. Having control over work processes might also help employees reduce frustration or work more efficiently, addressing negative emotional or cognitive activation issues and work-time interference problems mentioned earlier (Barnes et al., 2012; Sonnentag, 2018). Perceived control is modestly associated with better sleep quality in meta-analysis research, but not sleep quantity (Litwiller et al., 2017). Poor schedule control may be especially relevant given that unpredictable schedules (even when accounting for shift work) are strongly related to negative sleep-quality indicators (Harknett et al., 2020). Although subsequent research will elucidate these relationships further, there is some evidence for control or autonomy benefiting employee sleep.

Although social support is also a key work resource that can reduce work demands and experiences of strains arising from demands (Viswesvaran et al., 1999), surprisingly, meta-analysis findings suggest that work support in general is unrelated to employees' sleep quality or quantity (Litwiller et al., 2017). However, the specific types of social support, especially from leaders, may be most critical. For example, one intervention used both family-supportive supervisor behavior (a more targeted and specific measurement) and personal control over work time to improve both employee sleep quality and quantity (Olson et al., 2015). A similar intervention improved objective and subjective sleep duration among information technology workers (Crain et al., 2019). Training leaders on interactional justice—treating employees with dignity and respect—also appears to improve employee sleep based on intervention work (Greenberg, 2006). Another longitudinal study from Finland suggests that sleep may explain the relationship between organizational justice and employee health (Elovainio et al., 2003).

Combining leader influence with specific forms of support has resulted in the idea of sleep leadership. Sleep leadership encapsulates supervisor behaviors that seek to improve employees' sleep, such as showing concern for healthy sleep habits as well as role modeling and discussing effective sleep practices. Deployed military members in high-risk occupations show improved sleep with sleep leadership even when accounting for general leadership style (Gunia et al., 2015). More recently, a large study using actigraph measurements reported that higher employee ratings of family-supportive supervisor behavior were unexpectedly associated with shortened objective sleep time, but higher sleep leadership did predict less sleep disturbance and sleep-related impairment. Alternatively, supervisors' self-ratings of family-supportive supervisor behaviors did significantly predict better employee sleep hygiene and less sleep-related employee impairment (Sianoja et al., 2020).

Work-design or work-organization issues can also be a key organizational risk factor for sleep. Most applied studies of work-design issues surrounding sleep and fatigue have focused on nonstandard work schedules, especially shift work. Sleep problems often arise from circadian issues related to working night shifts (i.e., mismatch in typical sleep/wake cycle with daylight) and irregular shifts that make it difficult to adhere to a stable sleep schedule (Åkerstedt, 2003). Intervention work in this area suggests a few adjustments to shift-work characteristics can be effective for reducing sleep issues and fatigue (among other negative well-being indicators). These strategies include using faster rotations with fewer consecutive days working the night shift, forward rotations that move from early shifts followed by later shifts, as well as allowing some control over self-scheduling shifts in terms of timing or rest days (Bambra et al., 2008).

Last, it is important to consider ethical issues related to both sleep measurement and sleep interventions. Workers may feel coerced into providing personal health information that affects their privacy in the workplace (i.e., "paycheck vulnerability"; Rose & Pietri, 2002). Therefore, protecting employee confidentiality and choice to participate freely is critical. Additionally, researchers need to consider all potential sleep harm risks and side effects in field research, as well as maximizing benefits for all employees who participate (Barber, 2017).

Addressing Sleep-Related Fatigue Issues in Organizations

Organizations can also help employees cope with sleep's negative impact on work fatigue using fatigue management programs (also known as fatigue training or fatigue education). These programs often include a mix of educational activities about sleep and strategies for minimizing fatigue due to poor sleep, which is a secondary intervention point in the sleep and fatigue process (see Figure 12.1). They often target occupational settings with some level of unavoidable sleep disruption, such as transcontinental flight crews, nurses, medical residents, and other positions entailing irregular shifts or demanding hours. Meta-analytic results suggest fatigue training improves patient/personal safety, acute fatigue ratings, and sleep quality while reducing stress and burnout (Barger et al., 2018). Other systematic reviews of these programs show alertness, reaction time, sleep knowledge, and error prevention improvements (Redeker et al., 2019).

Programs that also include sleep hygiene education represent a primary prevention strategy oriented toward directly addressing poor sleep habits that may contribute to sleep problems (i.e., an individual behavior risk factor approach to improving sleep rather than the organizational risk approach discussed in the prior section). However, secondary prevention strategies that focus on managing fatigue arising from poor sleep are also a key component of these programs. Common training elements include work environment countermeasures focused on physical surroundings, napping, and caffeine use.

Creating the right conditions in the work environment can help employees manage fatigue. Broadly, organizations might focus on increasing employees' arousal levels to facilitate increased alertness when sleepiness or fatigue is high. One strategy is adjusting lighting levels. Increasing light intensity during night shifts helps individuals match their circadian cycles to the work environment. However, this approach might also have drawbacks in terms of subsequently disrupted sleep, and studies have predominantly focused on shift workers (Bonnefond et al., 2004; Hilditch et al., 2016). Noise can also improve alertness levels. White noise and pink noise (i.e., static noise) can improve alertness, but too high intensity noise could result in hearing damage or other negative outcomes (Bonnefond et al., 2004). Both light and noise effects on employee alertness are not well understood in field work (Bonnefond et al., 2004; Hilditch et al., 2016), thus creating a valuable opportunity for future research.

Providing employees opportunities to nap may also be useful for coping with fatigue from poor sleep. Shift workers exhibit better vigilance after a shift involving a 20-minute nap, although there were no effects of that nap on subjective sleepiness, fatigue, sleep duration, or sleep quality (Purnell et al., 2002). Yet other work suggests otherwise: medical interns working overnight increased their total sleep duration and reduce overall fatigue when on a nap schedule compared with a standard schedule (Arora et al., 2006). More recent reviews confirm such findings, suggesting that scheduled naps during work shifts improved performance and decreased fatigue for shift workers (Martin-Gill et al., 2018). Still, most work on naps has focused on shift workers, leaving much room for future research on daytime worker fatigue and performance, as well as the potential impact of naps on subsequent evening sleep behaviors and next-day fatigue.

Last, many fatigue management programs include pharmacological interventions, or drug use related to stimulants that increase alertness. Such strategies are often fraught with ethical concerns that need to balance individual health with relative errors in high-risk occupations, given that many of these medications can be habit-forming (Bonnet et al., 2005; Russo, 2007). Therefore, many programs focus on caffeine use and low-dose patterns that will be maximally effective for fatigue without creating future sleep or other health issues. Caffeine use can improve alertness and performance even with doses as low as 75 to 150 milligrams for well-rested individuals and 200 to 600 milligrams after one or more nights of sleep loss. Importantly, caffeine is unlikely to seriously disrupt sleep if sleep onset occurs 8 or more hours after consumption, although frequent consumption poses the risk of increased tolerance and potential withdrawal effects (Bonnet et al., 2005). Meta-analysis research also suggests that caffeine buffers against behavioral fatigue among shift workers but can also negatively affect subsequent sleep (Temple et al., 2018). Therefore, caffeine may be an effective short-term solution that is counterproductive for improving sleep and fatigue in the long run.

Future Considerations for Addressing Sleep and Fatigue in Organizational Research

We have learned much about how to improve sleep from intervention research related to organizational risk factors and fatigue management strategies. Other examples of exciting future directions we can take based on initial findings are discussed in this section.

Technological Aspects of Work-Design Risk Factors

Technological aspects of work design are also producing both nonstandard work schedules (unpredictability) and continuous work access (connectivity) with important implications for worker sleep. The traditional notion of a work shift may be disappearing with more online access to work. Constant access to others using electronic communications has facilitated workers' switching between work and home tasks quickly throughout the day (Kossek, 2016). In particular, using electronic devices to monitor and respond to work communications during nonwork hours has important implications for sleep. After-hours work communications through electronic devices (e.g., smartphones, computers) undermine sleep quality (Lanaj et al., 2014; Schieman & Young, 2013), and elicit pressure to respond immediately to work-related messages during both work and nonwork hours (Barber & Santuzzi, 2015). Studies point to issues surrounding heightened social expectations or norms for connectivity in the organization as risk factors that could serve as an intervention point, as well as individual tactics that might help protect sleep (Barber & Jenkins, 2014; Barber & Santuzzi, 2015). However, we still need intervention work to determine how to address sleep issues arising from high work connectivity while balancing electronic communication's benefits and costs.

Motivational Perspectives on Fatigue Management

Fatigue management strategies, to date, appear to mostly emphasize physical work environment factors (e.g., light, temperature) and physiological processes (e.g., napping, caffeine). However, psychosocial work environment factors and psychological processes related to motivation may also be worth investigating. Evidence suggests that at least some aspects of fatigue might be motivational in nature, especially in nonclinical settings (i.e., no clinical disorders in sleep or fatigue). Early laboratory research demonstrated an "incentive effect" with respect to sleep and behavioral indicators of fatigue (Haslam, 1983; Horne & Pettitt, 1985; Wilkinson, 1964). Even sleep-deprived individuals could compensate for short periods of poor sleep under some environmental reward conditions, like better pay or more interesting tasks. A similar pattern in self-regulation research indicates incentives can help manage self-regulatory fatigue (Masicampo et al., 2014). For example, perceptions of control and rewarding work among nurses during a 12-hour shift were more predictive of lower levels of fatigue than workload demands or the physical energy expended based on an activity monitor (Johnston et al., 2019). Similarly, it is worth investigating whether fatigue arising from relatively minor deviations in good sleep quantity or quality can be overcome with work environment changes that increase interest and attention (e.g., rewarding social interaction or meaningful/engaging tasks).

Individual Vulnerability to Fatigue From Poor Sleep
People may differ on their vulnerability to fatigue from sleep issues. Individual vulnerabilities to sleep issues and effects on fatigue have also not yet received much attention in applied research on sleep in organizations outside of clinical sleep disorders and tolerance for shift work (Saksvik et al., 2011). For example, some organizational research has targeted sleep apnea treatments to improve sleep quality, and subsequently work exhaustion (Carleton & Barling, 2020). Cognitive behavior therapy treatments for workers also appear to reduce negative affect (which includes fatigue), which subsequently predicts both helpful and counterproductive behavior at work (Barnes et al., 2017). Additionally, research on shift-work tolerance often focuses on demographic factors (age, gender) and circadian rhythm factors (morningness/eveningness, rigidity/ flexibility). Yet demographic factors such as age, gender, and marital status tend not to be associated with worker sleep issues in applied research overall (Litwiller et al., 2017).

Understanding worker preferences about sleep timing (chronotypes) may be useful given people with later sleep/wake cycles (i.e., eveningness) report more work exhaustion/burnout (Waleriańczyk et al., 2020). Yet aside from research demonstrating negative effects of circadian mismatches and rotating shift work's contribution to shift-work disorder (for a review, see Wickwire et al., 2017), less applied research in organizations examines circadian effects on nonshift workers' daily fatigue or performance. Still, researchers propose that evening chronotypes may struggle with work demands that are outside their preferred cycle, often referred to as circadian misalignment (i.e., social jetlag or sleep debt; Wittmann et al., 2006). For example, shifts that are aligned with employee chronotypes help employees sleep better in terms of both quality and quantity (Juda et al., 2013). Other work finds that evening types, unstable daily activity and sleep levels, and work habit differences each contribute to weekday sleep debt (Goto et al., 2021). Moreover, evening types were at an increased risk of sleep and psychological problems during the COVID-19 lockdown in Italy compared with morning types (Salfi et al., 2021). Thus, poor sleep quantity and quality may impact worker fatigue the most when employees are working outside their preferred sleep/wake cycles.

CONCLUSION

Applied organizational research has provided compelling evidence for why organizations should be concerned about employee sleep and fatigue—both of which have detrimental impacts on employee health and performance. Measuring sleep and fatigue in applied research can be challenging, but there are promising strategies for exploring these issues in complex and dynamic work settings outside of the controlled laboratory environment. Future occupational health research is needed to tease apart nuances in sleep and fatigue conceptualization as well as assessment strategies that can enhance or undermine the observed link between them in field studies. Additionally, research suggests organizations have major roles to play in reducing sleep and fatigue issues among their workers. These roles include intervening on organizational risk factors that contribute to worker sleep problems, and helping employees manage fatigue at work when they inevitably encounter sleep issues. We hope to see more applied intervention research in a variety of occupational settings (outside of shift work) that tackle work environment changes and fatigue management strategies that could help employees sleep well and be well.

REFERENCES

Åkerstedt, T. (2003). Shift work and disturbed sleep/wakefulness. *Occupational Medicine*, 53(2), 89–94. https://doi.org/10.1093/occmed/kqg046

Åkerstedt, T., Hume, K., Minors, D., & Waterhouse, J. (1994). The subjective meaning of good sleep, an intraindividual approach using the Karolinska Sleep Diary. *Perceptual and Motor Skills*, 79(1), 287–296. https://doi.org/10.2466/pms.1994.79.1.287

Åkerstedt, T., Nilsson, P. M., & Kecklund, G. (2009). Sleep and recovery. In S. Sonnentag, P. L. Perrewé, & D. C. Ganster (Eds.), *Current perspectives on job-stress recovery* (pp. 205–247). JAI Press/Emerald Group Publishing. https://doi.org/10.1108/S1479-3555(2009)0000007009

Arora, V., Dunphy, C., Chang, V. Y., Ahmad, F., Humphrey, H. J., & Meltzer, D. (2006). The effects of on-duty napping on intern sleep time and fatigue. *Annals of Internal Medicine*, 144(11), 792–798. Advance online publication. https://doi.org/10.7326/0003-4819-144-11-200606060-00005

Asgari Mehrabadi, M., Azimi, I., Sarhaddi, F., Axelin, A., Niela-Vilén, H., Myllyntausta, S., Stenholm, S., Dutt, N., Liljeberg, P., & Rahmani, A. M. (2020). Sleep tracking of a commercially available smart ring and smartwatch against medical-grade actigraphy in everyday settings: Instrument validation study. *JMIR mHealth and uHealth*, 8(10), e20465. https://mhealth.jmir.org/2020/11/e20465

Bakker, A. B., & Demerouti, E. (2017). Job demands–resources theory: Taking stock and looking forward. *Journal of Occupational Health Psychology, 22*(3), 273–285. https://doi.org/10.1037/ocp0000056

Bambra, C. L., Whitehead, M. M., Sowden, A. J., Akers, J., & Petticrew, M. P. (2008). Shifting schedules: The health effects of reorganizing shift work. *American Journal of Preventive Medicine, 34*(5), 427–434.e30. https://doi.org/10.1016/j.amepre.2007.12.023

Banks, S., & Dinges, D. F. (2007). Behavioral and physiological consequences of sleep restriction. *Journal of Clinical Sleep Medicine, 3*(5), 519–528. https://doi.org/10.5664/jcsm.26918

Barber, L. K. (2017). Ethical considerations for sleep intervention in organizational psychology research. *Stress and Health, 33*(5), 691–698. https://doi.org/10.1002/smi.2745

Barber, L. K., & Budnick, C. J. (2015). Turning molehills into mountains: Sleepiness increases workplace interpretive bias. *Journal of Organizational Behavior, 36*(3), 360–381. https://doi.org/10.1002/job.1992

Barber, L. K., & Jenkins, J. S. (2014). Creating technological boundaries to protect bedtime: Examining work–home boundary management, psychological detachment and sleep. *Stress and Health, 30*(3), 259–264. https://doi.org/10.1002/smi.2536

Barber, L. K., & Santuzzi, A. M. (2015). Please respond ASAP: Workplace telepressure and employee recovery. *Journal of Occupational Health Psychology, 20*(2), 172–189. https://doi.org/10.1037/a0038278

Barger, L. K., Runyon, M. S., Renn, M. L., Moore, C. G., Weiss, P. M., Condle, J. P., Flickinger, K. L., Divecha, A. A., Coppler, P. J., Sequeira, D. J., Lang, E. S., Higgins, J. S., & Patterson, P. D. (2018). Effect of fatigue training on safety, fatigue, and sleep in emergency medical services personnel and other shift workers: A systematic review and meta-analysis. *Prehospital Emergency Care, 22*(Suppl. 1), 58–68. https://doi.org/10.1080/10903127.2017.1362087

Barnes, C. M. (2012). Working in our sleep: Sleep and self-regulation in organizations. *Organizational Psychology Review, 2*(3), 234–257. https://doi.org/10.1177/2041386612450181

Barnes, C. M., Lucianetti, L., Devasheesh, B. P., & Christian, M. S. (2015). "You wouldn't like me when I'm sleepy": Leaders' sleep, daily abusive supervision, and work unit engagement. *Academy of Management Journal, 58*(5). https://doi.org/10.5465/amj.2013.1063

Barnes, C. M., Miller, J. A., & Bostock, S. (2017). Helping employees sleep well: Effects of cognitive behavioral therapy for insomnia on work outcomes. *Journal of Applied Psychology, 102*(1), 104–113. https://doi.org/10.1037/apl0000154

Barnes, C. M., Wagner, D. T., & Ghumman, S. (2012). Borrowing from sleep to pay work and family: Expanding time-based conflict to the broader nonwork domain. *Personnel Psychology, 65*(4), 789–819. https://doi.org/10.1111/peps.12002

Barnes, C. M., & Watson, N. F. (2019). Why healthy sleep is good for business. *Sleep Medicine Reviews, 47*, 112–118. https://doi.org/10.1016/j.smrv.2019.07.005

Baron, K. G., & Reid, K. J. (2014). Circadian misalignment and health. *International Review of Psychiatry, 26*(2), 139–154. https://doi.org/10.3109/09540261.2014.911149

Baumeister, R. F. (2002). Ego depletion and self-control failure: An energy model of the self's executive function. *Self and Identity, 1*(2), 129–136. https://doi.org/10.1080/152988602317319302

Bonnefond, A., Tassi, P., Roge, J., & Muzet, A. (2004). A critical review of techniques aiming at enhancing and sustaining worker's alertness during the night shift. *Industrial Health, 42*(1), 1–14. https://doi.org/10.2486/indhealth.42.1

Bonnet, M. H., Balkin, T. J., Dinges, D. F., Roehrs, T., Rogers, N. L., & Wesensten, N. J. (2005). The use of stimulants to modify performance during sleep loss: A review by the Sleep Deprivation and Stimulant Task Force of the American Academy of Sleep Medicine. *Sleep, 28*(9), 1163–1187. https://doi.org/10.1093/sleep/28.9.1163

Borbély, A. A., Daan, S., Wirz-Justice, A., & Deboer, T. (2016). The two-process model of sleep regulation: A reappraisal. *Journal of Sleep Research, 25*(2), 131–143. https://doi.org/10.1111/jsr.12371

Buysse, D. J., Reynolds, C. F., III, Monk, T. H., Berman, S. R., & Kupfer, D. J. (1989). The Pittsburgh Sleep Quality Index: A new instrument for psychiatric practice and research. *Psychiatry Research, 28*(2), 193–213. https://doi.org/10.1016/0165-1781(89)90047-4

Carleton, E. L., & Barling, J. (2020). Indirect effects of obstructive sleep apnea treatments on work withdrawal: A quasi-experimental treatment outcome study. *Journal of Occupational Health Psychology, 25*(6), 426–438. https://doi.org/10.1037/ocp0000183

Carskadon, M. A., & Dement, W. C. (2005). Normal human sleep overview. In M. H. Kryger, T. Roth, & W. C. Dement (Eds.), *Principles and practice of sleep medicine* (4th ed., pp. 13–23). Elsevier/Saunders. https://doi.org/10.1016/B0-72-160797-7/50009-4

Carskadon, M. A., Dement, W. C., Mitler, M. M., Roth, T., Westbrook, P. R., & Keenan, S. (1986). Guidelines for the multiple sleep latency test (MSLT): A standard measure of sleepiness. *Sleep, 9*(4), 519–524. https://doi.org/10.1093/sleep/9.4.519

Christian, M. S., & Ellis, A. P. J. (2011). Examining the effects of sleep deprivation on workplace deviance: A self-regulatory perspective. *Academy of Management Journal, 54*(5), 913–934. https://doi.org/10.5465/amj.2010.0179

Crain, T. L., Hammer, L. B., Bodner, T., Olson, R., Kossek, E. E., Moen, P., & Buxton, O. M. (2019). Sustaining sleep: Results from the randomized controlled work, family, and health study. *Journal of Occupational Health Psychology, 24*(1), 180–197. https://doi.org/10.1037/ocp0000122

Dawson, D., & McCulloch, K. (2005). Managing fatigue: It's about sleep. *Sleep Medicine Reviews, 9*(5), 365–380. https://doi.org/10.1016/j.smrv.2005.03.002

de Zambotti, M., Goldstone, A., Claudatos, S., Colrain, I. M., & Baker, F. C. (2018). A validation study of Fitbit Charge 2™ compared with polysomnography in adults. *Chronobiology International, 35*(4), 465–476. https://doi.org/10.1080/07420528.2017.1413578

Demerouti, E., Bakker, A. B., Vardakou, I., & Kantas, A. (2003). The convergent validity of two burnout instruments: A multitrait-multimethod analysis. *European Journal of Psychological Assessment, 19*(1), 12–23. https://doi.org/10.1027/1015-5759.19.1.12

Eatough, E., Shockley, K., & Yu, P. (2016). A review of ambulatory health data collection methods for employee experience sampling research. *Applied Psychology, 65*(2), 322–354. https://doi.org/10.1111/apps.12068

Eatough, E. M., & Spector, P. E. (2013). Quantitative self-report methods in occupational health psychology research. In M. Wang, R. Sinclair, & L. Tetrick (Eds.), *Research methods in occupational health psychology* (pp. 248–267). Taylor & Francis.

Elovainio, M., Kivimäki, M., Vahtera, J., Keltikangas-Järvinen, L., & Virtanen, M. (2003). Sleeping problems and health behaviors as mediators between organizational justice and health. *Health Psychology, 22*(3), 287–293. https://doi.org/10.1037/0278-6133.22.3.287

Evans, D. R., Boggero, I. A., & Segerstrom, S. C. (2016). The nature of self-regulatory fatigue and "ego depletion": Lessons from physical fatigue. *Personality and Social Psychology Review, 20*(4), 291–310. https://doi.org/10.1177/1088868315597841

Ferrara, M., & De Gennaro, L. (2001). How much sleep do we need? *Sleep Medicine Reviews, 5*(2), 155–179. https://doi.org/10.1053/smrv.2000.0138

Frone, M. R., & Tidwell, M. O. (2015). The meaning and measurement of work fatigue: Development and evaluation of the Three-Dimensional Work Fatigue Inventory (3D-WFI). *Journal of Occupational Health Psychology, 20*(3), 273–288. https://doi.org/10.1037/a0038700

Ganster, D. C., Crain, T. L., & Brossoit, R. M. (2018). Physiological measurement in the organizational sciences: A review and recommendations for future use. *Annual Review of Organizational Psychology and Organizational Behavior, 5*, 267–293. https://doi.org/10.1146/annurev-orgpsych-032117-104613

Gordon, A. M., Mendes, W. B., & Prather, A. A. (2017). The social side of sleep: Elucidating the links between sleep and social processes. *Current Directions in Psychological Science, 26*(5), 470–475. https://doi.org/10.1177/0963721417712269

Goto, Y., Fujiwara, K., Sumi, Y., Matsuo, M., Kano, M., & Kadotani, H. (2021). Work habit-related sleep debt: Insights from factor identification analysis and actigraphy data. *Frontiers in Public Health, 9,* 630640. Advance online publication. https://doi.org/10.3389/fpubh.2021.630640

Greenberg, J. (2006). Losing sleep over organizational injustice: Attenuating insomniac reactions to underpayment inequity with supervisory training in interactional justice. *Journal of Applied Psychology, 91*(1), 58–69. https://doi.org/10.1037/0021-9010.91.1.58

Gunia, B. C., Sipos, M. L., LoPresti, M., & Adler, A. B. (2015). Sleep leadership in high-risk occupations: An investigation of soldiers on peacekeeping and combat missions. *Military Psychology, 27*(4), 197–211. https://doi.org/10.1037/mil0000078

Harknett, K., Schneider, D., & Wolfe, R. (2020). Losing sleep over work scheduling? The relationship between work schedules and sleep quality for service sector workers. *SSM – Population Health, 12,* 100681. https://doi.org/10.1016/j.ssmph.2020.100681

Haslam, D. R. (1983). The incentive effect and sleep deprivation. *Sleep, 6*(4), 362–368. https://doi.org/10.1093/sleep/6.4.362

Henderson, A. A., & Horan, K. A. (2021). A meta-analysis of sleep and work performance: An examination of moderators and mediators. *Journal of Organizational Behavior, 42*(1), 1–19. https://doi.org/10.1002/job.2486

Hilditch, C. J., Dorrian, J., & Banks, S. (2016). Time to wake up: Reactive countermeasures to sleep inertia. *Industrial Health, 54,* 528–541. https://doi.org/10.2486/indhealth.2015-0236

Hockey, R. (2013). *The psychology of fatigue: Work, effort and control.* Cambridge University Press. https://doi.org/10.1017/CBO9781139015394

Horne, J. A., & Pettitt, A. N. (1985). High incentive effects on vigilance performance during 72 hours of total sleep deprivation. *Acta Psychologica, 58*(2), 123–139. https://doi.org/10.1016/0001-6918(85)90003-4

Inzlicht, M., Schmeichel, B. J., & Macrae, C. N. (2014). Why self-control seems (but may not be) limited. *Trends in Cognitive Sciences, 18*(3), 127–133. https://doi.org/10.1016/j.tics.2013.12.009

Johns, M. W. (1991). A new method for measuring daytime sleepiness: The Epworth sleepiness scale. *Sleep, 14*(6), 540–545. https://doi.org/10.1093/sleep/14.6.540

Johnston, D. W., Allan, J. L., Powell, D. J. H., Jones, M. C., Farquharson, B., Bell, C., & Johnston, M. (2019). Why does work cause fatigue? A real-time investigation of fatigue, and determinants of fatigue in nurses working 12-hour shifts. *Annals of Behavioral Medicine, 53*(6), 551–562. https://doi.org/10.1093/abm/kay065

Juda, M., Vetter, C., & Roenneberg, T. (2013). Chronotype modulates sleep duration, sleep quality, and social jet lag in shift-workers. *Journal of Biological Rhythms, 28*(2), 141–151. https://doi.org/10.1177/0748730412475042

Kim, S., & Kim, S. J. (2020). Psychometric properties of questionnaire for assessing chronotype. *Chronobiology in Medicine, 2*(1), 16–20. https://doi.org/10.33069/cim.2020.0003

Kossek, E. E. (2016). Managing work–life boundaries in the digital age. *Organizational Dynamics, 45*(3), 258–270. https://doi.org/10.1016/j.orgdyn.2016.07.010

Kristensen, T. S., Borritz, M., Villadsen, E., & Christensen, K. B. (2005). The Copenhagen Burnout Inventory: A new tool for the assessment of burnout. *Work & Stress, 19*(3), 192–207. https://doi.org/10.1080/02678370500297720

Lanaj, K., Johnson, R. E., & Barnes, C. M. (2014). Beginning the workday yet already depleted? Consequences of late-night smartphone use and sleep. *Organizational Behavior and Human Decision Processes, 124*(1), 11–23. https://doi.org/10.1016/j.obhdp.2014.01.001

Litwiller, B., Snyder, L. A., Taylor, W. D., & Steele, L. M. (2017). The relationship between sleep and work: A meta-analysis. *Journal of Applied Psychology, 102*(4), 682–699. https://doi.org/10.1037/apl0000169

Loeppke, R., Taitel, M., Richling, D., Parry, T., Kessler, R. C., Hymel, P., & Konicki, D. (2007). Health and productivity as a business strategy. *Journal of Occupational and Environmental Medicine, 49*(7), 712–721. https://doi.org/10.1097/JOM.0b013e318133a4be

Martin-Gill, C., Barger, L. K., Moore, C. G., Higgins, S., Teasley E. M., Weiss, P. M., Condle, J. P., Flickinger, K. L., Coppler, P. J., Sequeira, D. J., Divecha, A. A., Matthews, M. E., Lang, E. S., & Patterson, P. D. (2018). Effects of napping during shift work on sleepiness and performance in emergency medical services personnel and similar shift workers: A systematic review and meta-analysis. *Prehospital Emergency Care, 22*(Suppl. 1), 47–57. https://doi.org/10.1080/10903127.2017.1376136

Masicampo, E. J., Martin, S. R., & Anderson, R. A. (2014). Understanding and overcoming self-control depletion. *Social and Personality Psychology Compass, 8*(11), 638–649. https://doi.org/10.1111/spc3.12139

Maslach, C., Jackson, S. E., & Leiter, M. P. (1996). *Maslach Burnout Inventory manual* (3rd ed.). Mind Garden.

Meijman, T., & Mulder, G. (1998). Psychological aspects of workload. In C. J. de Wolff, P. J. D. Drenth, & T. Henk (Eds.), *Handbook of work and organizational psychology* (Vol. 2, pp. 5–34). Psychology Press.

Michielsen, H. J., De Vries, J., & Van Heck, G. L. (2003). Psychometric qualities of a brief self-rated fatigue measure: The Fatigue Assessment Scale. *Journal of Psychosomatic Research, 54*(4), 345–352. https://doi.org/10.1016/S0022-3999(02)00392-6

Mullins, H. M., Cortina, J. M., Drake, C. L., & Dalal, R. S. (2014). Sleepiness at work: A review and framework of how the physiology of sleepiness impacts the workplace. *Journal of Applied Psychology, 99*(6), 1096–1112. https://doi.org/10.1037/a0037885

Nixon, A. E., Mazzola, J. J., Bauer, J., Krueger, J. R., & Spector, P. E. (2011). Can work make you sick? A meta-analysis of the relationships between job stressors and physical symptoms. *Work and Stress, 25*(1), 1–22. https://doi.org/10.1080/02678373.2011.569175

Olson, R., Crain, T. L., Bodner, T. E., King, R., Hammer, L. B., Klein, L. C., Erickson, L., Moen, P., Berkman, L. F., & Buxton, O. M. (2015). A workplace intervention improves sleep: Results from the randomized controlled Work, Family, and Health Study. *Sleep Health, 1*(1), 55–65. https://doi.org/10.1016/j.sleh.2014.11.003

Pilcher, J. J., Burnett, M. L., & McCubbin, J. A. (2012). Measurement of sleep and sleepiness. In M. Wang, R. R. Sinclair, & L. Tetrick (Eds.), *Research methods in occupational health psychology: Measurement, design, and data analysis* (pp. 49–60). Routledge Taylor & Francis Group.

Purnell, M. T., Feyer, A. M., & Herbison, G. P. (2002). The impact of a nap opportunity during the night shift on the performance and alertness of 12-h shift workers. *Journal of Sleep Research, 11*(3), 219–227. https://doi.org/10.1046/j.1365-2869.2002.00309.x

Redeker, N. S., Caruso, C. C., Hashmi, S. D., Mullington, J. M., Grandner, M., & Morgenthaler, T. I. (2019). Workplace interventions to promote sleep health and an alert, healthy workforce. *Journal of Clinical Sleep Medicine, 15*(4), 649–657. https://doi.org/10.5664/jcsm.7734

Rose, S. L., & Pietri, C. E. (2002). Workers as research subjects: A vulnerable population. *Journal of Occupational and Environmental Medicine, 44*(9), 801–805. https://doi.org/10.1097/00043764-200209000-00001

Russo, M. B. (2007). Recommendations for the ethical use of pharmacologic fatigue countermeasures in the U.S. military. *Aviation, Space, and Environmental Medicine, 78*(5, Suppl.), B119–B127.

Sadeh, A. (2011). The role and validity of actigraphy in sleep medicine: An update. *Sleep Medicine Reviews, 15*(4), 259–267. https://doi.org/10.1016/j.smrv.2010.10.001

Sagherian, K., Geiger-Brown, J., Rogers, V. E., & Ludeman, E. (2019). Fatigue and risk of sickness absence in the working population: A systematic review and meta-analysis of longitudinal studies. *Scandinavian Journal of Work, Environment & Health, 45*(4), 333–345. https://doi.org/10.5271/sjweh.3819

Saksvik, I. B., Bjorvatn, B., Hetland, H., Sandal, G. M., & Pallesen, S. (2011). Individual differences in tolerance to shift work—A systematic review. *Sleep Medicine Reviews, 15*(4), 221–235. https://doi.org/10.1016/j.smrv.2010.07.002

Salfi, F., Lauriola, M., D'Atri, A., Amicucci, G., Viselli, L., Tempesta, D., & Ferrara, M. (2021). Demographic, psychological, chronobiological, and work-related predictors of sleep disturbances during the COVID-19 lockdown in Italy. *Scientific Reports, 11*(1), 11416. Advance online publication. https://doi.org/10.1038/s41598-021-90993-y

Schieman, S., & Young, M. C. (2013). Are communications about work outside regular working hours associated with work-to-family conflict, psychological distress and sleep problems? *Work and Stress, 27*(3), 244–261. https://doi.org/10.1080/02678373.2013.817090

Schiller, H., Lekander, M., Rajaleid, K., Hellgren, C., Åkerstedt, T., Barck-Holst, P., & Kecklund, G. (2017). The impact of reduced worktime on sleep and perceived stress— A group randomized intervention study using diary data. *Scandinavian Journal of Work, Environment & Health, 43*(2), 109–116. https://doi.org/10.5271/sjweh.3610

Shen, J., Barbera, J., & Shapiro, C. M. (2006). Distinguishing sleepiness and fatigue: Focus on definition and measurement. *Sleep Medicine Reviews, 10*(1), 63–76. https://doi.org/10.1016/j.smrv.2005.05.004

Shirom, A., & Melamed, S. (2006). A comparison of the construct validity of two burnout measures in two groups of professionals. *International Journal of Stress Management, 13*(2), 176–200. https://doi.org/10.1037/1072-5245.13.2.176

Sianoja, M., Crain, T. L., Hammer, L. B., Bodner, T., Brockwood, K. J., LoPresti, M., & Shea, S. A. (2020). The relationship between leadership support and employee sleep. *Journal of Occupational Health Psychology, 25*(3), 187–202. https://doi.org/10.1037/ocp0000173

Sonnentag, S. (2018). The recovery paradox: Portraying the complex interplay between job stressors, lack of recovery, and poor well-being. *Research in Organizational Behavior, 38*, 169–185. https://doi.org/10.1016/j.riob.2018.11.002

Taris, T. W. (2006). Is there a relationship between burnout and objective performance? A critical review of 16 studies. *Work and Stress, 20*(4), 316–334. https://doi.org/10.1080/02678370601065893

Techera, U., Hallowell, M., Stambaugh, N., & Littlejohn, R. (2016). Causes and consequences of occupational fatigue: Meta-analysis and systems model. *Journal of Occupational and Environmental Medicine, 58*(10), 961–973. https://doi.org/10.1097/JOM.0000000000000837

Temple, J. L., David Hostler, D., Martin-Gill, C., Moore, C. G., Weiss, P. M., Sequeira, D. J., Condle, J. P., Lang, E. S., Higgins, J. S., & Patterson, P. D. (2018). Systematic review and meta-analysis of the effects of caffeine in fatigues shift workers: Implications for emergency medical personnel services. *Prehospital Emergency Care, 22*(Suppl. 1). https://doi.org/10.1080/10903127.2017.1382624

Van de Water, A. T., Holmes, A., & Hurley, D. A. (2011). Objective measurements of sleep for non-laboratory settings as alternatives to polysomnography—A systematic review. *Journal of Sleep Research, 20*(1, Pt. 2), 183–200. https://doi.org/10.1111/j.1365-2869.2009.00814.x

Van Dijk, F. J., & Swaen, G. M. (2003). Fatigue at work. *Occupational and Environmental Medicine, 60*(Suppl. 1), i1–i2. https://doi.org/10.1136/oem.60.suppl_1.i1

van Hooff, M. L. M., Geurts, S. A. E., Kompier, M. A. J., & Taris, T. W. (2007). "How fatigued do you currently feel?" Convergent and discriminant validity of a single-item fatigue measure. *Journal of Occupational Health, 49*(3), 224–234. https://doi.org/10.1539/joh.49.224

Viswesvaran, C., Sanchez, J. I., & Fisher, J. (1999). The role of social support in the process of work stress: A meta-analysis. *Journal of Vocational Behavior, 54*(2), 314–334. https://doi.org/10.1006/jvbe.1998.1661

Waleriańczyk, W., Pruszczak, D., & Stolarski, M. (2020). Testing the role of midpoint sleep and social jetlag in the context of work psychology: An exploratory study. *Biological Rhythm Research, 51*(7), 1026–1043. https://doi.org/10.1080/09291016.2019.1571707

Wickwire, E. M., Geiger-Brown, J., Scharf, S. M., & Drake, C. L. (2017). Shift work and shift work disorder: Clinical and organizational perspectives. *Chest, 151*(5), 1156–1172. https://doi.org/10.1016/j.chest.2016.12.007

Wilkinson, R. T. (1964). Effects of up to 60 hours' sleep deprivation on different types of work. *Ergonomics, 7*(2), 175–186. https://doi.org/10.1080/00140136408930736

Winwood, P. C., Winefield, A. H., Dawson, D., & Lushington, K. (2005). Development and validation of a scale to measure work-related fatigue and recovery: The Occupational Fatigue Exhaustion/Recovery Scale (OFER). *Journal of Occupational and Environmental Medicine, 47*(6), 594–606. https://doi.org/10.1097/01.jom.0000161740.71049.c4

Wittmann, M., Dinich, J., Merrow, M., & Roenneberg, T. (2006). Social jetlag: Misalignment of biological and social time. *Chronobiology International, 23*(1–2), 497–509. https://doi.org/10.1080/07420520500545979

Zijlstra, F. R. H., Cropley, M., & Rydstedt, L. W. (2014). From recovery to regulation: An attempt to reconceptualize 'recovery from work.' *Stress and Health, 30*(3), 244–252. https://doi.org/10.1002/smi.2604

Zohar, D., Tzischinsky, O., Epstein, R., & Lavie, P. (2005). The effects of sleep loss on medical residents' emotional reactions to work events: A cognitive-energy model. *Sleep, 28*(1), 47–54. https://doi.org/10.1093/sleep/28.1.47

13

Taking a Broader View of Justice as a Component of Occupational Health

Moving Beyond Organizational Justice

M. Blake Hargrove

This chapter examines the relationship between justice and health and safety in the workplace. However, this chapter also intends to contribute by taking a larger look at justice than would normally be addressed in an organizational setting. As part of this handbook's overall goal, this chapter updates the reader on current streams of research and urges the scholars in our field to take a broader view of justice in organizations to better understand the connection between justice and occupational health and safety.

This chapter ambitiously seeks to push the closely related fields of *industrial and organizational* (I/O) psychology and organizational behavior[1] into some new directions, beginning with a review of justice in the organizational context including an explanation of the construct of *organizational justice* (OJ) over the past quarter of a century. This section includes an update of empirical work about the prevailing construct of OJ since the last publication of this handbook. Next, the chapter presents the probable etiology of justice as a universally held human value, relying primarily on the fields of evolutionary biology and primatology. Next, normative views of justice, with a principal focus on the work of John Rawls (1971), are described. The following section provides a glimpse of a few glaring injustices external to organizations and their potential impact upon occupational health and safety. The chapter concludes with a synthesis of the research presented and a call to action.

---

[1]For the sake of parsimony, these two closely related but perhaps distinct fields will be considered equivalent in this chapter and from this point in the chapter be referred to as "I/O."

https://doi.org/10.1037/0000331-013

Handbook of Occupational Health Psychology, Third Edition, L. E. Tetrick, G. G. Fisher, M. T. Ford, and J. C. Quick (Editors)

TRADITIONAL VIEWS OF ORGANIZATIONAL JUSTICE

While pioneers of I/O described the individual needs of workers to explain motivation, Fredrick Herzberg viewed needs-based theories skeptically and provided
an alternate perspective: Herzberg's motivator-hygiene theory (Herzberg, 1968;
Herzberg et al., 1959). In two-factor theory, workers require certain conditions
to be satisfied—these are called *hygiene factors*. Hygiene factors are necessary
but not sufficient conditions of motivation. Fairness is implicit among the most
common list of hygiene factors: compensation, policies, supervision, relationships, and relationships with peers. Additionally, work conditions and safety
are two hygiene factors explicitly connected to occupational health. Herzberg's
hygiene theory provides insight between subjective and objective views of
fairness to be subsequently discussed.

During the 1970s, I/O psychologists were beginning to employ the term *organizational justice*; however, many in I/O continued to follow Adams (1965), classical
economists, and Marxists by conceptualizing justice in the workplace as a fair
allocation of resources. During the 1980s, experimental and applied psychologists
along with their theoretical comrades in behavioral economy finalized the
dismantling of assumptions surrounding *Homo economicus* as a useful predictor
of individual human behavior. The OJ construct was, in part, reconceptualized as
emotional, perceptional, and attitudinal rather than mostly the cognitive bean-
counting suggested by early scholars. By the beginning of the 1990s, this more
socio-emotional concept of OJ guided I/O psychologists to build a body of empirical work (e.g., Greenberg, 1993) providing evidence that OJ and distributive justice were not interchangeable, that OJ was multidimensional, and that distributive
justice might well have the lowest effect size among the dimensions of OJ.

STABILIZATION OF OJ AS AN ATTITUDINAL CONSTRUCT WITHIN I/O

Two seminal meta-analyses conducted at the turn of the century stabilized the
understanding of OJ in the field of I/O (Cohen-Charash & Spector, 2001;
Colquitt et al., 2001). The two 2001 meta-analyses made an important contribution by confirming that OJ is dimensional. Colquitt et al. (2001) concluded
that OJ consists of three distinct dimensions: *distributive justice* (DJ), *procedural
justice* (PJ), and *interactional justice* (IJ). Although OJ has subsequently been
posited to have four or five dimensions, by separating interactional justice into
components (different explanations of IJ include *informational justice* and *interpersonal justice*), there emerged a broad consensus that continues to the present
that OJ has no fewer than three. Evaluating and analyzing mountains of
empirical evidence, both meta-analyses served to cement OJ as an attitude
formed by the affective and cognitive perception of stimuli. OJ, like all other
attitudes, is an internal individual mental state, rather than an objective appreciation of any given organizational situation. I/O psychology's choice to conceptualize OJ only as a perception creates a number of problems that will be
described in the next section.

A vast body of evidence suggests that each of the three dimensions is distinct, and all are connected to the allocation of resources. DJ concerns the quantity of resources allocated. For example, *ceteris paribus*, person A and person B perform identical work on identical tasks. Person A receives $2,000 for the work while person B receives $1,000. Person B would likely perceive unfairness—low DJ. PJ concerns the fairness or unfairness of the process of determining resource allocation. Returning to the example of persons A and B, imagine now that person A has 10 years of seniority over person B and that during those 10 years person B has received a series of raises. The difference in their pay may now be considered just because it is a well-understood process that wages increase over time. Therefore, in the identical distributive condition, person B may well perceive the difference as fair because an understood process was followed—high PJ. The third dimension, IJ, is the perceived quality of fairness of the interaction at the time resources are being allocated.

Significant evidence supports that the effect sizes PJ and IJ are greater than DJ. The most plausible explanation of this asymmetry is that PJ and IJ are attitudes resulting from an emotional response in the limbic system, while DJ has a much lower affective valence and relies principally on executive decision making. In other words, the asymmetry of effect size reflects findings in other realms of psychology that demonstrate that affect generally drives behavior more than cognition. Fascinating empirical work investigating DJ as cognitive and PJ as affective has been accomplished using functional magnetic resonance imaging (fMRI) technology. Dulebohn and his collaborators (2009) experimentally demonstrated that DJ primarily activates portions of the brain associated with cognitive processes including decision-making, while PJ activates portions of the brain associated with emotion and the limbic system.

This asymmetry of the effect size between the affective dimensions of PJ and IJ compared to DJ directly bears on health and safety. Workers who perceive high PJ and IJ regarding their working conditions may overpower their own perception of low DJ. In other words, workers may well accept unsafe conditions as high OJ if they perceive the processes and interactions under which they work fair. The long-running, popular television show presented on the Discovery Channel, *Deadliest Catch*, reminds us that even in popular culture, the objectively hazardous conditions in the Alaskan crab fishery do not appear to cause either a labor shortage or worker appeals for safer working conditions (Beers, 2005–2022).

CHALLENGES RESULTING FROM OJ BEING CONCEPTUALIZED AS AN ATTITUDE

Following the 2001 meta-analyses, I/O psychologists came to a consensus that OJ was an attitude and as such has almost always been measured by self-report surveys. The subjectivity poses at least four significant challenges impacting occupational health and safety.

First, the lack of objectivity in this definition of OJ presents a serious problem for those who believe workers are entitled to objective justice as a part of a basic schema of dignity and respect. Workers may well perceive sufficient OJ (fair enough supervision in the terms of Herzberg) even when conditions are demonstrably unfair. For example, undocumented workers may perceive their $10 per hour compensation at a pork-processing plant as sufficient (good OJ) when they are objectively being treated unfairly. The "legal" peers with whom they work side by side receive higher wages, overtime pay, and benefits (e.g., health care, retirement) from their employer (Gastón, 2011). In other words, sincere perceptions are often incorrect: Perceiving OJ cannot be equated with objective fairness. Incorrect perceptions of this type are a threat to occupational health due to the well-established negative mental health impacts resulting from abusive supervision.

Second, the conceptualization of OJ as a perception presents particular problems with regard to occupational health and safety. Workers may perceive sufficient OJ even when engaged in work that is demonstrably unsafe and predictably produces often untreatable and life-threatening disease. For example, surface/strip mining accounted for 62% of coal mining in the United States during 2019 (U.S. Energy Information Administration, 2020). The content of the dust that clouds around these operations includes respirable crystalline silica, a form of quartz that is more toxic than coal dust and regulated at one-twentieth the level; inhalation of silica can result in silicosis and other serious respiratory diseases that can be disabling or deadly (National Institute for Occupational Safety and Health, 2021). The Mine Safety and Health Administration (MSHA) requires surface-mining operators to take feasible engineering measures to reduce worker exposure to silica including enclosing cabs of heavy equipment (MSHA, n.d.) Nevertheless, a common complaint among miners is that enclosed cabs are not temperature controlled; when hot, workers presumably open windows and expose themselves to dust (MSHA, n.d.). MSHA requires reasonable engineering measures, but not air conditioners that cost from $2,500 to $4,500, equivalent to less than 4% of the average cost of one machine. Some operators are prepared to sacrifice workers' health to increase profit (MSHA, n.d.). For these operators, meeting minimal legal standards is fair enough. The surface miners working in objectively under-regulated, under-inspected, and potentially deadly conditions do not cry out for justice. Instead, coal miners cry out for more coal mining.

Third, subjective OJ does not incentivize organizations to maximize worker safety; this sensible obligation may be unnecessary for safety to be perceived as fair. In theory, unsafe workplaces would be predicted to violate safety needs and generate low OJ. It follows that employers who wish to motivate their workers should seek to make their workplaces safer so that workers will not feel treated unjustly; employers generally do want workplaces that are safe— but likely only safe enough. As a hygiene factor (à la Herzberg), safer work environments do not motivate. This means that organizations have little incentive to become safer. Because for most workers conditions must be "safe enough," employers lose their incentive to improve the safety of the workplace, even when such changes would be economically feasible. Simply put, many workers are willing to work under conditions that are not as safe as they could or should be because workers perceive the workplace to be sufficiently safe. This seems to be a strong argument for the passage of statutes requiring organizations to meet all reasonably feasible health and safety thresholds, and a robust schema of enforcement of the ensuing regulations. Safe enough for OJ does not mean safe enough for good public policy or a normatively just society, as discussed later in this chapter.

A fourth challenge with conceptualizing OJ as an attitude concerns the wide variance of perceptions and moral sensibilities that occur in different normative contexts. Meta-analytic evidence supports the assertion that OJ, as a perception, varies between individuals and groups, institutions and organizations, and national and regional cultures even when the objective conditions are identical (Fischer, 2013). Therefore, it is more than likely that diamond miners in South Africa report high OJ in objectively hazardous conditions compared with underground miners in the United Kingdom who work under objectively safer conditions that are strictly regulated by the British government.

THE IMPACT OF JUSTICE ON OCCUPATIONAL HEALTH

This section stands at the center of this chapter; it serves the core purpose of illuminating the relationship between justice and occupational health. Three subsections present the impact of injustice on health via the mechanism of distress, somatic health outcomes, and mental health outcomes relying on empirical studies since the publication of the handbook's last edition.

OJ and Distress

Entire chapters on the relationship between stress and occupational health and safety have been included in this handbook; this section concerning the relationships among justice, distress, and occupational health and safety is therefore intended to be brief. An explanation of the relationship cannot be overlooked, however, because one of the principal threats to occupational health in the workplace is distress and burnout resulting from the injustice of unsafe working conditions.

A consensus in the OJ literature supports a main effect relationship between injustice distress and other distress-related constructs. In a study of 432 Argentine workers, there was a strong, main effect relationship between DJ, PJ, IJ, and burnout, which mediated the effect of injustice on job satisfaction and turnover (Vaamonde et al., 2018). In a sample of Arab respondents, the expected main effect between low OJ and distress was found, but the study also found evidence that organizational citizenship mediated the relationship (Tziner & Sharoni, 2014). Another body of empirical work in the context of criminal justice and prison workers studied the relationship between OJ and distress. These studies confirm the high correlation of OJ to distress and of distress to negative occupational health outcomes (Boateng & Hsieh, 2019; Lambert et al., 2007, 2019; May et al., 2020). Taken together, recent empirical work supports the finding that injustice predicts distress.

Since the publication of the last edition of this handbook, there have been several relevant meta-analyses and reviews relevant to the pathway from OJ to distress to health. While the findings of the meta-analyses differed based on their research questions, both showed that injustice in the workplace as operationalized by low OJ (or one OJ's dimensions) was positively related to workplace distress (or closely related constructs). Findings provide evidence that distress mediates injustice's impact on negative health outcomes (Kivimaki et al., 2006; van der Molen et al., 2020; Zhang et al., 2019). In another comprehensive literature review, research demonstrated that the relationship between OJ and injustice has now been examined in a variety of industries and many work settings in developed countries; all provided evidence confirming distress as the most plausible mechanism for OJ to impact health (Elovainio et al., 2010). Finally, another review specifically investigated the relationship between OJ and coronary heart disease and found, once again, that distress was the principal mechanism through which injustice impacts health (Sara et al., 2018).

OJ and Somatic Health

In the period since the publication of the last edition of this handbook, there has not been a great deal of empirical research exploring the main effect of OJ on physical health outcomes in the United States. Instead, research on OJ and its relationship with somatic health has been primarily conducted in Europe and Japan. One area that has received significant attention is the relationship between injustice and sleep. A well-designed longitudinal study of 24,000 Finnish public sector employees (82% women) found an inverse relationship between OJ and persistent insomnia symptoms (Lallukka et al., 2017). Interestingly, the study found that the PJ dimension was not significantly related to insomnia symptoms. A study using a Swedish sample contradicted the Finnish study in part by providing evidence that sleep difficulties were predicted by low PJ (Bernhard-Oettel et al., 2020). Another study provided additional evidence that OJ has a primary effect on sleeping disorders (Manville et al., 2016). The study also found that time sleep-disorders completely mediated the relationship between OJ and musculoskeletal disorders. This suggests that the relationship between injustice and negative outcomes has multiple pathways. Finally, in another sample of European workers, Finnish nurses perceiving higher levels of OJ experienced fewer sleeping problems (Hietapakka et al., 2013). This study also provided evidence to support the most common IO meta-analytic finding that distress partially mediated the relationship between OJ and fewer sleeping problems, accounting for approximately 50% of the difference in sleep issues (Hietapakka et al., 2013).

One positive trend in empirical work concerning injustice and somatic health is that more researchers are using physiological objective measures rather than depending upon self-report measures to assess the impact of injustice on worker health. In a European study, 24-hour heart rate data were investigated comparing 222 blue-collar and 179 white-collar male workers (Herr et al., 2015). The researchers found evidence that IJ, and to a lesser extent PJ, impacted the 24-hour heart rate variability among white-collar workers but had no effect on blue-collar workers. Another physical measure used to operationalize health outcomes is low-density lipoprotein (LDL) cholesterol levels. Although LDL cholesterol levels are far less concerning than high-density lipoprotein levels, the National Institutes of Health (NIH; 2020) recommends LDL levels lower than 132 using the standard fasting cholesterol blood test. A study among a sample of Japanese workers found that low IJ among Japanese working men resulted in lower LDL cholesterol levels (Inoue et al., 2015).

Researchers also choose to take a more macro approach investigating justice and occupational health. In two separate studies of Japanese workers, evidence indicated that the levels of PJ and IJ impacted workers' willingness to report illness (Eguchi et al., 2019; Inoue et al., 2019). Generally, evidence showed that a higher perception of PJ and IJ had direct main effects, and that these effects were amplified among women workers. In a longitudinal Swedish study of 25,000 workers, higher OJ was associated with a lower risk for seeking disability pensions for musculoskeletal disorders (Juvani et al., 2016). In another well-designed longitudinal study among 7,011 European employed persons between the ages of 45 and 64, evidence indicated that both DJ and PJ contributed to lower productivity loss and lower illness-related absences (Ybema & van den Bos, 2010). These studies taken together suggest that under perceived fair conditions, workers may be both more likely to report illness and less likely to have unhealthy outcomes.

OJ and Mental Health

The study of health and safety in the workplace must obviously include mental health. Researchers have chosen a variety of mental illnesses to study utilizing a variety of research methods. In the same large longitudinal study used to examine reporting pensioning requests due to musculoskeletal causes, the investigators found that higher conditions of OJ were associated with lower levels of disability claims due to depression, suggesting that injustice might be a predictor of depression (Juvani et al., 2016). Other studies have also suggested that low PJ and IJ predict higher levels of depression (Lang et al., 2011; Wood et al., 2012). Unsurprisingly, given the evidence provided in the previous discussion of stress, studies have shown that the inverse relationship between PJ and IJ has a main effect relationship with psychological distress (Hietapakka et al., 2013; Inoue et al., 2016). This effect was found across diverse work contexts and among people of completely different cultural backgrounds.

Additionally, researchers have struggled about the potential bidirectionality of the relationship between perceptions of justice and mental health. This remains the case today. One ambitious study used three independent samples of U.S. military units and a longitudinal design; because perceptions of four dimensions of OJ lagged depressive symptoms, the evidence suggested that mental health might be an antecedent rather than an outcome of perceptions of justice (Lang et al., 2011). The direction of the relationship remains unresolved due to mixed results in a rigorous cross-lagged panel study conducted among 3,000 Swedish workers (Eib et al., 2018). Though this study was intentionally designed to help resolve the directionality question, the mixed results failed to produce conclusive evidence. The study found that PJ lagged depressive symptoms and illness-related absences but not self-reported health. The authors provided several possible explanations for the lack of definitive evidence. So, for now, the direction of the relationship between injustice and health remains an unresolved empirical question.

In the preceding paragraphs, justice and injustice have been operationalized in terms of OJ, a perception of fairness. As indicated from the prior discussion, there are significant problems, especially about occupational health arising from the disconnect between subjective perceptions and objective realities. The following section examines another approach to justice: the predisposition of workers to expect just conditions due to evolved neural anatomy.

FAIRNESS AS A BIOLOGICAL ADAPTATION

Developmental and evolutionary psychologists hold a strong, evidence-based consensus that sensitivity to fairness has a critical ontogenetic basis. Evidence indicates humans learn hard lessons about justice within their families of origin and peer groups. They adopt the norms of justice followed within their native cultures. Individuals' understanding of justice changes as they mature. Human understanding of fairness is not universal, and, in the beautiful diversity fundamental to humanity, different individuals from different cultures hold different notions of justice. Despite this variation, *Homo sapiens* also possess phylogenetic sensitivity to fairness, and each human possesses ancient alleles expressing themselves phenotypically in the anatomical structure of their brains; humans' neural anatomy predisposes each person to expect fairness (Wang et al., 2019).

From an evolutionary psychology perspective, fairness might be viewed as a critical adaptation to predispose people to engage in prosocial behavior (Decety & Yoder, 2017). Over the past decades, Frans de Waal and many other evolutionary psychologists, anthropologists, and primatologists have explored and documented a wide variety of what appear to be forms of morality in nonhuman animals (Brosnan & de Waal, 2014; de Waal, 2012). Studies have found evidence of moral ("right" or "wrong," "good" or "bad") behaviors in both mammals and birds (Laumer et al., 2019). However, for the purposes of brevity, this discussion of evolved morality will be (a) limited to the primates, our closest genetic cousins; and (b) to fairness, the subject of this chapter.

Through dozens of replicated experiments, de Waal and his collaborators have found that primates consistently demonstrate a sense of fairness (Campbell et al., 2020; Proctor et al., 2013). Like any other trait, fairness would have developed in primates via the process of natural selection. The prevailing theory is that fairness provided an advantage to early primates living in social groups. Those individuals that had the fairness phenotype, resulting from brain anatomy, had greater personal and inclusive fitness and their genes were more likely to pass to the subsequent generations than those individuals lacking the phenotype (Debove et al., 2017; Hall & Brosnan, 2016).

There is no plausible theory to suggest that humans alone among primates lack the fairness phenotype. To the contrary, an increasing body of experimental evidence using infants, toddlers, and young children provide support for a significant phylogenetic basis for a sensitivity to fairness and other pro-social behavior (Killen, 2018). *Homo sapiens*, like our primate cousins, possess neural anatomy that predisposes us to recognize and appreciate justice. De Waal and his colleagues never suggest that primates or humans ought or ought not be fair, nor are they asserting that every individual is naturally fair or behaves fairly. Instead, their work provides strong evidence that primate brains are morphologically predisposed to possess the phenotype of sensitivity to fairness.

The research from both primatology and developmental psychology support an understanding of fairness not as a value, but as a biological adaptation. *H. sapiens* possess the homeostatic expectation to be treated fairly (Gerdemann et al., 2022; Bjorklund, 2020). The essence of this handbook chapter concerns the potential negative impact of (in)justice on worker health and safety. This section seeks to help the reader better understand this impact by appreciating that justice is not just a personal or cultural expectation for workers; workers are biologically sensitive to fairness. Like all *Homo sapiens*, workers expect fair treatment, and occupational health and safety are central elements for worker justice. In the following section, we change course from an evolutionary perspective. We turn toward the moral and philosophical implications of justice as applied to workplace health and safety.

NORMATIVE JUSTICE

Long before Darwin and future biologists explored the mechanism by which animals evolved a sense of fairness and I/O theorists and researchers examined the impact of fairness and unfairness in the workplace, philosophers wrestled with concepts of justice. Over the past three millennia and among Asian, Near Eastern, and European contexts, great thinkers recognized the centrality of justice to the ethical systems they helped construct. Han Feizi, Confucius, Ibn Árabî, and many others over the centuries have struggled to define and explain fairness. Plato argued that justice is central to that which is good or bad: "of all things of a man's soul which he has within him, justice is the greatest good, and injustice the greatest evil" (Plato, c. 375 BCE). Augustine of Hippo, during the third century (CE), named justice as one of the four cardinal virtues.

Another seminal Christian ethicist, Thomas Aquinas, believed that morality was woven into the fabric of creation as part of the natural law. Great philosophers across civilizations have recognized justice as one of the keys to the timeless question "What is right and what is wrong?"

The ethical ramifications of justice continue to be explored in the modern era. Perhaps the most influential political philosopher in the past 50 years, John Rawls, lies at the center of philosophical discussions of justice today. Rawls first published *A Theory of Justice* in 1971, and in his paradigm-shifting book he proposes that a just society follow two principles:

1. Each person is to have an equal right to the most extensive total system of equal basic liberties compatible with a similar system of liberty for all.

2. Social and economic inequalities are to be arranged so that they are both: (a) to the greatest benefit of the least advantaged, consistent with the just savings principle, and (b) attached to offices and positions open to all under conditions of fair equality of opportunity. (Rawls, 1971, p.302)

Scholars from many disciplines analyzed, scrutinized, attacked, supported, lauded, and rejected these criteria. However, these criteria radically altered the discourse around justice when they were published and continue to do so today.

Perhaps the greatest ramification of these criteria about justice is that the impact of accident of birth should be minimized. Individuals have no control over what traits they will acquire, what gifts or disabilities they will possess, or to what geographic or socioeconomic status they might be assigned. In a fair world, accident of birth should not determine the path of lives. Whether born into privilege or poverty, a just society should be possible for all. Despite the admonitions of Rawls and his proponents, present economic and social systems fail to provide equal rights and opportunities and most certainly do not benefit the least advantaged.

IMPACT OF SOCIAL INJUSTICE ON OCCUPATIONAL HEALTH AND SAFETY

Though the title of this handbook chapter includes "justice," it might have been more accurate to focus on injustice. Humans, like the animals studied by de Waal and others, evolved to be especially sensitive to injustice. The followings subsections present a few of the many examples of human injustice related workers' health and safety.

The Globally Privileged Few and the Suffering Masses

This discussion of normative justice is not just a metaphysical exercise. Injustice in society directly impacts occupational health and safety, and the failure to put those principles into operation have been and will continue to be devastating. Enormous inequities in income and assets are taken for granted both within and across countries, and inequity directly impacts occupational health and safety. Simply put, rich people tend to work in safer spaces doing thought jobs, and poor people work under more dangerous conditions doing muscle jobs (Kim, 2018). Rich people are less likely to be injured or become ill at work than poor people (Rosenthal, 2021), and the most dangerous jobs are almost never done by the most privileged people (Kim, 2018). Ultimately, rich people live longer and healthier lives than poor people, and much of this variance can be explained by places and types of work (Crimmens et al., 2011). For most people, accident of birth likely predicts both safe working conditions and length of life under the current system. At work, it is the least advantaged who are put in the worst health and safety conditions—a reality 180° in opposition to Rawls's proposed just society.

Working conditions vary across the globe. At the rich end of the spectrum, EU workers are legally entitled to safe working conditions (European Commission, 2021). For the most part, governments enforce these regulations and even punish some of those responsible for unsafe workplaces. Unlike the EU, most global citizens have few rights and virtually no enforcement. For hundreds of millions, occupational health and safety are fully ignored. This, of course, leads to millions of unnecessary work-related deaths and injuries for exploited adult and child workers; figures must be estimated due to complete lack of reporting in most lesser developed countries. However, these estimates are staggering. Agencies of the UN estimate more than 2.3 million work-related deaths (ILO, 2021; LaDou et al., 2018). How many more workers will be made ill or injured? People working in often despicable conditions lose lives, limbs, sight, hearing, and suffer untold consequences to their mental health. One doesn't need to agree with Rawls to recognize gross injustice. By any definition of justice, a system that consistently generates unnecessary injuries and deaths is unfair and morally impermissible (Carbo et al., 2017). Yet this corporatist system dominates the economic activity of this planet. Not only does this system ignore unfair and unsafe working conditions for hundreds of millions of disadvantaged people; it also depends upon these conditions (Faber, 2018). Stated plainly, most citizens of wealthy nations turn a blind eye to the sickening working conditions under which hundreds of millions of working children and adults toil and ignore the fact that this suffering and deprivation of human rights produce cheap consumer goods sold to produce revenue for corporations. To efficiently maximize profitability, hundreds of millions endure unacceptably unsafe and unhealthy workplaces (Carbo et al., 2017).

Injustice in the United States

In the wealthiest country in the world, serious problems with occupational health and safety persist. However, these problems are not evenly distributed in the United States. They are unfairly distributed by the same unjust rule that separates the EU from Bangladesh: The rich are largely sheltered from exposure to the unsafe and unhealthy workplaces, while many poor Americans are not. One clear example of social injustice is the inverse relationship between worker safety and wages in the United States. Low-paying, blue-collar work tends to be far more dangerous than higher paying, white-collar work. For example, in 2020 the median hourly wage for a miner (including many highly skilled workers, such as master electricians) was $28.95 (Bureau of Labor Statistics [BLS], 2020), while the median hourly wage for a worker in the computer industry was $44.65 (BLS, 2021a). In 2020, there were 102,760 blue-collar workers in coal mining (BLS, 2020) and 362,580 white-collar workers in the computer industry (BLS, 2021a). During 2018, eleven coal miners were killed on the job (BLS, 2021b). It is important to note that this figure does not include the many hundreds of former miners that died from occupationally related respiratory disease. Also during 2018, fifteen computer workers were killed on the job (BLS, 2021b). The workplace fatality rate for coal miners was a little above 11 out of 100,000, and for computer workers was four out of 100,000. American coal miners take more than twice the fatality risk for 65% of the wages of a computer worker.

Another connection between occupational health and social injustice occurs in the endemic sexism in the United States. Sexism is more than just male supremacy in the United States; it is a serious health problem. It has been estimated that only 30% of rapes go reported, which is staggering given the Federal Bureau of Investigation's (FBI's; 2021) 2019 estimate of about 140,000 rapes. Another significant threat to women's health due to social injustice is the endemic sexual harassment experienced by most women, often at work. As with sexual assault, it is difficult to estimate how many millions of women suffer from harassment annually because the least likely action of a victim of sexual harassment is to report it (Feldblum & Lipnic, 2016). Other studies have produced evidence that severe forms of injustice, such as harassment and bullying, contribute to other dangerous mental health conditions, such as depression and posttraumatic stress disorder (Newins et al., 2021). This prolonged social injustice directed against women contributes to their sense of physical safety, psychological stability, and long-term mental health. Women don't stop being women at work; social injustice makes a clear impact on occupational health and safety.

The impact of "America's original sin," racism (Wallis, 2016), is well studied and well understood: Black Americans have different economic and health outcomes. Black workers (11.2%) are more than twice as likely to report being discriminated against "regularly" than Whites (3.8%; Lee et al., 2019), and the median income of Black Americans ($30,000) is $12,000 or 29% less than the national median ($42,000; McKinsey Global Institute, 2021). Black Americans' proportion of the population is not evident in the work they do. Black Americans make up roughly 13% of the U.S. population, 5.8% of physicians, 36.6% of home health care workers, and 35.5% of nursing assistants (McKinsey Global Institute, 2021). As previously established, there is an inverse relationship between wages and occupational health and safety, and Black Americans are highly clustered in low-wage jobs (McKinsey Global Institute, 2021). Overall, Black Americans' health outcomes (a part of which is occupational health) differ significantly from those of other Americans: Black male life expectancy is 6.3 years shorter on average (72.2) than that of the U.S. population (78.6; Arias & Xu, 2020), and Black Americans of working age are 14% more likely to report

12-month major depressions (8.85%) than Whites (7.75%; Dunlop et al., 2003). As usual, racism in America is not all that complicated, one just has to count. Racial injustice impacts the economic and health outcomes of every Black American worker. When Black Americans come to work, they don't stop being Black. To return to the I/O OJ framework, how could it be possible for Black Americans to perceive high DJ or PJ while living in a systematically unjust society and working in (mostly) unfair organizations?

CONCLUSION

For psychologists to bring their full set of tools to bear on worker safety, they must reassess the conceptualization of organizational justice beyond OJ. Objective justice matters to workers; in many contexts perceiving a high level of OJ provides little insight into objective working conditions. Conceptualizing justice as subjective attitude comes at a high human cost when it ignores the negative impact of objectively unsafe working conditions, economic disparity, and social injustice.

Justice demands that all workers have the right to a safe environment in which to earn their living. Psychologists studying the relationship between justice and occupational health and safety must broaden their concern across the globe, giving the same attention to worker safety in least developed countries that they do in their own safe corners in rich nations. A safe workplace is a human right, not a privilege for the relatively wealthy or the systematically privileged; having a safe and healthy place to work should not be an accident of birth. There is simply no justification for a person who happens to be born in the United States or France to have safer and healthier places to work than for their fellow human beings born in Bangladesh or Myanmar. Similarly systemic injustice—economic, sex-based, or ethnicity-based—can neither be permitted to determine the safety conditions of workers nor be ignored as a health risk-factor in the workplace.

Human neural anatomy is to some degree determinative; humans are born with the expectation of fair treatment. Rawls provides one framework for this expectation to be made into reality. A Rawlsian society obliges organizations to provide all workers with the fairness to which they are entitled, and this emphatically includes an objectively safe and healthy work environment. The next decade brings practitioners and scholars the opportunity to help build organizations in which accident of birth does not predict the standards of fairness, safety, or health. Together, we need to study, practice, and advocate for workers to have a fairer, safer, and healthier world—a world that they expect and a world to which they are entitled.

REFERENCES

Adams, J. S. (1965). Inequity in social exchange. *Advances in Experimental Social Psychology, 2*, 267–299. https://doi.org/10.1016/S0065-2601(08)60108-2

Arias, E., & Xu, J. (2020). *United States life tables, 2018.* Centers for Disease Control and Prevention. https://www.cdc.gov/nchs/data/nvsr/nvsr69/nvsr69-12-508.pdf

Bernhard-Oettel, C., Eib, C., Griep, Y., & Leineweber, C. (2020). How do job insecurity and organizational justice relate to depressive symptoms and sleep difficulties: A multilevel study on immediate and prolonged effects in Swedish workers. *Applied Psychology, 69*(4),1271–1300. https://doi.org/10.1111/apps.12222

Beers, T. (Executive Producer). (2005–2022). *Deadliest catch* [TV series]. Discovery Channel.

Bjorklund, D.F. (2020). *Child development in evolutionary perspective.* Cambridge University Press. https://doi.org/10.1017/9781108866187

Boateng, F. D., & Hsieh, M.-L. (2019). Misconduct within the "four walls": Does organizational justice matter in explaining prison officers' misconduct and job stress? *International Journal of Offender Therapy and Comparative Criminology, 63*(2), 289–308. https://doi.org/10.1177/0306624X18780941

Brosnan, S. F., & de Waal, F. B. (2014). Evolution of responses to (un)fairness. *Science, 346*(6207). https://www.science.org/doi/10.1126/science.1251776

Bureau of Labor Statistics. (2020). *May 2020, National industry-specific occupational employment and wage estimates, NAICS 212100—Coal mining.* https://www.bls.gov/oes/2020/may/naics4_212100.htm#49-0000

Bureau of Labor Statistics. (2021a). *Occupational employment and wages, May 2021, 15–1299 Computer occupations, all other.* https://www.bls.gov/oes/current/oes151299.htm

Bureau of Labor Statistics. (2021b). *Occupational injuries, illnesses, and fatalities profiles.* [Data table]. Bureau of Labor Statistics. https://data.bls.gov/gqt/ProfileData

Campbell, M. W., Wazeck, J., Suchak, M., Berman, S. M., & de Waal, F. B. M. (2020). Chimpanzees (*Pan troglodytes*) tolerate some degree of inequity while cooperating but refuse to donate effort for nothing. *American Journal of Primatology, 82*(1), 1–32. https://doi.org/10.1002/ajp.23084

Carbo, J. A., Dao, V. T., Haase, S. J., Hargrove, M. B., & Langella, I. M. (2017). *Social sustainability for business.* Routledge. https://doi.org/10.4324/9781315641980

Cohen-Charash, Y., & Spector, P. E. (2001). The role of justice in organizations: A meta-analysis. *Organizational Behavior and Human Decision Processes, 86*(2), 278–321. https://doi.org/10.1006/obhd.2001.2958

Colquitt, J. A., Conlon, D. E., Wesson, M. J., Porter, C. O., & Ng, K. Y. (2001). Justice at the millennium: A meta-analytic review of 25 years of organizational justice research. *Journal of Applied Psychology, 86*(3), 425–445. https://doi.org/10.1037/0021-9010.86.3.425

Crimmens, E., Preston, S. H., & Coen, B. (2011). Explaining divergent levels of longevity in high-income countries. In E. Crimmens, S. H. Preston, & B. Coen (Eds.), *National Research Council (US) Panel on Understanding Divergent Trends in Longevity in High-Income Countries* (117–141). National Academies Press. https://www.ncbi.nlm.nih.gov/books/NBK62362/

de Waal, F. B. (2012). The antiquity of empathy. *Science, 336*(6083), 874–876. https://doi.org/10.1126/science.1220999

Debove, S., Baumard, N., & André, J. B. (2017). On the evolutionary origins of equity. *PLOS ONE, 12*(3), e0173636. https://doi.org/10.1371/journal.pone.0173636

Decety, J., & Yoder, K. J. (2017). The emerging social neuroscience of justice motivation. *Trends in Cognitive Sciences, 21*(1), 6–14. https://doi.org/10.1016/j.tics.2016.10.008

Dulebohn, J. H., Conlon, D. E., Sarinopoulos, I., Davison, R. B., & McNamara, G. (2009). The biological bases of unfairness: Neuroimaging evidence for the distinctiveness of procedural and distributive justice. *Organizational Behavior and Human Decision Processes, 110*(2), 140–151. https://doi.org/10.1016/j.obhdp.2009.09.001

Dunlop, D. D., Song, J., Lyons, J. S., Mannheim, L. M., & Chang, R. W. (2003). Racial/ethnic differences in rates of depression among pre-retirement adults. *American Journal of Public Health, 93*(11), 1945–1952. https://doi.org/10.2105/ajph.93.11.1945

Eguchi, H., Tsutsumi, A., Inoue, A., & Kachi, Y. (2019). Organizational justice and illness reporting among Japanese employees with chronic diseases. *PLOS ONE, 14*(10), e0223595. https://doi.org/10.1371/journal.pone.0223595

Eib, C., Bernhard-Oettel, C., Magnusson Hanson, L. L., & Leineweber, C. (2018). Organizational justice and health: Studying mental preoccupation with work and social support as mediators for lagged and reversed relationships. *Journal of Occupational Health Psychology, 23*(4), 553–567. https://doi.org/10.1037/ocp0000115

Elovainio, M., Heponiemi, T., Sinervo, T., & Magnavita, N. (2010). Organizational justice and health; review of evidence. *Giornale italiano di medicina del lavoro ed ergonomia, 32*(3, Supp. B), B5–9. https://pubmed.ncbi.nlm.nih.gov/21299075/

European Commission. (2021). *The European Pillar of Social Rights Action Plan.* European Commission. https://ec.europa.eu/info/strategy/priorities-2019-2024/economy-works-people/jobs-growth-and-investment/european-pillar-social-rights/european-pillar-social-rights-action-plan_en

Faber, D. (2018). Global capitalism, reactionary neoliberalism, and the deepening of environmental injustices. *Capitalism Nature Socialism, 29*(2), 8–28. https://doi.org/10.1080/10455752.2018.1464250

Federal Bureau of Investigation. (2021, July 29). *Crime in the U.S. 2019: Rape.* https://ucr.fbi.gov/crime-in-the-u.s/2019/crime-in-the-u.s.-2019/topic-pages/rape

Feldblum, C. R., & Lipnic, V. (2016). *Select Task Force on the Study of Harassment in the Workplace.* US Equal Employment Opportunity Commission. https://www.eeoc.gov/select-task-force-study-harassment-workplace#_Toc453686298

Fischer, R. (2013). Belonging, status, or self-protection? Examining justice motives in a three-level cultural meta-analysis of organizational justice effects. *Cross-Cultural Research, 47*(1), 3–41. https://doi.org/10.1177/1069397112470424

Gastón, M. T. (2011). *Meatpacking workers' perceptions of working conditions, psychological contracts and organizational justice.* University of Nebraska.

Gerdemann, S. C., McAuliffe, K., Blake, P. R., Haun, D. B., & Hepach, R. (2022). The ontogeny of children's social emotions in response to (un) fairness. *Royal Society Open Science, 9*(8), pp. 1–24. https://doi.org/10.1098/rsos.191456

Greenberg, J. (1993). Stealing in the name of justice: Informational and interpersonal moderators of theft reactions to underpayment inequality. *Organizational Behavior and Human Decision Processes, 54*(1), 81–103. https://doi.org/10.1006/obhd.1993.1004

Hall, K., & Brosnan, S. F. (2016). A comparative perspective on the evolution of moral behavior. In T. K. Shackelford & R. D. Hansen (Eds.), *The evolution of morality* (pp. 157–176). Springer International. https://doi.org/10.1007/978-3-319-19671-8_8

Herr, R. M., Bosch, J. A., van Vianen, A. E., Jarczok, M. N., Thayer, J. F., Li, J., Schmidt, B., Fischer, J. E., & Loerbroks, A. (2015). Organizational justice is related to heart rate variability in white-collar workers, but not in blue-collar workers—Findings from a cross-sectional study. *Annals of Behavioral Medicine, 49*(3), 434–448. https://doi.org/10.1007/s12160-014-9669-9

Herzberg, F. I., Mausner, B., & Snyderman, B. (1959). *The motivation to work.* Wiley.

Herzberg, F. I. (1968). One more time: How do you motivate employees? *Harvard Business Review 81*(1), 87–96.

Hietapakka, L., Elovainio, M., Heponiemi, T., Presseau, J., Eccles, M., Aalto, A.-M., Pekkarinen, L., Kuokkanen, L., & Sinervo, T. (2013). Do nurses who work in a fair organization sleep and perform better and why? Testing potential psychosocial mediators of organizational justice. *Journal of Occupational Health Psychology, 18*(4), 481–491. https://doi.org/10.1037/a0033990

Inoue, A., Kawakami, N., Eguchi, H., Miyaki, K., & Tsutsumi, A. (2015). Organizational justice and physiological coronary heart disease risk factors in Japanese employees: A cross-sectional study. *International Journal of Behavioral Medicine, 22*(6), 775–785. https://doi.org/10.1007/s12529-015-9480-4

Inoue, A., Kawakami, N., Eguchi, H., & Tsutsumi, A. (2016). Modifying effect of ciga-rette smoking on the association of organizational justice with serious psychological distress in Japanese employees: A cross-sectional study. *International Archives of Occupational and Environmental Health, 89*(6), 901–910. https://doi.org/10.1007/s00420-016-1128-4

Inoue, A., Tsutsumi, A., Eguchi, H., & Kawakami, N. (2019). Organizational justice and refraining from seeking medical care among Japanese employees: A 1-year pro-spective cohort study. *International Journal of Behavioral Medicine, 26*(1), 76–84. https://doi.org/10.1007/s12529-018-9756-6

International Labour Organization. (2021, July 29). *World Statistic.* https://www.ilo.org/moscow/areas-of-work/occupational-safety-and-health/WCMS_249278/lang--en/index.htm

Juvani, A., Oksanen, T., Virtanen, M., Elovainio, M., Salo, P., Pentti, J., Vahtera, J. (2016). Organizational justice and disability pension from all-causes, depression and musculoskeletal diseases: A Finnish cohort study of public sector employees. *Scandinavian Journal of Work, Environment & Health, 45*(2), 395–404. https://doi.org/10.5271/sjweh.3582

Killen, M. (2018). The origins of morality: Social equality, fairness, and justice. *Philosophical Psychology, 31*(5), 767–803, https://doi.org/10.1080/09515089.2018.1486612

Kim, J. Y. (2018, April 10). *Rich and poor: Opportunities and challenges in an age of disruptions.* [Transcript: 2018 World Bank Group Spring Meeting positioning speech]. American University, Washington, DC. https://www.worldbank.org/en/news/speech/2018/04/10/rich-and-poor-opportunities-and-challenges-in-an-age-of-disruption

Kivimaki, M., Virtanen, M., Elovainio, M., Kouvonen, A., Vanaanen, A., & Vahtera, J. (2006). Work stress in the etiology of coronary heart disease—A meta-analysis. *Scandanavian Journal of Work, Environment & Health, 32*(6), 431–442. https://doi.org/10.5271/sjweh.1049

LaDou, J., London, L., & Watterson, A. (2018). Occupational health: A world of false promises. *Environmental Health, 17,* 81. https://doi.org/10.1186/s12940-018-0422-x

Lallukka, T., Halonen, J. I., Sivertsen, B., Pentti, J., Stenholm, S., Virtanen, M., Salo, P., Oksanen, T., Elovainio, M., Vahtera, J., & Kivimäki, M. (2017). Change in organi-zational justice as a predictor of insomnia symptoms: Longitudinal study analysing observational data as a non-randomized pseudo-trial. *International Journal of Epidemiology, 46*(4), 1277–1284. https://doi.org/10.1093/ije/dyw293

Lambert, E. G., Hogan, N. L., & Griffin, M. L. (2007). The impact of distributive and procedural justice on correctional staff job stress, job satisfaction, and organizational commitment. *Journal of Criminal Justice, 35*(6), 644–656. https://doi.org/10.1016/j.jcrimjus.2007.09.001

Lambert, E. G., Keena, L. D., Haynes, S. H., May, D., Ricciardelli, R., & Leone, M. (2019). Testing a path model of organizational justice and correctional staff job stress among Southern correctional staff. *Criminal Justice and Behavior, 46*(10), 1367–1384. https://doi.org/10.1177/0093854819843336

Lang, J., Bliese, P. D., Lang, J. W., & Adler, A. B. (2011). Work gets unfair for the depressed: Cross-lagged relations between organizational justice perceptions and depressive symptoms. *Journal of Applied Psychology, 96*(3), 602–618. https://doi.org/10.1037/a0022463

Laumer, I. B., Massen, J. J., Wakonig, B., Lorck-Tympner, M., Carminito, C., & Auersperg, A. M. (2019). Tentative evidence for inequity aversion to unequal work-effort but not to unequal reward distribution in Goffin's cockatoos. *Ethology, 126*(2), 185–194. https://doi.org/10.1111/eth.12947

Lee, R. T., Perez, A. T., Boykin, C. M., & Mendoze-Denton, R. (2019). On the prevalence of racial discrimination in the United States. *PLOS ONE, 14*(1), e0210698. https://doi.org/10.1371/journal.pone.0210698

Manville, C., El Akremi, A., Niezborala, M., & Mignonac, K. (2016). Injustice hurts, literally: The role of sleep and emotional exhaustion in the relationship between organization justice and musculoskeletal disorders. *Human Relations, 69*(9), 1315–1339. https://doi.org/10.1177/0018726715615927

May, D. C., Lambert, E. G., Leone, M. C., Keena, L. D., & Haynes, H. S. (2020). Stress among correctional officers: An organizational justice approach. *American Journal of Criminal Justice, 45*, 454–473. https://doi.org/10.1007/s12103-020-09520-w

McKinsey Global Institute. (2021). *The economic state of Black America: What is and what could be.* McKinsey & Company. https://www.mckinsey.com/featured-insights/diversity-and-inclusion/the-economic-state-of-black-america-what-is-and-what-could-be#

Mine Safety Health Administration, United States Department of Labor. (n.d.) *Program policy manual: Vol. 4. Metal and Nonmetal mines—Interpretation, application, and guidelines on enforcement of 30 CFR.* https://arlweb.msha.gov/regs/complian/ppm/PMVOL4F.htm

National Institute for Occupational Safety and Health. (2021, September 3). *Mining topic: Respiratory diseases.* https://www.cdc.gov/niosh/mining/topics/respiratorydiseases.html

National Institutes of Health. (2020). *Detection, evaluation, and treatment of high blood cholesterol in adults (Adult treatment panel III): Executive summary* (NIH Pub. No. 01-3670). https://www.nhlbi.nih.gov/files/docs/guidelines/atp3xsum.pdf

Newins, A. R., Glenn, J. J., Wilson, L. C., Wilson, S. M., Kimbrel, N. A., Beckham, J. C., VA Mid-Atlantic MIRECC Workgroup, & Calhoun, P. S. (2021). Psychological outcomes following sexual assault: Differences by sexual assault setting. *Psychological Services, 18*(4), 504–511. https://doi.org/10.1037/ser0000426

Plato. (ca. 375 BCE). *Plato: The Republic—Book II (continued).* http://www.literaturepage.com/read/therepublic-68.html

Proctor, D., Brosnan, S. F., & de Waal, F. B. (2013). How fairly do chimpanzees play the ultimatum game? *Communicative & Integrative Biology, 6*(3). https://doi.org/10.4161/cib.23819

Rawls, J. (1971). *A theory of justice.* Belknap Press, Harvard University Press. https://doi.org/10.4159/9780674042605

Rosenthal, A. (2021, April 19). Death by inequality: How workers' lack of power harms their health and safety. *Unequal Power Project, Economic Policy Institute.* https://www.epi.org/unequalpower/publications/death-by-inequality-how-workers-lack-of-power-harms-their-health-and-safety/

Sara, J. D., Prasad, M., Eleid, M. F., Zhang, M., Widmer, R. J., & Lerman, A. (2018). Association between work-related stress and coronary heart disease: A review of prospective studies through the job strain, effort-reward balance, and organizational justice models. *Journal of the American Heart Association, 7*(9), 1–18. https://doi.org/10.1161/JAHA.117.008073

Tziner, A., & Sharoni, G. (2014). Organizational citizenship behavior, organizational justice, job stress, and work family conflict: Examination of their interrelationships with respondents from a non-Western culture. *Journal of Work and Organizational Psychology, 30*(1), 35–42. https://doi.org/10.5093/tr2014a5

U.S. Energy Information Administration. (2020, December 1). *Coal explained: Coal and the environment.* https://www.eia.gov/energyexplained/coal/coal-and-the-environment.php

Vaamonde, J. D., Omar, A., & Salessi, S. (2018). From organizational justice perceptions to turnover intentions: The mediating effects of burnout and job satisfaction. *Europe's Journal of Psychology, 14*(3), 554–570. https://doi.org/10.5964/ejop.v14i3.1490

van der Molen, H. F., Nieuwenhuijsen, K., Frings-Desen, M. H., & de Groene, G. (2020). Work-related psychosocial risk factors for stress-related mental disorders: An updated systematic review and meta-analysis. *BMJ Open, 10*, e034849. https://doi.org/10.1136/bmjopen-2019-034849

Wallis, J. (2016). *America's original sin: Racism, White privilege, and the bridge to a new America.* Brazos Press.

Wang, Y., Zheng, D., Chen, J., Rao, L.-L., Li, S., & Zhou, Y. (2019). Born for fairness: Evidence of genetic contribution to a neural basis of fairness intuition. *Social Cognitive and Affective Neuroscience, 14*(5), 539–548. https://doi.org/10.1093/scan/nsz031

Wood, S., Braeken, J., & Niven, K. (2012). Discrimination and well-being in organizations: Testing the differential power and organizational justice theories of workplace aggression. *Journal of Business Ethics, 115*(3), 617–634. https://doi.org/10.1007/s10551-012-1404-5

Ybema, J. F., & van den Bos, K. (2010). Effects of organizational justice on depressive symptoms and sickness absence: A longitudinal perspective. *Social Science & Medicine, 70*(10), 1609–1617. https://doi.org/10.1016/j.socscimed.2010.01.027

Zhang, Y., Liu, X., Xu, S., Yang, L.-Q., & Bednall, T. C. (2019). Why abusive supervision impacts employee OCB and CWB: A meta-analytic review of competing mediating mechanisms. *Journal of Management, 45*(6), 2474–2497. https://doi.org/10.1177/0149206318823935

14

Mistreatment in Organizations

Where Are We, and Where Are We Going?

Liu-Qin Yang, Stefanie Fox, and Katharine McMahon

Workplace mistreatment,[1] sometimes labeled abuse, aggression, or harassment, is a prevalent issue in workplaces. It represents interpersonal interactions during which one (or more) social partner initiates negative, counternormative actions or stops positive, normative actions toward another social partner in the workplace (Cortina & Magley, 2003, as cited in Yang et al., 2014). It manifests in many forms among the broad worker population, ranging in intensity, frequency, and focus. The estimated prevalence rate for workplace mistreatment is high. For example, 98% of workers reported experiencing incivility at least once and 50% reported weekly experiences as a target (Porath & Pearson, 2012, as cited in Schilpzand et al., 2016), and about 15% of workers reported experiencing bullying (Nielsen et al., 2010). Workplace mistreatment is consequential for workers and their organizations. Estimates of annual organizational costs attributable to workplace mistreatment have been reported to range from billions for bullying to $14,000 per employee for incivility (Kline & Lewis, 2019; Pearson & Porath, 2009, as cited in Cortina et al., 2017).

Workplace mistreatment research has reached a consensus about a longstanding challenge about the conceptual distinction between different forms of mistreatment, which mainly stems from the overlap between commonly used measures of different forms of mistreatment as well as the imprecise operationalization of these mistreatment constructs during measurement (Bowling

---

[1]We omitted some reviews on mistreatment from this chapter, due to space limitation and the fact that they largely overlap with and are less comprehensive than those included here.

https://doi.org/10.1037/0000331-014
Handbook of Occupational Health Psychology, Third Edition, L. E. Tetrick, G. G. Fisher, M. T. Ford, and J. C. Quick (Editors)

et al., 2015; Hershcovis, 2011). In this chapter, we highlight the theoretical frameworks and empirical evidence of the nomological networks common to all forms of workplace mistreatment, as well as the findings unique to each commonly studied form of mistreatment, in hopes of making two new contributions to the field. First, we offer a comprehensive account of the current state of science for the entire workplace mistreatment literature, synthesizing the large body of existing literature over the past two decades including target, perpetrator, and witness perspectives as well as in-person and online forms of workplace mistreatment, which goes beyond prior reviews on this topic. Second, we put forth systematic empirical evidence on the perspectives unique to the most widely studied forms of workplace mistreatment, which should enrich the ongoing scholarly conversation on the conceptual distinction between different forms of mistreatment that has been argued primarily at the theoretical and methodological levels (Bowling et al., 2015; Hershcovis, 2011). Figure 14.1 shows the multilevel and multilens framework that our review uses.

There have been at least 30 reviews on this topic published since the early 2000s, the vast majority of which are meta-analytical reviews. These reviews cover the following forms of workplace mistreatment: incivility (rude behavior with ambiguous intent), ostracism (explicit exclusion or implicit avoidance), abusive supervision (sustained aggressive behavior from a supervisor), bullying (repeated and enduring hostile acts toward an individual with less power), physical aggression (aggressive physical acts), interpersonal deviance (enacted aggression toward other individuals), sexual/gender harassment (gender-specific mistreatment), and racial/ethnic harassment (race-specific mistreatment). Four of the 30 reviews were solely focused on workplace mistreatment in health care. In this chapter, we focus primarily on these published reviews and illustrate our observations and conclusions with some applicable empirical studies that may or may not be included in these reviews. We organize the chapter into several sections: general workplace mistreatment and commonality across forms, the most commonly studied forms of mistreatment, common challenges in studying general workplace mistreatment, future directions in studying general workplace mistreatment, and other considerations and findings on gender- or ethnicity-specific mistreatment.

GENERAL WORKPLACE MISTREATMENT AND COMMONALITY ACROSS FORMS

In this section, we summarize the theoretical and empirical perspectives applicable to all forms of workplace mistreatment. Although we extracted the theories from various sources of the literature (the reviews we included and empirical studies within or outside these reviews), we summarized the empirical findings on antecedents, consequences, mediators, and moderators common across forms of workplace mistreatment solely based on the reviews we included. We present a succinct summary of the current state of empirical research focused on target perspectives in Figure 14.1 and include evidence

FIGURE 14.1. Conceptual Model for General Workplace Mistreatment Across Forms (Target Perspective)

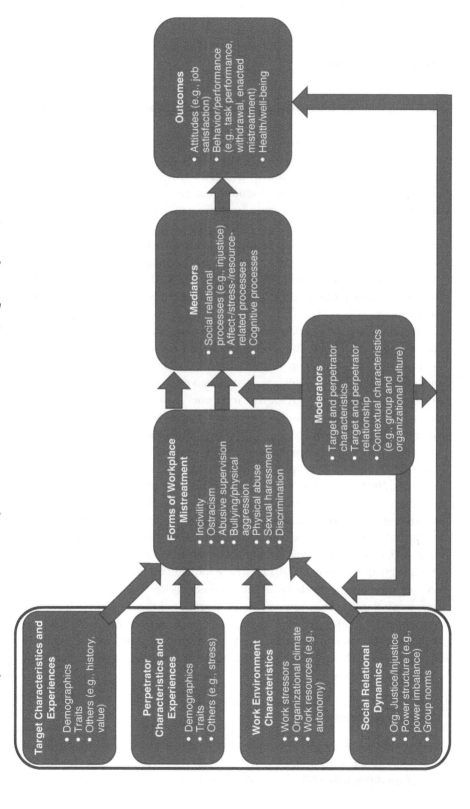

from both target and perpetrator perspectives throughout, with the target perspective making up the majority of the literature.

Theoretical Frameworks

In this subsection, we summarize the commonly used theoretical frameworks in the hope of offering a strong theoretical foundation to guide future progress in the literature of workplace mistreatment. The first category of theories commonly used is *person–environment interaction theories*, such as affective events theory (Weiss & Cropanzano, 1996, as cited in Schilpzand et al., 2016) and the transactional stress model (Lazarus & Folkman, 1984, as cited in Schilpzand et al., 2016), where individuals' emotional and cognitive responses (e.g., appraisal) to environmental events, or the match between individuals' needs and environmental demands, are key mechanisms underlying the antecedents and consequences of workplace mistreatment. The second category of theories is *social relational theories*, such as social exchange theory (Blau, 1964), where individuals' social relationships at work (e.g., dyadic or group level) are key mechanisms underlying the antecedents and consequences of workplace mistreatment.

The third category is *resource-focused theories*, such as conservation of resources theory (Hobfoll, 1989), the job demands and resources model (Bakker & Demerouti, 2007, as cited in Yang et al., 2020), and the integrated self-control model (Baumeister et al., 1998, as cited in Lian et al., 2017), where individuals' available personal and job resources (e.g., energy, self-control) relative to the amount of job demands and stressors are key mechanisms underlying the antecedents and consequences of workplace mistreatment. The fourth category of theories is *motivation-focused theories*, such as self-determination theory (Deci & Ryan, 2000, as cited in Yang et al., 2020) and group engagement theory (Tyler & Blader, 2003, as cited in Yang et al., 2020), where individuals' motivational processes (e.g., need satisfaction, group identification) are key mechanisms underlying the antecedents and consequences of workplace mistreatment.

The fifth category of theories is *physiology-focused stress theories*, such as allostatic load model (McEwen & Stellar, 1993) and stress reaction model (Zapf et al., 1996, as cited in Yang et al., 2012), where individuals' physiological processes are key mechanisms underlying the antecedents and consequences of mistreatment. Based on our review, these categories of theories were all applied in empirical research on various forms of work mistreatment, except that social relational theories and physiology-focused theories were more commonly applied in research on abusive supervision and physical aggression, respectively, than other categories.

Common Antecedents

In this subsection, we describe four categories of antecedents, among which individual characteristics and individual work experiences include the target's and perpetrator's characteristics and experiences.

Individual Characteristics

Consistent evidence has shown that target traits (e.g., negative affectivity, Big Five personalities), demographics (e.g., gender, race), and other characteristics (e.g., past history, personal values) are significantly linked to workers' exposure to workplace mistreatment (e.g., Bowling et al., 2015; Howard et al., 2020; Zhang & Bednall, 2016). For example, target negative affectivity has been consistently associated with more exposure to workplace mistreatment, whereas agreeableness has been consistently associated with less exposure (e.g., Bowling et al., 2015; Dhanani et al., 2020). As another example, women reported being exposed to more overall workplace mistreatment than men, and ethnic minorities (e.g., Hispanic workers) reported more exposure to overall workplace mistreatment than Caucasians (McCord et al., 2018). Last, individuals' past history of exposure to mistreatment (at work or outside of work) and their personal value of power distance can increase their susceptibility to more exposure at work (Bowling et al., 2015; Zhang & Bednall, 2016).

From perpetrators' perspectives, perpetrator traits (e.g., narcissism) and demographics (e.g., job tenure) are significantly linked to workers' enacted aggression or interpersonal deviance (e.g., Carpenter & Berry, 2017; Mackey et al., 2021). For example, neurotic, narcissist, and Machiavellian individuals are more likely to enact interpersonal aggression at work compared with agreeable, conscientious, and honest-humble individuals (Mackey et al., 2021; Pletzer et al., 2019). As another example, men and younger employees are more likely to enact interpersonal aggression than women and older employees, respectively (Hershcovis et al., 2007; Mackey et al., 2021).

Work Environment Characteristics

Cumulative evidence to date has suggested that work environment characteristics account for more variance in targets' exposure to workplace mistreatment, relative to target characteristics (e.g., negative affectivity, Big Five personalities; McCord et al., 2018). There are three commonly studied types of work environment characteristics as antecedents of exposure to and/or enacted interpersonal aggression: stressors, work resources, and organizational climate (e.g., Bowling & Beehr, 2006). Role stressors (e.g., role conflict) are related to more exposure to aggression, and organizational constraints are positively related to more exposure to and enacted aggression (Bowling & Beehr, 2006; Hershcovis et al., 2007). In contrast, work autonomy is related to less exposure to aggression (Bowling & Beehr, 2006). Mistreatment prevention climate and broader organizational climate (e.g., aggressive norms) are significantly related to mistreatment exposure (Yang et al., 2014).

Individual Work Experiences

Job dissatisfaction and individuals' negative emotions and stress are the two most studied types of work experiences contributing to exposure to and/or enacted interpersonal aggression. Dissatisfaction with one's job relates significantly to more exposure to incivility and bullying, as well as more enacted interpersonal aggression (Mackey et al., 2021; Salin, 2003), though job dissatisfaction can also be an outcome of mistreatment (Cortina et al., 2017). Negative emotions and stress (e.g., burnout), significantly predict more exposure to and enacted interpersonal aggression (Cortina et al., 2017; Mackey et al., 2021). More positive work experiences (e.g., perceived organizational support) relate to less enacted interpersonal aggression (Mackey et al., 2021).

Social Dynamics

Given the social relational nature of interpersonal mistreatment, social dynamics serve as an important category of antecedents for interpersonal mistreatment experiences. From the past reviews, we have identified four types of social dynamics: power structure, group norms, workplace mistreatment exposure, and organizational justice. In terms of power structure, target's low social power, perceived power imbalance, and flatter organizational structure were positively linked to more exposure to workplace mistreatment (e.g., Cortina et al., 2017; Salin, 2003). Group norms (e.g., norms for respect/civility) were significantly linked to exposure to incivility (Cortina et al., 2017; Schilpzand et al., 2016). Last, lower organizational justice (e.g., procedural justice) experienced by perpetrators has been consistently linked to enacted interpersonal aggression (e.g., Cortina et al., 2017; Zhang & Bednall, 2016).

Common Outcomes

Similar to past reviews (e.g., Bowling & Beehr, 2006), we focus on the following three categories of work outcomes from target, witness, and perpetrator perspectives: attitudes, behavior and performance, and health/well-being. In terms of attitudes toward work, cumulative evidence has supported the adverse relations of workplace mistreatment experiences with a variety of attitudes (e.g., turnover intentions, organizational commitment) with all attitudinal outcomes but psychological safety and work motivation established for the target's and perpetrator's perspectives (e.g., Lanctôt & Guay, 2014; Mackey et al., 2021).

With respect to behavioral and performance outcomes, cumulative evidence has supported the adverse relations of workplace mistreatment experiences with a variety of behaviors and performance types, including task performance, interpersonal helping behavior, deviance, and withdrawal, with all outcomes but deviance (for target and witness perspectives only) and ability to work (for target perspectives only) all established for all three perspectives (target, witness, and perpetrator; e.g., Carpenter & Berry, 2017; Cortina et al., 2017). There are two important observations about these outcomes: first, prior workplace mistreatment exposure (e.g., ostracism), either as a target or witness, has been consistently linked with the same employee's instigation of aggression toward others or enacted interpersonal deviance (e.g., Howard et al., 2020; Mackey et al., 2021), which evidences the "negative spiral" effect in the mistreatment development process as proposed by Andersson and Pearson (1999, as cited in Cortina et al., 2017). Second, the relation between ostracism exposure and interpersonal helping behavior can be positive (Robinson et al.,

2013). In terms of health and well-being outcomes, cumulative evidence has supported the adverse relations of workplace mistreatment experiences with a variety of outcomes, including more negative affect, less positive affect, more lasting stress symptoms (e.g., burnout), worse mental health, and worse physical health, with all outcomes but positive affect and physical health established for the target and witness perspectives (e.g., Cortina et al., 2017; Howard et al., 2020). In summary, workplace mistreatment has negative consequences for the target, witness(es), and perpetrator.

Common Mediators

Scholars have examined various cognitive, affective and stress/resource-focused, and social-relational mediational processes through which the target experiences attitudinal, behavioral, and well-being outcomes upon exposure to various forms of mistreatment. The cumulative evidence to date indicates three major categories of mediators in the relations between mistreatment exposure and target outcomes: (a) cognitive processes (e.g., rumination), (b) affective and stress/resource-focused processes (e.g., negative affect, resource depletion), and (c) social relational processes (e.g., perceived organizational injustice; see Hershcovis, 2011; Nielsen et al., 2020). Theoretically, it is conceivable that many (if not all) of these mediational processes would apply to the witness's perspective to explain why witnessed mistreatment accounts for the witness's attitudinal, behavioral, and well-being outcomes.

Common Moderators

The body of literature on contingent factors that moderate the antecedent–mistreatment and/or mistreatment–outcome relations is largely focused on the target's perspectives. There are two main categories of moderators: (a) individual differences (demographics and psychological characteristics) of the target; and (b) the group-, organization-, and societal-level contexts. In terms of demographics, cumulative evidence indicates that age, gender, and race can worsen or buffer the effects of mistreatment exposure on target stress reactions and/or coping strategies (e.g., to distance oneself versus respond aggressively; Cortina et al., 2017; Zhang & Liao, 2015). In terms of psychological characteristics, the target's positive and negative affectivity can buffer and worsen the mistreatment exposure–well-being relation, respectively (Nielsen et al., 2020; Tepper, 2007). With respect to the group-, organization-, and societal-level context, the length of relationship between the target and the perpetrator, the power status of the target, and the national culture (e.g., power distance) can moderate the mistreatment exposure and outcome relations (Robinson et al., 2013; Zhang & Liao, 2015).

Current State of Science

The vast majority of the reviews summarized in this section were solely focused on the target's perspectives; a few of them were solely focused on the perpetrator's perspectives (e.g., Mackey et al., 2021; Pletzer et al., 2019); and a few did explicitly include more than one perspective (e.g., Cortina et al., 2017). Overall, the literature has established the antecedent–mistreatment and mistreatment–outcome relations from target, witness, and perpetrator perspectives. Furthermore, theoretical and empirical work has examined the underlying mechanisms (mediators, moderators) from primarily the target's perspective, yet little empirical work (with some exceptions; e.g., Tepper, 2007) has been done to understand the mediational and moderational processes underlying either witnessed or enacted mistreatment or aggression.

SPECIFIC FORMS OF WORKPLACE MISTREATMENT

The most commonly studied forms of workplace mistreatment have also demonstrated unique findings that provide nuance between them. This section reviews specific perspectives for incivility, ostracism, abusive supervision, bullying, and physical aggression. Their particular relationships with variables present further distinction between the different types of mistreatment.

Incivility

The lowest intensity form of aggression, *incivility*, features ambiguous intent to harm (Andersson & Pearson, 1999, as cited in Cortina et al., 2017) and has garnered much attention in recent years of research due to results consistently demonstrating its insidious nature. Although there has been a large body of empirical evidence on the nomological network of incivility, particularly its outcomes, the literature has yet to establish an integrated theoretical framework (Schilpzand et al., 2016).

Despite this limitation, the incivility literature is exceptional compared with other forms of aggression research due to its evidence on multiple perspectives (i.e., target, perpetrator, witness experiences; Cortina et al., 2017), though it mostly focuses on the target. Antecedents unique to incivility include personal characteristics of a dominant conflict-management style (e.g., confrontational style with a focus on personal goals) and obsessive passion over one's work, and contextual factors of an environment tolerant of disrespectful behavior and passive managers (Cortina et al., 2017). Regarding outcomes, exposure to incivility uniquely predicts emotional labor (Cortina et al., 2017). Furthermore, cumulative evidence suggests that incivility is positively linked to more enacted incivility (Park & Martinez, 2021). Cyber incivility represents an area of research examining how technological advances influence expressions of incivility. Within this literature, many studies focus on how uncivil emails from supervisors influence the targets' job attitudes, strain, and performance (Lim & Teo, 2009; McCarthy et al., 2020), and there is conflicting evidence for whether in-person or cyber incivility has a greater impact on the targets (see Heischman et al., 2019; McCarthy et al., 2020).

Ostracism

Recently conceptualized as a form of incivility (Howard et al., 2020), *ostracism* occurs when an individual or group does not take actions that would include or engage another individual or group when socially they are expected to do so. This can take the form of explicit exclusion or implicit avoidance, may be viewed as deliberate or unintentional, and may be an acute experience or sustained treatment. Much existent research on ostracism examines the experience of the target, though some recent work integrates both target and perpetrator perspectives (e.g., Robinson et al., 2013). From the targets' perspectives, ostracism can be explained through Williams's (2009, as cited in Bilal et al., 2021) temporal need threat model, in which ostracism elicits short- and long-term reactions as responses to threatened need fulfillment. Additionally, the target-centric victimization framework utilizes characteristics regarding the target and the context to explain how targets react to perceived ostracism (Bilal et al., 2021; Howard et al., 2020). Furthermore, Robinson and colleagues (2013) created an empirically based conceptual model to examine the factors that predict and influence the presence of ostracism, and to conceptualize intentions such that purposeful and nonpurposeful ostracism arise from different combinations of contexts and lead to differential outcomes. In terms of antecedents, there are unique factors that predict ostracism. Regarding contextual characteristics, relationships with leaders predict exposure to ostracism such that higher leader–member exchange reduces ostracism and supervisory mistreatment (e.g., abusive supervision) predicts more ostracism (Howard et al., 2020). As leaders represent the opinions of the group, the way a leader treats a worker indicates how others should treat and value them. Furthermore, purposeful and nonpurposeful ostracism have different constellations of antecedents. Purposeful ostracism is influenced by the perceived cost of the behavior to the perpetrator and limitation of alternative mechanisms for social interaction (e.g., lack of tolerance for interpersonal aggression); nonpurposeful ostracism may occur as a result of a lack of oversight (e.g., among geographically dispersed workers) as well as disagreements on social norms and appropriateness (Robinson et al., 2013).

Ostracism affects targets such that they feel a lower sense of belonging, are more likely to be silent, and experience worsened self-perceptions (Howard et al., 2020). Interestingly, ostracized workers may respond to the experience in different forms: They may withdraw, increase their interpersonal interaction and helping colleagues, or become aggressive (Bilal et al., 2021). If the worker is motivated to end the ostracism, they are more likely to temporarily improve their performance and increase their helping behaviors (Robinson et al., 2013).

Abusive Supervision

Abusive supervision is experienced through sustained hostile verbal and nonverbal behaviors from a supervisor. Although rates of abusive supervision are assumed to be low—about 10% of employees experience it—perceptions of victimization and fears of retaliation may respectively inflate and underestimate the occurrence (Tepper et al., 2017). The existing literature on abusive supervision highlights the target's perspectives, as abusive supervision is experienced subjectively by the target. Social learning theory is uniquely fitted to guide examination of abusive supervision, offering an explanation for the perpetuation of abusive supervision through modeled abusive behaviors by influential and high-status individuals and organizational interpersonal norms (Tepper et al., 2017). Tepper and colleagues (2017) also examined identity threat as an explanation for the antecedents of abusive supervision (e.g., supervisors use hostility to cope with identity threat or employees' threat to their leader identity).

The antecedents of abusive supervision include experiences and characteristics of both perpetrators and targets. For example, supervisor well-being, emotional intelligence, and supportive leadership styles (e.g., transformational leadership) are negatively related to perpetration, while negative leadership styles are associated with increased perpetration (e.g., Li et al., 2016; Zhang & Bednall, 2016). Additionally, target narcissism is related to increased perceptions of abusive supervision (Zhang & Bednall, 2016), though it is important to note that narcissism may be related to inflated mistreatment perceptions (overreporting).

Bullying

Repeated and enduring acts toward an individual(s) with lower power status, which in turn form a hostile environment, embody the expression of *bullying*. The unique aspects of repetition and power imbalance differentiate bullying from other mistreatment forms. Although the cognitive activation theory of stress (i.e., there are both general stress responses [alarm] and subjective experiences of the stress responses [exhaustion]; Ursin & Eriksen, 2004, as cited in Nielsen et al., 2020) is commonly used to examine the bullying–sleep relation, some researchers opt to create their own framework of bullying. For example, Salin (2003) identified three major areas that interact and prompt bullying: enabling structures and processes that are seen as necessary (e.g., power imbalance), motivating structures and incentives (e.g., internal competition), and precipitating processes or triggering circumstances (e.g., organizational restructuring).

The persistence of bullying provokes issues with health outcomes such as sleep, and various sleep problems (e.g., insomnia) have been consistently associated with exposure to bullying, resulting from reactions to exposure (e.g., rumination; Nielsen et al., 2020). Similar to incivility, the nature of bullying allows it to appear online in addition to in person. Cyberbullying is a well-known issue in other contexts (e.g., among teenagers, on social media) and warrants attention in the workplace. Common manifestations of cyberbullying include withholding information and spreading gossip (Privitera & Campbell, 2009). One way to identify the unique characteristics of cyberbullying is to examine in-person and cyberbullying simultaneously (e.g., Privitera & Campbell,

2009). Characteristics of the online form (e.g., boundarylessness, invisibility) allow for an extended reach through pervasiveness, vindictiveness, feeling haunted, and settlement of disputes, enabling the avoidance of in-person two-way dialogue (D'Cruz & Noronha, 2013).

Physical Aggression

Also called physical violence and physical abuse, *physical aggression* includes all aggressive physical contact, whether or not injuries result. The vast majority of organizational physical aggression research is conducted in the medical industry, focusing on mistreatment from clients, coworkers, and supervisors, and featuring the target's perspective with some focus on the perpetrator. Some of the literature examines other industries where workers have contact with clients (e.g., transportation, education). Research on physical aggression often utilizes physiology-focused stress theories, such as cognitive activation theory of stress (Morphet et al., 2018).

Workplace physical aggression can be predicted by unique organizational and perpetrator characteristics. Industries where employees interact with clients (e.g., medical and service sectors) and work alone or at night see a higher rate of physical aggression from clients (Hogh & Viitasara, 2005). In the medical industry, training and policies meant to prevent violence help to reduce the occurrence (e.g., Yang et al., 2012). Furthermore, clients who perpetrate physical aggression may do so when provoked or mocked (Hogh & Viitasara, 2005).

In addition to consistent findings of negative well-being and health that physical aggression shares with other forms of mistreatment, targets of physical aggression also experience posttraumatic stress disorder and can develop injuries and musculoskeletal disorders as a result of physical aggression (e.g., Lanctôt & Guay, 2014; Yang et al., 2012). Furthermore, they may fear their attacker, which can be particularly problematic if the mistreatment source is a colleague or regular client (Hogh & Viitasara, 2005; Lanctôt & Guay, 2014).

CHALLENGES, SOLUTIONS, AND FUTURE DIRECTIONS

The extensive workplace mistreatment literature has identified numerous themes, trends, and explanations across situations. Despite this, research on this sensitive topic has encountered theoretical, methodological, and practical challenges. Addressing these weaknesses, enhancing scientific practices, and adapting to modern circumstances will advance the understanding and management of workplace mistreatment.

Theoretical Coherence

The many categories of theories used to examine workplace mistreatment, as observed by Schilpzand and colleagues (2016), contribute to a lack of theoretical coherence in the literature. In other words, different streams of empirical studies using different categories of theoretical frameworks (e.g., social relational theories, affective and stress-focused theories) generate different bodies of evidence supporting different theoretical processes leading to or resulting from workplace mistreatment. To address this issue, one viable future course of action for workplace mistreatment researchers is to explicitly operationalize the theoretical processes of the focal theoretical framework (e.g., group identification as a mediator of the abusive supervision–target performance relations to represent group engagement theory, a motivational framework), and test them against the mechanisms posited by other equally plausible theoretical frameworks. For example, psychological distress and perceived injustice as alternate mediators representing stress/resource-focused and social relational frameworks, respectively. Such efforts will facilitate integration of the understanding and evidence on different theoretical processes, leading to better theoretical coherence for research on specific forms of workplace mistreatment and for the field as a whole (e.g., Liang et al., 2016, as cited in Lian et al., 2017; Yang et al., 2020).

Another strategy for workplace mistreatment research is to systematically examine the causality of the relations between workplace mistreatment and other phenomena in its nomological network, to better understand the etiology of workplace mistreatment and its progression. For example, Howard and colleagues' (2020) meta-analytical review showed that the magnitude of the ostracism-deviance relation was about the same (population-level effect size of 0.34 vs. 0.37), regardless of whether deviance was measured before or after ostracism; workplace deviance can be an antecedent and/or outcome of ostracism exposure, and stress/resource-focused and/or social relation-focused theoretical processes can explain such reciprocal relations. More systematic causal evidence could inform the theoretical processes underlying workplace mistreatment and facilitate future theoretical coherence.

Unbalanced Perspectives

In the workplace mistreatment literature, there seems to be an imbalance in the effort toward understanding target, perpetrator, and witness perspectives, neglecting the accounts of the perpetrator, and even more so those of the witness. The sensitivity of conducting research from the perpetrator's perspective might account for the relatively few empirical studies (especially field studies), as perpetrators may hesitate to honestly report their aggressive behavior at work. Indeed, the social desirability issue in field survey research focused on enacted interpersonal aggression or deviance has been argued to be responsible for the low base rate of this phenomena in self-report data (Slora, 1989). As for the witness's perspective, it can be quite complex to choose appropriate timing and measurement tools to assess observation of the progression of workplace mistreatment. Not all forms of mistreatment or various manifestations of the same form (e.g., incivility, abusive supervision) can be observed by witnesses in the work setting. For example, some subtle manifestations of incivility may be conveyed through nonverbal cues from the perpetrator, and thus only observable by a witness who was at the right time and right place. Closely related to the timing issue, researchers are also advised to reexamine established scales of mistreatment (that are often focused on target perspectives), ensuring that all scale items are observable by witnesses while maintaining validity and reliability in assessing the focal mistreatment construct.

Measurement Issues

Measurement issues have been a long-standing challenge in the field of workplace mistreatment, especially in the measurement of workplace mistreatment and its different forms (Bowling et al., 2015; Hershcovis, 2011; Yang et al., 2014). Based on our review, there are three major issues that are all essential to the construct validity of mistreatment. First, the existent mistreatment measures do not precisely reflect key assumptions and distinguishing characteristics in the focal mistreatment construct (e.g., the "persistent" and "power imbalance" characteristics of bullying are not reflected in the most commonly used measure by Einarsen and Raknes, 1997; Hershcovis, 2011). Hershcovis (2011) suggested that researchers separate the measurement of defining characteristics (e.g., frequency, intent, perpetrator–target relationship) from that of the focal mistreatment construct itself, and possibly use these characteristics as moderators of the mistreatment–outcome relations. Second, specific time frames (e.g., over the past month) are not consistently utilized across studies for researchers' between-person research (with typically cross-sectional or time-lagged designs) representing the vast majority of the literature. This partially contributes to the lack of conceptual clarity in the mistreatment construct, where workplace mistreatment is sometimes measured and studied as a more transient phenomenon (e.g., discrete behavioral events within a specified period of time) but other times as a more chronic phenomenon without a time frame (Howard et al., 2020). Researchers typically do not explicitly recognize such key conceptual distinctions in their research conclusions. Howard and colleagues (2020) found that the relations of ostracism exposure with antecedents (e.g., tenure) and consequences (e.g., helping behavior) were stronger (vs. weaker) when ostracism was measured with a specific time frame (vs. without).

Third, there are significant overlaps between measures of workplace mistreatment, even if many of them are purported to assess conceptually distinct forms of mistreatment (Bowling et al., 2015; Hershcovis, 2011). To address the second and third issues, future researchers can be strategic in choosing measures to study broader versus narrower constructs of workplace mistreatment (e.g., use Einarsen & Raknes's, 1997, scale for broad mistreatment, develop and validate a new scale to study a new narrower construct such as lying), and in ensuring that the design of the measure (e.g., with or without a specific time frame in the instructions) is consistent with the mistreatment conceptualization and theoretical questions they focus on. We agree with Bowling and colleagues (2015) that broader mistreatment constructs may have stronger effect sizes in relating to broader target outcome variables (e.g., job attitudes, well-being), whereas narrower constructs may have stronger effect sizes with narrower and unique outcome variables (e.g., reduced popularity among coworkers resulting from lying).

More research on broad mistreatment from the perpetrator's and witness's perspectives is needed to shed light on theoretical processes leading to or resulting from enacting interpersonal deviance and witnessing mistreatment at work. On the other hand, opportunities for discovery remain wide open for examining narrower mistreatment constructs with unique defining characteristics, such as ostracism—a specific form of incivility (Howard et al., 2020)—or social manipulation (Bowling et al., 2015). Regardless of future research's focus on broader or narrower mistreatment constructs, effort to (re)validate measures may prove to be fruitful, considering the frequent overlaps between items of established measures (Bowling et al., 2015; Hershcovis, 2011). Specifically, it may be beneficial to measure more than one mistreatment construct simultaneously within the same empirical study. First, it can help differentiate similar constructs and measures. Second, it can help establish nomological networks unique to distinct forms of mistreatment (e.g., assessing ostracism along other subtypes of incivility, such as invasion of privacy; Bowling et al., 2015).

Challenges and Developments in Research Design

To date, most empirical studies on workplace mistreatment used cross-sectional designs, partially because it is challenging to study a sensitive topic like workplace mistreatment in field settings. The literature is moving toward using more sophisticated designs that allow stronger causal inference, such as mixed methods and experimental designs in the lab or field (e.g., Leiter et al., 2011; Yang et al., 2014; Zheng & van Dijke, 2020). Relatedly, the workplace mistreatment research seems to be headed in the direction of triangulation and replication, such as triangulating via experimental and field studies, or replicating study results with more than one independent sample (e.g., Hershcovis & Bhatnagar, 2017; Yang et al., 2020). Furthermore, as evidenced by a recent review (McCormick et al., 2020), experience sampling methods are being used to examine mistreatment incidents, such as uncivil events, as they unfold in situ. Last, it is extremely challenging to conduct field interventions to prevent or reduce workplace mistreatment—often termed *violence prevention*. The vast majority of the published intervention work to date has focused on health care settings (e.g., Leiter et al., 2011; for a review, see Morphet et al., 2018). Cumulative evidence suggests that consumer risk assessment, staff education, aggression management teams, and integrative efforts from first-line employees and management of different levels are generally effective in reducing workplace aggression in health care. However, it is unclear whether such evidence from health care settings will be generalizable to other industries; it is also unclear the extent to which (benefits of) these interventions will sustain themselves in the longer term. More future effort is needed to develop and evaluate intervention programs that account for social relational contexts and are effective, sustainable, and generalizable across industries.

Considering the Implications of Remote Work

As technology-assisted work processes become increasingly common, it is critical to consider modality of work in future research on workplace mistreatment (Barber & Santuzzi, 2015). One direction of research is to more systematically examine the similarities and differences between in-person and online workplace mistreatment (e.g., cyber incivility, cyberbullying); indeed, some recent research has begun to do so (e.g., Heischman et al., 2019; McCarthy et al., 2020). Another promising direction is to explore more innovative ways of investigating the perpetrator's and witness's perspectives with workplace mistreatment in field research, through utilizing technology-assisted research methods (e.g., to code mistreatment behaviors displayed in Zoom video recordings of team meetings).

OTHER CONSIDERATIONS: GENDER AND ETHNICITY MISTREATMENT AS HARASSMENT

When examining mistreatment in organizations, we noted that many studies identified social identities as antecedents and moderators of mistreatment experiences (e.g., Howard et al., 2020). Although the findings are noteworthy, these studies lack the consideration of workplace mistreatment due to a worker's social identity in the form of interpersonal behaviors (e.g., hostility), social exclusion, or fewer learning and advancement opportunities. We briefly highlight gender/sexual harassment and racial/ethnic harassment. For a more thorough examination of workplace discrimination and harassment, we recommend consulting the workplace diversity literature (e.g., Colella et al., 2017; Hebl et al., 2020).

Perspectives underpinning examination of gender and racial harassment are distinct from those applied in the general workplace mistreatment literature and encompass multiple frameworks including stereotype-based theories (e.g., stereotype content model), perpetrator traits (e.g., social dominance orientation), and motivations to reduce discrimination (e.g., tokenism; McCord et al., 2018). From the target's perspective, Crosby's relative deprivation theory (1976; cited in Triana et al., 2019) explains that marginalized workers perceive deprivation and discrimination when their treatment does not meet a standard (e.g., the treatment of other workers).

Although these forms of mistreatment are based on social identities, organizational factors can also predict their occurrence. Social identities predict corresponding forms of mistreatment (e.g., racial/ethnic minorities experience more racial harassment than White workers; McCord et al., 2018). Interestingly, though women experience a higher degree of gender harassment overall, men in certain industries (e.g., nursing) can experience a higher rate of gender harassment than women (Berdahl & Raver, 2011). Organizational climate (e.g., positive diversity climate or overall climate) predicts less racial harassment and/or gender harassment (McCord et al., 2018). Additionally, job–gender incongruence (e.g., women financial advisors) increases the occurrence of gender harassment (McCord et al., 2018). In addition to outcomes (e.g., job attitudes, health, work behaviors) shared with other forms of mistreatment, harassment uniquely affects performance appraisals (distinct from performance), career paths, promotions, and relationship quality with supervisors (e.g., leader–member exchange; Triana et al., 2021). Personal and organizational characteristics also influence the effects of identity-based mistreatment on target outcomes. For example, a target's lowered self-esteem mediates the relation between experienced harassment and lowered target performance. Further, an organization's high-quality diversity management buffers the harassment–performance relation (Triana et al., 2021).

An important consideration regarding gender and racial harassment is the legal ramification of these forms of mistreatment. Both of these identities are recognized as protected classes by the U.S. Equal Employment Opportunity Commission, making mistreatment based on these identities illegal and punishable by sanctions, fines, and legal suits (Raver & Nishii, 2010). A fine distinction should be made between identity-based harassment or mistreatment and prevalence of mistreatment by social identity. The former assumes the motivation for the mistreatment is related to the social identity of the target and is thus illegal. The latter is messier as differences in mistreatment prevalence may be due to a variety of factors and interpersonal mistreatment can be enacted to serve as an undetectable, socially acceptable form of discrimination with fewer legal risks (see Hebl et al., 2020; Raver & Nishii, 2010). For example, Cortina and colleagues (2017) pioneered the theory of selective incivility, positing that incivility can act as a covert, socially acceptable manifestation of gender and racial harassment.

Holistically, the existing literature on gender and racial harassment differs from general workplace mistreatment due to the described identity associations. Furthermore, the majority of empirical research on perpetration of gender and racial harassment includes lab experiments, interventions, and anonymous survey data to reduce the strong influence of external reasons to appear nonprejudiced (e.g., socially desirable responding). Overall, the body of research on identity-based workplace mistreatment is vital, impressive, and ever-growing, and we repeat the suggestion for further reading in the workplace diversity literature. Importantly, we want to note that the challenges we discussed about the general workplace mistreatment literature apply to the gender and racial harassment literature and that the future directions we suggested also apply to the gender and racial harassment research.

CONCLUSION

We summarized the mistreatment research evidence from the past 2 decades. We underscore that workplace mistreatment is consequential for the target, witness, and perpetrator, as well as work groups and the organizational bottom line, and that it is crucial to prevent and reduce occurrences of mistreatment at work using an integrated approach—based on strategies to be employed at the organizational, workgroup, and individual-worker levels. Future research can enhance theoretical coherence, expending targeted efforts to ensure precise operationalization of focal mistreatment constructs in chosen measures, examining the mistreatment processes that are unique to the future of work (e.g., remote work), and employing more rigorous research designs, such as replications and field intervention work.

REFERENCES

* denotes the reviews we included on the topic of workplace mistreatment

Barber, L. K., & Santuzzi, A. M. (2015). Please respond ASAP: Workplace telepressure and employee recovery. *Journal of Occupational Health Psychology, 20*(2), 172–189. https://doi.org/10.1037/a0038278

Berdahl, J. L., & Raver, J. L. (2011). Sexual harassment. In S. Zedeck (Ed.), *APA handbook of industrial and organizational psychology: Vol. 3. Maintaining, expanding, and contracting the organization* (pp. 641–669). American Psychological Association. https://doi.org/10.1037/12171-018

Bilal, A. R., Fatima, T., Imran, M. K., & Iqbal, K. (2021). Is it my fault and how will I react? A phenomenology of perceived causes and consequences of workplace ostracism. *European Journal of Management and Business Economics, 30*(1), 36–54. https://doi.org/10.1108/EJMBE-03-2019-0056

Blau, P. M. (1964). Justice in social exchange. *Sociological Inquiry, 34*, 193-206. https://doi.org/10.1111/j.1475-682X.1964.tb00583.x

*Bowling, N. A., & Beehr, T. A. (2006). Workplace harassment from the victim's perspective: A theoretical model and meta-analysis. *Journal of Applied Psychology, 91*(5), 998–1012. https://doi.org/10.1037/0021-9010.91.5.998

Bowling, N. A., Camus, K. A., & Blackmore, C. E. (2015). Conceptualizing and measuring workplace abuse: Implications for the study of abuse's predictors and consequences. In P. L. Perrewé, J. R. B. Halbesleben, & C. C. Rosen (Eds.), *Mistreatment in organizations* (Vol. 13, pp. 225–263). Emerald Group Publishing Limited. https://doi.org/10.1108/S1479-355520150000013008

*Carpenter, N. C., & Berry, C. M. (2017). Are counterproductive work behavior and withdrawal empirically distinct? A meta-analytic investigation. *Journal of Management, 43*(3), 834–863. https://doi.org/10.1177/0149206314544743

Colella, A., Hebl, M., & King, E. (2017). One hundred years of discrimination research in the *Journal of Applied Psychology*: A sobering synopsis. *Journal of Applied Psychology, 102*(3), 500–513. https://doi.org/10.1037/apl0000084

*Cortina, L. M., Kabat-Farr, D., Magley, V. J., & Nelson, K. (2017). Researching rudeness: The past, present, and future of the science of incivility. *Journal of Occupational Health Psychology, 22*(3), 299–313. https://doi.org/10.1037/ocp0000089

D'Cruz, P., & Noronha, E. (2013). Navigating the extended reach: Target experiences of cyberbullying at work. *Information and Organization, 23*(4), 324–343. https://doi.org/10.1016/j.infoandorg.2013.09.001

*Dhanani, L. Y., Main, A. M., & Pueschel, A. (2020). Do you only have yourself to blame? A meta-analytic test of the victim precipitation model. *Journal of Organizational Behavior, 41*(8), 706–721. https://doi.org/10.1002/job.2413

Einarsen, S., & Raknes, B. I. (1997). Harassment in the workplace and the victimization of men. *Violence and Victims, 12*(3), 247–263. https://doi.org/10.1891/0886-6708.12.3.247

Hebl, M., Cheng, S. K., & Ng, L. C. (2020). Modern discrimination in organizations. *Annual Review of Organizational Psychology and Organizational Behavior, 7*(1), 257–282. https://doi.org/10.1146/annurev-orgpsych-012119-044948

Heischman, R. M., Nagy, M. S., & Settler, K. J. (2019). Before you send that: Comparing the outcomes of face-to-face and cyber incivility. *The Psychologist Manager Journal, 22*(1), 1–23. https://doi.org/10.1037/mgr0000081

*Hershcovis, M. S. (2011). "Incivility, social undermining, bullying . . . oh my!": A call to reconcile constructs within workplace aggression research. *Journal of Organizational Behavior, 32*(3), 499–519. https://doi.org/10.1002/job.689

Hershcovis, M. S., & Bhatnagar, N. (2017). When fellow customers behave badly: Witness reactions to employee mistreatment by customers. *Journal of Applied Psychology, 102*(11), 1528–1544. https://doi.org/10.1037/apl0000249

*Hershcovis, M. S., Turner, N., Barling, J., Arnold, K. A., Dupré, K. E., Inness, M., LeBlanc, M. M., & Sivanathan, N. (2007). Predicting workplace aggression: A meta-analysis. *Journal of Applied Psychology, 92*(1), 228–238. https://doi.org/10.1037/0021-9010.92.1.228

Hobfoll, S. E. (1989). Conservation of resources: A new attempt at conceptualizing stress. *American Psychologist, 44*(3), 513–524. https://doi.org/10.1037/0003-066X.44.3.513

*Hogh, A., & Viitasara, E. (2005). A systematic review of longitudinal studies of nonfatal workplace violence. *European Journal of Work and Organizational Psychology, 14*(3), 291–313. https://doi.org/10.1080/13594320500162059

*Howard, M. C., Cogswell, J. E., & Smith, M. B. (2020). The antecedents and outcomes of workplace ostracism: A meta-analysis. *Journal of Applied Psychology, 105*(6), 577–596. https://doi.org/10.1037/apl0000453

Kline, R., & Lewis, D. (2019). The price of fear: Estimating the financial cost of bullying and harassment to the NHS in England. *Public Money & Management, 39*(3), 166–174. https://doi.org/10.1080/09540962.2018.1535044

*Lanctôt, N., & Guay, S. (2014). The aftermath of workplace violence among healthcare workers: A systematic literature review of the consequences. *Aggression and Violent Behavior, 19*(5), 492–501. https://doi.org/10.1016/j.avb.2014.07.010

Leiter, M. P., Laschinger, H. K. S., Day, A., & Oore, D. G. (2011). The impact of civility interventions on employee social behavior, distress, and attitudes. *Journal of Applied Psychology, 96*(6), 1258–1274. https://doi.org/10.1037/a0024442

Li, Y., Wang, Z., Yang, L.-Q., & Liu, S. (2016). The crossover of psychological distress from leaders to subordinates in teams: The role of abusive supervision, psychological capital, and team performance. *Journal of Occupational Health Psychology, 21*(2), 142–153. https://doi.org/10.1037/a0039960

Lian, H., Yam, K. C., Ferris, D. L., & Brown, D. (2017). Self-control at work. *The Academy of Management Annals, 11*(2), 703–732. https://doi.org/10.5465/annals.2015.0126

Lim, V. K. G., & Teo, T. S. H. (2009). Mind your E-manners: Impact of cyber incivility on employees' work attitude and behavior. *Information & Management, 46*(8), 419–425. https://doi.org/10.1016/j.im.2009.06.006

*Mackey, J. D., McAllister, C. P., Ellen, B. P., III, & Carson, J. E. (2021). A meta-analysis of interpersonal and organizational workplace deviance research. *Journal of Management, 47*(3), 597–622. https://doi.org/10.1177/0149206319862612

McCarthy, K., Pearce, J. L., Morton, J., & Lyon, S. (2020). Do you pass it on? An examination of the consequences of perceived cyber incivility. *Organizational Management Journal, 17*(1), 43–58. https://doi.org/10.1108/OMJ-12-2018-0654

*McCord, M. A., Joseph, D. L., Dhanani, L. Y., & Beus, J. M. (2018). A meta-analysis of sex and race differences in perceived workplace mistreatment. *Journal of Applied Psychology, 103*(2), 137–163. https://doi.org/10.1037/apl0000250

McCormick, B. W., Reeves, C. J., Downes, P. E., Li, N., & Ilies, R. (2020). Scientific contributions of within-person research in management: Making the juice worth the squeeze. *Journal of Management, 46*(2), 321–350. https://doi.org/10.1177/0149206318788435

McEwen, B. S., & Stellar, E. (1993). Stress and the individual: Mechanisms leading to disease. *Archives of Internal Medicine, 153*(18), 2093–2101. https://doi.org/10.1001/archinte.1993.00410180039004

*Morphet, J., Griffiths, D., Beattie, J., Velasquez Reyes, D., & Innes, K. (2018). Prevention and management of occupational violence and aggression in healthcare: A scoping review. *Collegian (Royal College of Nursing, Australia), 25*(6), 621–632. https://doi.org/10.1016/j.colegn.2018.04.003

*Nielsen, M. B., Harris, A., Pallesen, S., & Einarsen, S. V. (2020). Workplace bullying and sleep – A systematic review and meta-analysis of the research literature. *Sleep Medicine Reviews, 51,* 101289. https://doi.org/10.1016/j.smrv.2020.101289

Nielsen, M. B., Matthiesen, S. B., & Einarsen, S. (2010). The impact of methodological moderators on prevalence rates of workplace bullying. A meta-analysis. *Journal of Occupational and Organizational Psychology, 83*(4), 955–979. https://doi.org/10.1348/096317909X481256

*Park, L., & Martinez, L (2021). An "I" for an "I": A systematic review and meta-analysis of instigated and reciprocal incivility. *Journal of Occupational Health Psychology, 27*(1), 7–21. https://doi.org/10.1037/ocp0000293.

*Pletzer, J. L., Bentvelzen, M., Oostrom, J. K., & de Vries, R. E. (2019). A meta-analysis of the relations between personality and workplace deviance: Big Five versus HEXACO. *Journal of Vocational Behavior, 112,* 369–383. https://doi.org/10.1016/j.jvb.2019.04.004

Privitera, C., & Campbell, M. A. (2009). Cyberbullying: The new face of workplace bullying? *Cyberpsychology & Behavior, 12*(4), 395–400. https://doi.org/10.1089/cpb.2009.0025

Raver, J. L., & Nishii, L. H. (2010). Once, twice, or three times as harmful? Ethnic harassment, gender harassment, and generalized workplace harassment. *Journal of Applied Psychology, 95*(2), 236–254. https://doi.org/10.1037/a0018377

*Robinson, S. L., O'Reilly, J., & Wang, W. (2013). Invisible at work: An integrated model of workplace ostracism. *Journal of Management, 39*(1), 203–231. https://doi.org/10.1177/0149206312466141

*Salin, D. (2003). Ways of explaining workplace bullying: A review of enabling, motivating and precipitating structures and processes in the work environment. *Human Relations, 56*(10), 1213–1232. https://doi.org/10.1177/00187267035610003

*Schilpzand, P., De Pater, I. E., & Erez, A. (2016). Workplace incivility: A review of the literature and agenda for future research. *Journal of Organizational Behavior, 37*(S1), S57–S88. https://doi.org/10.1002/job.1976

Slora, K. B. (1989). An empirical approach to determining employee deviance base rates. *Journal of Business and Psychology, 4*(2), 199–219. https://doi.org/10.1007/BF01016441

*Tepper, B. J. (2007). Abusive supervision in work organizations: Review, synthesis, and research agenda. *Journal of Management, 33*(3), 261–289. https://doi.org/10.1177/0149206307300812

*Tepper, B. J., Simon, L., & Park, H. M. (2017). Abusive supervision. *Annual Review of Organizational Psychology and Organizational Behavior, 4*(1), 123–152. https://doi.org/10.1146/annurev-orgpsych-041015-062539

*Triana, M. del C., Gu, P., Chapa, O., Richard, O., & Colella, A. (2021). Sixty years of discrimination and diversity research in human resource management: A review with suggestions for future research directions. *Human Resource Management, 60*(1), 145–204. https://doi.org/10.1002/hrm.22052

*Triana, M. del C., Jayasinghe, M., Pieper, J. R., Delgado, D. M., & Li, M. (2019). Perceived workplace gender discrimination and employee consequences: A meta-analysis and complementary studies considering country context. *Journal of Management, 45*(6), 2419–2447. https://doi.org/10.1177/0149206318776772

*Yang, L.-Q., Caughlin, D. E., Gazica, M. W., Truxillo, D. M., & Spector, P. E. (2014). Workplace mistreatment climate and potential employee and organizational outcomes: A meta-analytic review from the target's perspective. *Journal of Occupational Health Psychology, 19*(3), 315–335. https://doi.org/10.1037/a0036905

Yang, L.-Q., Spector, P. E., Chang, C.-H., Gallant-Roman, M., & Powell, J. (2012). Psychosocial precursors and physical consequences of workplace violence towards nurses: A longitudinal examination with naturally occurring groups in hospital settings. *International Journal of Nursing Studies, 49*(9), 1091–1102. https://doi.org/10.1016/j.ijnurstu.2012.03.006

Yang, L.-Q., Zheng, X., Liu, X., Lu, C. Q., & Schaubroeck, J. M. (2020). Abusive supervision, thwarted belongingness, and workplace safety: A group engagement perspective. *Journal of Applied Psychology, 105*(3), 230–244. https://doi.org/10.1037/apl0000436

*Zhang, Y., & Bednall, T. C. (2016). Antecedents of abusive supervision: A meta-analytic review. *Journal of Business Ethics, 139*(3), 455–471. https://doi.org/10.1007/s10551-015-2657-6

*Zhang, Y., & Liao, Z. (2015). Consequences of abusive supervision: A meta-analytic review. *Asia Pacific Journal of Management, 32*(4), 959–987. https://doi.org/10.1007/s10490-015-9425-0

Zheng, M. X., & van Dijke, M. (2020). Expressing forgiveness after interpersonal mistreatment: Power and status of forgivers influence transgressors' relationship restoration efforts. *Journal of Organizational Behavior, 41*(8), 782–796. https://doi.org/10.1002/job.2432

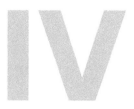

IV

SYMPTOMS, DISORDERS, AND CONSEQUENCES

INTRODUCTION: SYMPTOMS, DISORDERS, AND CONSEQUENCES

Part IV of this handbook contains chapters that draw upon the effects of conditions in the work environment and describe how those conditions relate to employees' health and well-being. Four of the chapters focus on negative aspects, and three of the chapters integrate positive aspects of the work environment on employees and organizations.

Chapter 15 discusses burnout, focusing on the effects of the occupational context in which relationships between people and the workplace are not aligned. Chapter 16 integrates psychosocial working conditions with mechanisms as to how stress affects individuals based on the results of intervention studies and describes risk factors for cardiovascular disease. Chapter 17 follows with a description of pain and musculoskeletal injuries and presents guidance on job accommodations and return to work. Chapter 18 provides an overview of the prevalence of substance use and impairment in the workplace, focusing on causes that are internal to the workplace. It will be noted that many of these topics have also been identified in earlier chapters in discussions of workplace stressors. In addition, this chapter addresses the organizational consequences of substance use and the effects of employee assistance programs in addressing substance use in the workplace. Chapter 24 provides more information on employee assistance programs.

At this point in Part IV, the chapters shift their focus from the more negative aspects of occupational health psychology to a positive perspective. Chapter 19 integrates existing definitions of well-being into an occupational context, thus providing ties between several of the earlier chapters that focus more on negative occupational health issues. Chapter 20 describes the theoretical approaches to recovery from work demands and relates recovery to employee well-being. Chapter 21 concludes this section of the handbook by discussing meaningful work and calling as they pertain to occupational health and worker well-being.

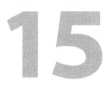

Job Burnout

Michael P. Leiter and Christina Maslach

Job burnout is an enduring focus of research, with the term eliciting over a million citations on Google Scholar in mid-2021. A consequence of the breadth of work on burnout is that reviews of the research literature tend to focus on distinct professions (e.g., physicians, West et al., 2020; nurses, Rushton et al., 2015; or teachers, Van Droogenbroeck et al., 2014). This chapter does not intend to conduct a similar review but instead presents the major conceptual developments regarding burnout.

As with many psychological terms, there has been debate on its precise definition as well as options for its operationalization. The World Health Organization (WHO) provided clarity while developing the 11th edition of the *International Classification of Diseases (ICD-11)*. Based on reviewing 40 years of research, WHO defined *burnout* as follows:

> Burn-out is a syndrome conceptualized as resulting from chronic workplace stress that has not been successfully managed. It is characterized by three dimensions:
>
> - feelings of energy depletion or exhaustion
> - increased mental distance from one's job, or feelings of negativism or cynicism related to one's job
> - reduced professional efficacy
>
> Burn-out refers specifically to phenomena in the occupational context and should not be applied to describe experiences in other areas of life. (WHO, 2019)

https://doi.org/10.1037/0000331-015
Handbook of Occupational Health Psychology, Third Edition, L. E. Tetrick, G. G. Fisher, M. T. Ford, and J. C. Quick (Editors)

WHO also stated that burnout was an occupational phenomenon; it is not classified as a medical condition. This statement contradicts approaches that have attempted to medicalize the syndrome or to make it synonymous with depression (e.g., Bianchi et al., 2015). Burnout can increase the extent to which workers are vulnerable to subsequent mental and physical disorders, and for which the workers might contact health services, but it is not an illness in and of itself. Rather, WHO positions burnout as an occupational condition (parallel to other such conditions, like chronic unemployment), in which stress "has not been successfully managed." That is, burnout pertains to the context in which work occurs (an occupational phenomenon), not to personal weaknesses of individuals. It follows that any actions to alleviate or to prevent burnout should focus on addressing shortcomings in the occupational context in order to make work more fulfilling, or at least more manageable. It does not follow that such actions should only have a limited focus on fixing shortcomings in workers in order to increase their resilience. The definition further emphasizes that burnout, so defined, pertains to work life. Other uses of the term, such as *parental burnout* (e.g., Mikolajczak et al., 2018), lie outside the domain defined by WHO.

BURNOUT AS A RELATIONSHIP CRISIS

An alternative to locating burnout as a disorder within people is to consider burnout as a crisis in the relationships of people with their workplaces. Neither the person nor the workplace is necessarily flawed, but they are not aligned well with one another. Employment is a relationship with expectations, obligations, and demands in both directions. Workplaces expect a lot from their people; people expect a lot from their workplaces. At times, those expectations are thwarted.

Over 3 decades of research on burnout have identified a plethora of organizational risk factors across many occupations in various countries. An analysis of this research literature identified six key areas of work life: workload, control, reward, community, fairness, and values (Leiter & Maslach, 2004). The first two areas are reflected in the demand–control model of job stress (Karasek & Theorell, 1990), and reward refers to the power of reinforcements to shape behavior. Community captures all the work on social support and interpersonal conflict, while fairness emerges from the literature on equity and social justice. Finally, the area of values includes the cognitive–emotional power of job goals and expectations.

One dynamic aggravating burnout comes from excessive demands. To a large extent the exhaustion dimension of burnout reflects people making unsustainable efforts to meet demands that exceed their capacity. In some instances, people compensate for insufficient resources, knowledge, or assistance to fulfill their workplace's demands by committing additional personal effort or time. The extra effort disrupts their capacity for recovery, perpetuating a cycle of diminishing returns as they begin the next workday already exhausted. People may overextend themselves out of dedication, believing that they are making a distinct and necessary contribution to a workplace they cherish. Or they may overextend themselves out of fear, believing that they will receive reprimands or even dismissal from their position if they fail to meet expectations. In either case, they expend an unsustainable amount of their energy to their jobs.

A second dynamic aggravating burnout comes from people feeling frustrated. People expect their workplaces to provide opportunities to fulfill psychological needs for belonging, autonomy, and competence (Ryan & Deci, 2017), as well as other core motives (Maslach & Banks, 2017). In fulfilling workplaces, people are valued by their colleagues, have the freedom to show initiative, receive confirmation as being effective contributors to the workplace, experience psychological safety, are treated fairly, do meaningful work, and have positive experiences on the job. The frustration arising from the thwarting of any or all of these motives represents a mismatch in the relationships of people with their workplaces. Research has confirmed inverse relationships of social support and burnout (Halbesleben, 2006; Maslach et al., 2001; Van Droogenbroeck et al., 2014) and has found that improving social encounters at work is associated with reductions in burnout (Leiter et al., 2011). Low levels of work-related efficacy are a defining feature of burnout (Maslach et al., 2017; Shoji et al., 2016), and improvements in efficacy are a pathway to reducing burnout (Bresó et al., 2011). Interventions to manage workload and to increase physicians' autonomy have been associated with increased work engagement and reduced burnout (Shirom et al., 2010; DeChant et al., 2019). Environments that frustrate psychological motives contribute to stress "that has not been successfully managed."

To the extent that members of work groups share similar aspirations and are subject to similar levels of demands, burnout may become a characteristic of the setting. Multilevel analysis has provided evidence of burnout having both individual- and work group–level qualities (Consiglio et al., 2013; González-Morales et al., 2012; Halbesleben & Leon, 2014). These analyses propose that, in addition to sharing similar motives and environmental parameters, people may also be subject to contagion by resonating with their colleagues' experiences of exhaustion, cynicism, and/or inefficacy.

ASSESSMENT OF BURNOUT

Early qualitative research about the burnout phenomenon was done in the 1970s by two psychologists (Freudenberger, 1974; Maslach, 1976); their findings were widely reported in newspapers and magazines. This early work was based on people's descriptions of their work experience, rather than being derived from some scholarly theory. The term *burnout* is a very evocative one, and people can easily relate to it as a response to job stressors. It can also be applied to other kinds of experiences (e.g., boredom, workaholism, laziness), so its actual meaning can be unclear and vague. Thus, there have been many subsequent attempts to establish a clear and consensual definition of this colloquial term and a corresponding method to assess it.

Several themes characterize the measurement work that has been conducted on burnout for more than 40 years. First, there is a major contrast between popular and academic measures of the burnout experience. In the 1970s, "do-it-yourself" tests, often published in popular media, purported to tell people whether they were burned out or not, based on nothing more than an intuitive judgment about what questions to ask. This do-it-yourself approach has continued over the decades, often by using a few items from one or more established measures and then adding some new ones. Despite the lack of supporting evidence for these measures, they are sometimes used by organizations in their annual staff surveys. In contrast, by the 1980s more substantive burnout measures were developed, based on psychometric research, in order to establish valid and reliable methods for assessing this phenomenon. A second wave of research-based measures were developed and published during the first 2 decades of the 21st century.

Second, there is a major contrast between research and clinical intervention as the intended goals of using a burnout measure. Research measures are designed to be used for *discovery* (the correlates of burnout as well as its causes and effects). In contrast, clinical measures are designed for *diagnosis* (who is suffering from burnout and thus needs treatment). Most of the academic measures were designed for discovery, not diagnosis, but sometimes they have been utilized for clinical purposes as well, which has posed some significant challenges. In particular, the clinical use usually presumes that burnout is a health or medical condition (and thus an individual person problem, rather than a situational job problem). In addition, the measures designed for research do not have the clinical database to support their being used for individual diagnosis.

Research Measures

On the research side, several measures have been developed. One of the first was the Maslach Burnout Inventory (MBI; Maslach & Jackson, 1981), which assesses the three dimensions of exhaustion, cynicism (or depersonalization), and efficacy (or personal accomplishment). The content of the scale items was drawn from prior qualitative research interviews and observations, and the subsequent testing and refinement of these items were based on an extensive program of psychometric research to establish the validity and reliability of the final measure. Research has confirmed these three dimensions as being interrelated (Taris et al., 2005). Reviews have established, as well as through meta-analysis, that the three subscales have distinct predictors and outcomes (Lee & Ashforth, 1996). The response format of frequency, which ranges from never to daily, conveys that the defining question for burnout is *how often* people are experiencing the impact of the chronic job stressors. For example, starting a workday already exhausted a few times a year is within normal bounds, but doing so a few times a week indicates difficulties. Other measures developed in the 1980s focused on just the single dimension of exhaustion (Freudenberger & Richelson, 1980; Pines et al., 1981).

Much of the conceptual underpinning for these initial measures came from then-current work on organizational stress and job–person fit (see Kahn & Byosiere, 1992). There was a focus on the process of how burnout developed over time. Some stage models were proposed, such as the transactional model with its three stages of imbalance between work demands and individual resources, the emotional response of exhaustion and anxiety, and then changes in attitudes and behavior, such as greater cynicism (Cherniss, 1980). Because much of the early research focused on burnout within human service occupations, the wording of the items reflected that origin. A general version of the MBI, which could be used for any occupation, was developed in the 1990s (MBI-GS; MBI; Schaufeli et al., 1996), and subsequent burnout measures were designed to be more occupation-neutral from the outset.

Several new burnout measures were developed in the first 2 decades of the 2000s and were characterized by underlying theory, multiple dimensions, quantitative research, and correlation with the MBI. Some measures continued to have a primary focus on the concept of exhaustion (which is usually viewed as the human stress response). The Shirom-Melamed Burnout Measure (SMBM; Shirom & Melamed, 2006) distinguished between three types of exhaustion (physical fatigue, emotional exhaustion, and cognitive weariness), and the Copenhagen Burnout Inventory (Kristensen et al., 2005) made a distinction between physical and psychological exhaustion. The SMBM has its conceptual roots in the conservation of resources theory (Hobfoll, 1989), which proposes the management of personal resources, including various forms of energy, as a central construct. The measure conceptualizes burnout as resulting from difficulties in managing those resources.

The Oldenburg Burnout Inventory (OLBI; Demerouti et al., 2003) assesses burnout with two dimensions: exhaustion and disengagement. Disengagement shares features with cynicism or depersonalization. This measure was developed within the framework of the job demands–resources model (Demerouti et al., 2001). This framework depicts exhaustion as arising from excessive demands; in contrast, disengagement arises from resource shortfalls.

Subsequent burnout measures have provided a new version of the three basic dimensions, such as the Bergen Burnout Inventory (Feldt et al., 2014), which assesses exhaustion at work, cynicism toward the meaning of work, and sense of inadequacy at work. Other measures have added new concepts—for example, the Spanish Burnout Inventory (Gil-Monte & Figueiredo-Ferraz, 2013) has four dimensions: enthusiasm toward the job, psychological exhaustion, indolence, and guilt.

In addition to the presence of multiple measures being used in burnout research, there are other problems in consolidating the empirical findings because of inconsistencies in how researchers score the measures and the information they publish (Eckleberry-Hunt et al., 2018). For example, the tendency to shorten the MBI to fewer items has been shown to lead to overestimates of the prevalence of burnout (Lim et al., 2019). Despite these challenges, there seems to be enough shared similarity to generate consistent patterns of research findings (rather than distinctly different ones), so the resulting aggregated body of evidence that was reviewed by WHO is quite substantial.

Clinical Measures

In contrast to research studies, in which measures are used to collect aggregated data from large numbers of participants, the goal of clinical diagnosis is to identify an individual's unique pattern of responses for a defined health condition. For example, earlier work focused on distinguishing three different clinical subtypes of burnout: frenetic, underchallenged, and worn out (Montero-Marín & García-Campayo, 2010). More recently, there has been a general societal trend toward wanting to diagnose individuals who experience burnout, thus treating it as some sort of personal medical disease (which is contrary to the WHO definition). As a result, some of the research measures, as well as some of the popular homegrown ones, have been adapted, changed, or even misused to serve as a diagnostic tool for individual burnout (see Maslach & Leiter, 2021, for a discussion of this issue). In most cases, the intent is a good one—namely, to identify people who are experiencing a health problem and to then provide some sort of treatment or cure. However, the negative stigma that is often attached to burnout means that many people will resist being identified by that term and will not seek out help, even if they could benefit from it.

Although job burnout itself is not considered to be a medical condition, it has clearly been linked to several health problems, such as psychosomatic disorders, sleep disruptions, and depression. It is possible to identify and treat such problems on their own—a prior diagnosis of burnout is not required. However, some new work is being done to develop a burnout measure that includes these health problems within its definition of burnout (Burnout Assessment Tool; BAT; Schaufeli et al., 2020). In addition to subscales measuring exhaustion and psychological distancing, the BAT has subscales on impaired cognition, depressed mood, psychological distress, and psychosomatic complaints, all of which combine to yield a single binary cut-off score. It is not yet clear what the clinical value will be of such a single-score measure, but the explicit objective is to be able to differentiate people experiencing burnout from people who are not.

Person-Oriented Analyses

In contrast to this simpler, single-score approach, more recent work has been focusing on using multiple indicators to identify a broader range of job-related experiences beyond just burnout. Person-oriented approaches begin with the proposition that people comprise a multiplicity of elements and processes that become integrated into systems, the components of which interact with one another. Correlations among measures of these elements indicate their usual mode of interaction, but the approach recognizes that people combine elements in different ways. Person-oriented analyses, such as cluster analysis or latent profile analysis (LPA), assist in identifying distinct patterns of combinations. That is, these approaches use an iterative process to identify profiles of scores that are shared among a meaningful proportion of a sample. Somewhere between the idea that every person is unique and the idea that everyone is the same lies the concept that there are a finite number of profiles that describe the combinations of the elements.

Person-oriented analyses have identified various profiles based on LPA (Mäkikangas et al., 2021). Other studies have used LPA with the OLBI, in combination with the Utrecht Work Engagement scale (Timms et al., 2012). These analyses have shared the identification of two profiles: one with positive scores on the three subscales and a second with negative scores on all three. But they have also found intermediate profiles on which the subscales are not consistent with one another. An analysis of two large health care samples identified five profiles (Leiter & Maslach, 2016). In addition to the all-positive and all-negative profiles (labeled *engagement* and *burnout,* respectively), three additional profiles had negative scores on only one of the three subscales: overextended (negative on exhaustion), disengaged (negative on cynicism), and ineffective (negative on efficacy). An LPA of 45,000 cases in a normative data base (Maslach et al., 2017) found the largest profile to be engaged (36%), with nearly equal frequencies of people in the other four profiles, ranging from 14% in burnout to 18% in overextended.

The relationship of these five profiles with the six areas of work life (based on data from 235 health care providers) is displayed in Figure 15.1. Scores above the midline are in the match direction (a good job–person fit) while scores below the midline are in the mismatch direction (a poor job–person

FIGURE 15.1. Areas of Work Life Across Profiles

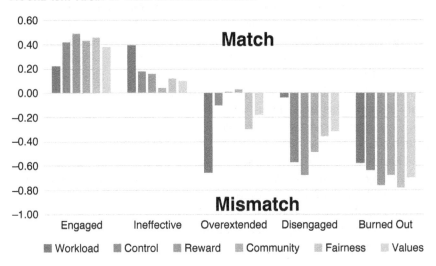

fit). This analysis suggests that burnout, as a syndrome of three interrelated dimensions, differs from states with only one dimension being problematic. The practice of equating burnout with "just exhaustion" obscures the differences between people with excessive work overload and those experiencing a wide range of mismatches across social and ethical domains. For example, the over-extended profile (high exhaustion combined with moderate to positive scores on the other two burnout dimensions) shows a strong mismatch on workload with moderate scores in the other five areas of work life. The overextended pro-file has a major issue with workload but does not report significant mismatches in the other areas of work life. Efforts to alleviate work overload would be wel-comed, as they would address the points of major concern for these people. In contrast, the burnout profile (high exhaustion, high cynicism, low efficacy) has mismatches in all six areas of work life. Efforts to address work overload may be welcomed, but they would leave much unresolved. The disengaged profile con-trasts with the overextended profile in that workload is near the midline, indi-cating a neutral view of work overload, but mismatches across the other five areas of work life. Efforts to address workload would miss issues that are important to these people. These distinctions between the profiles can inform action to alleviate challenges that people experience in their work.

INTERVENTION

Studies have looked time and again at the conditions related to burnout. This work has produced a wealth of knowledge about causes and effects of burnout, although it has not always sorted out what functions as a cause from what is an effect of burnout. Often, the pathways go in reciprocal patterns: for example, people find unpleasant social interactions as exhausting, and then when people feel exhausted, they may behave unpleasantly in their social interactions. Exam-ining causal models has supported causal paths occurring in multiple directions between employees' experiences and aspects of work life. A meta-analysis of structural equation analyses containing at least two time points (Guthier et al., 2020) found evidence of work–life areas affecting the three aspects of burnout, as well as evidence of employees' experience of exhaustion, cynicism, and effi-cacy affecting their evaluations of their work context. Overall, this analysis aligned with the view of multiple interdependencies of employees' personal experience and qualities of their work environments. The review noted that the rarity of studies that tracked individuals more than twice prevented addressing many questions about the development and alleviation of burnout. Two time points do not adequately define a trend.

What would help sort out these pathways is the most neglected part of the research agenda for burnout: testing methods for preventing burnout and alleviating burnout after it settles in. Although the world is awash in research on burnout, the surveys continue to rework ground that has already been har-vested. Few studies attempt to tackle the thornier question of how to make an enduring difference.

Starting from the idea that burnout rests upon mismatches between people and their work situations, intervention means changing that relationship. One potential quality that could make a difference is flexibility regarding how, when, and where to do the job, along with a sense of agency to help people maintain constructive and fulfilling relationships with work (Halpern, 2005). That is, flexible policies open more possibilities for fulfillment at work. In parallel, the same qualities offer new options for managers to support employees. In contrast, rigid centralized policies limit the options available to managers to create solutions within their work groups (Lee & Cummings, 2008). Ideally, that capacity would lie with immediate supervisors who could respond promptly and maintain ongoing support to assure that actions have the intended impact. Management is not an exact science: people cannot assume that every initiative will be well-received or effective. Searching for solutions always entails a bit of back and forth. There needs to be an ongoing dialogue.

Individual Intervention Approaches

A major focus of intervention research reflects an assumption that it is the individual employee who is not successfully managing stress on the job. With greater resilience in terms of physical health, fitness, and strength, individuals could withstand whatever stressors they encounter. With more effective coping skills and recovery strategies, people could manage those stressors successfully (Awa et al., 2010).

An example of this approach is mindfulness training (e.g., Luken & Sammons, 2016), which does not advocate changing the workplace or even individuals' behavior at work. Instead, it introduces routines, such as sitting meditation, that people practice away from the workplace. When effective, the technique can alleviate stress already developed at work and prevent the development of subsequent stress reactions. Meta-analyses of mindfulness studies related to burnout have confirmed that these approaches reduce exhaustion for participants, but have little or no impact on cynicism or inefficacy (Maricuţoiu et al., 2016). However, research also that found that participants who reported decreases in exhaustion when developing mindfulness skills were more likely to show additional benefits to well-being at an eight-month follow-up assessment (Kinnunen et al., 2020). Another study combined mindfulness training with Hatha yoga sessions to produce decreases in exhaustion (Sallon et al., 2017). Overall, these studies confirmed that people benefited from developing the capacity to relax deeply and to gain psychological distance from the demand of their jobs.

The general strategy in these approaches was increasing participants' capacity to withstand the demands of their jobs. Much of the activity (e.g., mindfulness, yoga, relaxation) occurred away from the workplace, improving employees' capacity to recover from demands and to approach subsequent demands with more equanimity. To the extent that these activities touched on job demands per se, it was to improve employees' capacity to think about those demands in less distressing ways. These interventions have implications for employees' relationships with their workplaces but do not change the workplace. Instead, they develop employees' reactions to the existing nature of the workplace in ways that reduce their distress.

Organizational Interventions

An alternative to improving employees' capacity to endure or cope with existing workplace stressors is to change the workplace. This approach entertains the idea that stressed employees may be sufficiently resilient and have adequate coping skills, but that their workplaces present them with excessive challenges. This strategy has the benefit of going to the root of the problem with direct implications for employees' relationships with their workplaces. It has the challenge of integrating workplace leadership into the intervention project to the extent that the process calls for changing management practices or structures. Although leadership may be committed to the goals of reducing burnout and promoting work engagement, they may not be committed to changing their basic operation.

Organizational interventions present challenges for evaluation that inhibit progress toward establishing evidence-based management practices. A meta-analysis of intervention research had trouble finding consistency across studies (McKinley et al., 2017). For example, many studies used workshop formats with similar themes, but their curriculum had few identifiable points in common. The gold standard of randomized controlled trials (RCTs) has little relevance to organizational interventions (Nielsen et al., 2008). Participants' active involvement in designing, implementing, and assessing interventions can be an important success factor (International Labor Organization, 2001; LeBlanc & Schaufeli, 2008; Tafvelin et al., 2019), but can prevent assessments that would keep participants and facilitators unaware of their status with regard to being in a test or control group. Successful interventions tend to include leaders who engage in close listening and who then modify processes in response to participants' experiences (DeJoy et al., 2010; Halbesleben et al., 2006). As a result, groups participating in the intervention lack consistency in what exactly the intervention entailed.

Further, studies would need to operate on a large scale to have the capacity to randomly assign work groups to test or control groups. Often, workplace leaders insist that the process include work groups with the greatest need rather than permit randomization. The intervention process may be difficult to replicate. As has been noted, descriptions of organizational interventions often lack distinctive information on the specific activities and on relevant contextual features that may influence the impact (Murta et al., 2007). Instead of attempting to shoehorn a study design into the RCT framework, researchers can establish valid findings by including multiple forms of assessment for which they have registered hypothesized outcomes, while providing more information on context and process to permit replication (Nielsen & Abildgaard, 2013).

In addition to being collaborative, it is important for organizational interventions to be targeted and strategic, such that they fit with the workplace's aspirations and values. Workplaces often lose the focus of an initiative through "mission creep," in which a project expands beyond its initial objectives or program design (DeJoy et al., 2010). Programs that align well with the workplace's strategic plans have a greater potential to sustain, because the workplaces have the personnel, facilities, and habits that fit with the new initiative. For example, large health care facilities often have in-house facilitators and trainers who have the space and responsibility to conduct ongoing sessions with work groups. This quality is especially important when addressing burnout because of its persistent nature. Sustaining the gains of interventions requires ongoing effort. Otherwise, conditions that aggravate burnout could reestablish themselves. This quality requires workplaces to have a long-term capacity to maintain critical support (e.g., Mommersteeg et al., 2006; Salmela-aro et al., 2004). To maintain credibility and support, it is important that interventions be evaluated with valid assessment instruments to determine the extent to which they are reaching their objectives (Moulding et al., 1999).

Job crafting provides a relatively straightforward approach to organizational intervention in that it coaches employees to change their work processes while keeping those changes within their range of control. That is, the process explores employees' latitude for modifying their work without requiring changes in workplace structures or policies. One application of job crafting (van den Heuvel et al., 2015) coached a group of police officers to shift some of their work time from activities they considered to be tedious to activities they found more enjoyable. By changing the police officers' regular work routines, job crafting generated more positive experiences at work. Participants reported, as well, an increase in goal attainment and more rewarding work experiences associated with the process.

A more interactive approach to changing work processes employed group problem solving to address problems that participants identified in their work life (Halbesleben et al., 2006). Rather than focus on the employees' mental or physical well-being, the project focused on the work itself and the management practices of the workplace. Managers participated in the sessions with members of their work groups. Although this model does not lend itself to addressing organization-wide policies and practices, it does contain the authority to modify how things are done on the level of the participating work groups. Similarly, a project in a Swedish hospital reported lower levels of exhaustion for nurses who developed individualized patient care models within their work groups (Berg et al., 1994). Again, the issue was not managing nurses' emotional response to existing work conditions but implementing processes that helped them change conditions to be less challenging.

Improving Work-Group Dynamics

People encounter their work-group cultures directly in their social interactions at work. Through interacting with others, people learn the norms of their work groups. They also experience the regard in which others view them. Research has confirmed that the quality of social relationships at work is closely connected to employees' experiences of all three aspects of burnout

(Halbesleben, 2006). Thus, improving social encounters has become a strategy for preventing and alleviating burnout. One approach has been civility, respect, and engagement with work (CREW), based upon facilitated sessions in which members of work groups reflect on their social encounters as a step toward developing more respectful ways of interacting (Osatuke et al., 2009). This study at Veterans Health Administration (VHA) settings in the United States demonstrated that the CREW process increased levels of civility among participating work groups while nontreatment control groups remained unchanged.

Applications of CREW in Canadian hospitals replicated the VHA findings of improved civility from CREW. These studies also found that improvements in civility mediated decreases in exhaustion and cynicism as well as improvements in respect, job satisfaction, and management trust (Leiter et al., 2011). Evaluation is a core component of the CREW approach, with surveys occurring at baseline to assess the groups' starting point. The surveys are repeated subsequently to determine the impact and to identify the need for additional support.

FUTURE DIRECTIONS

Despite inspiring global interest in job burnout and thousands of surveys across a wide range of occupations, much remains to be learned about this topic. The biggest gaps in knowledge pertain to process: how does burnout develop over time, both in terms of intensifying and subsiding? The research formats for addressing these questions are challenging. As burnout occurs as a relationship crisis, examining it requires ongoing assessment of the work context as well as the people interacting with that context. Simply tracking people over time does not suffice, as the sampling strategy may miss important changes in employees' experiences or fail to assess those aspects of work life that prompted those changes. Research that tracks the impact of theory-based interventions brings in the relevant time frame and tests theory-based hypotheses regarding the mechanisms through which change occurs.

After nearly half a century of research on job burnout, few surprises remain to be discovered about its correlations with work environments, health, or well-being. However, much remains to be understood about strategies to make deliberate, positive changes in the ways that people experience their jobs and careers. A practical challenge for researchers is enlisting the cooperation of people to participate in these studies, including the task of responding to surveys and interviews intended to tap into their experiences. There are additional challenges in enlisting the active participation of workplace leaders who are willing to explore innovative strategies for promoting constructive and fulfilling relationships of people with their work. Beyond these practical challenges, researchers must work to elaborate, test, and develop theoretical models that point toward intervention strategies with a potential for lasting change. It may be that interventions to address burnout operate more like an exercise program than a vaccine. It is likely that improvements will need ongoing attention, not simply to prevent backsliding but also to adapt to substantive changes in the nature of work (Maslach & Leiter, 2022).

Burnout as an occupational condition reflecting stress that has not been well managed reflects strains in the relationships of people with their workplaces. Despite workplaces being the sources of burnout, much of the advice on burnout ignores the context to encourage healthy lifestyles and time-management strategies (Lubbadeh, 2020). These sources of advice convey an assumption that workplaces cannot or will not change their practices.

However, major life disruptions will challenge that assumption, and the COVID-19 pandemic has been a clear example of that. The pandemic prompted abrupt transformations in where and when people worked, as well as the ways they communicated with colleagues while doing their job. It turns out that workplaces *can* change, and so the more relevant question for the future is: how can we redesign workplaces to be healthier, with a better fit between people and the job, so that workers can thrive and be engaged rather than being beaten down and burned out? A solution will not be a return to the "normal" of the past, but it will include fresh opportunities to make meaningful changes that will more successfully manage the impact of chronic job stressors.

REFERENCES

Awa, W. L., Plaumann, M., & Walter, U. (2010). Burnout prevention: A review of intervention programs. *Patient Education and Counseling*, 78(2), 184–190. https://doi.org/10.1016/j.pec.2009.04.008

Berg, A., Hansson, U. W., & Hallberg, I. R. (1994). Nurses' creativity, tedium and burnout during 1 year of clinical supervision and implementation of individually planned nursing care: Comparisons between a ward for severely demented patients and a similar control ward. *Journal of Advanced Nursing*, 20(4), 742–749. https://doi.org/10.1046/j.1365-2648.1994.20040742.x

Bianchi, R., Schonfeld, I. S., & Laurent, E. (2015). Burnout–depression overlap: A review. *Clinical Psychology Review*, 36, 28–41. https://doi.org/10.1016/j.cpr.2015.01.004

Bresó, E., Schaufeli, W. B., & Salanova, M. (2011). Can a self-efficacy-based intervention decrease burnout, increase engagement, and enhance performance? A quasi-experimental study. *Higher Education*, 61(4), 339–355. https://doi.org/10.1007/s10734-010-9334-6

Cherniss, C. (1980). *Staff burnout: Job stress in the human services*. Sage.

Consiglio, C., Borgogni, L., Alessandri, G., & Schaufeli, W. B. (2013). Does self-efficacy matter for burnout and sickness absenteeism? The mediating role of demands and resources at the individual and team levels. *Work and Stress*, 27(1), 22–42. https://doi.org/10.1080/02678373.2013.769325

Dechant, P. F., Acs, A., Rhee, K. B., Boulanger, T. S., Snowdon, J. L., Tutty, M. A., Sinsky, C. A., & Thomas Craig, K. J. (2019). Effect of Organization-Directed Workplace Interventions on Physician Burnout: A Systematic Review. *Mayo Clinic Proceedings: Innovations, Quality & Outcomes*, 3(4), 384-408. https://doi.org/10.1016/j.mayocpiqo.2019.07.006

DeJoy, D. M., Wilson, M. G., Vandenberg, R. J., McGrath-Higgins, A. L., & Griffin-Blake, C. S. (2010). Assessing the impact of healthy work organization intervention. *Journal of Occupational and Organizational Psychology*, 83(1), 139–165. https://doi.org/10.1348/096317908X398773

Demerouti, E., Bakker, A. B., Nachreiner, F., & Schaufeli, W. B. (2001). The job demands–resources model of burnout. *Journal of Applied Psychology, 86*(3), 499–512. https://doi.org/10.1037/0021-9010.86.3.499

Demerouti, E., Bakker, A. B., Vardakou, I., & Kantas, A. (2003). The convergent validity of two burnout instruments: A multitrait–multimethod analysis. *European Journal of Psychological Assessment, 19*(1), 12–23. https://psycnet.apa.org/doi/10.1027/1015-5759.19.1.12

Eckleberry-Hunt, J., Kirkpatrick, H., & Barbera, T. (2018). The problems with burnout research. *Academic Medicine, 93*(3), 367–370. https://doi.org/10.1097/ACM.0000000000001890

Feldt, T., Rantanen, J., Hyvönen, K., Mäkikangas, A., Huhtala, M., Pihlajasaari, P., & Kinnunen, U. (2014). The 9-item Bergen Burnout Inventory: Factorial validity across organizations and measurements of longitudinal data. *Industrial Health, 52*(2), 102–112.

Freudenberger, H. J. (1974). Staff burn-out. *Journal of Social Issues, 30*(1), 159–165. https://doi.org/10.1111/j.1540-4560.1974.tb00706.x

Freudenberger, H. J., & Richelson, G. (1980). *Burn-out: The high cost of high achievement.* Doubleday.

Gil-Monte, P. R., & Figueiredo-Ferraz, H. H. (2013). Psychometric properties of the 'Spanish Burnout Inventory' among employees working with people with intellectual disability. *Journal of Intellectual Disability Research, 57,* 959–968.

González-Morales, M. G., Peiró, J. M., Rodríguez, I., & Bliese, P. D. (2012). Perceived collective burnout: A multilevel explanation of burnout. *Anxiety, Stress, and Coping, 25*(1), 43–61. https://doi.org/10.1080/10615806.2010.542808

Guthier, C., Dormann, C., & Voelkle, M. C. (2020). Reciprocal effects between job stressors and burnout: A continuous time meta-analysis of longitudinal studies. *Psychological Bulletin, 146*(12), 1146–1173. https://doi.org/10.1037/bul0000304

Halbesleben, J. R. (2006). Sources of social support and burnout: A meta-analytic test of the conservation of resources model. *Journal of Applied Psychology, 91*(5), 1134–1145. https://doi.org/10.1037/0021-9010.91.5.1134

Halbesleben, J. R., & Leon, M. R. (2014). Multilevel models of burnout: Separating group level and individual level effects in burnout research. In A. B. Bakker, M. P. Leiter, & C. Maslach (Eds.), *Burnout at work* (pp. 130–152). Psychology Press.

Halbesleben, J. R., Osburn, H. K., & Mumford, M. D. (2006). Action research as a burnout intervention reducing burnout in the federal fire service. *The Journal of Applied Behavioral Science, 42*(2), 244–266. https://doi.org/10.1177/0021886305285031

Halpern, D. F. (2005). How time-flexible work policies can reduce stress, improve health, and save money. *Stress and Health, 21*(3), 157–168. https://doi.org/10.1002/smi.1049

Hobfoll, S. E. (1989). Conservation of resources: A new attempt at conceptualizing stress. *American Psychologist, 44*(3), 513–524. https://doi.org/10.1037/0003-066X.44.3.513

International Labor Organization. (2001). *Guidelines on occupational safety and health management systems.* International Labor Office. https://www.ilo.org/wcmsp5/groups/public/---ed_protect/---protrav/---safework/documents/normativeinstrument/wcms_107727.pdf

Kahn, R. L., & Byosiere, P. (1992). Stress in organizations. In M. D. Dunnette & L. M. Hough (Eds.), *Handbook of industrial and organizational psychology* (Vol. 3, pp. 571–650). Consulting Psychologists Press.

Karasek, R., & Theorell, T. (1990). *Stress, productivity, and the reconstruction of working life.* Basic Books.

Kristensen, T. S., Borritz, M., Villadsen, E., & Christensen, K. B. (2005). The Copenhagen Burnout Inventory: A new tool for the assessment of burnout. *Work and Stress, 19*(3), 192–207. https://doi.org/10.1080/02678370500297720

Kinnunen S. M., Puolakanaho A., Mäkikangas A., Tolvanen A., Lappalainen R. (2020). Does a mindfulness-, acceptance-, and value-based intervention for burnout have long-term effects on different levels of subjective well-being? *International Journal of Stress Management, 27*, 82–87. https://doi.org/10.1037/str0000132

Le Blanc, P. M., & Schaufeli, W. B. (2008). Burnout interventions: An overview and illustration. In J. R. Halbesleben (Ed.), *Handbook of stress and burnout in health care* (pp. 201–216). Nova Science Publishers.

Lee, H., & Cummings, G. G. (2008). Factors influencing job satisfaction of front line nurse managers: A systematic review. *Journal of Nursing Management, 16*(7), 768–783. https://doi.org/10.1111/j.1365-2834.2008.00879.x

Lee, R. T., & Ashforth, B. E. (1996). A meta-analytic examination of the correlates of the three dimensions of job burnout. *Journal of Applied Psychology, 81*(2), 123–133. https://doi.org/10.1037/0021-9010.81.2.123

Leiter, M. P., Laschinger, H. K. S., Day, A., & Gilin Oore, D. (2011). The impact of civility interventions on employee social behavior, distress, and attitudes. *Journal of Applied Psychology, 96*(6), 1258–1274. https://doi.org/10.1037/a0024442

Leiter, M. P., & Maslach, C. (2004). Areas of worklife: A structured approach to organizational predictors of job burnout. In P. L. Perrewe & D. C. Ganster (Eds.), *Research in occupational stress and well being* (Vol. 3, pp. 91–134). Elsevier Science.

Leiter, M. P., & Maslach, C. (2016). Latent burnout profiles: A new approach to understanding the burnout experience. *Burnout Research, 3*(4), 89–100. https://doi.org/10.1016/j.burn.2016.09.001

Lim, W. Y., Ong, J., Ong, S., Hao, Y., Abdullah, H. R., Koh, D. L., & Mok, U. S. M. (2019). The abbreviated Maslach Burnout Inventory can overestimate burnout: A study of anesthesiology residents. *Journal of Clinical Medicine, 9*(1), 61. https://doi.org/10.3390/jcm9010061

Lubbadeh, T. (2020). Job burnout: A general literature review. *International Review of Management and Marketing, 10*(3), 7–15. https://doi.org/10.32479/irmm.9398

Luken, M., & Sammons, A. (2016). Systematic review of mindfulness practice for reducing job burnout. *American Journal of Occupational Therapy, 70*(2). https://doi.org/10.5014/ajot.2016.016956

Mäkikangas, A., Leiter, M. P., Kinnunen, U., & Feldt, T. (2021). Profiling development of burnout over eight years: Relation with job demands and resources. *European Journal of Work and Organizational Psychology, 30*(5), 720–731. https://doi.org/10.1080/1359432X.2020.1790651

Maricuţoiu, L. P., Sava, F. A., & Butta, O. (2016). The effectiveness of controlled interventions on employees' burnout: A meta-analysis. *Journal of Occupational and Organizational Psychology, 89*(1), 1–27. https://doi.org/10.1111/joop.12099

Maslach, C. (1976). Burned-out. *Human Behavior, 5*, 16–22.

Maslach, C., & Banks, C. G. (2017). Psychological connections with work. In C. L. Cooper & M. P. Leiter (Eds.), *The Routledge companion to wellbeing at work* (pp. 37–54). Routledge. https://doi.org/10.4324/9781315665979-4

Maslach, C., & Jackson, S. E. (1981). The measurement of experienced burnout. *Journal of Organizational Behavior, 2*(2), 99–113. https://doi.org/10.1002/job.4030020205

Maslach, C., Jackson, S. E., Leiter, M. P., Schaufeli, W. B., & Schwab, R. L. (2017). *Maslach Burnout Inventory manual* (4th ed.). Mind Garden Publishing.

Maslach, C., & Leiter, M. P. (2021). Burnout: What it is and how to measure it. In *HBR guide to beating burnout* (pp. 211–221). Harvard Business Review Press.

Maslach, C., & Leiter, M. P. (2022). *The burnout challenge*. Harvard University Press.

Maslach, C., Schaufeli, W. B., & Leiter, M. P. (2001). Job burnout. *Annual Review of Psychology, 52*(1), 397–422. https://doi.org/10.1146/annurev.psych.52.1.397

McKinley, T. F., Boland, K. A., & Mahan, J. D. (2017). Burnout and interventions in pediatric residency: A literature review. *Burnout Research, 6*, 9–17. https://doi.org/10.1016/j.burn.2017.02.003

Mikolajczak, M., Raes, M. E., Avalosse, H., & Roskam, I. (2018). Exhausted parents: Sociodemographic, child-related, parent-related, parenting and family-functioning correlates of parental burnout. *Journal of Child and Family Studies, 27*(2), 602–614. https://doi.org/10.1007/s10826-017-0892-4

Mommersteeg, P. M., Heijnen, C. J., Verbraak, M. J., & van Doornen, L. J. (2006). A longitudinal study on cortisol and complaint reduction in burnout. *Psychoneuroendocrinology, 31*(7), 793–804. https://doi.org/10.1016/j.psyneuen.2006.03.003

Montero-Marín, J., & García-Campayo, J. (2010). A newer and broader definition of burnout: Validation of the "Burnout Clinical Subtype Questionnaire (BCSQ-36)." *BMC Public Health, 10*(1), 302–310. https://doi.org/10.1186/1471-2458-10-302

Moulding, N. T., Silagy, C. A., & Weller, D. P. (1999). A framework for effective management of change in clinical practice: Dissemination and implementation of clinical practice guidelines. *Quality in Health Care, 8*(3), 177–183. https://doi.org/10.1136/qshc.8.3.177

Murta, S. G., Sanderson, K., & Oldenburg, B. (2007). Process evaluation in occupational stress management programs: A systematic review. *American Journal of Health Promotion, 21*(4), 248–254. https://doi.org/10.4278/0890-1171-21.4.248

Nielsen, K., & Abildgaard, J. S. (2013). Organizational interventions: A research-based framework for the evaluation of both process and effects. *Work and Stress, 27*(3), 278–297. https://doi.org/10.1080/02678373.2013.812358

Nielsen, K., Randall, R., Yarker, J., & Brenner, S. O. (2008). The effects of transformational leadership on followers' perceived work characteristics and psychological well-being: A longitudinal study. *Work and Stress, 22*(1), 16–32. https://doi.org/10.1080/02678370801979430

Osatuke, K., Mohr, D., Ward, C., Moore, S. C., Dyrenforth, S., & Belton, L. (2009). Civility, respect, engagement in the workforce (CREW): Nationwide organization development intervention at Veterans Health Administration. *The Journal of Applied Behavioral Science, 45*(3), 384–410. https://doi.org/10.1177/0021886309335067

Pines, A., Aronson, E., & Kafry, D. (1981). *Burnout: From tedium to personal growth.* Free Press.

Rushton, C. H., Batcheller, J., Schroeder, K., & Donohue, P. (2015). Burnout and resilience among nurses practicing in high-intensity settings. *American Journal of Critical Care, 24*(5), 412–420. https://doi.org/10.4037/ajcc2015291

Ryan, R. M., & Deci, E. D. (2017). *Self-determination theory: Basic needs in motivation, development, and wellness.* Guilford Press. https://doi.org/10.1521/978.14625/28806

Sallon, S., Katz-Eisner, D., Yaffe, H., & Bdolah-Abram, T. (2017). Caring for the caregivers: Results of an extended, five-component stress-reduction intervention for hospital staff. *Behavioral Medicine, 43*(1), 47–60. https://doi.org/10.1080/08964289.2015.1053426

Salmela-aro, K., Näätänen, P., & Nurmi, J. E. (2004). The role of work-related personal projects during two burnout interventions: A longitudinal study. *Work and Stress, 18*(3), 208–230. https://doi.org/10.1080/02678370412331317480

Schaufeli, W. B., Desart, S., & De Witte, H. (2020). Burnout Assessment Tool (BAT)—Development, validity, and reliability. *International Journal of Environmental Research and Public Health, 17*(24), 9495. https://doi.org/10.3390/ijerph17249495

Schaufeli, W. B., Leiter, M. P., Maslach, C., & Jackson, S. E. (1996). Maslach Burnout Inventory—General Survey (MBI-GS). In C. Maslach, S. E. Jackson, M. P. Leiter, W. B. Schaufeli, & R. L. Schwab (Eds.), *Maslach Burnout Inventory manual* (4th ed., pp. 19–26). Mind Garden Publishing.

Shirom, A., & Melamed, S. (2006). A comparison of the construct validity of two burnout measures in two groups of professionals. *International Journal of Stress Management, 13*(2), 176–200. https://doi.org/10.1037/1072-5245.13.2.176

Shirom, A., Nirel, N., & Vinokur, A. D. (2010). Work hours and caseload as predictors of physician burnout: The mediating effects by perceived workload and by autonomy. *Applied Psychology*, *59*(4), 539–565. https://doi.org/10.1111/j.1464-0597.2009.00411.x

Shoji K., Cieslak R., Smoktunowicz E., Rogala A., Benight C.C., Luszczynska A. (2016). Associations between job burnout and self-efficacy: A meta-analysis. *Anxiety, Stress, & Coping. 29*(4), 367–386.

Tafvelin, S., von Thiele Schwarz, U., Nielsen, K., & Hasson, H. (2019). Employees' and line managers' active involvement in participatory organizational interventions: Examining direct, reversed, and reciprocal effects on well-being. *Stress and Health*, *35*(1), 69–80. https://doi.org/10.1002/smi.2841

Taris, T. W., Le Blanc, P. M., Schaufeli, W. B., & Schreurs, P. J. G. (2005). Are there causal relationships between the dimensions of the Maslach Burnout Inventory? A review and two longitudinal tests. *Work and Stress*, *19*(3), 238–255. https://doi.org/10.1080/02678370500270453

Timms, C., Brough, P., & Graham, D. (2012). Burnt-out but engaged: The co-existence of psychological burnout and engagement. *Journal of Educational Administration*, *50*(3), 327–345. https://doi.org/10.1108/09578231211223338

van den Heuvel, M., Demerouti, E., & Peeters, M. C. W. (2015). The job crafting intervention: Effects on job resources, self-efficacy, and affective well-being. *Journal of Occupational and Organizational Psychology*, *88*(3), 511–532. https://doi.org/10.1111/joop.12128

Van Droogenbroeck, F., Spruyt, B., & Vanroelen, C. (2014). Burnout among senior teachers: Investigating the role of workload and interpersonal relationships at work. *Teaching and Teacher Education*, *43*, 99–109. https://doi.org/10.1016/j.tate.2014.07.005

West, C. P., Dyrbye, L. N., Sinsky, C., Trockel, M., Tutty, M., Nedelec, L., Carlasare, L. E., & Shanafelt, T. D. (2020). Resilience and burnout among physicians and the general US working population. *JAMA Network Open*, *3*(7), e209385. https://doi.org/10.1001/jamanetworkopen.2020.9385

World Health Organization. (2019). Burn-out an "occupational phenomenon." *International Classification of Diseases*. https://www.who.int/mental_health/evidence/burn-out/en/

16

Occupational Psychosocial Factors and Cardiovascular Disease

Paul Landsbergis, Javier García-Rivas, Arturo Juárez-García, BongKyoo Choi, Marnie Dobson Zimmerman, Viviola Gomez Ortiz, Niklas Krause, Jian Li, and Peter Schnall

Cardiovascular disease (CVD) is the leading cause of death globally, representing 32% of all deaths (World Health Organization [WHO], 2021a), and a major contributor to disability (Roth et al., 2020). Hypertension (high blood pressure), the leading cause of CVD globally (Roth et al., 2020), affects an estimated 1.28 billion adults aged 30 to 79 years worldwide, two thirds living in low- and middle-income countries (WHO, 2021b). Other CVD risk factors, including obesity, diabetes, and metabolic syndrome, have also become global epidemics (Virani et al., 2021). However, inadequate attention has been paid to occupational risk factors for CVD, particularly psychosocial factors and workplace-based interventions and policy, which we discuss in this chapter. This chapter updates our previous, more comprehensive reviews (Landsbergis et al., 2017; Schnall et al., 2016, 2017).

Decades of research have enabled us to formulate a social–ecological model of occupational psychosocial factors and CVD, including social determinants of health; political, economic, social, labor market, and workplace-level risk factors; and biopsychosocial mechanisms (see Figure 16.1). We first discuss recent trends in CVD and work-related risk factors, then we review the risk factors at various levels of our model, intervention research, and recommendations for research and policy.

https://doi.org/10.1037/0000331-016
Handbook of Occupational Health Psychology, Third Edition, L. E. Tetrick, G. G. Fisher, M. T. Ford, and J. C. Quick (Editors)

FIGURE 16.1. Social–Ecological Model of Occupational Psychosocial Factors and Cardiovascular Disease (CVD)

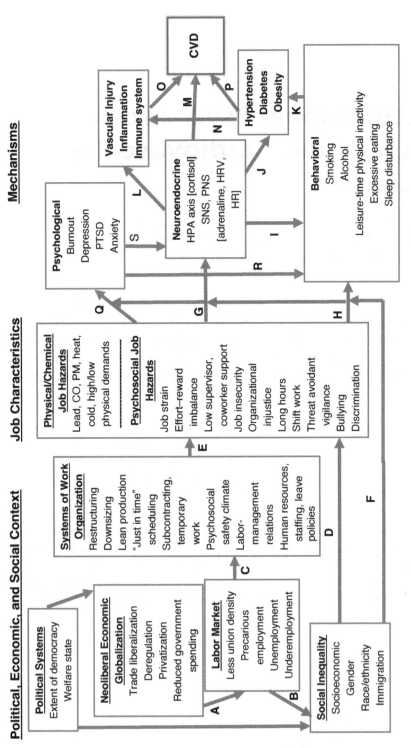

Note. We omitted potential double-direction arrows in this model for the sake of parsimony. CO = carbon monoxide; PM = particulate matter; PTSD = posttraumatic stress disorder; HPA axis = hypothalamic–pituitary–adrenal axis; SNS = sympathetic nervous system; PNS = parasympathetic nervous system; HRV = heart rate variability; HR = heart rate; CVD = cardiovascular disease. Adapted from "Globalization, Work, and Cardiovascular Disease," by P. L. Schnall, M. Dobson, and P. Landsbergis, 2016, *International Journal of Health Services, 46*(4), pp. 659 & 661 (https://doi.org/10.1177/0020731416664687). Copyright 2016 by SAGE Publications. Adapted with permission.

RECENT TRENDS IN CARDIOVASCULAR DISEASE AND ITS "STANDARD" RISK FACTORS

The rate of decline in CVD mortality has slowed considerably in most developed countries in recent years, particularly in working-age groups, and CVD death rates rose in seven countries for at least one sex in 2017 (Lopez & Adair, 2019). Between 2000 and 2015, the CVD mortality gap between the United States and its peer countries widened (National Academies of Sciences, 2021). In the United States, life expectancy had increased for the past century but declined between 2015 and 2017 due mainly to an increase in death rates in working-age adults (25–64 years) from stress-related causes, including drug poisoning; alcohol-induced causes; suicide; and diabetes, obesity, and CVD (Harris et al., 2021, p. e1). A National Academy of Sciences report points out that "social, economic, and cultural changes that have undermined economic security, intergenerational mobility, and social support networks can adversely affect cardiometabolic health through stress-mediated biological pathways and reduced access to care" (Harris et al., 2021, p. e2).

Related explanations for CVD trends are increases in the prevalence of other stress-related conditions such as obesity, diabetes, and metabolic syndrome (Virani et al., 2021), short sleeping hours (Sheehan et al., 2019), and limited future gains from further reducing already low smoking rates (Lopez & Adair, 2019). The age-adjusted prevalence of hypertension increased in the United States between 1988 and 2010 and increased again between 2010 and 2018 for most gender and race groups (Virani et al., 2021). Mental health disorders, including depression and anxiety, are becoming more common globally, and depression is the leading cause of disability worldwide (WHO, 2017).

CVD mortality inequalities by socioeconomic status (SES) persist internationally (Lopez & Adair, 2019), with increasing inequalities seen in some countries or time periods (Tüchsen & Endahl, 1999). In the United States, small increases in SES inequalities in hypertension prevalence occurred between 2010 and 2014 (Centers for Disease Control and Prevention, 2021). The most recent U.S. study of CVD SES inequalities (by county-level SES) showed increasing relative SES inequalities within the context of declines in all SES groups (Singh et al., 2015).

RECENT TRENDS IN PSYCHOSOCIAL WORKING CONDITIONS IN THE UNITED STATES

Labor market and socioeconomic factors, which help shape work organization and psychosocial job hazards (see arrows A–E in Figure 16.1), have been worsening in the United States. For example, income inequality has increased since about 1980, mirroring declines in union membership (Shierholz, 2019), and social mobility has declined (Chetty et al., 2017). A system of work organization, lean production (a newer version of Taylorism), developed originally for manufacturing, is associated with higher work stressors and psychological distress (arrow E; Landsbergis et al., 1999; Toivanen & Landsbergis, 2013). Several studies of "lean health care" in Northern Europe had mixed findings on job characteristics and worker health (Benders et al., 2017; Lindskog et al., 2016). Lean methods in the public sector have been labeled "new public management" (NPM) in countries where the welfare state is largely public, and "managerialism" in countries like the United States, which "calls on the private market to serve public purposes and favors running human service agencies like a business" (Lewiskin et al., 2021, p. 260).

Work hours increased 14% between 1982 and 2016 from 1,652 to 1,883 hours per year (Economic Policy Institute, 2019). Job stressors, such as low job control, job strain, and work–family conflict, increased in the United States between 2002 and 2014 (Myers et al., 2019) in addition to previous work–family conflict increases between 1977 and 1997 (Nomaguchi, 2009). There has been little change in some definitions of contingent work. However, the proportion of "standard part-time workers" increased from 11.9% to 16.2% from 2006 to 2010, resulting in an increase of all workers in "alternative work arrangements" from 35.3% to 40.4% (Government Accountability Office, 2015). A broader measure of precarious employment, including inadequate material rewards, stability, working-time arrangements, workers' rights, collective organization, interpersonal relations, and training, increased by 9% in the United States between 1988 and 2016 (Oddo et al., 2021). Also, journalistic exposés have focused on work intensification in some major employers' workplaces, including Amazon (Long & Evans, 2021), Federal Express (Thomas, 2020), and oil refineries (Monforton, 2015). Work intensification has typically been studied in relation to higher injury rates (Strategic Organizing Center, 2021), but it should also be studied for its effect on CVD risk.

HISTORICAL CONTEXT

These trends are the most recent manifestations of a long process of economic, political, and social development. Cross-cultural anthropological studies have consistently found that nonindustrial societies, such as hunter-gatherers, have a very low prevalence of hypertension and that blood pressure (BP) does not inevitably rise with age as in industrial societies (Waldron et al., 1982). CVD and its risk factors increased in prevalence with the "epidemiological transition" from agricultural to industrial production, resulting in urbanization and ensuing changes in the nature of work (e.g., longer work hours, the assembly line, the digital revolution), living conditions, diet, and physical activity. The transition first occurred in developed countries and continues now in developing countries with increases in smoking, sugar consumption, serum cholesterol, obesity, diabetes, and hypertension (Schnall et al., 2016).

Since the 1970s, the philosophy of neoliberalism has promoted not only "free trade" (e.g., reduced tariffs) but also conservative fiscal and economic policies, including reduction of government spending on education, welfare programs and health care, privatization of the public sector, and deregulation of occupational and environmental health and financial sectors (Schnall et al., 2016). Privatization, downsizing, restructuring, and a lower prevalence of unionized workers are factors that can increase precariousness and work stressors, such as job insecurity, time pressure, workload, low job control, and low workplace support (see Figure 16.1, arrows A, C, E), especially in the presence of an inadequate social safety-net and especially among the most vulnerable workers (arrow D; Muntaner et al., 2010).

PSYCHOSOCIAL WORK STRESSORS, CVD, AND CVD RISK FACTORS

The concept of *job strain*, a widely studied work stressor, defined as high psychological job demands combined with low job decision latitude or job control, was developed in the 1970s. Low social support was later added to the model (Karasek & Theorell, 1990). A newer work stressor model, *effort–reward imbalance* (ERI), was proposed in the 1990s and is defined as a "mismatch between high workload (high demand) and low control over long-term rewards" (Siegrist et al., 1990, p. 1128). Rewards include *esteem reward* (respect and support), job security, and promotion prospects.

Cardiovascular Disease

Studies have examined the relationship between CVD and psychosocial work stressors:

- *Job strain.* Most reviews and meta-analyses of research on job strain and CVD have found strong evidence of a positive relationship (Kivimäki et al., 2014, 2019; Theorell et al., 2016).

- *ERI.* A review of 14 prospective studies indicated that ERI at work was associated with 42% higher incident CVD (Siegrist & Li, 2020).

- *Bullying and violence.* Five prospective studies suggested that workplace bullying and violence increased risk of CVD by 25% to 59% (Romero Starke et al., 2020; Xu et al., 2019).

- *Long work hours.* A series of major reviews coordinated by the WHO and the International Labour Organization (ILO) concluded that working more than 55 hours per week had "sufficient evidence of harmfulness" for ischemic heart disease (IHD) and stroke with an estimated 745,194 deaths and 23.3 million disability-adjusted life years from CVD attributable to long work hours in 2016 (Descatha et al., 2020; J. Li et al., 2020; Pega et al., 2021).

- *Shift work.* A meta-analysis found the risk of any CVD event to be 17% higher and the risk of IHD 26% higher among shift workers compared with day workers (Torquati et al., 2018).

- *Recurrent CVD.* Prospective studies have also found associations between returning to work in a position with job strain or ERI (J. Li et al., 2015) or long work hours (J. Li et al., 2015; Trudel, Brisson, et al., 2021) after having had a heart attack and a higher recurrence of IHD or myocardial infarction.

- *Attributable %.* The 6th International Conference on Work Environment and Cardiovascular Diseases ("The Tokyo Declaration") concluded that "about 10 to 20% of all causes of CVD deaths among the working age populations can be attributed to work" (Tsutsumi, 2015, p. 4).

- *Combined exposures.* A multicohort (Dragano et al., 2017) suggested that the effect of ERI and job strain on incident coronary heart disease (CHD) is additive rather than synergistic.

Blood Pressure and Hypertension

Ambulatory blood pressure (ABP) and heart rate measured with portable monitors are elevated during work (vs. nonwork) hours (del Arco-Galán et al., 1994; Pickering et al., 1982; Pieper et al., 1993). Work activities that are demanding and over which workers have little control or autonomy can provoke sharp rises in BP under experimental conditions (James et al., 1986; Steptoe et al., 1999; Tobe et al., 2007). ABP is a much better predictor than casual clinic BP of target organ damage (Sega et al., 2001; Verdecchia et al., 1999), incident CVD (Brguljan-Hitij et al., 2014, Hansen et al., 2007; Ohkubo et al., 2005; Pierdomenico et al., 2005), and mortality (Dolan et al., 2005). As a result, masked hypertension (MH), defined as elevated ABP but normal casual clinic BP, is a risk factor for fatal and nonfatal cardiovascular events (Brguljan-Hitij et al., 2014; Zhang et al., 2019). MH occurs in 10% to 15% of people with normal clinic BP, and masked uncontrolled hypertension in treated hypertensive patients has a prevalence ranging from 30% to 50% (Zhang et al., 2019).

Job Strain

A quantitative meta-analysis of cross-sectional studies found that job strain is a risk factor for work, home, and sleep ABP, with an effect size of 3.4 mm Hg systolic work ABP (see Figure 16.1, arrows G–K; Landsbergis, Dobson, et al., 2013). In a prospective study of white-collar and blue-collar men in New York City, leaving a situation of job strain led to a drop in systolic ABP of 5.3 mm Hg at work and 4.7 mm Hg at home over three years (Schnall et al., 1998). However, in a prospective study of Quebec white-collar workers, in men no association was found between chronic high-strain exposure and ABP; however, high-strain, active, and passive jobs were associated with ABP using contemporaneous exposure (Trudel et al., 2016). Among women in the same study, no association was found between BP and job strain (Trudel et al., 2013). A different study found that, among 480 U.S. workers, associations between job strain and systolic and diastolic ABP were stronger among blue-collar workers compared with white-collar workers (Joseph et al., 2016), similar to the findings of the NYC ABP study (see Figure 16.1, interaction shown by arrows F–H)

(Landsbergis et al., 2003). In a study of 419 female Las Vegas hotel cleaners, higher job strain was associated with increased 18-hour systolic ABP, after work hours systolic ABP, and ambulatory pulse pressure (Feaster & Krause, 2018).

Effort–Reward Imbalance

Of one prospective and 11 cross-sectional studies, seven found significant associations of ERI with BP or hypertension (see Figure 16.1, arrows G–K; Gilbert-Ouimet et al., 2014). A more recent study of hotel room cleaners found a small effect of ERI on ABP (Feaster et al., 2019). In white-collar men in Quebec, associations were not seen between repeated ERI exposure and ABP. Women younger than 45 years old reporting ERI at baseline and 3 years later had significantly higher ABP at follow-up (122.2/78.9 mm Hg) than those unexposed (120.4/77.4 mm Hg). Three-year hypertension incidence was 2.78 (95% CI [1.26, 6.10]) times higher among women older than 45 exposed to ERI at both times (Gilbert-Ouimet et al., 2012).

Long Work Hours

White-collar women in Quebec working long (vs. regular) hours had higher diastolic ABP at 2.5-year follow-up (+1.8 mm Hg (95% CI [0.5, 3.1]). In men, increases were seen for systolic ABP (2.5 mm Hg [95% CI [0.5, 4.4]) and diastolic ABP (2.3 mm Hg [95% CI [1.0, 3.7]]; see Figure 16.1, arrows G–K). Associations were greater in workers with high family responsibilities (Gilbert-Ouimet et al., 2022).

Threat-Avoidant Vigilance

Threat-avoidant vigilance (TAV) is defined as a high level of alertness in order to avoid serious accidents and loss of human life, leading to increased levels of biological arousal (Belkic et al., 2000). Occupations with TAV, including urban bus drivers (Bushnell et al., 2011) and firefighters (Khaja et al., 2021), have some of the highest prevalence rates of hypertension (see Figure 16.1, arrows G–K).

Other Work Stressors

Associations with BP have also been made with negative supervisory interactions (Wong & Kelloway, 2016), domestic overload and job strain among nurses (Portela et al., 2013), "unpleasant" work schedules among call center workers (Maina et al., 2011), and additional 24-hour shifts among professional firefighters (Choi, Schnall, & Dobson, 2016; see Figure 16.1, arrows G–K).

Masked Hypertension

Shift work and the combination of job strain and ERI were associated with MH in a small cross-sectional study in NYC (Landsbergis, Travis, & Schnall, 2013). However, among Quebec white-collar workers, MH was not associated with job strain in women and only with high-demand/high-latitude ("active") jobs in men (Trudel et al., 2010). On the other hand, in Quebec, MH was associated with ERI (Boucher et al., 2017) and long working hours (Trudel et al., 2020).

Work Stressors and CVD Behavioral Risk Factors

Psychosocial work stressors can lead to CVD through direct activation of neuro-endocrine stress pathways (see Figure 16.1, arrows G, J, L–P), but also indirectly through health behaviors such as smoking, heavy alcohol use, unhealthy diet, physical inactivity, and sleeping problems (arrows H, K, N–P; Chandola et al., 2008; Niedhammer et al., 2022; O'Connor et al., 2021; Riopel et al., 2021). Therefore, adjusting for health behaviors in analysis may underestimate the total effect of work stressors on CVD (Choi et al., 2015; Riopel et al., 2021).

Smoking prevalence and intensity have been associated in cross-sectional studies with job strain and its components (Mattsson et al., 2021; Nyberg et al., 2013; Rugulies et al., 2008) as well as with ERI (Siegrist & Rödel, 2006). Prospective studies have shown that quitting smoking is more likely among workers facing less job strain (Heikkilä et al., 2012; Kouvonen et al., 2009), higher social support (Yasin et al., 2012) and job control, low physical demands, and day shift work (Sanderson et al., 2005).

Heavy alcohol use has also been associated with job strain (Allard et al., 2011; Azagba & Sharaf, 2011) and, partially, with job demands, low job control, and ERI (Siegrist & Rödel, 2006), although weak results for long work hours were seen in a recent meta-analysis (Pachito et al., 2021).

Unhealthy diet, including foods high in sugar and fat, has been associated with job demands, low job control, low social support (Buxton et al., 2009; Liu et al., 2017; Miyaki et al., 2012), and shift work (Souza et al., 2019). Further research is needed on other work stressors (Tanaka et al., 2019).

Leisure-time physical inactivity is associated with ERI (Kouvonen et al., 2006), job strain (Choi et al., 2010a; Nyberg et al., 2013; van Oostrom et al., 2021), and low job control (Allard et al., 2011).

Sleeping problems have been associated with job strain, heavy workload, low social support, ERI, work–family conflict, organizational injustice, and workplace bullying in a systematic review (Linton et al., 2015) and a meta-analysis (Yang et al., 2018). Some recent prospective studies also found reciprocal relationships—job stressors increase sleep problems, and sleep problems increase future job stressors (Cho & Chen, 2020; Johannessen & Sterud, 2017; Törnroos et al., 2017), although another study found only main effects of stressors (Nielsen et al., 2021).

Work Stressors and CVD Metabolic Risk Factors

Body mass index (BMI) and obesity have been associated with sedentary work (Choi et al., 2010b), long hours (Virtanen et al., 2020), shift work (Choi, Dobson, et al., 2016; Myers et al., 2021), and job strain, in some cases (Choi et al., 2014), but not ERI (Nordentoft et al., 2020). Job stressors may influence weight gain directly through circadian rhythm disturbances (e.g., sleep disturbances due to shift work or long work hours; see Figure 16.1, arrows H and K) and activation of the hypothalamic–pituitary–adrenocortical (HPA) axis and metabolic changes (neuroendocrine pathway; arrows G, I–K; Choi et al., 2011; Solovieva et al., 2013).

Diabetes and metabolic syndrome are associated with job strain (W. Li et al., 2021; Nyberg et al., 2014), ERI (Loerbroks et al., 2015; Mutambudzi et al., 2018), and long work hours (Kivimäki et al., 2015). Associations are plausible since cortisol (e.g., produced by job stressors) "stimulates glucose production in the liver and antagonizes the action of insulin in peripheral tissues" (Brunner & Kivimäki, 2013, p. 449; arrows G–K).

Work Stressors and CVD Psychological Risk Factors

Depression or depressive symptoms are linked by substantial evidence, including longitudinal studies, to job strain and its components (see Figure 16.1, arrows Q, R, S, I-P; Madsen et al., 2017), ERI (Rugulies et al., 2017), work–family conflict, and job insecurity (Duchaine et al., 2020; Nigatu & Wang, 2018; Theorell et al., 2015). There is "inadequate evidence," however, for a relationship between long work hours and depression (Rugulies et al., 2021). Work stressors account for 15% to 35% of depressive disorders (LaMontagne et al., 2008; Niedhammer et al., 2022). Depression, a CVD risk factor, may directly affect the development of CVD through activation of the HPA axis, low heart-rate variability, alteration of platelet receptors or reactivity, instability of the ventricles or myocardial ischemia (Musselman et al., 1998). Depression caused by work stressors may also increase unhealthy behaviors (Shirom et al., 2009).

Burnout, recognized by the WHO as an occupational phenomenon in the *ICD-11*, has been associated with high job demands, low job control, low support, low rewards, and job insecurity in a systematic review and meta-analysis (Aronsson et al., 2017). Recent evidence also suggested burnout is a significant predictor of CVD and metabolic disorders (Salvagioni et al., 2017).

Work Psychosocial Stressors and Physical Work Demands

Researchers have investigated acute injury risks and chronic musculoskeletal and CVD health effects of biomechanical forces, working postures, low and high physical activity at work (Holtermann et al., 2019), work–rest cycles, repetitiveness, and psychological factors (Kroemer & Grandjean, 1997). Prolonged standing (Krause et al., 2000; Waters & Dick, 2015) and sedentary work (Choi et al., 2010b; Eriksen et al., 2015) increase CVD risk. Evidence on detrimental health effects of occupational physical activity (OPA), in contrast to health-promoting leisure-time physical activity (the "physical activity health paradox"), has shown that health effects of physical activity depend, in part, on social context (work vs. leisure) and individual workers' physical capacities (Holtermann et al., 2018). High OPA levels are associated with an

18% to 25% *increased* CVD mortality risk (Coenen et al., 2018; J. Li et al., 2013). A cohort study of Italian men found increased CHD risk for high job strain and for low (vs. medium) OPA. However, low-OPA/high job-strain workers benefit from sport physical activity (SpPA), reducing their risk up to 90%. In contrast, the protective effect of SpPA on CHD in other OPA job-strain categories (e.g., high OPA) was modest or even absent (Ferrario et al., 2019).

Physical activity research would benefit if work exposures—such as work organization constraints, workstation design, physical activity opportunities and demands, recovery time, and lack of worker control—were better incorporated. They are causal determinants of either "sedentary lifestyle" (see Figure 16.1, arrows G–P) or high physical workload exceeding workers' cardiorespiratory capacities. Further, most of the detrimental health effects of high OPA are seen among workers with preexisting atherosclerosis or IHD (Krause et al., 2000, 2007, 2015; Wang et al., 2016). Thus, routine exclusion of workers with preexisting CVD from prospective epidemiologic studies is bound to mask those health effects in the most vulnerable aging worker populations, leading to a bias toward the null.

Both psychosocial and physical work factors are produced by the organization of work, and moderate to high correlations exist between some physical and psychosocial stressors, with the strongest covariation among blue-collar production and low-status office workers (MacDonald et al., 2001). Further research and primary prevention approaches are needed that consider both psychosocial and physical cardiovascular strains and take cardiorespiratory fitness and preexisting CVD into account.

Systems of Work Organization

As described in Figure 16.1, systems of work organization can increase work stressors, and thus risk of illness. For example, NYC social workers working under NPM (a form of public sector "lean production") had a greater risk of depression (odds ratio [OR] = 1.45), anxiety (OR = 1.59), hypertension (OR = 1.15), and sleeping problems (OR = 1.55; Zelnick et al., 2022). A 7.5-year follow-up of Finnish public employees found a relative risk (RR) of 2.0 for CVD mortality (95% CI [1.0, 3.9]) among survivors of major (vs. no) downsizing (Vahtera et al., 2005). Downsizing survivors often face a higher workload (Quinlan & Bohle, 2009), reduced job control, increased job strain, ERI, and job insecurity (Ferrie et al., 2008). It is therefore essential that systems of work organization, often implemented for business purposes, be evaluated for their impact on working conditions and on cardiovascular health. We also need to assess psychosocial safety climate (PSC), defined as the organizational policies, practices, and procedures for the protection of worker psychological health and safety, which has been associated with less job strain and less depression (Bailey et al., 2015) and with lowered risk of CVD (Becher et al., 2018).

Labor Market and Employment Relations

A meta-analysis of 17 cohort studies found a modestly increased risk of IHD due to job insecurity (RR = 1.32, 95% CI [1.09, 1.50]; Virtanen et al., 2013). Migration to find better work and living conditions, a form of precariousness, has also been linked to stress, and risk of hypertension, obesity, and diabetes (Rosenthal, 2014).

Employees of a UK government agency, privatized between 1990 and 1993, had greater increases in cardiac ischemia (based on abnormal electrocardiograms [ECGs] or angina), BMI, and BP (women only), compared with UK government employees whose agencies were not privatized (Ferrie et al., 1998b) despite the fact that the proportion of men working at sites undergoing privatization engaging in vigorous exercise was greater than for other government employees. Another analysis of UK civil servants found a higher prevalence of ischemia in women *anticipating* privatization. Men showed higher BP (but only in the privatized group) and greater BMI, but no change in exercise, which declined in women anticipating privatization (Ferrie et al., 1998a). Thus, the potential costs of privatization—increases in stressful working conditions and increases in CVD risk—need to be assessed *before* privatization decisions are made.

BIOPSYCHOSOCIAL MECHANISMS: HOW WORK STRESS "WORKS"

We have described a number of biopsychosocial mechanisms in the text and in Figure 16.1, although a comprehensive discussion of such mechanisms is beyond the scope of this chapter. In general, many work-related psychosocial stressors reflect either subjective perceptions of powerlessness or objective conditions of lack of control, both individual and collective, stemming from historical and current social and workplace transformations. For example, the job strain model's control dimension is operationalized as decision latitude over work processes; for ERI it is measured as control over job security and opportunities for advancement, while for bullying it is conceptualized as the inability to prevent bullying, all of which are hypothesized as significant causes of the stress response.

Two major physiological mechanisms mediate the relationships between stressors and illness (see Figure 16.1, arrows G, I–P): (1) adrenal medullary responses, involving adrenaline and noradrenaline, and sympathetic arousal of the cardiovascular system, reflecting an active response to demands, known as the "fight-or-flight" response; and (2) the HPA axis, involving cortisol, often activated in situations in which people face threats over which they have little control. The HPA axis mediates a behavioral response of defeat, withdrawal, and conservation of resources. Thus, these two pathways reflect the demands and low-control aspects of "job strain" (Landsbergis et al., 2017). The combination of adrenaline and cortisol (such as from high demands plus low control) is particularly damaging to the blood vessels and heart (Turner et al., 2020). A related way of conceptualizing the physiologic response due to repeated or chronic stress is "allostatic load," or "wear and tear on the body" (McEwen & Stellar, 1993), though there is limited consensus on methods to measure allostatic load (Mauss et al., 2015). Work stressors increase heart rate and decrease heart-rate variability (de Looff et al., 2018), two risk factors for CVD (Hillebrand et al., 2013; Perret-Guillaume et al., 2009; see Figure 16.1, arrows G, I–P). Work stressors, specifically low job control, can also inhibit anabolism (regeneration or growth of tissues; Theorell, 2008). Further research is needed on work stressors and anabolism, inflammation (Duchaine et al., 2021), immune system dysregulation (Fioranelli et al., 2018), and vascular injury (Thubrikar, 2007), and to what extent, and over what time period, the biological consequences of work stressors can be reversed.

INTERVENTION STUDIES

Common programs to reduce CVD risk have been worksite-based health promotion, wellness, or stress management. However, rigorous research has indicated minimal or null effects of such programs (Jones et al., 2019; Rongen et al., 2013). Organizational and group-level workplace interventions have been effective in reducing work stressors (Brisson et al., 2020; Fox et al., 2022; Karasek, 2004; Lamontagne et al., 2007; Montano et al., 2014). However, important organizational interventions, such as collective bargaining contracts, worker cooperatives, or legislative and regulatory-level interventions, are rarely evaluated and thus are not included in review articles. Examples include laws providing for better nurse–patient staffing ratios, bans on mandatory overtime, paid sick days, paid family leave, or retail worker schedule predictability (Healthy Work Campaign, 2021).

Unfortunately, no organizational intervention studies have been conducted on primary prevention of CVD, and few have been conducted on preventing CVD risk factors such as hypertension. We present three examples of organizational interventions to reduce BP. First, a small Swedish study found that systolic BP increased among workers on a traditional auto-assembly line but did *not* increase during a work shift among auto-assembly workers in a flexible team-based work organization (Melin et al., 1999).

Second, another small Swedish study examined the impact of a set of interventions in Stockholm, including separate bus lanes, a bus priority traffic signal system, passenger peninsulas, reducing illegally parked cars, and electronic information systems for passengers. The intervention was effective in reducing perceived workload, job hassles, systolic BP, heart rate, and distress after work among bus drivers. However, no significant change was seen for diastolic BP, fatigue, or psychosomatic symptoms (Evans et al., 1999; Rydstedt et al., 1998).

Third, an intervention among white-collar workers at an insurance services agency in Quebec involved surveys, focus groups, and meetings at work in order to "diagnose" problems and suggest changes in policies and procedures.

Managers made decisions about changes, specific to each department over 17 to 24 months. There were joint union-management committees in four of nine intervention departments. Changes implemented included regular employee/manager meetings on routine matters, group meetings with managers, organizational restructuring to reduce workload, slowing implementation of changes in work processes and computer software to allow adaptation, more flexible work hours, and career and skills development (Gilbert-Ouimet et al., 2015). Follow-up at 30 months showed lower psychological distress and lower job demands, and higher coworker support and respect/esteem, although there was no change in low job control, supervisor support or reward, in the intervention (vs. control) group (Gilbert-Ouimet et al., 2011). BP and hypertension significantly decreased in the intervention group, with no change in the control group. The differential decrease in systolic BP between the intervention and control group was 2.0 mm Hg 95% CI [3.0, 1.0], 1.0 mm Hg for diastolic BP [1.7, 0.3], and hypertension prevalence decreased by 15%, with a prevalence ratio of 0.85, 95% CI [0.74–0.98] (Trudel, Gilbert-Ouimet, et al., 2021).

RESEARCH DIRECTIONS AND RECOMMENDATIONS

Psychosocial working conditions influence CVD risk, and the "upstream" political and economic context and employment conditions help shape psychosocial working conditions (see Figure 16.1, arrows A–E). Thus, all these factors, especially work organization, should be key targets in the primary prevention of CVD and CVD risk. Further research is needed on the following topics:

- The specific causes of job strain, effort–reward imbalance, and other psychosocial work stressors, in order to ascertain potential "upstream" or distal intervention points. These may include informal (vs. formal) employment, privatization of public services, deregulation, inadequate public sector budgets, union density, precarious employment, social inequalities, lean production, downsizing, subcontracting, and PSC (see Figure 16.1, arrows A–E), as well as the relationships between these labor market and work organization factors and economic globalization and international trade deals

- The potential joint effects or interaction between physical and psychosocial job demands and CVD risk, including relationships between psychosocial work stressors, OPA, and leisure-time physical activity

- The cardiovascular effects of understudied work stressors, such as TAV, organizational or workplace injustice (discrimination, harassment, or bullying), workplace violence, electronic performance monitoring, emotional demands/labor, contingent or "gig" work, nonstandard work arrangements, and digital platforms

- The specific, modifiable working conditions among vulnerable worker populations at high risk of CVD, such as cleaners or professional drivers, low-wage workers, immigrant workers, older workers, workers with preexisting CVD, and workers exposed to psychosocial stressors combined with high levels of physical job demands, such as prolonged standing, heavy lifting, or environmental heat (e.g., retail, warehouse, farm, and construction workers)

- The effectiveness of organizational-level workplace interventions in reducing CVD risk, including evaluation of rarely studied interventions, such as collective bargaining, worker cooperatives, and legislation and regulation. In workplace-based studies, participatory action research (PAR) is a valuable process for intervention effectiveness and evaluation (Punnett et al., 2013; Rosskam, 2009)

- The differences in work stressors and health between countries, both developed countries (Niedhammer et al., 2022) and developing countries (Kortum et al., 2010)

- The economic costs of work-related CVD. Recent estimates of the costs of 10 workplace stressors include more than 120,000 U.S. deaths each year and 5% to 8% of health care costs (Goh et al., 2015)

- The impact of climate change and rising environmental temperatures on increasing key hemodynamic CVD risk factors, such as working and resting heart rates and BP (Levi et al., 2018)

The following approaches are recommended to facilitate such research:

- Adding work organization questions to ongoing prospective CVD studies funded by the National Institutes of Health (Landsbergis et al., 2015)

- Further development of expert- or observer-based measures of work stressors (Greiner et al., 2004) in addition to current self-report survey instruments

- Create job exposure matrixes based on data from national surveys to impute exposure to job stressors to individuals and groups within occupational categories when data on job characteristics for individual workers is not available but occupational title is available (Choi, 2020; Schwartz et al., 1988)

We also recommend surveillance of the prevalence of exposures and outcomes and trends over time. U.S. national surveillance systems have little data on work psychosocial or physical stressors. The U.S. National Institute for Occupational Safety and Health (NIOSH) conducted national Quality of Work Life (QWL) surveys in 2002, 2006, 2010, 2014, and 2018. However, much larger QWL sample sizes are needed in order to provide more precise estimates by work exposure, outcome, industry, occupation, gender, and race/ethnicity. Only one current U.S. psychosocial working conditions survey, the Healthy Work Survey, based in part on national NIOSH QWL survey questions, provides users with an automated report comparing individual or group scores to national survey distributions (Choi et al., 2019).

PRIMARY PREVENTION OF CVD: WORKPLACE AND EMPLOYMENT POLICY INTERVENTIONS AND PROGRAMS

Efforts to reduce CVD and its risk factors have focused mainly on diagnosis and medical treatment, and, to a lesser extent, public health promotion interventions, such as anti-smoking campaigns. In the United States, CVD costs were $363 billion in 2016–2017 or 13% of all U.S. health care costs (Virani et al., 2021). Given the increase in CVD mortality in the United States despite all these efforts and the evidence presented, it is clear that more attention needs to be paid to workplace and policy interventions to reduce occupational risk factors, particularly occupational psychosocial factors, and their upstream causes.

Integrating Workplace Health Promotion and Work Organization Change

Workplace health promotion focused solely on individuals has shown limited effectiveness (Jones et al., 2019; Rongen et al., 2013). One upstream approach has been legislation or regulation ultimately still aimed at individual behavior change, such as cigarette taxes, labeling of caloric, fat, salt, and sugar food content, or promoting physical activity through changing the built environment (Gaziano, 2005; Institute of Medicine, 2010). We recommend a more comprehensive framework for primary prevention of CVD that focuses on upstream socioeconomic factors, and the need to transform employment and working conditions that are either directly detrimental to health or promote unhealthy behaviors. NIOSH recommends a *Total Worker Health®* approach, which includes integrating health promotion and disease management with changes to the work environment and the creation of a "culture of health," with a focus on "worker well-being." Limitations of such an approach have been described (Lax, 2016). Further research is needed to assess the effectiveness of such integrated models.

Legislative Models of Work Organization Reform at Regional, National, and International Levels

Since the 1970s, in Northern and Western Europe there have been concerted efforts to prevent work psychosocial stressors through national laws (e.g., Swedish Work Environment Act, 1991) and international agreements (e.g., European Framework Directive on Safety and Health at Work, 89/391 EEC), which likely account for the lower prevalence of job strain and other job stressors in some European countries (Niedhammer et al., 2022). Dollard and Neser (2013) found that the most important factors explaining better worker self-reported health between European nations were union density and PSC. The majority of countries with the highest levels of union density and PSC had social democratic political systems, such as in the Scandinavian countries. However, workers in many nations face weaker bargaining positions relative to employers due to economic globalization. Declining union density in the United States has led to limited success in enacting national legislation or regulations to improve psychosocial working conditions or even address traditional occupational safety and health hazards. However, greater success in improving psychosocial working conditions has been achieved in the United States through state and municipal level legislative campaigns, such as mandating staffing levels or banning mandatory overtime for nurses (Aiken et al., 2010), paid sick days or paid family leave, retail worker schedule predictability, and workplace violence prevention in health care (Healthy Work Campaign, 2021), or increasing rewards for work through minimum- and living-wage ordinances in major cities.

CONCLUSION

Recent increases in CVD mortality rates, widening inequalities in working-age populations, the continuing global rank of CVD as the top cause of mortality, the high costs of medical treatment, and the substantial burden of CVD associated with environmental factors including the workplace, make the development of effective primary interventions an urgent and promising goal. Greater efforts are needed to educate health professionals and the public about how improving employment and working conditions are key to preventing the epidemic of CVD. A major effort to reduce psychosocial hazards due to employment and working conditions, through a variety of strategies, is essential.

REFERENCES

Aiken, L. H., Sloane, D. M., Cimiotti, J. P., Clarke, S. P., Flynn, L., Seago, J. A., Spetz, J., & Smith, H. L. (2010). Implications of the California nurse staffing mandate for other states. *Health Services Research, 45*(4), 904–921. https://doi.org/10.1111/j.1475-6773.2010.01114.x

Allard, K. O., Thomsen, J. F., Mikkelsen, S., Rugulies, R., Mors, O., Kærgaard, A., Kolstad, H. A., Kaerlev, L., Andersen, J. H., Hansen, Å. M., & Bonde, J. P. (2011). Effects of psychosocial work factors on lifestyle changes: A cohort study. *Journal of Occupational and Environmental Medicine, 53*(12), 1364–1371. https://doi.org/10.1097/JOM.0b013e3182363bda

Aronsson, G., Theorell, T., Grape, T., Hammarström, A., Hogstedt, C., Marteinsdottir, I., Skoog, I., Träskman-Bendz, L., & Hall, C. (2017). A systematic review including meta-analysis of work environment and burnout symptoms. *BMC Public Health, 17*(264). https://doi.org/10.1186/s12889-017-4153-7

Azagba, S., & Sharaf, M. F. (2011). The effect of job stress on smoking and alcohol consumption. *Health Economics Review, 1*(15). https://doi.org/10.1186/2191-1991-1-15

Bailey, T. S., Dollard, M. F., & Richards, P. A. (2015). A national standard for psychosocial safety climate (PSC): PSC 41 as the benchmark for low risk of job strain and depressive symptoms. *Journal of Occupational Health Psychology, 20*(1), 15–26. https://doi.org/10.1037/a0038166

Becher, H., Dollard, M. F., Smith, P., & Li, J. (2018). Predicting circulatory diseases from psychosocial safety climate: A prospective cohort study from Australia. *International*

Journal of Environmental Research and Public Health, 15(3), 415. https://doi.org/10.3390/ijerph15030415

Belkic, K., Landsbergis, P. A., Schnall, P., Baker, D., Theorell, T., Siegrist, J., Peter, R., & Karasek, R. (2000). Psychosocial factors: Review of the empirical data among men. In P. Schnall, K. Belkic, P. A. Landsbergis, & D. Baker (Eds.), *The workplace and cardiovascular disease: Occupational medicine: State of the art reviews* (Vol. 15, pp. 24–46). Hanley and Belfus.

Benders, J., Bleijerveld, H., Schouteten, R. (2017) Continuous improvement, burnout and job engagement: A study in a Dutch nursing department. *International Journal of Health Planning and Management, 32*(4), 481–491. https://doi.org/10.1002/hpm.2355

Boucher, P., Gilbert-Ouimet, M., Trudel, X., Duchaine, C. S., Milot, A., & Brisson, C. (2017). Masked hypertension and effort–reward imbalance at work among 2369 white-collar workers. *Journal of Human Hypertension, 31*(10), 620–626. https://doi.org/10.1038/jhh.2017.42

Brguljan-Hitij, J., Thijs, L., Li, Y., Hansen, T. W., Boggia, J., Liu, Y. P., Asayama, K., Wei, F. F., Bjorklund-Bodegard, K., Gu, Y. M., Ohkubo, T., Jeppesen, J., Torp-Pedersen, C., Dolan, E., Kuznetsova, T., Katarzyna, S. S., Tikhonoff, V., Malyutina, S., Casiglia, E., . . . Staessen, J. A. (2014). Risk stratification by ambulatory blood pressure monitoring across JNC classes of conventional blood pressure. *American Journal of Hypertension, 27*(7), 956–965. https://doi.org/10.1093/ajh/hpu002

Brisson, C., Aubé, K., Gilbert-Ouimet, M., Duchaine, C., Trudel, X., & Vézina, M. (2020). Organizational-level interventions and occupational health. In T. Theorell (Ed.), *Handbook of socioeconomic determinants of occupational health* (pp. 1–32). Springer Nature. https://doi.org/10.1007/978-3-030-05031-3_22-1

Brunner, E. J., & Kivimäki, M. (2013). Epidemiology: Work-related stress and the risk of type 2 diabetes mellitus. *Nature Reviews. Endocrinology, 9*(8), 449–450. https://doi.org/10.1038/nrendo.2013.124

Bushnell, P. T., Li, J., & Landen, D. (2011). Group medical claims as a source of information on worker health and potentially work-related diseases. *Journal of Occupational and Environmental Medicine, 53*(12), 1430–1441. https://doi.org/10.1097/JOM.0b013e3182363bbe

Buxton, O. M., Quintiliani, L. M., Yang, M. H., Ebbeling, C. B., Stoddard, A. M., Pereira, L. K., & Sorensen, G. (2009). Association of sleep adequacy with more healthful food choices and positive workplace experiences among motor freight workers. *American Journal of Public Health, 99*(S3, Suppl. 3), S636–S643. https://doi.org/10.2105/AJPH.2008.158501

Centers for Disease Control and Prevention. (2021). *About underlying cause of death, 1999–2019.* https://wonder.cdc.gov/ucd-icd10.html

Chandola, T., Britton, A., Brunner, E., Hemingway, H., Malik, M., Kumari, M., Badrick, E., Kivimaki, M., & Marmot, M. (2008). Work stress and coronary heart disease: What are the mechanisms? *European Heart Journal, 29*(5), 640–648. https://doi.org/10.1093/eurheartj/ehm584

Chetty, R., Grusky, D., Hell, M., Hendren, N., Manduca, R., & Narang, J. (2017). The fading American dream: Trends in absolute income mobility since 1940. *Science, 356*(6336), 398–406. https://doi.org/10.1126/science.aal4617

Cho, E., & Chen, T.-Y. (2020). The bidirectional relationships between effort–reward imbalance and sleep problems among older workers. *Sleep Health, 6*(3), 299–305. https://doi.org/10.1016/j.sleh.2020.01.008

Choi, B. (2020). Developing a job exposure matrix of work organization hazards in the United States: A review on methodological issues and research protocol. *Safety and Health at Work, 11*(4), 397–404. https://doi.org/10.1016/j.shaw.2020.05.007

Choi, B., Dobson, M., Landsbergis, P., Ko, S., Yang, H., Schnall, P., & Baker, D. (2014). Job strain and obesity [Letter to the editor]. *Journal of Internal Medicine, 275*(4), 438–440. https://doi.org/10.1111/joim.12173

Choi, B., Dobson, M., Landsbergis, P., & Schnall, P. (2019). *Developing a short on-line standard questionnaire for work organization risk assessment in the United States: The Healthy Work Survey (HWS) Project.* APA-NIOSH Work, Stress and Health Conference, Philadelphia, PA, United States.

Choi, B., Dobson, M., Schnall, P., & Garcia-Rivas, J. (2016). 24-hour work shifts, sedentary work, and obesity in male firefighters. *American Journal of Industrial Medicine, 59*(6), 486–500. https://doi.org/10.1002/ajim.22572

Choi, B., Schnall, P., & Dobson, M. (2016). Twenty-four-hour work shifts, increased job demands, and elevated blood pressure in professional firefighters. *International Archives of Occupational and Environmental Health, 89*(7), 1111–1125. https://doi.org/10.1007/s00420-016-1151-5

Choi, B., Schnall, P., Dobson, M., Israel, L., Landsbergis, P., Galassetti, P., Pontello, A., Kojaku, S., & Baker, D. (2011). Exploring occupational and behavioral risk factors for obesity in firefighters: A theoretical framework and study design. *Safety and Health at Work, 2*(4), 301–312. https://doi.org/10.5491/SHAW.2011.2.4.301

Choi, B., Schnall, P., Landsbergis, P., Dobson, M., Ko, S., Gómez-Ortiz, V., Juárez-Garcia, A., & Baker, D. (2015). Recommendations for individual participant data meta-analyses on work stressors and health outcomes: Comments on IPD-Work Consortium papers. *Scandinavian Journal of Work, Environment, and Health, 41*(3), 299–311. https://doi.org/10.5271/sjweh.3484

Choi, B., Schnall, P. L., Yang, H., Dobson, M., Landsbergis, P., Israel, L., Karasek, R., & Baker, D. (2010a). Psychosocial working conditions and active leisure-time physical activity in middle-aged U.S. workers. *International Journal of Occupational Medicine and Environmental Health, 23*(3), 239–253. https://psycnet.apa.org/record/2011-05089-003

Choi, B., Schnall, P. L., Yang, H., Dobson, M., Landsbergis, P., Israel, L., Karasek, R., & Baker, D. (2010b). Sedentary work, low physical job demand, and obesity in US workers. *American Journal of Industrial Medicine, 53*(11), 1088–1101. https://doi.org/10.1002/ajim.20886

Coenen, P., Huysmans, M. A., Holtermann, A., Krause, N., van Mechelen, W., Straker, L. M., & van der Beek, A. J. (2018). Do highly physically active workers die early? A systematic review with meta-analysis of data from 193 696 participants. *British Journal of Sports Medicine, 52*(20), 1320–1326. https://doi.org/10.1136/bjsports-2017-098540

de Looff, P. C., Cornet, L. J. M., Embregts, P. J. C. M., Nijman, H. L. I., & Didden, H. C. M. (2018). Associations of sympathetic and parasympathetic activity in job stress and burnout: A systematic review. *PLOS ONE, 13*(10), e0205741. https://doi.org/10.1371/journal.pone.0205741

del Arco-Galán, C., Súarez-Fernández, C., & Gabriel-Sánchez, R. (1994). What happens to blood pressure when on-call? *American Journal of Hypertension, 7*(5), 396–401. https://doi.org/10.1093/ajh/7.5.396

Descatha, A., Sembajwe, G., Pega, F., Ujita, Y., Baer, M., Boccuni, F., Di Tecco, C., Duret, C., Evanoff, B. A., Gagliardi, D., Godderis, L., Kang, S. K., Kim, B. J., Li, J., Magnusson Hanson, L. L., Marinaccio, A., Ozguler, A., Pachito, D., Pell, J., . . . Iavicoli, S. (2020). The effect of exposure to long working hours on stroke: A systematic review and meta-analysis from the WHO/ILO Joint Estimates of the Work-related Burden of Disease and Injury. *Environment International, 142*, 105746. https://doi.org/10.1016/j.envint.2020.105746

Dolan, E., Stanton, A., Thijs, L., Hinedi, K., Atkins, N., McClory, S., Den Hond, E., McCormack, P., Staessen, J. A., & O'Brien, E. (2005). Superiority of ambulatory over clinic blood pressure measurement in predicting mortality: The Dublin outcome study. *Hypertension, 46*(1), 156–161. https://doi.org/10.1161/01.HYP.0000170138.56903.7a

Dollard, M. F., & Neser, D. Y. (2013). Worker health is good for the economy: Union density and psychosocial safety climate as determinants of country differences in worker health and productivity in 31 European countries. *Social Science & Medicine*, *92*, 114–123. https://doi.org/10.1016/j.socscimed.2013.04.028

Dragano, N., Siegrist, J., Nyberg, S. T., Lunau, T., Fransson, E. I., Alfredsson, L., Bjorner, J. B., Borritz, M., Burr, H., Erbel, R., Fahlén, G., Goldberg, M., Hamer, M., Heikkilä, K., Jöckel, K. H., Knutsson, A., Madsen, I. E. H., Nielsen, M. L., Nordin, M., . . . Kivimäki, M. (2017). Effort–reward imbalance at work and incident coronary heart disease: A multicohort study of 90,164 individuals. *Epidemiology, 28*(4), 619–626. https://doi.org/10.1097/EDE.0000000000000666

Duchaine, C. S., Aubé, K., Gilbert-Ouimet, M., Vézina, M., Ndjaboué, R., Massamba, V., Talbot, D., Lavigne-Robichaud, M., Trudel, X., Pena-Gralle, A. B., Lesage, A., Moore, L., Milot, A., Laurin, D., & Brisson, C. (2020). Psychosocial stressors at work and the risk of sickness absence due to a diagnosed mental disorder: A systematic review and meta-analysis. *JAMA Psychiatry, 77*(8), 842–851. https://doi.org/10.1001/jamapsychiatry.2020.0322

Duchaine, C. S., Brisson, C., Talbot, D., Gilbert-Ouimet, M., Trudel, X., Vézina, M., Milot, A., Diorio, C., Ndjaboué, R., Giguère, Y., Mâsse, B., Dionne, C. E., Maunsell, E., & Laurin, D. (2021). Psychosocial stressors at work and inflammatory biomarkers: PROspective Quebec Study on Work and Health. *Psychoneuroendocrinology, 133*, 105400. https://doi.org/10.1016/j.psyneuen.2021.105400

Economic Policy Institute. (2019). *Annual wages and work hours.* State of Working America Data Library.

Eriksen, D., Rosthoj, S., Burr, H., & Holtermann, A. (2015). Sedentary work—Associations between five-year changes in occupational sitting time and body mass index. *Preventive Medicine, 73*, 1–5. https://doi.org/10.1016/j.ypmed.2014.12.038

Evans, G. W., Johansson, G., & Rydstedt, L. (1999). Hassles on the job: A study of a job intervention with urban bus drivers. *Journal of Organizational Behavior, 20*(2), 199–208. https://doi.org/10.1002/(SICI)1099-1379(199903)20:2<199::AID-JOB939>3.0.CO;2-I

Feaster, M., Arah, O. A., & Krause, N. (2019). Effort-reward imbalance and ambulatory blood pressure among female Las Vegas hotel room cleaners. *American Journal of Industrial Medicine, 62*(6), 523–534. https://doi.org/10.1002/ajim.22980

Feaster, M., & Krause, N. (2018). Job strain associated with increases in ambulatory blood and pulse pressure during and after work hours among female hotel room cleaners. *American Journal of Industrial Medicine, 61*(6), 492–503. https://doi.org/10.1002/ajim.22837

Ferrario, M. M., Veronesi, G., Roncaioli, M., Holtermann, A., Krause, N., Clays, E., Borchini, R., Grassi, G., Cesana, G., & the Cohorts Collaborative Study in Northern Italy (CCSNI) Research Group. (2019). Exploring the interplay between job strain and different domains of physical activity on the incidence of coronary heart disease in adult men. *European Journal of Preventive Cardiology, 26*(17), 1877–1885. https://doi.org/10.1177/2047487319852186

Ferrie, J., Westerlund, H., Virtanen, M., Vahtera, J., & Kivimaki, M. (2008). Flexible labor markets and employee health. *Scandinavian Journal of Work, Environment & Health Supplements* (6), 98–110. https://www.sjweh.fi/article/1257

Ferrie, J. E., Shipley, M. J., Marmot, M. G., Stansfeld, S., & Smith, G. D. (1998a). The health effects of major organisational change and job insecurity. *Social Science & Medicine, 46*(2), 243–254. https://doi.org/10.1016/S0277-9536(97)00158-5

Ferrie, J. E., Shipley, M. J., Marmot, M. G., Stansfeld, S. A., & Smith, G. D. (1998b). An uncertain future: The health effects of threats to employment security in white-collar men and women. *American Journal of Public Health, 88*(7), 1030–1036. https://doi.org/10.2105/AJPH.88.7.1030

Fioranelli, M., Bottaccioli, A. G., Bottaccioli, F., Bianchi, M., Rovesti, M., & Roccia, M. G. (2018). Stress and inflammation in coronary artery disease: A review psychoneuroendocrineimmunology-based. *Frontiers in Immunology, 9*, 2031. https://doi.org/10.3389/fimmu.2018.02031

Fox, K., Johnson, S., Berkman, L., Sianoja, M., Soh, Y., Kubzansky, L., & Kelly, E. (2022). Organisational- and group-level workplace interventions and their effect on multiple domains of worker well-being: A systematic review. *Work and Stress*, *36*(1), 1–30. https://doi.org/10.1080/02678373.2021.1969476

Gaziano, T. A. (2005). Cardiovascular disease in the developing world and its cost-effective management. *Circulation*, *112*(23), 3547–3553. https://doi.org/10.1161/CIRCULATIONAHA.105.591792

Gilbert-Ouimet, M., Baril-Gingras, G., Cantin, V., Leroux, I., Vézina, M., Trudel, L., Bourbonnais, R., & Brisson, C. (2015). Changes implemented during a workplace psychosocial intervention and their consistency with intervention priorities. *Journal of Occupational and Environmental Medicine*, *57*(3), 251–261. https://doi.org/10.1097/JOM.0000000000000252

Gilbert-Ouimet, M., Brisson, C., Vézina, M., Milot, A., & Blanchette, C. (2012). Repeated exposure to effort–reward imbalance, increased blood pressure, and hypertension incidence among white-collar workers: Effort–reward imbalance and blood pressure. *Journal of Psychosomatic Research*, *72*(1), 26–32. https://doi.org/10.1016/j.jpsychores.2011.07.002

Gilbert-Ouimet, M., Brisson, C., Vézina, M., Trudel, L., Bourbonnais, R., Masse, B., Baril-Gingras, G., & Dionne, C. E. (2011). Intervention study on psychosocial work factors and mental health and musculoskeletal outcomes. *Healthcare Papers*, *11*, 47–66. https://doi.org/10.12927/hcpap.2011.22410

Gilbert-Ouimet, M., Trudel, X., Brisson, C., Milot, A., & Vézina, M. (2014). Adverse effects of psychosocial work factors on blood pressure: Systematic review of studies on demand–control–support and effort–reward imbalance models. *Scandinavian Journal of Work, Environment & Health*, *40*(2), 109–132. https://doi.org/10.5271/sjweh.3390

Gilbert-Ouimet, M., Trudel, X., Talbot, D., Vezina, M., Milot, A., & Brisson, C. (2022). Long working hours associated with elevated ambulatory blood pressure among female and male white-collar workers over a 2.5-year follow-up. *Journal of Human Hypertension*, *36*(2), 207–217. https://doi.org/10.1038/s41371-021-00499-3

Goh, J., Pfeffer, J., & Zenios, S. A. (2015). The relationship between workplace stressors and mortality and health costs in the United States. *Management Science*, *62*(2), 608–628. https://doi.org/10.1287/mnsc.2014.2115

Government Accountability Office. (2015). *Contingent workforce* (GAO-15-168R Contingent Workforce). Washington, DC.

Greiner, B. A., Krause, N., Ragland, D., & Fisher, J. M. (2004). Occupational stressors and hypertension: A multi-method study using observer-based job analysis and self-reports in urban transit operators. *Social Science & Medicine*, *59*(5), 1081–1094. https://doi.org/10.1016/j.socscimed.2003.12.006

Hansen, T. W., Kikuya, M., Thijs, L., Björklund-Bodegård, K., Kuznetsova, T., Ohkubo, T., Richart, T., Torp-Pedersen, C., Lind, L., Jeppesen, J., Ibsen, H., Imai, Y., Staessen, J. A. (2007). Prognostic superiority of daytime ambulatory over conventional blood pressure in four populations: A meta-analysis of 7030 individuals. *Journal of Hypertension*, *25*(8), 1554–1564. https://doi.org/10.1097/HJH.0b013e3281c49da5

Harris, K. M., Woolf, S. H., & Gaskin, D. J. (2021). High and rising working-age mortality in the US: A report from the National Academies of Sciences, Engineering, and Medicine. *JAMA*, *325*(20), 2045–2046. https://doi.org/10.1001/jama.2021.4073

Healthy Work Campaign. (2021). *Healthy work strategies*. https://healthywork.org/resources/healthy-work-strategies/

Heikkilä, K., Nyberg, S. T., Fransson, E. I., Alfredsson, L., De Bacquer, D., Bjorner, J. B., Bonenfant, S., Borritz, M., Burr, H., Clays, E., Casini, A., Dragano, N., Erbel, R., Geuskens, G. A., Goldberg, M., Hooftman, W. E., Houtman, I. L., Joensuu, M., Jöckel, K. H., . . . Kivimäki, M. (2012). Job strain and tobacco smoking: An individual-participant data meta-analysis of 166,130 adults in 15 European studies. *PLOS ONE, 7*(7), e35463. https://doi.org/10.1371/journal.pone.0035463

Hillebrand, S., Gast, K. B., de Mutsert, R., Swenne, C. A., Jukema, J. W., Middeldorp, S., Rosendaal, F. R., & Dekkers, O. M. (2013). Heart rate variability and first cardiovascular event in populations without known cardiovascular disease: Meta-analysis and dose–response meta-regression. *Europace, 15*(5), 742–749. https://doi.org/10.1093/europace/eus341

Holtermann, A., Krause, N., van der Beek, A. J., & Straker, L. (2018). The physical activity paradox: Six reasons why occupational physical activity (OPA) does not confer the cardiovascular health benefits that leisure time physical activity does. *British Journal of Sports Medicine, 52*(3), 149–150. https://doi.org/10.1136/bjsports-2017-097965

Holtermann, A., Mathiassen, S. E., & Straker, L. (2019). Promoting health and physical capacity during productive work: The Goldilocks Principle. *Scandinavian Journal of Work, Environment & Health, 45*(1), 90–97. https://doi.org/10.5271/sjweh.3754

Institute of Medicine. (2010). *Promoting cardiovascular health in the developing world: A critical challenge to achieve global health*. The National Academies Press.

James, G. D., Yee, L. S., Harshfield, G. A., Blank, S. G., & Pickering, T. G. (1986). The influence of happiness, anger, and anxiety on the blood pressure of borderline hypertensives. *Psychosomatic Medicine, 48*(7), 502–508. https://doi.org/10.1097/00006842-198609000-00005

Johannessen, H. A., & Sterud, T. (2017). Psychosocial factors at work and sleep problems: A longitudinal study of the general working population in Norway. *International Archives of Occupational and Environmental Health, 90*(7), 597–608. https://doi.org/10.1007/s00420-017-1222-2

Jones, D., Molitor, D., & Reif, J. (2019). What do workplace wellness programs do? Evidence from the Illinois workplace wellness study. *The Quarterly Journal of Economics, 134*(4), 1747–1791. https://doi.org/10.1093/qje/qjz023

Joseph, N. T., Muldoon, M. F., Manuck, S. B., Matthews, K. A., MacDonald, L. A., Grosch, J., & Kamarck, T. W. (2016). The role of occupational status in the association between job strain and ambulatory blood pressure during working and nonworking days. *Psychosomatic Medicine, 78*(8), 940–949. https://doi.org/10.1097/PSY.0000000000000349

Karasek, R. (2004). An analysis of 19 international case studies of stress prevention through work reorganization using the demand/control model. *Bulletin of Science, Technology & Society, 24*(5), 446–456. https://doi.org/10.1177/0270467604269583

Karasek, R. A., & Theorell, T. (1990). *Healthy work: Stress, productivity, and the reconstruction of working life*. Basic Books.

Khaja, S. U., Mathias, K. C., Bode, E. D., Stewart, D. F., Jack, K., Moffatt, S. M., & Smith, D. L. (2021). Hypertension in the United States Fire Service. *International Journal of Environmental Research and Public Health, 18*(10), 5432. https://doi.org/10.3390/ijerph18105432

Kivimäki, M., Batty, G. D., Ferrie, J. E., & Kawachi, I. (2014). Cumulative meta-analysis of job strain and CHD. *Epidemiology, 25*(3), 464–465. https://doi.org/10.1097/EDE.0000000000000087

Kivimäki, M., Nyberg, S. T., Pentti, J., Madsen, I. E. H., Hanson, L. L. M., Rugulies, R., Vahtera, J., & Coggon, D. (2019). Individual and combined effects of job strain components on subsequent morbidity and mortality. *Epidemiology, 30*(4), e27–e29. https://doi.org/10.1097/EDE.0000000000001020

Kivimäki, M., Virtanen, M., Kawachi, I., Nyberg, S. T., Alfredsson, L., Batty, G. D., Bjorner, J. B., Borritz, M., Brunner, E. J., Burr, H., Dragano, N., Ferrie, J. E., Fransson, E. I., Hamer, M., Heikkila, K., Knutsson, A., Koskenvuo, M., Madsen, I. E. H., Nielsen, M. L., . . . Jokela, M. (2015). Long working hours, socioeconomic status, and the risk of incident type 2 diabetes: A meta-analysis of published and unpublished data from 222 120 individuals. *Lancet Diabetes Endocrinol, 3*(1), 27–34. https://doi.org/10.1016/S2213-8587(14)70178-0

Kortum, E., Leka, S., & Cox, T. (2010). Psychosocial risks and work-related stress in developing countries: Health impact, priorities, barriers and solutions. *International Journal of Occupational Medicine and Environmental Health, 23*(3), 225–238.

Kouvonen, A., Kivimäki, M., Virtanen, M., Heponiemi, T., Elovainio, M., Pentti, J., Linna, A., & Vahtera, J. (2006). Effort-reward imbalance at work and the co-occurrence of lifestyle risk factors: Cross-sectional survey in a sample of 36,127 public sector employees. *BMC Public Health, 6*(1), 24. https://doi.org/10.1186/1471-2458-6-24

Kouvonen, A., Vahtera, J., Väänänen, A., De Vogli, R., Heponiemi, T., Elovainio, M., Virtanen, M., Oksanen, T., Cox, S. J., Pentti, J., & Kivimäki, M. (2009). Relationship between job strain and smoking cessation: The Finnish Public Sector Study. *Tobacco Control, 18*(2), 108–114. https://doi.org/10.1136/tc.2008.025411

Krause, N., Brand, R. J., Arah, O. A., & Kauhanen, J. (2015). Occupational physical activity and 20-year incidence of acute myocardial infarction: Results from the Kuopio Ischemic Heart Disease Risk Factor Study. *Scandinavian Journal of Work, Environment & Health, 41*(2), 124–139. https://doi.org/10.5271/sjweh.3476

Krause, N., Brand, R. J., Kaplan, G. A., Kauhanen, J., Malla, S., Tuomainen, T. P., & Salonen, J. T. (2007). Occupational physical activity, energy expenditure and 11-year progression of carotid atherosclerosis. *Scandinavian Journal of Work, Environment & Health, 33*(6), 405–424. https://doi.org/10.5271/sjweh.1171

Krause, N., Lynch, J. W., Kaplan, G. A., Cohen, R. D., Salonen, R., & Salonen, J. T. (2000). Standing at work and progression of carotid atherosclerosis. *Scandinavian Journal of Work, Environment & Health, 26*(3), 227–236. https://doi.org/10.5271/sjweh.536

Kroemer, K., & Grandjean, E. (1997). *Fitting the task to the human: A textbook of occupational ergonomics* (5th ed.). Taylor & Francis. https://doi.org/10.1201/9780367807337

LaMontagne, A. D., Keegel, T., Louie, A. M., Ostry, A., & Landsbergis, P. A. (2007). A systematic review of the job-stress intervention evaluation literature, 1990–2005. *International Journal of Occupational and Environmental Health, 13*(3), 268–280. https://doi.org/10.1179/oeh.2007.13.3.268

LaMontagne, A. D., Keegel, T., Vallance, D., Ostry, A., & Wolfe, R. (2008). Job strain— Attributable depression in a sample of working Australians: Assessing the contribution to health inequalities. *BMC Public Health, 8*, 181. https://doi.org/10.1186/1471-2458-8-181

Landsbergis, P. A., Cahill, J., Schnall, P. (1999). The impact of lean production and related new systems of work organization on worker health. *Journal of Occupational Health Psychology, 4*(2), 108–130.

Landsbergis, P. A., Diez-Roux, A. V., Fujishiro, K., Baron, S., Kaufman, J. D., Meyer, J. D., Koutsouras, G., Shimbo, D., Shrager, S., Stukovsky, K. H., & Szklo, M. (2015). Job strain, occupational category, systolic blood pressure, and hypertension prevalence: The multi-ethnic study of atherosclerosis. *Journal of Occupational and Environmental Medicine, 57*(11), 1178–1184. https://doi.org/10.1097/JOM.0000000000000533

Landsbergis, P. A., Dobson, M., Koutsouras, G., & Schnall, P. (2013). Job strain and ambulatory blood pressure: A meta-analysis and systematic review. *American Journal of Public Health, 103*(3), e61–e71. https://doi.org/10.2105/AJPH.2012.301153

Landsbergis, P. A., Dobson, M., LaMontagne, A. D., Choi, B., Schnall, P., & Baker, D. B. (2017). Occupational stress. In B. S. Levy, D. H. Wegman, S. L. Baron, & R. K. Sokas (Eds.), *Occupational and environmental health* (7th ed., pp. 325–343). Oxford University Press. https://doi.org/10.1093/oso/9780190662677.003.0017

Landsbergis, P. A., Schnall, P. L., Pickering, T. G., Warren, K., & Schwartz, J. E. (2003). Lower socioeconomic status among men in relation to the association between job strain and blood pressure. *Scandinavian Journal of Work, Environment & Health, 29*(3), 206–215. https://doi.org/10.5271/sjweh.723

Landsbergis, P. A., Travis, A., & Schnall, P. L. (2013). Working conditions and masked hypertension. *High Blood Pressure & Cardiovascular Prevention: The Official Journal of the Italian Society of Hypertension, 20*(2), 69–76. https://doi.org/10.1007/s40292-013-0015-2

Lax, M. B. (2016). The perils of integrating wellness and safety and health and the possibility of a worker-oriented alternative. *New Solutions, 26*(1), 11–39. https://doi.org/10.1177/1048291116629489

Levi, M., Kjellstrom, T., & Baldasseroni, A. (2018). Impact of climate change on occupational health and productivity: A systematic literature review focusing on workplace heat. *La Medicina del Lavoro, 109*(3), 163–179. https://doi.org/10.23749/mdl.v109i3.6851

Lewiskin, J., Abramovitz, M., & Zelnick, J. (2021). On the front lines: The impact of Managerialism on the New York City addiction treatment workforce. *New Solutions, 31*(3), 259–270. https://doi.org/10.1177/10482911211041615

Li, J., Loerbroks, A., & Angerer, P. (2013). Physical activity and risk of cardiovascular disease: What does the new epidemiological evidence show? *Current Opinion in Cardiology, 28*(5), 575–583. https://doi.org/10.1097/HCO.0b013e328364289c

Li, J., Pega, F., Ujita, Y., Brisson, C., Clays, E., Descatha, A., Ferrario, M. M., Godderis, L., Iavicoli, S., Landsbergis, P. A., Metzendorf, M. I., Morgan, R. L., Pachito, D. V., Pikhart, H., Richter, B., Roncaioli, M., Rugulies, R., Schnall, P. L., Sembajwe, G., . . . Siegrist, J. (2020). The effect of exposure to long working hours on ischaemic heart disease: A systematic review and meta-analysis from the WHO/ILO Joint Estimates of the Work-related Burden of Disease and Injury. *Environment International, 142*, 105739. https://doi.org/10.1016/j.envint.2020.105739

Li, J., Zhang, M., Loerbroks, A., Angerer, P., & Siegrist, J. (2015). Work stress and the risk of recurrent coronary heart disease events: A systematic review and meta-analysis. *International Journal of Occupational Medicine and Environmental Health, 28*(1), 8–19. https://doi.org/10.2478/s13382-014-0303-7

Li, W., Yi, G., Chen, Z., Dai, X., Wu, J., Peng, Y., Ruan, W., Lu, Z., & Wang, D. (2021). Is job strain associated with a higher risk of Type 2 diabetes mellitus? A systematic review and meta-analysis of prospective cohort studies. *Scandinavian Journal of Work, Environment & Health, 47*(4), 249–257. https://doi.org/10.5271/sjweh.3938

Lindskog, P., Hemphälä, J., Eklund, J., Eriksson, A. (2016). Lean in healthcare: Engagement in development, job satisfaction or exhaustion? *Journal of Hospital Administration, 5*(5), 91–105. https://doi.org/10.5430/jha.v5n5p91

Linton, S. J., Kecklund, G., Franklin, K. A., Leissner, L. C., Sivertsen, B., Lindberg, E., Svensson, A. C., Hansson, S. O., Sundin, Ö., Hetta, J., Björkelund, C., & Hall, C. (2015). The effect of the work environment on future sleep disturbances: A systematic review. *Sleep Medicine Reviews, 23*, 10–19. https://doi.org/10.1016/j.smrv.2014.10.010

Liu, Y., Song, Y., Koopmann, J., Wang, M., Chang, C. D., & Shi, J. (2017). Eating your feelings? Testing a model of employees' work-related stressors, sleep quality, and unhealthy eating. *Journal of Applied Psychology, 102*(8), 1237–1258. https://doi.org/10.1037/apl0000209

Loerbroks, A., Shang, L., Angerer, P., & Li, J. (2015). Effort–reward imbalance at work increases the risk of the metabolic syndrome: A prospective study in Chinese university staff. *International Journal of Cardiology, 182*, 390–391. https://doi.org/10.1016/j.ijcard.2015.01.030

Long, K. A., & Evans, W. (2021, May 25). Amazon's relentless pace is injuring warehouse workers and violating the law, Washington state regulator says. *The Seattle Times and Reveal from The Center for Investigative Reporting.* https://www.seattletimes.com/business/amazon/amazons-relentless-pace-is-violating-the-law-and-injuring-warehouse-workers-washington-state-regulator-says/

Lopez, A. D., & Adair, T. (2019). Is the long-term decline in cardiovascular-disease mortality in high-income countries over? Evidence from national vital statistics.

International Journal of Epidemiology, 48(6), 1815–1823. https://doi.org/10.1093/ije/dyz143

MacDonald, L. A., Karasek, R. A., Punnett, L., & Scharf, T. (2001). Covariation between workplace physical and psychosocial stressors: Evidence and implications for occupational health research and prevention. *Ergonomics, 44*(7), 696–718. https://doi.org/10.1080/00140130119943

Madsen, I. E. H., Nyberg, S. T., Magnusson Hanson, L. L., Ferrie, J. E., Ahola, K., Alfredsson, L., Batty, G. D., Bjorner, J. B., Borritz, M., Burr, H., Chastang, J. F., de Graaf, R., Dragano, N., Hamer, M., Jokela, M., Knutsson, A., Koskenvuo, M., Koskinen, A., Leineweber, C., . . . Kivimäki, M. (2017). Job strain as a risk factor for clinical depression: Systematic review and meta-analysis with additional individual participant data. *Psychological Medicine, 47*(8), 1342–1356. https://doi.org/10.1017/S003329171600355X

Maina, G., Bovenzi, M., Palmas, A., Prodi, A., & Filon, F. L. (2011). Job strain, effort-reward imbalance and ambulatory blood pressure: Results of a cross-sectional study in call handler operators. *International Archives of Occupational and Environmental Health, 84*(4), 383–391. https://doi.org/10.1007/s00420-010-0576-5

Mattsson, K., Hougaard, K. S., & Sejbaek, C. S. (2021). Exposure to psychosocial work strain and changes in smoking behavior during pregnancy—A longitudinal study within the Danish National Birth Cohort. *Scandinavian Journal of Work, Environment & Health, 47*(1), 70–77. https://doi.org/10.5271/sjweh.3921

Mauss, D., Li, J., Schmidt, B., Angerer, P., & Jarczok, M. N. (2015). Measuring allostatic load in the workforce: A systematic review. *Industrial Health, 53*(1), 5–20. https://doi.org/10.2486/indhealth.2014-0122

McEwen, B. S., & Stellar, E. (1993). Stress and the individual: Mechanisms leading to disease. *Archives of Internal Medicine, 153*(18), 2093–2101. https://doi.org/10.1001/archinte.1993.00410180039004

Melin, B., Lundberg, U., Soderlund, J., & Granqvist, M. (1999). Psychophysiological stress reactions of male and female assembly workers: A comparison between two different forms of work organization. *Journal of Organizational Behavior, 20*(1), 47–61. https://doi.org/10.1002/(SICI)1099-1379(199901)20:1<47::AID-JOB871>3.0.CO;2-F

Miyaki, K., Song, Y., Htun, N. C., Tsutsumi, A., Hashimoto, H., Kawakami, N., Takahashi, M., Shimazu, A., Inoue, A., Kurioka, S., & Shimbo, T. (2012). Folate intake and depressive symptoms in Japanese workers considering SES and job stress factors: J-HOPE study. *BMC Psychiatry, 12*, 33. https://doi.org/10.1186/1471-244X-12-33

Monforton, C. (2015). *Injuries and deaths on minds of striking Steelworkers.* https://scienceblogs.com/thepumphandle/2015/02/05/injuries-and-deaths-on-minds-of-striking-steelworkers/

Montano, D., Hoven, H., & Siegrist, J. (2014). Effects of organisational-level interventions at work on employees' health: A systematic review. *BMC Public Health, 14*(1), 135. https://doi.org/10.1186/1471-2458-14-135

Muntaner, C., Chung, H., Solar, O., Santana, V., Castedo, A., Benach, J., & the EMCONET Network. (2010). A macro-level model of employment relations and health inequalities. *International Journal of Health Services, 40*(2), 215–221. https://doi.org/10.2190/HS.40.2.c

Musselman, D. L., Evans, D. L., & Nemeroff, C. B. (1998). The relationship of depression to cardiovascular disease: Epidemiology, biology, and treatment. *Archives of General Psychiatry, 55*(7), 580–592. https://doi.org/10.1001/archpsyc.55.7.580

Mutambudzi, M., Siegrist, J., Meyer, J. D., & Li, J. (2018). Association between effort-reward imbalance and self-reported diabetes mellitus in older U.S. workers. *Journal of Psychosomatic Research, 104*, 61–64. https://doi.org/10.1016/j.jpsychores.2017.11.008

Myers, S., Govindarajulu, U., Joseph, M., & Landsbergis, P. (2019). Changes in work characteristics over 12 years: Findings from the 2002–2014 US National NIOSH

Quality of Work Life Surveys. *American Journal of Industrial Medicine, 62*(6), 511–522. https://doi.org/10.1002/ajim.22971

Myers, S., Govindarajulu, U., Joseph, M. A., & Landsbergis, P. (2021). Work characteristics, body mass index, and risk of obesity: The National Quality of Work Life Survey. *Annals of Work Exposures and Health, 65*(3), 291–306. https://doi.org/10.1093/annweh/wxaa098

National Academies of Sciences, Engineering, and Medicine. (2021). *Briefing slides: High and rising mortality rates among working-age adults.*

Niedhammer, I., Sultan-Taïeb, H., Parent-Thirion, A., & Chastang, J. F. (2022). Update of the fractions of cardiovascular diseases and mental disorders attributable to psychosocial work factors in Europe. *International Archives of Occupational and Environmental Health, 95*(1), 233–247. https://doi.org/10.1007/s00420-021-01737-4

Nielsen, M. B., Pallesen, S., Einarsen, S. V., Harris, A., Rajalingam, D., & Gjerstad, J. (2021). Associations between exposure to workplace bullying and insomnia: A cross-lagged prospective study of causal directions. *International Archives of Occupational and Environmental Health, 94*(5), 1003–1011. https://doi.org/10.1007/s00420-020-01618-2

Nigatu, Y. T., & Wang, J. (2018). The combined effects of job demand and control, effort–reward imbalance and work–family conflicts on the risk of major depressive episode: A 4-year longitudinal study. *Occupational and Environmental Medicine, 75*(1), 6–11. https://doi.org/10.1136/oemed-2016-104114

Nomaguchi, K. (2009). Change in work–family conflict among employed parents between 1977 and 1997. *Journal of Marriage and Family, 71*(1), 15–32. https://doi.org/10.1111/j.1741-3737.2008.00577.x

Nordentoft, M., Rod, N. H., Bonde, J. P., Bjorner, J. B., Cleal, B., Larsen, A. D., Madsen, I. E. H., Magnusson Hanson, L. L., Nexo, M. A., Pedersen, L. R. M., Sterud, T., Xu, T., & Rugulies, R. (2020). Effort–reward imbalance at work and weight changes in a nationwide cohort of workers in Denmark. *American Journal of Industrial Medicine, 63*(7), 634–643. https://doi.org/10.1002/ajim.23110

Nyberg, S. T., Fransson, E. I., Heikkilä, K., Ahola, K., Alfredsson, L., Bjorner, J. B., Borritz, M., Burr, H., Dragano, N., Goldberg, M., Hamer, M., Jokela, M., Knutsson, A., Koskenvuo, M., Koskinen, A., Kouvonen, A., Leineweber, C., Madsen, I. E., Magnusson Hanson, L. L., . . . Kivimäki, M. (2014). Job strain as a risk factor for Type 2 diabetes: A pooled analysis of 124,808 men and women. *Diabetes Care, 37*(8), 2268–2275. https://doi.org/10.2337/dc13-2936

Nyberg, S. T., Fransson, E. I., Heikkilä, K., Alfredsson, L., Casini, A., Clays, E., De Bacquer, D., Dragano, N., Erbel, R., Ferrie, J. E., Hamer, M., Jöckel, K. H., Kittel, F., Knutsson, A., Ladwig, K. H., Lunau, T., Marmot, M. G., Nordin, M., Rugulies, R., . . . Kivimäki, M. (2013). Job strain and cardiovascular disease risk factors: Meta-analysis of individual-participant data from 47,000 men and women. *PLOS ONE, 8*(6), e67323. https://doi.org/10.1371/journal.pone.0067323

O'Connor, D. B., Thayer, J. F., & Vedhara, K. (2021). Stress and health: A review of psychobiological processes. *Annual Review of Psychology, 72*(1), 663–688. https://doi.org/10.1146/annurev-psych-062520-122331

Oddo, V. M., Zhuang, C. C., Andrea, S. B., Eisenberg-Guyot, J., Peckham, T., Jacoby, D., & Hajat, A. (2021). Changes in precarious employment in the United States: A longitudinal analysis. *Scandinavian Journal of Work, Environment & Health, 47*(3), 171–180. https://doi.org/10.5271/sjweh.3939

Ohkubo, T., Kikuya, M., Metoki, H., Asayama, K., Obara, T., Hashimoto, J., Totsune, K., Hoshi, H., Satoh, H., & Imai, Y. (2005). Prognosis of "masked" hypertension and "white-coat" hypertension detected by 24-h ambulatory blood pressure monitoring 10-year follow-up from the Ohasama study. *Journal of the American College of Cardiology, 46*(3), 508–515. https://doi.org/10.1016/j.jacc.2005.03.070

Pachito, D. V., Pega, F., Bakusic, J., Boonen, E., Clays, E., Descatha, A., Delvaux, E., De Bacquer, D., Koskenvuo, K., Kröger, H., Lambrechts, M. C., Latorraca, C. O. C., Li, J., Cabrera Martimbianco, A. L., Riera, R., Rugulies, R., Sembajwe, G., Siegrist, J., Sillanmäki, L., . . . Godderis, L. (2021). The effect of exposure to long working hours on alcohol consumption, risky drinking and alcohol use disorder: A systematic review and meta-analysis from the WHO/ILO Joint Estimates of the Work-related Burden of Disease and Injury. *Environment International, 146*, 106205. https://doi.org/10.1016/j.envint.2020.106205

Pega, F., Náfrádi, B., Momen, N. C., Ujita, Y., Streicher, K. N., Prüss-Üstün, A. M., Technical Advisory Group, Descatha, A., Driscoll, T., Fischer, F. M., Godderis, L., Kiiver, H. M., Li, J., Magnusson Hanson, L. L., Rugulies, R., Sørensen, K., & Woodruff, T. J. (2021). Global, regional, and national burdens of ischemic heart disease and stroke attributable to exposure to long working hours for 194 countries, 2000–2016: A systematic analysis from the WHO/ILO Joint Estimates of the Work-related Burden of Disease and Injury. *Environment International, 154*, 106595. https://doi.org/10.1016/j.envint.2021.106595

Perret-Guillaume, C., Joly, L., & Benetos, A. (2009). Heart rate as a risk factor for cardiovascular disease. *Progress in Cardiovascular Diseases, 52*(1), 6–10. https://doi.org/10.1016/j.pcad.2009.05.003

Pickering, T. G., Harshfield, G. A., Kleinert, H. D., Blank, S., & Laragh, J. H. (1982). Blood pressure during normal daily activities, sleep, and exercise: Comparison of values in normal and hypertensive subjects. *JAMA, 247*(7), 992–996. https://doi.org/10.1001/jama.1982.03320320028025

Pieper, C., Warren, K., & Pickering, T. G. (1993). A comparison of ambulatory blood pressure and heart rate at home and work on work and non-work days. *Journal of Hypertension, 11*(2), 177–183. https://doi.org/10.1097/00004872-199302000-00010

Pierdomenico, S. D., Lapenna, D., Bucci, A., Di Tommaso, R., Di Mascio, R., Manente, B. M., Caldarella, M. P., Neri, M., Cuccurullo, F., & Mezzetti, A. (2005). Cardiovascular outcome in treated hypertensive patients with responder, masked, false resistant, and true resistant hypertension. *American Journal of Hypertension, 18*(11), 1422–1428. https://doi.org/10.1016/j.amjhyper.2005.05.014

Portela, L. F., Rotenberg, L., Almeida, A. L., Landsbergis, P., & Griep, R. H. (2013). The influence of domestic overload on the association between job strain and ambulatory blood pressure among female workers. *International Journal of Environmental Research and Public Health, 10*(12), 6397–6408. https://doi.org/10.3390/ijerph10126397

Punnett, L., Warren, N., Henning, R., Nobrega, S., & Cherniack, M. (2013). Participatory ergonomics as a model for integrated programs to prevent chronic disease. *Journal of Occupational and Environmental Medicine, 55*(12, Suppl.).

Quinlan, M., & Bohle, P. (2009). Overstretched and unreciprocated commitment: Reviewing research on the occupational health and safety effects of downsizing and job insecurity. *International Journal of Health Services, 39*(1), 1–44. https://doi.org/10.2190/HS.39.1.a

Riopel, C., Lavigne-Robichaud, M., Trudel, X., Milot, A., Gilbert-Ouimet, M., Talbot, D., Aubé, K., & Brisson, C. (2021). Job strain and incident cardiovascular disease: The confounding and mediating effects of lifestyle habits. An overview of systematic reviews. *Archives of Environmental & Occupational Health, 76*(6), 330–337. https://doi.org/10.1080/19338244.2020.1828244

Romero Starke, K., Hegewald, J., Schulz, A., Garthus-Niegel, S., Nübling, M., Wild, P. S., Arnold, N., Latza, U., Jankowiak, S., Liebers, F., Rossnagel, K., Riechmann-Wolf, M., Letzel, S., Beutel, M., Pfeiffer, N., Lackner, K., Münzel, T., & Seidler, A. (2020). Cardiovascular health outcomes of mobbing at work: Results of the population-based, five-year follow-up of the Gutenberg health study. *Journal of Occupational Medicine and Toxicology, 15*(1), 15. https://doi.org/10.1186/s12995-020-00266-z

Rongen, A., Robroek, S. J. W., van Lenthe, F. J., & Burdorf, A. (2013). Workplace health promotion: A meta-analysis of effectiveness. *American Journal of Preventive Medicine, 44*(4), 406–415. https://doi.org/10.1016/j.amepre.2012.12.007

Rosenthal, T. (2014). The effect of migration on hypertension and other cardiovascular risk factors: A review. *Journal of the American Society of Hypertension, 8*(3), 171–191. https://doi.org/10.1016/j.jash.2013.12.007

Rosskam, E. (2009). Using participatory action research methodology to improve worker health. In P. Schnall, M. Dobson, & E. Rosskam (Eds.), *Unhealthy work: Causes, consequences, cures* (pp. 211–228). Baywood.

Roth, G. A., Mensah, G. A., Johnson, C. O., Addolorato, G., Ammirati, E., Baddour, L. M., Barengo, N. C., Beaton, A. Z., Benjamin, E. J., Benziger, C. P., Bonny, A., Brauer, M., Brodmann, M., Cahill, T. J., Carapetis, J., Catapano, A. L., Chugh, S. S., Cooper, L. T., Coresh, J., . . . Fuster, V. (2020). Global burden of cardiovascular diseases and risk factors, 1990–2019: Update from the GBD 2019 Study. *Journal of the American College of Cardiology, 76*(25), 2982–3021. https://doi.org/10.1016/j.jacc.2020.11.010

Rugulies, R., Aust, B., & Madsen, I. E. (2017). Effort–reward imbalance at work and risk of depressive disorders: A systematic review and meta-analysis of prospective cohort studies. *Scandinavian Journal of Work, Environment & Health, 43*(4), 294–306. https://doi.org/10.5271/sjweh.3632

Rugulies, R., Scherzer, T., & Krause, N. (2008). Associations between psychological demands, decision latitude, and job strain with smoking in female hotel room cleaners in Las Vegas. *International Journal of Behavioral Medicine, 15*(1), 34–43. https://doi.org/10.1007/BF03003072

Rugulies, R., Sørensen, K., Di Tecco, C., Bonafede, M., Rondinone, B. M., Ahn, S., Ando, E., Ayuso-Mateos, J. L., Cabello, M., Descatha, A., Dragano, N., Durand-Moreau, Q., Eguchi, H., Gao, J., Godderis, L., Kim, J., Li, J., Madsen, I. E. H., Pachito, D. V., . . . Pega, F. (2021). The effect of exposure to long working hours on depression: A systematic review and meta-analysis from the WHO/ILO Joint Estimates of the Work-related Burden of Disease and Injury. *Environment International, 155*, 106629. https://doi.org/10.1016/j.envint.2021.106629

Rydstedt, L. W., Johansson, G., & Evans, G. W. (1998). The human side of the road: Improving the working conditions of urban bus drivers. *Journal of Occupational Health Psychology, 3*(2), 161–171. https://doi.org/10.1037/1076-8998.3.2.161

Salvagioni, D. A. J., Melanda, F. N., Mesas, A. E., González, A. D., Gabani, F. L., & Andrade, S. M. (2017). Physical, psychological and occupational consequences of job burnout: A systematic review of prospective studies. *PLOS ONE, 12*(10), e0185781. https://doi.org/10.1371/journal.pone.0185781

Sanderson, D. M., Ekholm, O., Hundrup, Y. A., & Rasmussen, N. K. (2005). Influence of lifestyle, health, and work environment on smoking cessation among Danish nurses followed over 6 years. *Preventive Medicine, 41*(3–4), 757–760. https://doi.org/10.1016/j.ypmed.2005.06.002

Schnall, P., Dobson, M., & Landsbergis, P. (2017). Work, stress and cardiovascular disease. In J. Quick & C. Cooper (Eds.), *Handbook of stress and health* (pp. 97–124). Wiley. https://doi.org/10.1002/9781118993811.ch6

Schnall, P. L., Dobson, M., & Landsbergis, P. (2016). Globalization, work, and cardiovascular disease. *International Journal of Health Services, 46*(4), 656–692. https://doi.org/10.1177/0020731416664687

Schnall, P. L., Schwartz, J. E., Landsbergis, P. A., Warren, K., & Pickering, T. G. (1998). A longitudinal study of job strain and ambulatory blood pressure: Results from a three-year follow-up. *Psychosomatic Medicine, 60*(6), 697–706. https://doi.org/10.1097/00006842-199811000-00007

Schwartz, J. E., Pieper, C. F., & Karasek, R. A. (1988). A procedure for linking psychosocial job characteristics data to health surveys. *American Journal of Public Health, 78*(8), 904–909. https://doi.org/10.2105/AJPH.78.8.904

Sega, R., Trocino, G., Lanzarotti, A., Carugo, S., Cesana, G., Schiavina, R., Valagussa, F., Bombelli, M., Giannattasio, C., Zanchetti, A., & Mancia, G. (2001). Alterations of cardiac structure in patients with isolated office, ambulatory, or home hypertension: Data from the general population (Pressione Arteriose Monitorate E Loro Associazioni [PAMELA] Study). *Circulation, 104*(12), 1385–1392. https://doi.org/10.1161/hc3701.096100

Sheehan, C. M., Frochen, S. E., Walsemann, K. M., & Ailshire, J. A. (2019). Are U.S. adults reporting less sleep?: Findings from sleep duration trends in the National Health Interview Survey, 2004–2017. *Sleep, 42*(2), 1–8. https://doi.org/10.1093/sleep/zsy221

Shierholz, H. (2019). *Working people have been thwarted in their efforts to bargain for better wages by attacks on unions.* https://www.epi.org/publication/labor-day-2019-collective-bargaining/

Shirom, A., Armon, G., Berliner, S., Shapira, I., & Melamed, S. (2009). The effects of job strain on risk factors for cardiovascular disease. In C. Cooper, J. Quick, & M. Schabracq (Eds.), *International handbook of work and health psychology* (pp. 49–75). Wiley Blackwell. https://doi.org/10.1002/9780470682357.ch4

Siegrist, J., & Li, J. (2020). Effort-reward imbalance and occupational health. In T. Theorell (Ed.), *Handbook of socioeconomic determinants of occupational health* (pp. 355–382). Springer.

Siegrist, J., Peter, R., Junge, A., Cremer, P., & Seidel, D. (1990). Low status control, high effort at work and ischemic heart disease: Prospective evidence from blue-collar men. *Social Science & Medicine, 31*(10), 1127–1134. https://doi.org/10.1016/0277-9536(90)90234-J

Siegrist, J., & Rödel, A. (2006). Work stress and health risk behavior. *Scandinavian Journal of Work, Environment & Health, 32*(6), 473–481. https://doi.org/10.5271/sjweh.1052

Singh, G. K., Siahpush, M., Azuine, R. E., & Williams, S. D. (2015). Increasing area deprivation and socioeconomic inequalities in heart disease, stroke, and cardiovascular disease mortality among working age Populations, United States, 1969–2011. *International Journal of MCH and AIDS, 3*(2), 119–133. https://www.ncbi.nlm.nih.gov/pubmed/27621992

Solovieva, S., Lallukka, T., Virtanen, M., & Viikari-Juntura, E. (2013). Psychosocial factors at work, long work hours, and obesity: A systematic review. *Scandinavian Journal of Work, Environment & Health, 39*(3), 241–258. https://doi.org/10.5271/sjweh.3364

Souza, R. V. d., Sarmento, R. A., Almeida, J. C. d., & Canuto, R. (2019). The effect of shift work on eating habits: A systematic review. *Scandinavian Journal of Work, Environment and Health, 45*(1), 7–21.

Steptoe, A., Cropley, M., & Joekes, K. (1999). Job strain, blood pressure and response to uncontrollable stress. *Journal of Hypertension, 17*(2), 193–200. https://doi.org/10.1097/00004872-199917020-00003

Strategic Organizing Center. (2021). *Primed for pain: Amazon's epidemic of workplace injuries.* https://thesoc.org/amazon-primed-for-pain/

Swedish Working Environment Act. Amending the Working Environment Act, No. 1160 of 1977 (Svensk författningssamling). Stockholm, Sweden. 1991.

Tanaka, R., Tsuji, M., Tsuchiya, T., & Kawamoto, T. (2019). Association between work-related factors and diet: A review of the literature. *Workplace Health & Safety, 67*(3), 137–145. https://doi.org/10.1177/2165079918812481

Theorell, T. (2008). Anabolism and catabolism—Antagonistic partners in stress and strain. *Scandinavian Journal of Work, Environment and Health Supplements* (6), 136–143. https://www.sjweh.fi/article/1260

Theorell, T., Hammarström, A., Aronsson, G., Träskman Bendz, L., Grape, T., Hogstedt, C., Marteinsdottir, I., Skoog, I., & Hall, C. (2015). A systematic review including meta-analysis of work environment and depressive symptoms. *BMC Public Health, 15*(1), 738. https://doi.org/10.1186/s12889-015-1954-4

Theorell, T., Jood, K., Järvholm, L. S., Vingård, E., Perk, J., Östergren, P. O., & Hall, C. (2016). A systematic review of studies in the contributions of the work environment to ischaemic heart disease development. *European Journal of Public Health, 26*(3), 470–477. https://doi.org/10.1093/eurpub/ckw025

Thomas, W. (2020, December 22, 2020). A temp worker died on the job after FedEx didn't fix a known hazard. The fine: $7000. *MLK50: Justice Through Journalism.* https://mlk50.com/2020/12/22/fedex-prioritizes-packages-over-employee-safety-workers-and-experts-say/

Thubrikar, M. (2007). *Vascular mechanics and pathology.* Springer. https://doi.org/10.1007/978-0-387-68234-1

Tobe, S. W., Kiss, A., Sainsbury, S., Jesin, M., Geerts, R., & Baker, B. (2007). The impact of job strain and marital cohesion on ambulatory blood pressure during 1 year: The double exposure study. *American Journal of Hypertension, 20*(2), 148–153. https://doi.org/10.1016/j.amjhyper.2006.07.011

Toivanen, S., Landsbergis, P. (2013). Lean och arbetstagarnas hälsa [Lean and worker health]. In P. Sederblad & L. Abrahamsson (Eds.), *Lean i arbetslivet.* Liber.

Törnroos, M., Hakulinen, C., Hintsanen, M., Puttonen, S., Hintsa, T., Pulkki-Råback, L., Jokela, M., Lehtimäki, T., Raitakari, O. T., & Keltikangas-Järvinen, L. (2017). Reciprocal relationships between psychosocial work characteristics and sleep problems: A two-wave study. *Work and Stress, 31*(1), 63–81. https://doi.org/10.1080/02678373.2017.1297968

Torquati, L., Mielke, G. I., Brown, W. J., & Kolbe-Alexander, T. (2018). Shift work and the risk of cardiovascular disease. A systematic review and meta-analysis including dose–response relationship. *Scandinavian Journal of Work, Environment & Health, 44*(3), 229–238. https://doi.org/10.5271/sjweh.3700

Trudel, X., Brisson, C., Gilbert-Ouimet, M., Vézina, M., Talbot, D., & Milot, A. (2020). Long working hours and the prevalence of masked and sustained hypertension. *Hypertension, 75*(2), 532–538. https://doi.org/10.1161/HYPERTENSIONAHA.119.12926

Trudel, X., Brisson, C., & Milot, A. (2010). Job strain and masked hypertension. *Psychosomatic Medicine, 72*(8), 786–793. https://doi.org/10.1097/PSY.0b013e3181eaf327

Trudel, X., Brisson, C., Milot, A., Masse, B., & Vézina, M. (2013). Psychosocial work environment and ambulatory blood pressure: Independent and combined effect of demand-control and effort-reward imbalance models. *Occupational and Environmental Medicine, 70*(11), 815–822. https://doi.org/10.1136/oemed-2013-101416

Trudel, X., Brisson, C., Milot, A., Masse, B., & Vézina, M. (2016). Adverse psychosocial work factors, blood pressure and hypertension incidence: Repeated exposure in a 5-year prospective cohort study. *Journal of Epidemiology and Community Health, 70*(4), 402–408. https://doi.org/10.1136/jech-2014-204914

Trudel, X., Brisson, C., Talbot, D., Gilbert-Ouimet, M., & Milot, A. (2021). Long working hours and risk of recurrent coronary events. *Journal of the American College of Cardiology, 77*(13), 1616–1625. https://doi.org/10.1016/j.jacc.2021.02.012

Trudel, X., Gilbert-Ouimet, M., Vézina, M., Talbot, D., Mâsse, B., Milot, A., & Brisson, C. (2021). Effectiveness of a workplace intervention reducing psychosocial stressors at work on blood pressure and hypertension. *Occupational and Environmental Medicine, 78*(10), 738–744. https://doi.org/10.1136/oemed-2020-107293

Tsutsumi, A. (2015). Prevention and management of work-related cardiovascular disorders. *International Journal of Occupational Medicine and Environmental Health, 28*(1), 4–7. https://doi.org/10.2478/s13382-014-0319-z

Tüchsen, F., & Endahl, L. A. (1999). Increasing inequality in ischaemic heart disease morbidity among employed men in Denmark 1981–1993: The need for a new preventive policy. *International Journal of Epidemiology, 28*(4), 640–644. https://doi.org/10.1093/ije/28.4.640

Turner, A. I., Smyth, N., Hall, S. J., Torres, S. J., Hussein, M., Jayasinghe, S. U., Ball, K., & Clow, A. J. (2020). Psychological stress reactivity and future health and disease outcomes: A systematic review of prospective evidence. *Psychoneuroendocrinology*, *114*, 104599. https://doi.org/10.1016/j.psyneuen.2020.104599

Vahtera, J., Kivimäki, M., Forma, P., Wikström, J., Halmeenmäki, T., Linna, A., & Pentti, J. (2005). Organisational downsizing as a predictor of disability pension: The 10-town prospective cohort study. *Journal of Epidemiology and Community Health*, *59*(3), 238–242. https://doi.org/10.1136/jech.2004.021824

van Oostrom, S. H., Nachat, A., Loef, B., & Proper, K. I. (2021). The mediating role of unhealthy behaviors and body mass index in the relationship between high job strain and self-rated poor health among lower educated workers. *International Archives of Occupational and Environmental Health*, *94*(1), 95–105. https://doi.org/10.1007/s00420-020-01565-y

Verdecchia, P., Clement, D., Fagard, R., Palatini, P., & Parati, G. (1999). Task force III: Target-organ damage, morbidity and mortality. *Blood Pressure Monitoring*, *4*(6), 303–318. https://doi.org/10.1097/00126097-199912000-00004

Virani, S. S., Alonso, A., Aparicio, H. J., Benjamin, E. J., Bittencourt, M. S., Callaway, C. W., Carson, A. P., Chamberlain, A. M., Cheng, S., Delling, F. N., Elkind, M. S. V., Evenson, K. R., Ferguson, J. F., Gupta, D. K., Khan, S. S., Kissela, B. M., Knutson, K. L., Lee, C. D., Lewis, T. T., . . . Tsao, C. W. (2021). Heart disease and stroke statistics—2021 update: A report from the American Heart Association. *Circulation*, *143*(8), e254–e743. https://doi.org/10.1161/CIR.0000000000000950

Virtanen, M., Jokela, M., Lallukka, T., Magnusson Hanson, L., Pentti, J., Nyberg, S. T., Alfredsson, L., Batty, G. D., Casini, A., Clays, E., DeBacquer, D., Ervasti, J., Fransson, E., Halonen, J. I., Head, J., Kittel, F., Knutsson, A., Leineweber, C., Nordin, M., . . . Kivimäki, M. (2020). Long working hours and change in body weight: Analysis of individual-participant data from 19 cohort studies. *International Journal of Obesity*, *44*(6), 1368–1375. https://doi.org/10.1038/s41366-019-0480-3

Virtanen, M., Nyberg, S. T., Batty, G. D., Jokela, M., Heikkilä, K., Fransson, E. I., Alfredsson, L., Bjorner, J. B., Borritz, M., Burr, H., Casini, A., Clays, E., De Bacquer, D., Dragano, N., Elovainio, M., Erbel, R., Ferrie, J. E., Hamer, M., Jöckel, K. H., . . . Kivimäki, M. (2013). Perceived job insecurity as a risk factor for incident coronary heart disease: Systematic review and meta-analysis. *BMJ*, *347*(1), f4746. https://doi.org/10.1136/bmj.f4746

Waldron, I., Nowotarski, M., Freimer, M., Henry, J. P., Post, N., & Witten, C. (1982). Cross-cultural variation in blood pressure: A quantitative analysis of the relationships of blood pressure to cultural characteristics, salt consumption and body weight. *Social Science & Medicine*, *16*(4), 419–430. https://doi.org/10.1016/0277-9536(82)90050-8

Wang, A., Arah, O. A., Kauhanen, J., & Krause, N. (2016). Shift work and 20-year incidence of acute myocardial infarction: Results from the Kuopio Ischemic Heart Disease Risk Factor Study. *Occupational and Environmental Medicine*, *73*(9), 588–594. https://doi.org/10.1136/oemed-2015-103245

Waters, T. R., & Dick, R. B. (2015). Evidence of health risks associated with prolonged standing at work and intervention effectiveness. *Rehabilitation Nursing*, *40*(3), 148–165. https://doi.org/10.1002/rnj.166

Wong, J. H., & Kelloway, E. K. (2016). What happens at work stays at work? Workplace supervisory social interactions and blood pressure outcomes. *Journal of Occupational Health Psychology*, *21*(2), 133–141. https://doi.org/10.1037/a0039900

World Health Organization. (2017). *Depression and other common mental disorders: Global health estimates.*

World Health Organization. (2021a). *Cardiovascular diseases.* https://www.who.int/news-room/fact-sheets/detail/cardiovascular-diseases-(cvds)

World Health Organization. (2021b). *Hypertension.* https://www.who.int/news-room/fact-sheets/detail/hypertension

Xu, T., Magnusson Hanson, L. L., Lange, T., Starkopf, L., Westerlund, H., Madsen, I. E. H., Rugulies, R., Pentti, J., Stenholm, S., Vahtera, J., Hansen, A. M., Virtanen, M., Kivimäki, M., & Rod, N. H. (2019). Workplace bullying and workplace violence as risk factors for cardiovascular disease: A multi-cohort study. *European Heart Journal*, *40*(14), 1124–1134. https://doi.org/10.1093/eurheartj/ehy683

Yang, B., Wang, Y., Cui, F., Huang, T., Sheng, P., Shi, T., Huang, C., Lan, Y., & Huang, Y.-N. (2018). Association between insomnia and job stress: A meta-analysis. *Sleep and Breathing*, *22*(4), 1221–1231. https://doi.org/10.1007/s11325-018-1682-y

Yasin, S. M., Retneswari, M., Moy, F.-M., Darus, A., & Koh, D. (2012). Job stressors and smoking cessation among Malaysian male employees. *Occupational Medicine*, *62*(3), 174–181. https://doi.org/10.1093/occmed/kqs005

Zelnick, J., Abramovitz, M., & Pirutinsky, S. (2022). Managerialism: A workforce health hazard in human service settings. *American Journal of Industrial Medicine*. https://doi.org/10.1002/ajim.23395

Zhang, D. Y., Guo, Q. H., An, D. W., Li, Y., & Wang, J. G. (2019). A comparative meta-analysis of prospective observational studies on masked hypertension and masked uncontrolled hypertension defined by ambulatory and home blood pressure. *Journal of Hypertension*, *37*(9), 1775–1785. https://doi.org/10.1097/HJH.0000000000002109

17

Pain, Musculoskeletal Injuries, and Return to Work

William S. Shaw, Alicia G. Dugan, and Jennifer Garza

Musculoskeletal pain and injury are experienced by workers across nearly all industries and occupations. How employers respond to prevent worker pain and injury has important implications for worker health and well-being as well as significant financial and organizational implications for employers. Musculoskeletal pain and injury is a major contributor to the global burden of disease (Safiri et al., 2021), and these disorders have contributed to a sizable increase in the number of Americans out of work due to disability (Franklin et al., 2015). Work-related musculoskeletal disorders (MSDs) alone have been estimated to cost from $45 billion to $54 billion annually in the United States (National Research Council and Institute of Medicine Panel on Musculoskeletal Disorders in the Workplace, 2001). In this chapter, we review issues and trends related to the prevention and management of pain and disability in the workplace, with a special emphasis on chronic and intermittent pain, organizational support and communication, job accommodation, return-to-work processes, and the changing nature of work.

MSDs generally include all medical conditions affecting muscles, bones, and joints, including tendinitis, sprains and strains, osteoarthritis, carpal tunnel syndrome, neck and back pain, and other specific diagnoses and conditions. MSDs are quite common, and they increase in prevalence with age. The predominant symptom is pain, but MSDs can also cause joint stiffness, swelling, dull aches, and restricted movement. Back and neck symptoms are most common, but MSDs can also impact the upper and lower extremities.

https://doi.org/10.1037/0000331-017
Handbook of Occupational Health Psychology, Third Edition, L. E. Tetrick, G. G. Fisher, M. T. Ford, and J. C. Quick (Editors)

Work-related musculoskeletal disorders (WMSDs) generally include only those MSDs where the work environment or performance of work contributes significantly to onset or exacerbation. Both rates of WMSDs and time away from work vary by industry (see Figure 17.1), with the highest prevalence among occupations involving lifting heavy objects, daily exposure to whole-body vibration, routine overhead work, work with the neck in chronic flexion, or repetitive tasks (U.S. Bureau of Labor Statistics, 2020). Occupational ergonomics has contributed to reducing awkward postures, repetitive movements, and other ergonomic risk factors in the workplace, but challenges remain in construction, warehousing, nursing, and other occupations requiring heavy physical demands. (See Chapter 29 of this handbook for a description and summary of occupational ergonomics.) Workplace injuries, however, represent only a fraction of musculoskeletal pain, and 40% of U.S. workers report pain (occupational or nonoccupational) that limits their ability to work (Burton et al., 2004; Ricci et al., 2006).

Higher income countries have reported gradual declines in workplace injuries for the past 3 decades (Marcum & Adams, 2017; Mustard et al., 2003), but these gains have been offset by an aging workforce (Berecki-Gisolf et al., 2012), higher rates of obesity and chronic musculoskeletal pain among new and existing workers (Ward & Schiller, 2013), and longer work absences after pain episodes (Ricci et al., 2006). Thus, while workers have benefited from fewer ergonomic exposures in the workplace and fewer occupational injuries on average, they are increasingly challenged to manage work limitations associated with pain and to return to usual job responsibilities after injury (see Figure 17.2).

On the employer side, the challenges are many: (a) managing sickness absence and functional limitation while maintaining productivity; (b) facilitating adequate leeway and accommodation to workers while applying fairness and consistency; (c) providing adequate health and disability benefits; (d) integrating health promotion programs with injury prevention; (e) keeping older, more experienced workers on the job; and (f) coordinating organizational efforts with multiple health care, insurance, and disability systems (Gignac et al., 2021; Gould-Werth et al., 2018; Kaye et al., 2011; Varekamp & van Dijk, 2010; Wynne-Jones et al., 2011). There is accumulating evidence to guide employer decision making in these areas, but the organizational complexity of the problem makes this fertile ground for occupational health psychology and one with important theoretical and practical implications for worker health and safety. In the following sections, we summarize evidence of physical, psychological, and organizational risk factors for pain and best employer strategies for worker support and accommodation.

WORK-RELATED FACTORS ASSOCIATED WITH MUSCULOSKELETAL DISORDERS

Several categories of work-related factors, including physical as well as psychosocial factors, have been associated with MSDs in epidemiologic studies. Consensus evidence of the associations between physical and psychosocial

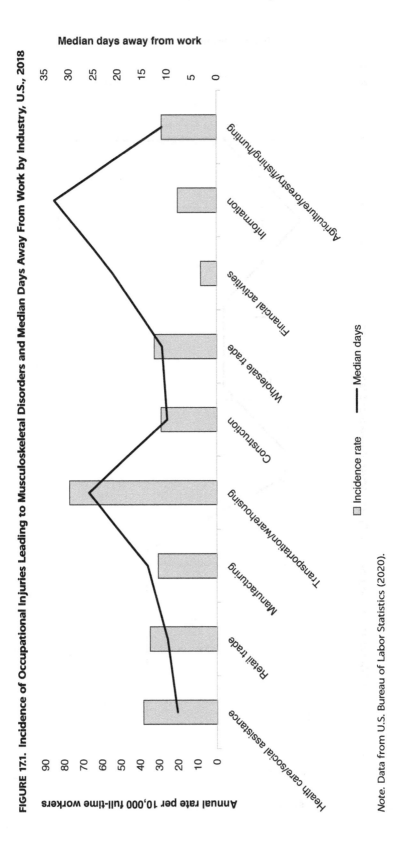

FIGURE 17.1. Incidence of Occupational Injuries Leading to Musculoskeletal Disorders and Median Days Away From Work by Industry, U.S., 2018

Note. Data from U.S. Bureau of Labor Statistics (2020).

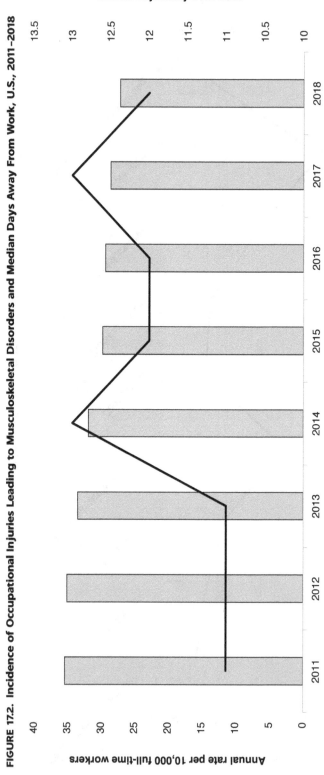

FIGURE 17.2. Incidence of Occupational Injuries Leading to Musculoskeletal Disorders and Median Days Away From Work, U.S., 2011–2018

Note. Data from U.S. Bureau of Labor Statistics (2020).

factors and musculoskeletal pain was summarized in a 2001 publication by the National Academies Panel on Musculoskeletal Disorders and the Workplace (National Research Council and Institute of Medicine Panel on Musculoskeletal Disorders in the Workplace, 2001). Since that time, additional research and several systematic reviews have provided further support for associations between workplace physical and psychosocial factors and MSDs.

MSDs have well-documented associations with workplace physical risk factors such as repetitive motion, heavy lifting, nonneutral postures, and vibration (IJmker et al., 2007; Mayer et al., 2012; van Rijn et al., 2010). Studies have typically measured physical risk factors via self-reports or by estimated workloads. Recently, some studies have also sought to link direct measurements of physical risk factors to musculoskeletal symptoms and disorders. For example, Balogh and colleagues (2019) reported associations between directly measured head velocity, trapezius activity, upper arm velocity, forearm extensor activity, and wrist posture and velocity as well as most neck/shoulder and elbow/hand complaints and diagnoses. Merkus et al. (2021) found connections between directly measured upper arm elevation and trapezius muscle activity and neck and shoulder pain among construction and healthcare employees. In a meta-analysis of pooled data sets including quantitative measurements across various occupations, Nordander et al. (2016) observed associations between head inclination, upper arm elevation, muscle activity of the trapezius and forearm extensors, and wrist posture and angular velocity with neck and shoulder musculoskeletal symptoms. Several systematic reviews have shown links between workplace psychosocial factors including decision latitude, quantitative job demands, and social support and MSDs (Bongers et al., 2002; da Costa & Vieira, 2010; van den Heuvel et al., 2005). Certain physical and psychosocial factors have been differentially associated with various body regions, as described in the following section.

Work Factors for Neck and Shoulder Pain

Several previous studies have found associations between various physical factors and symptoms or disorders in the neck or shoulder regions. Van Rijn et al. (2010) observed associations between shoulder symptoms and disorders and high force, lifting, repetitive motions, high psychosocial job demands. Da Costa and Vieira (2010) found evidence of links between heavy physical work and shoulder symptoms. Arvidsson et al. (2016) observed associations between pain in the neck and shoulders and a high mechanical exposure index as well as high job demands. Van den Heuvel et al. (2005) also reported associations between neck/shoulder symptoms and high job demands. Psychosocial job demands have also been associated with neck/shoulder symptoms and disorders (Arvidsson et al., 2020; da Costa & Vieira, 2010; van Rijn et al., 2010).

Work Factors for Elbow Pain

Elbow symptoms have been associated with physical factors such as repetitive motions, job control, social support, vibration, and static postures (van Rijn et al., 2010). Van den Heuvel et al. (2005) reported an association between elbow symptoms, high job demands, and low social support.

Work Factors for Hand and Wrist Pain

Hand and wrist symptoms have been associated with physical factors such as computer work, heavy physical work, and awkward posture (da Costa & Vieira, 2010). Van den Heuvel et al. (2005) reported associations between hand or wrist symptoms, high job demands, and low social support.

Work Factors for Low Back Pain

Low back symptoms have been associated with heavy physical work, awkward postures, and lifting (da Costa & Vieira, 2010). Arvidsson et al. (2016) reported associations between back pain and a high mechanical exposure index and high job demands. Da Costa and Vieira (2010) also reported associations between back pain and psychosocial factors.

Work Factors for Leg and Foot Pain

Da Costa and Vieira (2010) reported associations between heavy physical work and lifting, and hip pain, awkward postures, lifting, repetition, and knee pain. Arvidsson et al. (2016) reported associations between foot pain and a high physical exposure index.

CHRONICITY OF PAIN AND DISABILITY

Defining the word *disability* can be problematic, as the word has many definitions depending on whether it is being used for legislative mandates, social experiences, corporate benefits, or self-identification. According to the World Health Organization (WHO; 2001), disability has three dimensions: (a) *impairment* in bodily structures or physiological capacities; (b) *limitation* in functional activities like walking, hearing, or problem solving; and (c) *loss of participation* in normal daily social and occupational roles and activities. The International Classification of Functioning, Disability, and Health (ICF) framework (WHO, 2001) describes disability as encompassing all three dimensions of impairment, limitation, and decreased participation. Disability can be associated with an injury, a condition since childhood, the development of a chronic condition, or episodic, progressive, or static symptoms. The phrase *work disability* is often used to refer specifically to decreased participation in occupational roles and activities in the workplace. It occurs along a continuum from minor functional difficulties to sickness absence to permanent departure from the workforce.

Few studies have examined separately the risk factors for transitions between different stages of musculoskeletal symptoms and disability. Evanoff and colleagues (2014) proposed a model in which physical factors were more strongly associated with initial incidence of MSDs among asymptomatic workers, while psychological factors were more strongly associated with chronic disorders and disability. This framework has been supported by several research studies as well. For instance, Miranda et al. (2005) reported different determinants of specific MSDs compared with subjective complaints without clinical findings in a large Finnish study.

While several prospective studies have been conducted in recent years, and other recent studies have addressed some methodological concerns regarding the collection of data on workplace physical and psychosocial risk factors and MSDs, more research is needed to fully understand the relationship between work and MSDs, especially studies that describe the transition from discomfort to pain to disability. Randomized clinical trials have not been a feasible study design for determining the health effects of nontherapeutic risk factors, so much of the available evidence is based on observational cohorts (Punnett, 2014). Future studies should consider improved classification of physical and psychosocial exposures as well as musculoskeletal outcomes and assess interactions between work and out-of-work factors (Hagberg et al., 2012).

Return-to-work programs in the employment setting enable workers to gradually resume normal job responsibilities after an injury, illness, or medical procedure while they continue to participate in medical rehabilitation. In the case of musculoskeletal conditions, a gradual return to work may help improve physical and social activity, often with medical restrictions implemented to avoid pain flare-ups and reinjuries. Even with medical restrictions in place to prevent serious harm, individuals can display different tolerances to performing work tasks with functional difficulties, residual symptoms, or fear of severe pain exacerbations (Bunzli et al., 2017). For employers, a successful return to work may reduce disability payments, restore productivity output, and avoid rehiring and training; thus, many employers strive for a proactive approach to coordinating return-to-work arrangements with workers and their physicians. Still, the process of returning to work can vary substantially by job type, severity of illness or injury, organizational or workplace constraints, and individual-level concerns. Identifying individual-level barriers and involving workers in collaborative problem-solving may be necessary when simple administrative processes fail.

JOB ACCOMMODATION AND RETURN TO WORK

An important responsibility mandated for employers in most regions and jurisdictions is to facilitate return-to-work arrangements for workers after a sickness absence and to provide reasonable accommodation to workers with disabling or limiting health conditions. Though randomized trials of accommodation are largely impractical in the occupational context, there is moderate scientific support that a routine employer offer of job modification reduces the duration of sickness absence and decreases employer and insurer costs after musculoskeletal pain (Cullen et al., 2018; van Vilsteren et al., 2015; Wong et al., 2021). Workplace accommodations may also help improve worker retention (Jonsson et al., 2019; Stynen et al., 2016), convey a positive message of diversity and inclusion, and satisfy regulatory requirements of employers pertaining to job accommodation and equal opportunity. While most medium- and large-sized employers have written policies and procedures around return-to-work facilitation and job accommodation, the literature continues to cite a lack of organizational support, mistrust, and miscommunication from workers seeking needed job modifications or accommodations to stay at work or return to work (Kensbock et al., 2017; MacEachen et al., 2006). Only one in five older workers with a disabling MSD report ever receiving a workplace accommodation (Hill et al., 2016).

Organizational Challenges

Several circumstances can make the process of returning to work or requesting accommodations a challenge for workers and employers. One system-level factor is the heavy reliance on information and recommendations from physicians as the sole basis for accommodations and return-to-work arrangements. This places a large responsibility on physicians to understand the details of a job, understand how functional limitations of the patient might intersect with job demands, consider the individual concerns and suggestions of patients, and be knowledgeable about job flexibility and availability of accommodations within a wide range of occupational, industry, and company settings. Most accommodations reported by workers involve some element of modified job responsibilities, including making exceptions to usual policies, assistance from coworkers, changes in working hours, changing the work environment, modifying physical workloads, or providing assistive technology (Shaw et al., 2014; Wong et al., 2021). Having a clearly defined organizational process for return-to-work planning and accommodation that incorporates input from the worker, supervisor, and clinician is a fundamental step for employers to improve pain and disability outcomes (Main & Shaw, 2016; Main, Shaw, & Hopkinton Conference Working Group on Workplace Disability Prevention, 2016; Schandelmaier et al., 2012; Shaw et al., 2016; Williams & Westmorland, 2002).

Individual Factors

A second challenge for return-to-work planning and accommodation for pain disorders is the wide variation of worker experiences in terms of functional limitations, coping, pain beliefs, and perceived need for accommodation. Efforts to apply strict uniform policies for accommodation and return to work can be difficult to enforce across organizations when individual workers with similar diagnoses report different needs for support and accommodation. Hence, two employees experiencing low back pain in the same working group may experience variable trajectories of recovery and return to work, and this can be a puzzle for human resources professionals who are trying to maintain fair practices and consistency across the organization. Psychosocial aspects of pain that are especially pertinent to return to work include pain self-efficacy, pain catastrophizing, recovery expectations, perceived functional limitations, and psychological distress (Gray et al., 2011; Nicholas et al., 2011; Steenstra et al., 2017).

Creating a return-to-work planning process that is sensitive to individual differences in these factors while still maintaining a fair and objective organizational process can pose significant challenges for human resources professionals, policy makers, and frontline supervisors. General recommendations for a successful employer-based return-to-work program include: (a) a strong organizational commitment to health and safety, (b) a routine offer of modified or alternate work, (c) support to injured or disabled workers without disadvantaging coworkers and supervisors, (d) training and inclusion of frontline supervisors, (e) early and considerate contact with employees who are out of work, (f) a designated individual to coordinate return-to-work efforts, and (g) a plan for facilitating communication with health care providers when needed (Cullen et al., 2018; Main, Shaw, & Mitchell, 2016).

Supervisor Support

The role of supervisors in supporting return-to-work planning, facilitating job modifications, and providing appropriate communication and follow-up with workers has been a regular theme in return-to-work and job accommodation research. In larger organizations, human resources professionals may be the central organizational contact for processing, managing, and documenting return-to-work arrangements and requests for job accommodation, but supervisors' knowledge of individual workers and workplace factors may be critical to identify specific return-to-work barriers and opportunities for an individual worker (Buys et al., 2019; Lappalainen et al., 2021). Communication bottlenecks between disability case managers and frontline supervisors have been cited as a significant problem in the disability management process (Jetha et al., 2019; Lappalainen et al., 2019). The supervisor's actual role in facilitating return-to-work arrangements may vary by industry context and corporate structures, but workers often report that their supervisor played an important role in a sustainable return to work, and lack of communication and support from a supervisor has been shown to be a common detriment to resuming work (Corbière et al., 2017; Sears et al., 2021; Smith et al., 2020). Measures of supervisor support for return-to-work and job accommodation efforts are frequent predictors of reduced disability duration (Jetha et al., 2018; Kristman et al., 2017). Many supervisors, however, cite a lack of training in this area and frequent frustration with an iterative process in which their organizational autonomy for decision-making seems uncertain (Williams-Whitt et al., 2016). More transformative and considerate leadership styles and better knowledge of organizational policies are correlated with stronger supervisor accommodation efforts (Kristman et al., 2017). Interactive and peer-based training programs designed to improve supervisor responses to injuries and disabilities have shown promise in reducing injury rates and lost workdays (Schreuder et al., 2013; Spector & Reul, 2017).

EMERGING TOPICS

The modern workplace is undergoing many transformations in both high- and low-income countries, and these are changing exposures to risk factors and circumstances surrounding musculoskeletal pain and disability. These include changing work arrangements, altered work environments, changes in the nature of work, and changes in the base health of workers themselves.

Changing Work Arrangements

New technologies, globalization, and an on-demand economy are changing the nature of work, and organizations and workers are attempting to adapt while also maintaining optimal occupational health and safety (Tamers et al., 2020). The prevalence of precarious employment is rising, characterized by work that is insecure, temporary, and may offer insufficient hours to earn a living wage (Blustein et al., 2020; Vives et al., 2013). There is growing evidence that workers with precarious work arrangements in various occupations and geographies experience increased exposure to occupational and ergonomic hazards, as well as psychosocial and economic stressors that may result in musculoskeletal symptoms (Min et al., 2013; Park & Lee, 2021; Sargeant, 2014). This situation is exacerbated by workers having inadequate benefits such as paid work leave for the purposes of recovering from injury, and affordable, quality health insurance.

Working time arrangements can also be precarious. Precarious schedules, defined as having long shifts, nondaytime hours, and irregular and unpredictable hours, are increasingly prevalent, even for workers with nonprecarious employment in occupations that have traditionally been stable, secure, and unionized (Härmä et al., 2015). A recent study on working time characteristics on musculoskeletal symptoms showed that low schedule control was associated with neck/shoulder musculoskeletal symptoms, while frequently working long hours (over 48 per week) was associated with leg/foot musculoskeletal symptoms (Garza et al., 2022). Precarious schedule characteristics are linked to fatigue, insufficient recovery time, and poor sleep, which may pose risks to safety and musculoskeletal health resulting from decreased cognitive functioning, impaired performance, and increased errors (Dawson & McCulloch, 2005). Additionally, long work hours and irregular or unpredictable schedules can reduce health behaviors needed to maintain good musculoskeletal health, such as leisure time, physical activity, and healthy diet (Artazcoz et al., 2009; Wong et al., 2019).

Changing Work Environments

The coronavirus (COVID-19) pandemic caused dramatic changes to the work environments of millions of workers across the globe who, due to social distancing measures, began to work from home in early 2020, remained working at home for over a year, and may continue to work from home, to some degree, permanently. This development is critical for musculoskeletal health in terms of both the challenges and opportunities it poses. However, it is premature to draw conclusions as the evidence regarding health effects of working from home is early and mixed, and the impact of working at home on the mental and physical health of workers varies considerably based on numerous situational factors. For instance, an evaluation of the health effects of teleworking in Japan during COVID-19 found that teleworkers experienced increased eye/shoulder/back strain and stress resulting from the introduction of a new work system (Nagata et al., 2021). During the COVID-19 shelter-at-home period, desk workers in the United States showed declines in physical functioning, increased (nonworkday) sedentary behavior, and worse sleep quality and mood (Barone Gibbs et al., 2021). Links between lockdown conditions and pain/functioning need further examination, but one study found pandemic-related stress and related factors (e.g., compromised sleep, disruption of daily life routines, anxiety, worry, and isolation, greater family and work stress, excessive screen time) were associated with a variety of physical symptoms (i.e., headaches, insomnia, digestive problems, hormonal imbalances, and fatigue; Majumdar et al., 2020). Another study found that anxiety regarding health during COVID-19 was related to musculoskeletal symptoms (Kirmizi et al., 2021).

Changing Work

The information age brought with it numerous changes to job demands within many occupations. In particular, the use of computers with visual display units and keyboards is increasingly common and requires employees to work in prolonged postures of forward flexion of head, neck and trunk, anterior shoulder rotation, and non-neutral arm reaching, often from static sitting postures (Madeleine et al., 2013). Musculoskeletal pain is commonly reported by workers who use computers, particularly in the upper extremities (neck/shoulder area; Waersted et al., 2010), and load is affected by the computer's location, height, and angle in relation to the body (Punnett & Bergqvist, 1997). In addition to workstations, the development of pain in computer users is related to interacting factors (i.e., individual, physical, psychosocial, organizational; Madeleine et al., 2013).

While office workers are a group at obvious risk of musculoskeletal pain due to computer use, even occupations that have historically been associated with manual, labor-intensive physical demands (e.g., manufacturing), due to technological advances, now increasingly require workers to staff computer workstations to operate automated machines in prolonged sitting or standing postures. This illustrates how workers in all types of jobs have musculo-skeletal job demands and ergonomic risks, though they may have different configurations of demands. While the musculoskeletal risks of some jobs may be due to excessive activity/dynamic postures (overload), the musculoskeletal risks of other jobs may be due to insufficient activity/static postures (under-load). An additional concern also highlighted by the shift toward computer-aided machining jobs in manufacturing is that such jobs have increasing cognitive demands (e.g., tasks require technical skills and critical thinking) that pose their own risk to musculoskeletal health. Combined with the increased use of computers and mobile devices in the personal lives of individuals from all sociodemographic backgrounds, the cumulative strain that technology poses across life domains is heavy for many people, but this is an under-researched area (Borhany et al., 2018). Further research is needed to assess the full range of MSDs and occupational and nonoccupational risk factors, as well as to clarify specific dose relationships and thresholds of exposure for specific disorders.

Changing Workforce

Demographic and socioeconomic changes, as well as recent social movements (e.g., #MeToo, Black Lives Matter), have highlighted the need for increased attention to vulnerable populations of workers who may be at higher risk of exposure to physical and psychosocial stressors at work, and more vulnerable to work-related illness and injury, including MSDs. For example, the mean age of workers is rising, and by 2024 the proportion of workers 55+ years old in the U.S. workforce is estimated to increase to 25% (Toossi, 2015). Workers are retiring later due to economic pressures and an increased age of eligibility for receiving full social security benefits.

It is advantageous for older workers to remain working for as long as pos-sible, as there are insufficient younger workers to replace older workers exiting the workforce; older workers also have a strong work ethic as well as high levels of autonomy, flexibility, and efficiency (Loeppke et al., 2013; Shultz & Adams, 2012). However, older workers have more numerous health challenges compared to younger workers, including a higher prevalence of MSDs, in addi-tion to decreases in physical capacity, cognition, memory, vision, and hearing (Loeppke et al., 2013; National Research Council and Committee on the Health and Safety Needs of Older Workers, 2004; Silverstein, 2008). Excessive job demands can lead to greater risk, and recovery from illness and injury requires a greater length of time (Loeppke et al., 2013; Silverstein, 2008).

Older individuals, and those who experience high physical demands and psychological distress, have a higher prevalence of musculoskeletal pain overall (McBeth & Jones, 2007). Work-related activities may initiate or aggravate existing MSDs, and older workers may be at particular risk due to tissue changes and slower tissue healing (National Research Council and Com-mittee on the Health and Safety Needs of Older Workers, 2004). Work-place challenges described by workers with chronic or episodic pain include self-doubt and other negative self-perceptions, interpersonal conflicts or other problems coordinating workload with coworkers, as well as the inflexibility of job tasks or lack of accommodation (Tveito et al., 2010). Workers manage these challenges by modifying work activities and routines on their own, finding ways to reduce discomfort, using cognitive strategies to overcome negative beliefs, preparing for pain flare-ups, increasing regular movement, and searching for job leeway (Tveito et al., 2010). Disclosure of health concerns to an employer, however, can be a difficult decision for many workers (Gignac et al., 2021). Finding effective pathways for workers and employers to discuss ongoing health-related functional limitations remains an important organizational challenge for the future.

CONCLUSION

The changing nature of work has reduced some physical risk factors for MSDs in the workplace, but organizational shifts and the declining health of the workforce have presented other musculoskeletal challenges for workers. Issues of return-to-work coordination, health disclosure, supervisor support, and job accommodation remain significant factors for employers. Future research might focus on the most vulnerable workers, on episodic and intermittent sources of musculoskeletal disability, and identification of workplace policies that allow for early intervention before musculoskeletal discomfort leads to chronic pain and disability.

REFERENCES

Artazcoz, L., Cortès, I., Escribà-Agüir, V., Cascant, L., & Villegas, R. (2009). Understanding the relationship of long working hours with health status and health-related behaviours. *Journal of Epidemiology and Community Health, 63*(7), 521–527. https://doi.org/10.1136/jech.2008.082123

Arvidsson, I., Gremark Simonsen, J., Dahlqvist, C., Axmon, A., Karlson, B., Björk, J., & Nordander, C. (2016). Cross-sectional associations between occupational factors and musculoskeletal pain in women teachers, nurses and sonographers. *BMC Musculoskeletal Disorders, 17*(1), 35. https://doi.org/10.1186/s12891-016-0883-4

Arvidsson, I., Gremark Simonsen, J., Lindegård-Andersson, A., Björk, J., & Nordander, C. (2020). The impact of occupational and personal factors on musculoskeletal pain—A cohort study of female nurses, sonographers and teachers. *BMC Musculoskeletal Disorders, 21*(1), 621. https://doi.org/10.1186/s12891-020-03640-4

Balogh, I., Arvidsson, I., Björk, J., Hansson, G. Å., Ohlsson, K., Skerfving, S., & Nordander, C. (2019). Work-related neck and upper limb disorders—quantitative exposure–response relationships adjusted for personal characteristics and psychosocial conditions. *BMC Musculoskeletal Disorders, 20*(1), 139. https://doi.org/10.1186/s12891-019-2491-6

Barone Gibbs, B., Kline, C. E., Huber, K. A., Paley, J. L., & Perera, S. (2021). Covid-19 shelter-at-home and work, lifestyle and well-being in desk workers. *Occupational Medicine, 71*(2), 86–94. https://doi.org/10.1093/occmed/kqab011

Berecki-Gisolf, J., Clay, F. J., Collie, A., & McClure, R. J. (2012). The impact of aging on work disability and return to work: Insights from workers' compensation claim records. *Journal of Occupational and Environmental Medicine, 54*(3), 318–327. https://doi.org/10.1097/JOM.0b013e31823fdf9d

Blustein, D. L., Perera, H. N., Diamonti, A. J., Gutowski, E., Meerkins, T., Davila, A., Erby, W., & Konowitz, L. (2020). The uncertain state of work in the U.S.: Profiles of decent work and precarious work. *Journal of Vocational Behavior, 122,* 103481. https://doi.org/10.1016/j.jvb.2020.103481

Bongers, P. M., Kremer, A. M., & ter Laak, J. (2002). Are psychosocial factors, risk factors for symptoms and signs of the shoulder, elbow, or hand/wrist?: A review of the epidemiological literature. *American Journal of Industrial Medicine, 41*(5), 315–342. https://doi.org/10.1002/ajim.10050

Borhany, T., Shahid, E., Siddique, W. A., & Ali, H. (2018). Musculoskeletal problems in frequent computer and internet users. *Journal of Family Medicine and Primary Care,* 7(2), 337–339. https://doi.org/10.4103/jfmpc.jfmpc_326_17

Bunzli, S., Singh, N., Mazza, D., Collie, A., Kosny, A., Ruseckaite, R., & Brijnath, B. (2017). Fear of (re)injury and return to work following compensable injury: Qualitative insights from key stakeholders in Victoria, Australia. *BMC Public Health,* 17(1), 313. https://doi.org/10.1186/s12889-017-4226-7

Burton, W. N., Pransky, G., Conti, D. J., Chen, C. Y., & Edington, D. W. (2004). The association of medical conditions and presenteeism. *Journal of Occupational and Environmental Medicine,* 46(6, Suppl.), S38–S45. https://doi.org/10.1097/01.jom.0000126687.49652.44

Buys, N. J., Selander, J., & Sun, J. (2019). Employee experience of workplace supervisor contact and support during long-term sickness absence. *Disability and Rehabilitation,* 41(7), 808–814. https://doi.org/10.1080/09638288.2017.1410584

Corbière, M., Negrini, A., Durand, M. J., St-Arnaud, L., Briand, C., Fassier, J. B., Loisel, P., & Lachance, J. P. (2017). Development of the Return-to-Work Obstacles and Self-Efficacy Scale (ROSES) and validation with workers suffering from a common mental disorder or musculoskeletal disorder. *Journal of Occupational Rehabilitation,* 27(3), 329–341. https://doi.org/10.1007/s10926-016-9661-2

Cullen, K. L., Irvin, E., Collie, A., Clay, F., Gensby, U., Jennings, P. A., Hogg-Johnson, S., Kristman, V., Laberge, M., McKenzie, D., Newnam, S., Palagyi, A., Ruseckaite, R., Sheppard, D. M., Shourie, S., Steenstra, I., Van Eerd, D., & Amick, B. C., III. (2018). Effectiveness of workplace interventions in return-to-work for musculoskeletal, pain-related and mental health conditions: An update of the evidence and messages for practitioners. *Journal of Occupational Rehabilitation,* 28(1), 1–15. https://doi.org/10.1007/s10926-016-9690-x

da Costa, B. R., & Vieira, E. R. (2010). Risk factors for work-related musculoskeletal disorders: A systematic review of recent longitudinal studies. *American Journal of Industrial Medicine,* 53(3), 285–323. https://doi.org/10.1002/ajim.20750

Dawson, D., & McCulloch, K. (2005). Managing fatigue: It's about sleep. *Sleep Medicine Reviews,* 9(5), 365–380. https://doi.org/10.1016/j.smrv.2005.03.002

Evanoff, B., Dale, A. M., & Descatha, A. (2014). A conceptual model of musculoskeletal disorders for occupational health practitioners. *International Journal of Occupational Medicine and Environmental Health,* 27(1), 145–148. https://doi.org/10.2478/s13382-014-0232-5

Franklin, G. M., Wickizer, T. M., Coe, N. B., & Fulton-Kehoe, D. (2015). Workers' compensation: Poor quality health care and the growing disability problem in the United States. *American Journal of Industrial Medicine,* 58(3), 245–251. https://doi.org/10.1002/ajim.22399

Garza, J. L., Ferguson, J. M., Dugan, A. G., Decker, R. E., Laguerre, R. A., Suleiman, A. O., & Cavallari, J. M. (2022). Investigating the relationship between working time characteristics on musculoskeletal symptoms: A cross sectional study. *Archives of Environmental & Occupational Health,* 77(2), 141–148. https://doi.org/10.1080/19338244.2020.1860878

Gignac, M. A. M., Bowring, J., Jetha, A., Beaton, D. E., Breslin, F. C., Franche, R. L., Irvin, E., Macdermid, J. C., Shaw, W. S., Smith, P. M., Thompson, A., Tompa, E., Van Eerd, D., & Saunders, R. (2021). Disclosure, privacy and workplace accommodation of episodic disabilities: Organizational perspectives on disability communication-support processes to sustain employment. *Journal of Occupational Rehabilitation, 31*(1), 153–165. https://doi.org/10.1007/s10926-020-09901-2

Gould-Werth, A., Morrison, K., & Ben-Shalom, Y. (2018). Employers' perspectives on accommodating and retaining employees with newly acquired disabilities: An exploratory study. *Journal of Occupational Rehabilitation, 28*(4), 611–633. https://doi.org/10.1007/s10926-018-9806-6

Gray, H., Adefolarin, A. T., & Howe, T. E. (2011). A systematic review of instruments for the assessment of work-related psychosocial factors (Blue Flags) in individuals with non-specific low back pain. *Manual Therapy, 16*(6), 531–543. https://doi.org/10.1016/j.math.2011.04.001

Hagberg, M., Violante, F. S., Bonfiglioli, R., Descatha, A., Gold, J., Evanoff, B., & Sluiter, J. K. (2012). Prevention of musculoskeletal disorders in workers: Classification and health surveillance—statements of the Scientific Committee on Musculoskeletal Disorders of the International Commission on Occupational Health. *BMC Musculoskeletal Disorders, 13*(1), 109. https://doi.org/10.1186/1471-2474-13-109

Härmä, M., Ropponen, A., Hakola, T., Koskinen, A., Vanttola, P., Puttonen, S., Sallinen, M., Salo, P., Oksanen, T., Pentti, J., Vahtera, J., & Kivimäki, M. (2015). Developing register-based measures for assessment of working time patterns for epidemiologic studies. *Scandinavian Journal of Work, Environment & Health, 41*(3), 268–279. https://doi.org/10.5271/sjweh.3492

Hill, M. J., Maestas, N., & Mullen, K. J. (2016). Employer accommodation and labor supply of disabled workers. *Labour Economics, 41*, 291–303.

IJmker, S., Huysmans, M. A., Blatter, B. M., van der Beek, A. J., van Mechelen, W., & Bongers, P. M. (2007). Should office workers spend fewer hours at their computer? A systematic review of the literature. *Occupational and Environmental Medicine, 64*(4), 211–222. https://doi.org/10.1136/oem.2006.026468

Jetha, A., LaMontagne, A. D., Lilley, R., Hogg-Johnson, S., Sim, M., & Smith, P. (2018). Workplace social system and sustained return-to-work: A study of supervisor and co-worker supportiveness and injury reaction. *Journal of Occupational Rehabilitation, 28*(3), 486–494. https://doi.org/10.1007/s10926-017-9724-z

Jetha, A., Yanar, B., Lay, A. M., & Mustard, C. (2019). Work disability management communication bottlenecks within large and complex public service organizations: A sociotechnical systems study. *Journal of Occupational Rehabilitation, 29*(4), 754–763. https://doi.org/10.1007/s10926-019-09836-3

Jonsson, R., Dellve, L., & Halleröd, B. (2019). Work despite poor health? A 14-year follow-up of how individual work accommodations are extending the time to retirement for workers with poor health conditions. *SSM—Population Health, 9*, 100514. https://doi.org/10.1016/j.ssmph.2019.100514

Kaye, H. S., Jans, L. H., & Jones, E. C. (2011). Why don't employers hire and retain workers with disabilities? *Journal of Occupational Rehabilitation, 21*(4), 526–536. https://doi.org/10.1007/s10926-011-9302-8

Kensbock, J. M., Boehm, S. A., & Bourovoi, K. (2017). Is there a downside of job accommodations? An employee perspective on individual change processes. *Frontiers in Psychology, 8*, 1536. https://doi.org/10.3389/fpsyg.2017.01536

Kirmizi, M., Yalcinkaya, G., & Sengul, Y. S. (2021). Gender differences in health anxiety and musculoskeletal symptoms during the COVID-19 pandemic. *Journal of Back and Musculoskeletal Rehabilitation, 34*(2), 161–167. https://doi.org/10.3233/BMR-200301

Kristman, V. L., Shaw, W. S., Reguly, P., Williams-Whitt, K., Soklaridis, S., & Loisel, P. (2017). Supervisor and organizational factors associated with supervisor support of job accommodations for low back injured workers. *Journal of Occupational Rehabilitation, 27*(1), 115–127. https://doi.org/10.1007/s10926-016-9638-1

Lappalainen, L., Liira, J., & Lamminpää, A. (2021). Work disability negotiations between supervisors and occupational health services: Factors that support supervisors in work disability management. *International Archives of Occupational and Environmental Health, 94*(4), 689–697. https://doi.org/10.1007/s00420-020-01623-5

Lappalainen, L., Liira, J., Lamminpää, A., & Rokkanen, T. (2019). Work disability negotiations: Supervisors' view of work disability and collaboration with occupational health services. *Disability and Rehabilitation, 41*(17), 2015–2025. https://doi.org/10.1080/09638288.2018.1455112

Loeppke, R. R., Schill, A. L., Chosewood, L. C., Grosch, J. W., Allweiss, P., Burton, W. N., Barnes-Farrell, J. L., Goetzel, R. Z., Heinen, L., Hudson, T. W., Hymel, P., Merchant, J., Edington, D. W., Konicki, D. L., & Larson, P. W. (2013). Advancing workplace health protection and promotion for an aging workforce. *Journal of Occupational and Environmental Medicine, 55*(5), 500–506. https://doi.org/10.1097/JOM.0b013e31829613a4

MacEachen, E., Clarke, J., Franche, R. L., Irvin, E., & the Workplace-based Return to Work Literature Review Group. (2006). Systematic review of the qualitative literature on return to work after injury. *Scandinavian Journal of Work, Environment & Health, 32*(4), 257–269. https://doi.org/10.5271/sjweh.1009

Madeleine, P., Vangsgaard, S., Hviid Andersen, J., Ge, H. Y., & Arendt-Nielsen, L. (2013). Computer work and self-reported variables on anthropometrics, computer usage, work ability, productivity, pain, and physical activity. *BMC Musculoskeletal Disorders, 14*(1), 226. https://doi.org/10.1186/1471-2474-14-226

Main, C. J., & Shaw, W. S. (2016). Conceptual, methodological, and measurement challenges in addressing return to work in workers with musculoskeletal disorders. In I. Z. Schultz & R. J. Gatchel (Eds.), *Handbook of return to work* (pp. 423–438). Springer. https://doi.org/10.1007/978-1-4899-7627-7_24

Main, C. J., Shaw, W. S., & the Hopkinton Conference Working Group on Workplace Disability Prevention. (2016). Employer policies and practices to manage and prevent disability: Conclusion to the special issue. *Journal of Occupational Rehabilitation, 26*(4), 490–498. https://doi.org/10.1007/s10926-016-9655-0

Main, C. J., Shaw, W. S., & Mitchell, J. (2016). Towards an approach to return to work interventions in musculoskeletal disorders. In I. Z. Schultz & R. J. Gatchel (Eds.), *Handbook of return to work* (pp. 439–457). Springer. https://doi.org/10.1007/978-1-4899-7627-7_25

Majumdar, P., Biswas, A., & Sahu, S. (2020). COVID-19 pandemic and lockdown: Cause of sleep disruption, depression, somatic pain, and increased screen exposure of office workers and students of India. *Chronobiology International, 37*(8), 1191–1200. https://doi.org/10.1080/07420528.2020.1786107

Marcum, J., & Adams, D. (2017). Work-related musculoskeletal disorder surveillance using the Washington state workers' compensation system: Recent declines and patterns by industry, 1999–2013. *American Journal of Industrial Medicine, 60*(5), 457–471. https://doi.org/10.1002/ajim.22708

Mayer, J., Kraus, T., & Ochsmann, E. (2012). Longitudinal evidence for the association between work-related physical exposures and neck and/or shoulder complaints: A systematic review. *International Archives of Occupational and Environmental Health, 85*(6), 587–603. https://doi.org/10.1007/s00420-011-0701-0

McBeth, J., & Jones, K. (2007). Epidemiology of chronic musculoskeletal pain. *Best Practice & Research Clinical Rheumatology, 21*(3), 403–425. https://doi.org/10.1016/j.berh.2007.03.003

Merkus, S. L., Mathiassen, S. E., Lunde, L. K., Koch, M., Wærsted, M., Forsman, M., Knardahl, S., & Veiersted, K. B. (2021). Can a metric combining arm elevation and trapezius muscle activity predict neck/shoulder pain? A prospective cohort study in construction and healthcare. *International Archives of Occupational and Environmental Health, 94*(4), 647–658. https://doi.org/10.1007/s00420-020-01610-w

Min, K. B., Park, S. G., Song, J. S., Yi, K. H., Jang, T. W., & Min, J. Y. (2013). Subcontractors and increased risk for work-related diseases and absenteeism. *American Journal of Industrial Medicine, 56*(11), 1296–1306. https://doi.org/10.1002/ajim.22219

Miranda, H., Viikari-Juntura, E., Heistaro, S., Heliövaara, M., & Riihimäki, H. (2005). A population study on differences in the determinants of a specific shoulder disorder versus nonspecific shoulder pain without clinical findings. *American Journal of Epidemiology, 161*(9), 847–855. https://doi.org/10.1093/aje/kwi112

Mustard, C., Cole, D., Shannon, H., Pole, J., Sullivan, T., & Allingham, R. (2003). Declining trends in work-related morbidity and disability, 1993–1998: A comparison of survey estimates and compensation insurance claims. *American Journal of Public Health, 93*(8), 1283–1286. https://doi.org/10.2105/AJPH.93.8.1283

Nagata, T., Ito, D., Nagata, M., Fujimoto, A., Ito, R., Odagami, K., Kajiki, S., Uehara, M., Oyama, I., Dohi, S., Fujino, Y., & Mori, K. (2021). Anticipated health effects and proposed countermeasures following the immediate introduction of telework in response to the spread of COVID-19: The findings of a rapid health impact assessment in Japan. *Journal of Occupational Health, 63*(1), e12198. https://doi.org/10.1002/1348-9585.12198

National Institute for Occupational Safety and Health. (2015). *Musculoskeletal disorders. NIOSH Program Portfolio.* Retrieved from https://www.cdc.gov/niosh/programs/msd/

National Research Council, Committee on the Health and Safety Needs of Older Workers. (2004). *Health and safety needs of older workers.* National Academies Press.

National Research Council and Institute of Medicine Panel on Musculoskeletal Disorders in the Workplace. (2001). *Musculoskeletal disorders and the workplace: Low back and upper extremities.* National Academies Press.

Nicholas, M. K., Linton, S. J., Watson, P. J., Main, C. J., & the "Decade of the Flags" Working Group. (2011). Early identification and management of psychological risk factors ("yellow flags") in patients with low back pain: A reappraisal. *Physical Therapy, 91*(5), 737–753. https://doi.org/10.2522/ptj.20100224

Nordander, C., Hansson, G. Å., Ohlsson, K., Arvidsson, I., Balogh, I., Strömberg, U., Rittner, R., & Skerfving, S. (2016). Exposure–response relationships for work-related neck and shoulder musculoskeletal disorders—Analyses of pooled uniform data sets. *Applied Ergonomics, 55,* 70–84. https://doi.org/10.1016/j.apergo.2016.01.010

Park, S., & Lee, J. H. (2021). Precarious employment and increased incidence of musculoskeletal pain among wage workers in Korea: A cross-sectional study. *International Journal of Environmental Research and Public Health, 18*(12), 6299. https://doi.org/10.3390/ijerph18126299

Punnett, L. (2014). Musculoskeletal disorders and occupational exposures: How should we judge the evidence concerning the causal association? *Scandinavian Journal of Public Health, 42*(13, Suppl.), 49–58. https://doi.org/10.1177/1403494813517324

Punnett, L., & Bergqvist, U. (1997). *Visual display unit work and upper extremity musculoskeletal disorders: A review of epidemiological findings.* National [Sweden] Institute for Working Life. https://core.ac.uk/download/pdf/16312236.pdf

Ricci, J. A., Stewart, W. F., Chee, E., Leotta, C., Foley, K., & Hochberg, M. C. (2006). Back pain exacerbations and lost productive time costs in United States workers. *Spine, 31*(26), 3052–3060. https://doi.org/10.1097/01.brs.0000249521.61813.aa

Safiri, S., Kolahi, A. A., Cross, M., Hill, C., Smith, E., Carson-Chahhoud, K., Mansournia, M. A., Almasi-Hashiani, A., Ashrafi-Asgarabad, A., Kaufman, J., Sepidarkish, M., Shakouri, S. K., Hoy, D., Woolf, A. D., March, L., Collins, G., & Buchbinder, R. (2021). Prevalence, deaths, and disability-adjusted life years due to musculoskeletal disorders for 195 countries and territories 1990–2017. *Arthritis & Rheumatology, 73*(4), 702–714. https://doi.org/10.1002/art.41571

Sargeant, M. (2014). Domestic workers: Vulnerable workers in precarious work. *E-Journal of International and Comparative Labour Studies, 3*(1). https://ejcls.adapt.it/index.php/ejcls_adapt/article/view/152

Schandelmaier, S., Ebrahim, S., Burkhardt, S. C., de Boer, W. E., Zumbrunn, T., Guyatt, G. H., Busse, J. W., & Kunz, R. (2012). Return to work coordination programmes for work disability: A meta-analysis of randomised controlled trials. *PLOS ONE, 7*(11), e49760. https://doi.org/10.1371/journal.pone.0049760

Schreuder, J. A., Groothoff, J. W., Jongsma, D., van Zweeden, N. F., van der Klink, J. J., & Roelen, C. A. (2013). Leadership effectiveness: A supervisor's approach to manage return to work. *Journal of Occupational Rehabilitation, 23*(3), 428–437. https://doi.org/10.1007/s10926-012-9409-6

Sears, J. M., Schulman, B. A., Fulton-Kehoe, D., & Hogg-Johnson, S. (2021). Workplace organizational and psychosocial factors associated with return-to-work interruption and reinjury among workers with permanent impairment. *Annals of Work Exposures and Health, 65*(5), 566–580. https://doi.org/10.1093/annweh/wxaa133

Shaw, W. S., Kristman, V. L., Williams-Whitt, K., Soklaridis, S., Huang, Y. H., Côté, P., & Loisel, P. (2014). The Job Accommodation Scale (JAS): Psychometric evaluation of a new measure of employer support for temporary job modifications. *Journal of Occupational Rehabilitation, 24*(4), 755–765. https://doi.org/10.1007/s10926-014-9508-7

Shaw, W. S., Main, C. J., Pransky, G., Nicholas, M. K., Anema, J. R., Linton, S. J., & the Hopkinton Conference Working Group on Workplace Disability Prevention. (2016). Employer policies and practices to manage and prevent disability: Foreword to the special issue. *Journal of Occupational Rehabilitation, 26*(4), 394–398. https://doi.org/10.1007/s10926-016-9658-x

Shultz, K. S., & Adams, G. A. (2012). *Aging and work in the 21st century.* Psychology Press.

Silverstein, M. (2008). Meeting the challenges of an aging workforce. *American Journal of Industrial Medicine, 51*(4), 269–280. https://doi.org/10.1002/ajim.20569

Smith, P., LaMontagne, A. D., Lilley, R., Hogg-Johnson, S., & Sim, M. (2020). Are there differences in the return to work process for work-related psychological and musculoskeletal injuries? A longitudinal path analysis. *Social Psychiatry and Psychiatric Epidemiology, 55*(8), 1041–1051. https://doi.org/10.1007/s00127-020-01839-3

Spector, J. T., & Reul, N. K. (2017). Promoting early, safe return to work in injured employees: A randomized trial of a supervisor training intervention in a healthcare setting. *Journal of Occupational Rehabilitation, 27*(1), 70–81. https://doi.org/10.1007/s10926-016-9633-6

Steenstra, I. A., Munhall, C., Irvin, E., Oranye, N., Passmore, S., Van Eerd, D., Mahood, Q., & Hogg-Johnson, S. (2017). Systematic review of prognostic factors for return to work in workers with sub acute and chronic low back pain. *Journal of Occupational Rehabilitation, 27*(3), 369–381. https://doi.org/10.1007/s10926-016-9666-x

Stynen, D., Jansen, N. W., Slangen, J. J., & Kant, I. (2016). Impact of development and accommodation practices on older workers' job characteristics, prolonged fatigue, work engagement, and retirement intentions over time. *Journal of Occupational and Environmental Medicine, 58*(11), 1055–1065. https://doi.org/10.1097/JOM.0000000000000853

Tamers, S. L., Streit, J., Pana-Cryan, R., Ray, T., Syron, L., Flynn, M. A., Castillo, D., Roth, G., Geraci, C., Guerin, R., Schulte, P., Henn, S., Chang, C. C., Felknor, S., & Howard, J. (2020). Envisioning the future of work to safeguard the safety, health, and well-being of the workforce: A perspective from the CDC's National Institute for Occupational Safety and Health. *American Journal of Industrial Medicine, 63*(12), 1065–1084. https://doi.org/10.1002/ajim.23183

Toossi, M. (2015). Labor force projections to 2024: The labor force is growing, but slowly. *Monthly Labor Review.* U.S. Bureau of Labor Statistics. https://doi.org/10.21916/mlr.2015.48

Tveito, T. H., Shaw, W. S., Huang, Y. H., Nicholas, M., & Wagner, G. (2010). Managing pain in the workplace: A focus group study of challenges, strategies and what matters most to workers with low back pain. *Disability and Rehabilitation, 32*(24), 2035–2045. https://doi.org/10.3109/09638281003797398

U.S. Bureau of Labor Statistics. (2020). *Fact sheet: Occupational injuries and illnesses resulting in musculoskeletal disorders (MSDs), May 2020*. https://www.bls.gov/iif/oshwc/case/msds.htm

van den Heuvel, S. G., van der Beek, A. J., Blatter, B. M., Hoogendoorn, W. E., & Bongers, P. M. (2005). Psychosocial work characteristics in relation to neck and upper limb symptoms. *Pain, 114*(1), 47–53. https://doi.org/10.1016/j.pain.2004.12.008

van Rijn, R. M., Huisstede, B. M., Koes, B. W., & Burdorf, A. (2010). Associations between work-related factors and specific disorders of the shoulder—A systematic review of the literature. *Scandinavian Journal of Work, Environment & Health, 36*(3), 189–201. https://doi.org/10.5271/sjweh.2895

van Vilsteren, M., van Oostrom, S. H., de Vet, H. C., Franche, R. L., Boot, C. R., & Anema, J. R. (2015). Workplace interventions to prevent work disability in workers on sick leave. *Cochrane Database of Systematic Reviews*. https://doi.org/10.1002/14651858.CD006955.pub3

Varekamp, I., & van Dijk, F. J. (2010). Workplace problems and solutions for employees with chronic diseases. *Occupational Medicine, 60*(4), 287–293. https://doi.org/10.1093/occmed/kqq078

Vives, A., Amable, M., Ferrer, M., Moncada, S., Llorens, C., Muntaner, C., Benavides, F. G., & Benach, J. (2013). Employment precariousness and poor mental health: Evidence from Spain on a new social determinant of health. *Journal of Environmental and Public Health, 2013*, 978656. https://doi.org/10.1155/2013/978656

Wærsted, M., Hanvold, T. N., & Veiersted, K. B. (2010). Computer work and musculoskeletal disorders of the neck and upper extremity: A systematic review. *BMC Musculoskeletal Disorders, 11*(1), 79. https://doi.org/10.1186/1471-2474-11-79

Ward, B. W., & Schiller, J. S. (2013). Prevalence of multiple chronic conditions among US adults: Estimates from the National Health Interview Survey, 2010. *Preventing Chronic Disease, 10*, 120203. https://doi.org/10.5888/pcd10.120203

Williams, R. M., & Westmorland, M. (2002). Perspectives on workplace disability management: A review of the literature. *Work, 19*(1), 87–93.

Williams-Whitt, K., Kristman, V., Shaw, W. S., Soklaridis, S., & Reguly, P. (2016). A model of supervisor decision-making in the accommodation of workers with low back pain. *Journal of Occupational Rehabilitation, 26*(3), 366–381. https://doi.org/10.1007/s10926-015-9623-0

Wong, J., Kallish, N., Crown, D., Capraro, P., Trierweiler, R., Wafford, Q. E., Tiema-Benson, L., Hassan, S., Engel, E., Tamayo, C., & Heinemann, A. W. (2021). Job accommodations, return to work and job retention of people with physical disabilities: A systematic review. *Journal of Occupational Rehabilitation, 31*(3), 474–490. https://doi.org/10.1007/s10926-020-09954-3

Wong, K., Chan, A. H. S., & Ngan, S. C. (2019). The effect of long working hours and overtime on occupational health: A meta-analysis of evidence from 1998 to 2018. *International Journal of Environmental Research and Public Health, 16*(12), 2102. https://doi.org/10.3390/ijerph16122102

World Health Organization. (2001). *International classification of functioning, disability, and health (ICF)*.

Wynne-Jones, G., Buck, R., Porteous, C., Cooper, L., Button, L. A., Main, C. J., & Phillips, C. J. (2011). What happens to work if you're unwell? Beliefs and attitudes of managers and employees with musculoskeletal pain in a public sector setting. *Journal of Occupational Rehabilitation, 21*(1), 31–42. https://doi.org/10.1007/s10926-010-9251-7

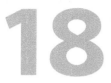

Alcohol and Illicit Drug Involvement in the Workforce and Workplace

Michael R. Frone and Peter A. Bamberger

Substance involvement[1] (SI) represents a significant public and occupational health issue that imposes economic and health-related societal costs (Davenport et al., 2019; Hedegaard et al., 2020; National Drug Intelligence Center, 2011; Office of the Surgeon General, 2016; Sacks et al., 2015). Moreover, employee SI is of interest to managers, unions, and policy makers because it may lead to adverse effects in the workplace, and the workplace may cause or exacerbate employee SI (Frone, 2019). Despite the importance of these general issues, occupational health psychologists have devoted little systematic attention to employee SI. Therefore, we briefly summarize the literature on this issue. We begin by exploring the prevalence of alcohol and illicit drug involvement among employees. Next, we turn to the leading causes and consequences of employee SI and conclude with an overview of work-based interventions. Before turning to these issues, we should note that this chapter

---

[1]We use the broad term *substance involvement* to acknowledge the importance of viewing the consumption of psychoactive substances as a multidimensional construct and to refer to all dimensions involving their consumption collectively. See Frone (2013, 2019) for a discussion of substance involvement's key dimensions and their definitions.

Portions of this chapter are adapted from "Alcohol, Drugs, and Workplace Safety Outcomes: A View From a General Model of Employee Substance Use and Productivity," by M. R. Frone, in J. Barling & M. R. Frone (Eds.), *The Psychology of Workplace Safety* (pp. 127–156), 2004, American Psychological Association (https://doi.org/10.1037/10662-007). Copyright 2004 by the American Psychological Association; and adapted from *Alcohol and Illicit Drug Use in the Workforce and Workplace*, by M. R. Frone, 2013, American Psychological Association (https://doi.org/10.1037/13944-000). Copyright 2013 by the American Psychological Association.

https://doi.org/10.1037/0000331-018
Handbook of Occupational Health Psychology, Third Edition, L. E. Tetrick, G. G. Fisher, M. T. Ford, and J. C. Quick (Editors)

does not present a comprehensive overview of the association between SI and the workforce and workplace. Therefore, we refer the interested reader to two broader reviews (Frone, 2013, 2019).

PREVALENCE OF EMPLOYEE SI

We briefly summarize various U.S. prevalence data and trends based on three national surveys: National Survey on Drug Use and Health (NSDUH), National Survey Workplace Health and Safety (NSWHS), and National Survey of Work Stress and Health (NSWSH). Although little prevalence data exist for employee SI outside the United States, the available prevalence data suggest patterns similar to those found in the United States (for additional information, see Frone 2013).

We begin this section by presenting the prevalence of overall SI in the U.S. workforce, which primarily reflects SI away from the workplace and outside work hours (i.e., off-the-job involvement). We then turn to prevalence data that captures the temporal context of employee SI. As described by Frone (2019):

> Temporal context refers to EPSI [employee psychoactive substance involvement] in relation to the workday—(*a*) before work (i.e., within 2 h of starting one's work shift), (*b*) during the workday (i.e., while performing one's job and during lunch and other breaks), and (*c*) after work (i.e., within 2 h of leaving work). Any involvement (i.e., use or impairment) before or during the workday represents workplace involvement. Although substance involvement after work represents overall workforce (off-the-job) substance involvement, it may be more responsive to workplace experiences than are broader measures that also capture substance involvement on nonwork days. (p. 278)

Overall Employee SI

Table 18.1 presents prevalence estimates for several dimensions of overall SI based on 2019 NSDUH data (see the table notes for relevant variable definitions). As shown in the table, 77.3% of U.S. workers report any use of alcohol during the past year, and 62.7% report any use of alcohol during the past month. Binge drinking during the past month is prevalent among workers (31.1%), though heavy drinking (i.e., frequent binge drinking) occurs among a minority of workers (7.5%). The overall prevalence of any illicit substance use among workers is 20.4% and 14.4% during the past year and month, respectively. The most widely used illicit substance is cannabis (20.1% and 12.9% during the past year and past month, respectively), followed by any illicit use of prescription pain relievers (3.8% and 1% during the past year and past month, respectively). Moreover, Table 18.1 reveals that 6.5% of workers have a current alcohol use disorder and 2.9% have a current illicit drug use disorder. Although not shown in the table, 2019 NSDUH data reveal that 1.2% of employed adults receive treatment annually for these disorders, and 8.5% are in recovery or have recovered from an SI problem.

TABLE 18.1. Prevalence of Overall Substance Involvement in the U.S. Workforce

Substance	Past year use	Past month use	Past year substance use disorder[a]
Any alcohol use	77.3%	62.7%	6.5%
Binge drinking[b]	ND	31.1%	ND
Heavy drinking[c]	ND	7.5%	ND
Any illicit substance use[d]	20.4%	14.4%	2.9%
Cannabis	20.1%	12.9%	1.7%
Cocaine (crack)	2.3%	0.8%	0.3%
Hallucinogens	2.6%	0.8%	0.1%
Inhalants	0.6%	0.3%	0%
Methamphetamine	0.6%	0.4%	0.4%
Heroin (opioid)	0.2%	0.1%	0.1%
Pain relievers (opioids)	3.8%	1%	0.5%
Stimulants	2.3%	0.7%	0.2%
Tranquilizers	2.1%	0.7%	0.2%
Sedatives	0.5%	0.1%	0.04%

Note. Substance involvement estimates are from the 2019 National Survey of Drug Use and Health, calculated using the Substance Abuse and Mental Health Services Administration's (SAMHSA) public online data analysis system (PDAS; https://pdas.samhsa.gov/#/). ND = Not determined.
[a]*Substance use disorder* refers to meeting criteria for illicit drug or alcohol dependence or abuse based on definitions in the fourth edition of the *Diagnostic and Statistical Manual of Mental Disorders* (American Psychiatric Association, 2000). Also see Frone (2013, 2019).
[b]*Binge drinking* refers to drinking five or more drinks for males or four or more drinks for females on the same occasion (i.e., at the same time or within a couple of hours of each other) on at least one day in the past 30 days.
[c]*Heavy drinking* is defined as binge drinking on five or more days in the past 30 days.
[d]*Illicit substance use* refers to (a) the use of psychoactive substances that are illegal to possess and unavailable by medical prescription or (b) the illicit (i.e., recreational, nonmedical) use of any psychotherapeutic substance requiring a medical prescription, which occurs when used without a prescription or used with a prescription, but more frequently or in higher doses than prescribed.

Data on employee SI trends based on NSDUH data (Center for Behavioral Health Statistics & Quality, 2015) indicate a relatively stable overall prevalence of any past-month illicit drug use in the U.S. workforce between 1998 (9%) and 2004 (10%; Walsh, 2008). Between 2004 and 2016, the prevalence of any past-month illicit drug use remained relatively stable, increasing two percentage points from 10% to 12% (Frone, 2019). Furthermore, NSDUH data from 2002 to 2014 for the adult U.S. population suggest that this net increase in the prevalence of overall illicit drug use is primarily due to increased cannabis use (Frone, 2019), which is likely the result of growing state-level legalization. Canadian national data show an increase in overall cannabis use associated with nationwide legalization—14% pre-legalization in 2018 and 17.5% and 20% post-legalization in 2019 and 2020, respectively (Rotermann, 2021).

Temporal Context of Employee SI

The prevalence of employee SI by temporal context comes from the NSWHS (Frone, 2006a, 2006b, 2013) and NSWSH (Frone, 2019) and is shown in Table 18.2 (see the table notes for relevant definitions). Fewer than 2% of workers reported alcohol use before work and alcohol intoxication during the

TABLE 18.2. Prevalence of Contextual Substance Involvement in the U.S. Workforce

Substance and context of use	Survey years	Past year use	Monthly or more frequent use	Less than monthly use
Alcohol use before work	2002–2003	1.7%	0.5%	1.2%
	2008–2011	1.4%	0.4%	1%
Alcohol use during the workday	2002–2003	7%	2.6%	4.4%
	2008–2011	6%	1.9%	4.1%
Alcohol intoxication during the workday	2002–2003	1.7%	0.7%	1%
	2008–2011	1.4%	0.7%	0.7%
Alcohol hangover at work	2002–2003	9.1%	1.8%	7.3%
	2008–2011	8.8%	2.1%	6.8%
Any workplace alcohol use or impairment[a]	2002–2003	15.2%	4.5%	10.7%
	2008–2011	13.8%	3.6%	10.2%
Alcohol use after work	2002–2003	37.8%	24.7%	13.1%
	2008–2011	47.5%	28.1%	19.4%
Illicit drug use before work	2002–2003	2.7%	1.9%	0.8%
Illicit drug use during the workday	2002–2003	2.4%	1.7%	0.7%
Illicit drug intoxication during the workday	2002–2003	2.8%	1.8%	1%
Any workplace illicit drug use or impairment[a]	2002–2003	3.3%	2.4%	0.9%
Illicit drug use after work	2002–2003	5.7%	3.7%	2%

Note. Prevalence estimates for alcohol use were obtained from the National Survey of Workplace Health and Safety (Frone, 2006a, 2013; data collected from January 2002 to June 2003) and the National Survey of Work Stress and Health (Frone, 2019; data collected from December 2008 to April 2011). Prevalence estimates for illicit drug use were obtained from the National Survey of Workplace Health and Safety (Frone, 2006b, 2013; data collected from January 2002 to June 2003). From "Employee Psychoactive Substance Involvement: Historical Context, Key Findings, and Future Directions," by M. R. Frone, 2019, *Annual Review of Organizational Psychology and Organizational Behavior, 6*(1), pp. 273–297 (https://doi.org/10.1146/annurev-orgpsych-012218-015231). Copyright 2019 by Annual Reviews. Reprinted with permission.
[a]*Any workplace use or impairment* includes use before work, use during the workday, intoxication during the workday, or hangover during the workday.

workday. Roughly 6% to 7% of workers reported alcohol use during the workday (primarily during lunch breaks), with 9% of workers experiencing a hangover during the workday. The overall prevalence of any workplace alcohol use or impairment was 13.8% to 15.2%. Alcohol use after work was reported by 37.8% to 47.5% of workers. Workplace illicit drug use (before or during work) or impairment was reported by 2.4% to 2.8% of workers, with 3.3% reporting any workplace use or impairment. Illicit drug use after work was reported by 5.7% of workers.

Finally, the multidimensional nature of employee SI appears to be important. For example, Frone (2016a) found that during the 2008 recession, the proportion of drinkers increased compared to before the recession among middle-aged but not among young employees. Moreover, the recession was not related to drinkers' usual frequency or quantity of use. However, the recession was related to a higher frequency of heavy drinking and intoxication. Further, consistent with concerns over job security, the recession was negatively associated with the frequency and quantity of workday alcohol use and positively related to both dimensions of after-work alcohol use.

WORKPLACE CAUSES OF EMPLOYEE SI

The potential causes of employee SI can be classified along two primary dimensions (Frone, 2003, 2013): causes external to the workplace (e.g., demographic, genetic, personality, substance use outcome expectancies, environmental factors) and causes internal to the workplace (e.g., socialization and exposures at work). Because the latter tend to be of greater interest to occupational health psychologists, we focus on them in this chapter. For a summary of research on the key factors external to the workplace, see Frone (2013). The predictors of employee SI *internal* to the workplace represent four general dimensions: workplace substance use climate, workplace social control, work stressors, and chronic work-related pain.

Workplace Substance Use Climate

Workplace substance use climate represents employees' perceptions of the extent to which their work environment is supportive of SI at work (Frone, 2009, 2012). Ames and colleagues have suggested that workplace substance use climate comprises three dimensions (e.g., Ames & Grube, 1999; Ames & Janes, 1992). The first dimension is the perceived physical availability of alcohol and drugs at work, representing the ease of obtaining alcohol or other drugs at work and using them during work hours and breaks. Findings from the few studies that have examined the association of physical availability and employees' use of alcohol or illicit drugs are mixed. Macdonald et al. (1999) found that easy availability of substances was positively related to employee alcohol use problems. However, Ames and Grube (1999) failed to find an association between the physical availability of alcohol at work and drinking at work. Similarly, Frone (2003) found that the physical availability of alcohol and marijuana at work was unrelated to overall and workplace alcohol and marijuana use. However, more recently, Frone and Trinidad (2014) treated physical availability of alcohol at work and workplace alcohol use and impairment as multidimensional constructs and concluded that "perceived physical availability of alcohol at work is a risk factor for alcohol use and impairment during the workday, and that this association is more complex than previously hypothesized" (p. 1271).

The second and third dimensions of workplace substance use climate represent two types of social norms—descriptive and injunctive. Because these two constructs are related conceptually and empirically, they are discussed together. *Descriptive* workplace norms represent the extent to which members of an individual's workplace social network use or are impaired by alcohol or drugs at work. *Injunctive* norms represent the extent to which members of an individual's workplace social network approve of using or working under the influence of alcohol or drugs at work. Several studies collectively supported positive associations between descriptive or injunction workplace norms and overall or workplace SI (Ames & Grube, 1999; Bacharach et al., 2002; Bamberger & Cohen, 2015; Frone, 2003; Frone & Brown, 2010; Macdonald et al., 1999). For example, using a national sample of U.S. workers, Frone and Brown (2010) found that injunctive (but not descriptive) workplace alcohol norms were positively associated with more frequent overall alcohol use and intoxication. Both types of norms were positively associated with more frequent alcohol use before work, alcohol use and intoxication during the workday, and alcohol use after work. There were similar results for the associations of both types of workplace illicit substance use norms to overall and work-related illicit SI. Liu et al. (2015) found that in addition to descriptive norms held by organizational veterans, those held by clients were also associated with performance-oriented drinking motives and, as a result, hazardous alcohol consumption. Finally, Frone (2009, 2012) explored the association of workplace substance use climate to the work outcomes of most employees who do not use alcohol and drugs at work. The results revealed that all three dimensions of workplace substance use climate were negatively related to workplace safety and employee morale and positively related to work strain. These findings suggest that exposure to a permissive substance use climate at work may be relevant to the broader workforce that includes employees who do not use alcohol and drugs at work.

Workplace Social Control

SI may be higher among employees who are not integrated into or regulated by the work organization (Ames et al., 2000; Bacharach et al., 2002). Therefore, *workplace social control* refers to a broad set of work conditions that put employees at lower or higher risk of SI, such as levels of commitment or attachment to an organization, mobility during work hours, visibility of work behaviors, contact with or level of supervision, extent of formal and informal policies, and disciplinary actions regarding SI. Although several studies have shown a direct inverse association between workplace social control—in the form of supervisory policy enforcement—and employee SI (Ames et al., 2000; Bamberger & Cohen, 2015; Biron et al., 2011), others have suggested a more nuanced association. For example, using a national sample of 2,429 U.S. workers, Frone and Trinidad (2012) found no evidence linking the frequency of contact with supervisors with any of the 12 employee SI measures. In contrast, they found that supervisor enforcement of SI policies was inversely related to employee SI. However, the specific associations found were a joint function of the context of use (off the job vs. on the job) and the legality of the substance.

Workplace Stressors

Workplace stressors have received the most empirical attention as a risk factor for employee SI (for broader reviews, see Frone, 1999, 2013, 2019). It is widely believed that employee SI represents a strategy for coping with negative outcomes or strains resulting from exposure to aversive physical and psychosocial qualities of the work environment (Ames & Janes, 1992; Bacharach et al., 2002; Frone, 1999, 2019). This expectation derives from the notion of tension reduction developed in the literature on alcohol use (Conger, 1956). Generally stated, the tension-reduction hypothesis has two propositions. First, the *stress-response dampening proposition* posits that individuals will use substances before exposure to a stressor to avoid the experience of tension or strain resulting from the exposure (e.g., Sayette, 1999). Second, the *stress-induced substance use proposition* states that exposure to stressors will lead to substance use to mitigate the experienced tension and strain (e.g., Frone, 1999; Sayette, 1999).

Most work stress research has tested the stress-induced substance use proposition that more frequent or intense exposure to work stressors causes more frequent or heavier use of alcohol and drugs after exposure to the stressors. The general expectation that workplace stress is a cause of employee SI is consistent with several more recent conceptual frameworks positing that individuals self-medicate with psychoactive substances for affect regulation. These conceptual frameworks include affect regulation (Cooper et al., 1995), negative reinforcement (McCarthy et al., 2010), self-medication (Khantzian, 1997), and drug instrumentalization (Müller, 2020). In contrast, little research has tested the stress-response damping proposition that employees may use substances before exposure to work stressors to avoid anticipated negative affect.

Research testing the stress-induced substance use proposition regarding the link between work stressors and illicit substance use, although limited, suggests notable associations. Two studies found a positive association between job insecurity and overall illicit substance use (Colell et al., 2016; Kivimäki et al., 2007). Three studies found a positive association between aversive workplace conditions (e.g., high work demands, low decision latitude, workplace violence) and overall and workplace illicit substance use (Frone, 2008a; Madsen et al., 2011; Pelfrene et al., 2002).

More research has focused on the association between work-related stressors and alcohol use. Unfortunately, most research analyzing the direct association between work stressors and alcohol use has failed to support such an association (see Frone, 1999, 2019), although there are several notable exceptions. For instance, work–family conflict has been related to overall measures of employee alcohol use and misuse in cross-sectional and longitudinal studies (e.g., Frone, 2000; Frone et al., 1997). Similarly, aversive employment contexts such as a recession, downsizing, and perceived unfair treatment are positively associated with the frequency and quantity of consumption after work and heavy episodic (binge) drinking (Frone, 2016a, 2018).

One reason for the lack of a direct association between within-role work stressors and alcohol use may be that past research focused exclusively on measures of overall SI that assess consumption at times and in settings removed from the workday. Measures of SI that consider the temporal context of consumption may provide a more consistent link to work stressors (Frone, 1999). For instance, although Frone (2008a) failed to find support for a link between the within-role work stressors and measures of *overall* alcohol and illicit drug use, results indicated support for the associations of work stressors to alcohol and illicit drug use *before* work, *during* the workday, and *after* work. In addition, the temporal assessment of SI allowed tests of and provided support for both the stress-response dampening (i.e., SI before work) and stress-induced substance use (i.e., SI during and after work) propositions of the tension-reduction hypothesis (Frone, 2008a).

Another reason for the lack of a direct association between within-role work stressors and SI may be the focus on overall levels of stress and SI experienced over an extended period rather than on the direct effects of discrete work stressors (e.g., customer/client incivility) on contemporaneous (or near contemporaneous) SI. Demonstrating the efficacy of such an approach, Liu et al. (2009) found that for each unique stressful work event (assessed daily over 5 weeks), daily alcohol use increased by a factor of 1.21 later that same day.

Other researchers have begun to explore variables that may mediate or moderate the association between work stressors and SI. Although some studies of within-role work stressors failed to support the mediating role of negative affect (e.g., Cooper et al., 1990; Richman et al., 2002), other studies supported this indirect effect (e.g., Greenberg & Grunberg, 1995). In addition to negative affect, Delaney et al. (2002) found that the inability to unwind after work mediated the association between job problems and alcohol use. Several studies indicated a mediating role of negative affect in the association of work–family conflict and alcohol use (e.g., Frone et al., 1994). Additionally, building on self-medication models of SI, Bamberger and Cohen (2015) examined a mediational model among commercial truck drivers, finding that both role conflict and abusive supervision were positively associated with psychological distress, which was positively associated with the severity of alcohol misuse. Finally, Frone (2015) tested the mediating influence of negative and positive work rumination. The study found support for indirect positive associations between negative work conditions (e.g., work demands, emotionally unpleasant work) and both overall and workplace alcohol involvement via negative work rumination (i.e., negative work-related perseverative cognitions). In contrast, the findings revealed indirect negative associations between positive work conditions (e.g., distributive justice, emotionally pleasant work) and overall involvement via positive work rumination (i.e., positive work-related perseverative cognitions).

Several studies tested and provided support for *moderating* effects on the associations of both work stressors and work–family conflict to alcohol use (Bacharach et al., 2002; Frone et al., 1995; Grandey et al., 2019; Grunberg et al., 1999; Wang et al., 2010). For example, Frone et al. (1995) found that both job demands and role ambiguity were positively related to heavy drinking, but only among employees reporting that their work role was psychologically important for self-definition. Studies also suggested moderating effects for several of the

Big Five personality characteristics. Liu et al. (2009) found that a positive within-person association between negative work events and evening alcohol use was amplified among workers with high levels of neuroticism. Similarly, Bamberger and Bacharach (2006) observed that an association between abusive supervision and problem drinking was stronger among blue-collar workers low in conscientiousness.

Finally, several studies tested and supported moderated-mediation models of within-role work stressors and alcohol use. For example, Grunberg et al. (1998) found that work demands, interpersonal criticism from supervisors and coworkers, and feeling stuck in one's job were associated with job dissatisfaction, with the latter related to problem drinking (but only among those reporting drinking to reduce negative emotions). Wolff et al. (2013) demonstrated support for a moderated mediation model linking work–family conflict and the overall frequency of heavy alcohol use via negative affect, with the association between negative affect and heavy drinking being stronger among those maintaining strong tension-reduction alcohol expectancies. In a broader study, Frone (2016b) found that negative affect and work fatigue each mediated the association between a composite measure of work stressors and several dimensions of alcohol involvement—overall heavy use, workday use, and after-work use. In addition, the negative affect–mediated effects were strongest among men with strong tension-reduction alcohol expectancies, and the work fatigue–mediated effects were strongest among men with strong fatigue-reduction alcohol expectancies.

Work-Related Chronic Pain

In 2020, 2.7 million work injuries and illnesses were recorded in the United States (Bureau of Labor Statistics, 2021). Several studies have indicated that leading up to the opiate crisis, many employees experiencing chronic pain (e.g., back pain, carpal tunnel) were prescribed opiates. Indeed, a study in Washington state revealed 260 unintentional deaths from opioids prescribed to workers in that state's workers' compensation system between 1996 and 2002 (Franklin et al., 2005). Further evidence of a link between workplace injury and opioid fatalities can be found in cross-industry studies. Such studies have indicated that the rate of opioid overdose fatalities is up to 6 times higher than the national average in industries with high rates of work-related injuries and illnesses that lack paid sick leave policies (Harduar Morano et al., 2018; Massachusetts Department of Public Health, 2018).

ORGANIZATIONAL CONSEQUENCES OF EMPLOYEE SI

The organizational consequences of employee SI have received much attention and speculation in the literature. Although it is widely believed that employee use of psychoactive substances has a strong and consistent negative association with employee productivity, past research has suggested that these associations are neither consistent nor robust (Frone, 2004, 2013, 2019). After exploring the association of employee SI with three organizational consequences (i.e., attendance outcomes, task and contextual performance, and job accidents and injury outcomes), we describe a general model of SI and employee productivity, highlighting the potential complexity of these associations (Frone, 2004, 2013, 2019).

Attendance Outcomes

Sickness absenteeism represents the most frequently studied outcome of employee SI, with most studies finding a positive association between alcohol involvement and absenteeism (for a review, see Schou & Moan, 2016). Two likely mechanisms underlie this association: (a) poor health stemming from long-term heavy consumption and (b) heightened likelihood of impairment following episodes of heavy consumption. Consistent with this logic, Bacharach et al. (2010) found that the frequency of heavy episodic drinking (but not usual quantity and frequency of consumption) predicted absenteeism. Moreover, they found this association was weaker in contexts characterized by high levels of coworker support but amplified under conditions of high supervisor support. Still, findings regarding a link between illicit SI and absenteeism are more limited and mixed. On the one hand, Van Hasselt et al. (2015) found past-month illicit substance use was positively associated with the number of days absent in the past month, and that misuse of prescription medications significantly increases the probability of 1 or 2 missed workdays in the past month. On the other hand, Lim et al. (2000) saw no evidence of a link between a past-year illicit substance use disorder (SUD) and workdays missed.

Task and Contextual Performance

Basic laboratory research on the acute effects of alcohol suggest that blood alcohol concentrations (BAC) that are low (BAC $\leq$ .05%) to moderate (> .05%–.08%) do not impair simple dimensions of task performance (e.g., tracking, reaction, attention). However, low to moderate BACs may lead to psychomotor and cognitive deficits as task complexity increases. At high levels of BAC (> .08%), research more consistently reveals psychomotor and cognitive deficits. In general, impairment in cognitive and psychomotor performance increase as both the level of intoxication (BAC) and task complexity increase. Given the level of complexity and heterogeneity in the associations between other drugs and human performance, it is not possible to summarize that research literature. More detail can be found in Frone (2013).

Workplace simulation studies more directly mimic the tasks needed to perform specific jobs. A variety of workplace simulation studies have been conducted. However, these studies vary across several important dimensions, including sample size, sample type (e.g., those with experience in the simulated job vs. those with no experience), the simulated job (e.g., drill press operation, assembly jobs, welding, merchant ship power plant operation and piloting, managerial, and various surgical procedures), and the types of assessed outcomes. Given this heterogeneity and the fact that there is often only one study for a given job or task, it is challenging to provide generalizable conclusions. More detail on these workplace simulation studies can be found in Frone (2013).

Even though laboratory studies and workplace simulations often have strong internal validity, the statistically significant cognitive and psychomotor deficits may be weak in practical terms and offer limited external validity. Moreover, although field studies provide greater external validity than laboratory and simulation studies, research conducted over the past 30 years has mainly generated equivocal findings. For example, of the six studies conducted in the United States, the United Kingdom, China, and Australia since 2000, three (Kirkham et al., 2015; Shi et al., 2013; Yu et al., 2015) reported a significant positive association between alcohol involvement and presenteeism (self-reported unproductive time at work due to illness), whereas three found null effects (Boles et al., 2004; Burton et al., 2005; Lim et al., 2000). Additionally, studies examining the effects of alcohol consumption on supervisor-rated employee performance (Shi et al., 2013; Weiss et al., 2008), as well as illicit SI on self- and other-rated performance indicators (Lim et al., 2000; Wadsworth et al., 2006; Weiss et al., 2008), have also yielded null findings. However, considering the timing of cannabis use (i.e., during, after, or prior to the start of the workday), a study of 281 employee–supervisor dyads in the United States did find a significant, negative association between both the frequency of use before and during work and supervisor-rated task performance (Bernerth & Walker, 2020). Moreover, studies support an association between alcohol and illicit drug use and higher levels of counterproductive behavior, such as psychological and physical withdrawal at work and the perpetration of aggression and antagonistic behaviors at work (e.g., Bernerth & Walker, 2020). For example, using a sample of 1,301 U.S. blue-collar workers (262 women) from 58 workgroups, Bacharach et al. (2007) found a positive association between the proportion of men who drank heavily in a workgroup and women's reports of gender harassment by men in the group, with this association amplified in groups characterized by stronger injunctive alcohol norms.

Accident and Injury Outcomes

Data on employee SI and work injuries come from two sources: (a) postaccident and random SI testing (if SI underlies accidents, positivity rates for the former should be greater than the latter), and (b) epidemiological and organizational field studies. Regarding the first source, based on positivity rates from millions of urine and oral fluid tests for overall illicit drug use in the general workforce over the period 2005 to 2009 (published by Quest Diagnostics, 2010), Frone (2013) found no difference in the positivity rates for random versus postaccident urine tests, and positivity rates for oral fluid tests (better at detecting recent illicit drug use) were actually slightly higher for random (vs. postaccident) testing. Similarly, positivity rates for random breathalyzer testing for alcohol violations conducted by the Federal Transit Administration between 2006 and 2008 were slightly higher than postaccident breathalyzer testing (Frone, 2013). Therefore, these comparisons offer no support for an association between SI and workplace accidents, even in safety-sensitive transport occupations.

The evidence supporting a positive association between overall employee SI and workplace accidents and injuries is no stronger in epidemiologic field studies. Over a dozen reviews conducted through 2010 (for references, see Frone, 2013) failed to consistently support associations between employee alcohol use and workplace accidents, with any statistically significant positive associations having small effect sizes. Similarly, a 2018 literature review found that of 16 studies comparing work-related injuries among cannabis-consuming and non-cannabis-consuming workers, seven supported a positive association (although none could show evidence of pre-injury cannabis use or impairment at time of injury); one suggested a negative, protective effect; and eight indicated a null effect (Biasutti et al., 2020). Studies based on emergency room (Cherpitel, 2007; Taylor et al., 2010) and organizational data (Frone, 1998) suggest that to the extent that employee SI plays a role in workplace injuries, it does so only as a result of heavy consumption or use occurring no more than six hours prior to the accident (i.e., when the victim may be experiencing acute impairment). Such inconsistent findings and methodological weaknesses in epidemiological field studies make it premature to draw any conclusions regarding the causal role of employee SI in the etiology of workplace accidents.

A GENERAL MODEL OF EMPLOYEE SI AND PRODUCTIVITY

As should be clear from our review, there is substantial inconsistency in findings relating employee SI to various organizational outcomes. Some of the inconsistency is found across field studies exploring different outcomes (e.g., attendance, task performance, injuries), and some is found comparing laboratory studies of acute impairment with field studies of chronic patterns of use. These inconsistencies may not be surprising because many researchers seem to assume that the mere consumption of a psychoactive substance, regardless of its temporal context or the amount consumed, will have the same effect across all productivity outcomes for all employees. However, the general SI literature suggests that the underlying process linking employee SI to workplace productivity may be more complicated. Failing to account for this complexity may explain much of the inconsistency in past findings. To account for these inconsistencies and highlight the potential complexity in associations between employee SI and productivity outcomes, Frone (2004, 2013) developed the conceptual model depicted in Figure 18.1. A summary of the major features of this model follows; however, the reader is referred to the original source for a detailed discussion of relevant constructs, implications, and supporting evidence.

FIGURE 18.1. An Integrative Model of Employee Substance Involvement and Work Productivity

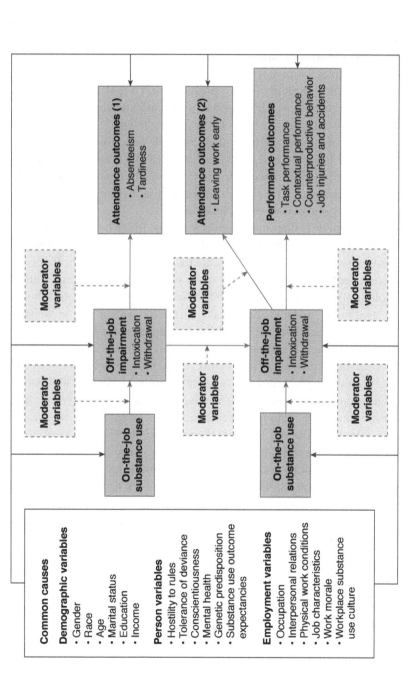

Note. Solid lines represent main (i.e., Direct) effects and dashed lines represent interaction (i.e., Moderator) effects. Adapted from *Alcohol and Illicit Drug Use in the Workforce and Workplace* (p. 133), by M. R. Frone, 2013, American Psychological Association (https://doi.org/10.1037/13944-000). Copyright 2013 by the American Psychological Association.

The first general feature of the model is that the temporal context of SI is matched to specific organizational outcomes. In past research, researchers typically assessed employees' overall SI, which primarily reflected SI off the job rather than workplace SI, which reflects use and impairment on the job. Thus, the model explicitly distinguishes between off-the-job and on-the-job substance use and impairment. It is also important to differentiate between attendance and performance outcomes. Attendance outcomes represent the failure to come to work on time (i.e., tardiness) or at all (i.e., absenteeism), as well as leaving work early. Performance outcomes represent behaviors and outcomes that occur on the job, such as accidents and injuries, task and contextual performance, and counterproductive behavior. As shown in Figure 18.1, the model proposes a correspondence between the temporal context of employee substance use and impairment and the type of productivity outcomes affected. In other words, off-the-job substance use and impairment primarily predict tardiness and absenteeism, and on-the-job substance use and impairment predict leaving work early and performance outcomes.

The second general feature of the model is distinguishing between substance use and substance impairment. The model proposes that substance impairment is the proximal cause of poor productivity outcomes and mediates the more distal effect of substance use. In other words, if substance use—either off the job or on the job—does not lead to significant impairment, it should not be related to the outcomes. Specifically, increased levels of off-the-job substance use are expected to cause higher levels of impairment and more severe withdrawal (when use is not possible or decreased among heavy users) off the job, which then causes poor attendance. Likewise, higher levels of off-the-job substance use may be related to intoxication at work because individuals may still have a nonzero blood level when they arrive at work, and withdrawal symptoms at work may be more severe among chronic, heavy off-the-job substance users if they do not consume the substance during their work shift. Also, higher levels of on-the-job substance use are expected to cause higher levels of on-the-job impairment. In turn, on-the-job impairment and withdrawal are expected to increase the likelihood of leaving work early and negatively affecting performance outcomes.

The third general feature of the model is that it calls attention to the need to control for common causes of employee SI and the various productivity outcomes. Care must be taken in interpreting some prior studies that have supported associations between employee SI and the various organizational outcomes. Much of this research has lacked adequate controls for common causes of substance use, substance impairment, and productivity. Differences across studies in the potential confounding variables that were modeled may partly explain inconsistencies across studies in the extent to which employee SI was related to specific outcomes.

Finally, the model highlights the need to consider variables potentially moderating the associations among substance use, substance impairment, and organizational outcomes. Notable moderators include pharmacological, dispositional, motivational, and situational influences discussed by Frone (2004). As shown in Figure 18.1, different variables may moderate the association between substance use and substance impairment and between substance impairment and productivity outcomes.

WORKPLACE PREVENTION AND REHABILITATION INTERVENTIONS

Efforts to leverage the workplace as a basis for employee substance misuse prevention and rehabilitation have taken several forms. Prevention and deterrence interventions include various types of alcohol and drug testing, as well as efforts to shift substance use norms. Rehabilitation efforts revolve around efforts to motivate employees with an SUD to seek appropriate, professional assistance and follow-up care. Studies indicate SUD treatment has beneficial productivity effects for employed individuals (Goplerud et al., 2017; Slaymaker & Owen, 2006).

Deterrence efforts in the United States have largely been shaped by various federal regulations (e.g., Drug-Free Workplace Act of 1988; Executive Order 12564 of 1986). Although not mandating nonfederal employers to engage in workforce drug testing, these regulations legitimized and encouraged such practices by larger enterprises. A 2018 HireRight Inc. survey (as cited in Real Reporting Foundation, 2022) indicated that 63% of employer survey respondents tested job applicants for illicit drugs, a substantial increase over the 55% prevalence estimate for 2004 reported by Frone (2013). According to Quest Diagnostics (2022), the illicit drug use positivity rate in 2021 was 2.2% for Federally Mandated Safety-Sensitive workers subjected to urine drug tests as a condition of employment and was 5.6% for the general U.S. workforce. Research on the deterrence efficacy of testing is equivocal at best (Frone, 2013). Studies, many of which have significant methodological limitations, have yet to clearly demonstrate that pre-employment and random testing reduce the use of illicit drugs or alcohol misuse (Frone, 2013; Joseph Rowntree Foundation, 2004; Macdonald et al., 2010). As for the productivity-related benefits of employee drug and alcohol testing, a qualitative review of 23 studies on testing and workplace safety published between 1990 and 2013 found none to include a randomized clinical trial, and only one as "demonstrating strong methodological rigor" (Pidd & Roche, 2014, p. 154). However, that study (Snowden et al., 2007) found random alcohol testing to be associated with a reduction in fatal accidents in the transport industry. Given the limitations of workforce testing for alcohol and illicit drugs, there is increasing employer interest in impairment testing that accounts for specific job skills and adjusts for learning from repeated uses. Because such tests are presumably sensitive to impairment from multiple causes, such as medical and nonmedical prescription drug use, illegal drug use, alcohol use, fatigue, and chronic medical conditions, preliminary and largely anecdotal evidence has suggested that they may have beneficial effects on workplace safety and be associated with diminished employee resistance (Maltby, n.d.).

Workplace alcohol prevention and rehabilitation interventions initially emerged in the 1940s, developing into more broad-brush programs addressing a wider variety of employee behavioral health problems under the label of employee assistance programs (EAPs; Steele, 1989, 1995; see Frone, 2013, for a review). These programs, some on-site (i.e., internal EAPs), but most accessible as off-site, external services, offer confidential screening, assessment, referral, and case management services to employees. Additionally, some offer brief interventions and postrehabilitation follow-up services. Although employees can self-refer to these services, they are usually motivated to seek the assistance of an EAP to avoid disciplinary proceedings for certain types of workplace performance issues such as absenteeism, tardiness, or a safety rule violation. Increasingly, peer assistance programs are working parallel to and often in cooperation with EAPs, such as Google's Blue Dot program and various union-based member assistance programs. These programs, staffed by employee volunteers who receive training in peer counseling and referral, facilitate employee help-seeking, assist with postrehabilitation aftercare, and, in more extreme cases, arrange for at-risk coworkers to get immediate care (Golan et al., 2010). Some of these programs, such as Operation RedBlock—a union-initiated, management-supported program in the railroad sector—engage in extensive, peer-based efforts both in the workplace and the community to shift substance-use norms (Bacharach et al., 1994, 2001). Although literature reviews suggest that systematic and robust research on EAPs is lacking (Csiernik, 2005; Joseph et al., 2018), studies evaluating the impact of EAPs suggest that they may have a beneficial impact on a variety of outcomes (Osilla et al., 2008; PricewaterhouseCoopers, 2014; Sieck & Heirich, 2010). For example, several studies indicate a positive association of EAP utilization and employee attendance (Li et al., 2015; Richmond et al., 2014; Sharar & Lennox, 2014), although others (Osilla et al., 2010; Spetch et al., 2011) suggest that this impact may be minimal at best. Similarly, studies examining the impact of EAP utilization indicate a beneficial decline in presenteeism (Li et al., 2015; Richmond et al., 2014; Sharar & Lennox, 2014) and enhanced workplace functioning (Dickerson et al., 2012; Jacobson et al., 2011). Internet-based brief interventions may also hold promise to prevent and address workforce substance misuse (Larimer et al., 2012). Finally, for a review of workplace EAP and workplace wellness interventions for SI, see Frone (2013).

CONCLUSION

This chapter briefly reviewed the literature on SI in the workforce and in the workplace for occupational health psychologists. The literature on the scope of employee alcohol and illicit drug use supports several general conclusions. First, despite the opioid crisis and the attention devoted to illicit drug involvement by employers, policymakers, and companies conducting drug tests, the use of alcohol by employees tends to be more problematic for employers than employee illicit drug involvement. Alcohol use, impairment, and disorders are more prevalent than illicit drug use, impairment, and disorders in the workforce and workplace. Second, comparing the prevalence of overall (i.e., workforce) SI with the prevalence of workplace SI shows that most use and impairment occur outside the workplace. Indeed, 79% of U.S. employees who use alcohol do not report any workplace alcohol use, and 78% of those who report illicit drug use do not report any workplace illicit drug use (Frone, 2008b). Finally, employee SI represents a multidimensional construct. Failing to assess multiple dimensions of alcohol or drug use simultaneously provides limited information on the association between the workplace and employee alcohol and drug use. For a more detailed discussion of this issue, see Frone (2013, 2019).

Research examining the causes and particularly the outcomes of employee SI is inconsistent and inconclusive. This is partly due to a lack of research in some areas and partly due to conceptual and measurement shortcomings. Future research needs to be much more nuanced and multidimensional if we are to better understand (a) the role of work-related risk factors (e.g., workplace substance use climate, work stressors), (b) how the effects of these workplace risk factors may be conditioned by various moderators, and (c) the complex association of employee SI to organizational outcomes.

Similarly, research on prevention and rehabilitation—focusing largely on the deterrence effects of drug testing and the efficacy of EAP utilization—has also suffered from methodological limitations. With limited evidence to suggest that applicant, random, and postaccident drug testing offer meaningful deterrence and productivity benefits, the evidence regarding the efficacy of work-based prevention and rehabilitation programs such as EAPs, peer assistance, and internet-based brief interventions is somewhat more encouraging. Still, in this domain as well, more rigorous evaluation efforts are needed.

To develop defensible and effective evidence-based policies and interventions regarding employee SI, relevant stakeholders will require more integrative and higher quality research. Occupational health psychologists are well positioned to provide such research, including a new generation of integrative, theoretically grounded studies exploring how extant findings may be transformed into more efficacious work-based interventions.

REFERENCES

American Psychiatric Association. (2000). *Diagnostic and statistical manual of mental disorders* (4th ed., text rev.).

Ames, G. M., & Grube, J. W. (1999). Alcohol availability and workplace drinking: Mixed method analyses. *Journal of Studies on Alcohol, 60*(3), 383–393. https://doi.org/10.15288/jsa.1999.60.383

Ames, G. M., Grube, J. W., & Moore, R. S. (2000). Social control and workplace drinking norms: A comparison of two organizational cultures. *Journal of Studies on Alcohol, 61*(2), 203–219. https://doi.org/10.15288/jsa.2000.61.203

Ames, G. M., & Janes, C. J. (1992). A cultural approach to conceptualizing alcohol and the workplace. *Alcohol Health and Research World, 16*(2), 112–119. https://psycnet.apa.org/record/1994-39390-001

Bacharach, S. B., Bamberger, P., & Biron, M. (2010). Alcohol consumption and workplace absenteeism: The moderating effect of social support. *Journal of Applied Psychology, 95*(2), 334–348. https://doi.org/10.1037/a0018018

Bacharach, S. B., Bamberger, P., & McKinney, V.M. (2007). Harassing under the influence: The prevalence of male heavy drinking, the embeddedness of permissive workplace drinking norms, and the gender harassment of female coworkers. *Journal of Occupational Health Psychology, 12*(3), 232–250. https://doi.org/10.1037/1076-8998.12.3.232

Bacharach, S. B., Bamberger, P., & Sonnenstuhl, W. J. (1994). *Member assistance programs in the workplace: The role of labor in the prevention & treatment of substance abuse.* Cornell University Press.

Bacharach, S. B., Bamberger, P., & Sonnenstuhl, W. J. (2001). *Mutual aid and union renewal: Cycles of logics of action.* Cornell University Press. https://doi.org/10.7591/9781501720789

Bacharach, S. B., Bamberger, P. A., & Sonnenstuhl, W. J. (2002). Driven to drink: Managerial control, work-related risk factors, and employee problem drinking. *Academy of Management Journal, 45*(4), 637–658. https://doi.org/10.5465/3069302

Bamberger, P. A., & Bacharach, S. B. (2006). Abusive supervision and subordinate problem drinking: Taking resistance, stress and subordinate personality into account. *Human Relations, 59*(6), 723–752. https://doi.org/10.1177/0018726706066852

Bamberger, P. A., & Cohen, A. (2015). Driven to the bottle: Work-related risk factors and alcohol misuse among commercial drivers. *Journal of Drug Issues, 45*(2), 180–201. https://doi.org/10.1177/0022042615575373

Bernerth, J. B., & Walker, H. J. (2020). Altered states or much to do about nothing? A study of when cannabis is used in relation to the impact it has on performance. *Group & Organization Management, 45*(4), 459–478. https://doi.org/10.1177/1059601120917590

Biasutti, W. R., Leffers, K. S. H., & Callaghan, R. C. (2020). Systematic review of cannabis use and risk of occupational injury. Advance online publication. *Substance Use & Misuse, 55*(11), 1733–1745. https://doi.org/10.1080/10826084.2020.1759643

Biron, M., Bamberger, P. A., & Noyman, T. (2011). Work-related risk factors and employee substance use: Insights from a sample of Israeli blue-collar workers. *Journal of Occupational Health Psychology, 16*(2), 247–263. https://doi.org/10.1037/a0022708

Boles, M., Pelletier, B., & Lynch, W. (2004). The relationship between health risks and work productivity. *Journal of Occupational and Environmental Medicine, 46*(7), 737–745. https://doi.org/10.1097/01.jom.0000131830.45744.97

Bureau of Labor Statistics. (2021). *Employer-reported workplace injuries & illnesses—2020.* USDOL-21-1927. https://www.bls.gov/news.release/pdf/osh.pdf

Burton, W. N., Chen, C.-Y., Conti, D. J., Schultz, A. B., Pransky, G., & Edington, D. W. (2005). The association of health risks with on-the-job productivity. *Journal of Occupational and Environmental Medicine, 47*(8), 769–777. https://doi.org/10.1097/01.jom.0000169088.03301.e4

Center for Behavioral Health Statistics & Quality. (2015). *Behavioral health trends in the United States: Results from the 2014 National Survey on Drug Use and Health.* Substance Abuse Mental Health Services Administration, U.S. Department of Health & Human Services.

Cherpitel, C. J. (2007). Alcohol and injuries: A review of international emergency room studies since 1995. *Drug and Alcohol Review, 26*(2), 201–214. https://doi.org/10.1080/09595230601146686

Colell, E., Sanchez-Niubo, A., Ferrer, M., & Domingo-Salvany, A. (2016). Gender differences in the use of alcohol and prescription drugs in relation to job insecurity. Testing a model of mediating factors. *The International Journal on Drug Policy, 37,* 21–30. https://doi.org/10.1016/j.drugpo.2016.07.002

Conger, J. J. (1956). Alcoholism: Theory, problem and challenge. II. Reinforcement theory and the dynamics of alcoholism. *Quarterly Journal of Studies on Alcohol, 17*(2), 296–305. https://doi.org/10.15288/qjsa.1956.17.296

Cooper, M. L., Frone, M. R., Russell, M., & Mudar, P. (1995). Drinking to regulate positive and negative emotions: A motivational model of alcohol use. *Journal of Personality and Social Psychology, 69*(5), 990–1005. https://doi.org/10.1037/0022-3514.69.5.990

Cooper, M. L., Russell, M., & Frone, M. R. (1990). Work stress and alcohol effects: A test of stress-induced drinking. *Journal of Health and Social Behavior, 31*(3), 260–276. https://doi.org/10.2307/2136891

Csiernik, R. (2005). A review of EAP evaluation in the 1990s. *Employee Assistance Quarterly, 19*(4), 21–37. https://doi.org/10.1300/J022v19n04_02

Davenport, S., Weaver, A., & Caverly, M. (2019). *Economic impact of non-medical opioid use in the United States: Annual estimates and projections for 2015–2019.* Society of Actuaries.

Delaney, W. P., Grube, J. W., Greiner, B., Fisher, J. M., & Ragland, D. R. (2002). Job stress, unwinding and drinking in transit operators. *Journal of Studies on Alcohol, 63*(4), 420–429. https://doi.org/10.15288/jsa.2002.63.420

Dickerson, S. J., Murphy, M. W., & Clavelle, P. R. (2012). Work adjustment and general level of functioning pre- and post-EAP counseling. *Journal of Workplace Behavioral Health, 27*(4), 217–226. https://doi.org/10.1080/15555240.2012.725586

Drug-Free Workplace Act, 41 U.S.C. § 8101 (1988).

Executive Order No. 12564, 51 Fed. Reg. 32889, 3 C.F.R. 224 (1986).

Franklin, G. M., Mai, J., Wickizer, T., Turner, J. A., Fulton-Kehoe, D., & Grant, L. (2005). Opioid dosing trends and mortality in Washington State workers' compensation, 1996–2002. *American Journal of Industrial Medicine, 48*(2), 91–99. https://doi.org/10.1002/ajim.20191

Frone, M. R. (1998). Predictors of work injuries among employed adolescents. *Journal of Applied Psychology, 83*(4), 565–576. https://doi.org/10.1037/0021-9010.83.4.565

Frone, M. R. (1999). Work stress and alcohol use. *Alcohol Research & Health, 23*(4), 284–291. https://www.ncbi.nlm.nih.gov/pmc/articles/PMC6760381/

Frone, M. R. (2000). Work–family conflict and employee psychiatric disorders: The National Comorbidity Survey. *Journal of Applied Psychology, 85*(6), 888–895. https://doi.org/10.1037/0021-9010.85.6.888

Frone, M. R. (2003). Predictors of overall and on-the-job substance use among young workers. *Journal of Occupational Health Psychology, 8*(1), 39–54. https://doi.org/10.1037/1076-8998.8.1.39

Frone, M. R. (2004). Alcohol, drugs, and workplace safety outcomes: A view from a general model of employee substance use and productivity. In J. Barling & M. R. Frone (Eds.), *The psychology of workplace safety* (pp. 127–156). American Psychological Association. https://doi.org/10.1037/10662-007

Frone, M. R. (2006a). Prevalence and distribution of alcohol use and impairment in the workplace: A U.S. national survey. *Journal of Studies on Alcohol, 67*(1), 147–156. https://doi.org/10.15288/jsa.2006.67.147

Frone, M. R. (2006b). Prevalence and distribution of illicit drug use in the workforce and in the workplace: Findings and implications from a U.S. national survey. *Journal of Applied Psychology, 91*(4), 856–869. https://doi.org/10.1037/0021-9010.91.4.856

Frone, M. R. (2008a). Are work stressors related to employee substance use? The importance of temporal context assessments of alcohol and illicit drug use. *Journal of Applied Psychology, 93*(1), 199–206. https://doi.org/10.1037/0021-9010.93.1.199

Frone, M. R. (2008b). Employee alcohol and illicit drug use: Scope, causes, and consequences. In J. Barling & C. L. Cooper (Eds.), *The SAGE handbook of organizational behavior: Vol. 1. Micro approaches* (pp. 519–540). Sage. https://doi.org/10.4135/9781849200448.n28

Frone, M. R. (2009). Does a permissive workplace substance use climate affect employees who do not use alcohol and drugs at work? A U.S. national study. *Psychology of Addictive Behaviors, 23*(2), 386–390. https://doi.org/10.1037/a0015965

Frone, M. R. (2012). Workplace substance use climate: Prevalence and distribution in the U.S. workforce. *Journal of Substance Use, 17*(1), 72–83. https://doi.org/10.3109/14659891.2010.531630

Frone, M. R. (2013). *Alcohol and illicit drug use in the workforce and workplace.* American Psychological Association. https://doi.org/10.1037/13944-000

Frone, M. R. (2015). Relations of negative and positive work experiences to employee alcohol use: Testing the intervening role of negative and positive work rumination. *Journal of Occupational Health Psychology, 20*(2), 148–160. https://doi.org/10.1037/a0038375

Frone, M. R. (2016a). The Great Recession and employee alcohol use: A U.S. population study. *Psychology of Addictive Behaviors, 30*(2), 158–167. https://doi.org/10.1037/adb0000143

Frone, M. R. (2016b). Work stress and alcohol use: Developing and testing a biphasic self-medication model. *Work and Stress, 30*(4), 374–394. https://doi.org/10.1080/02678373.2016.1252971

Frone, M. R. (2018). Organizational downsizing and alcohol use: A national study of U.S. workers during the Great Recession. *Addictive Behaviors, 77*, 107–113. https://doi.org/10.1016/j.addbeh.2017.09.016

Frone, M. R. (2019). Employee psychoactive substance involvement: Historical context, key findings, and future directions. *Annual Review of Organizational Psychology and Organizational Behavior, 6*(1), 273–297. https://doi.org/10.1146/annurev-orgpsych-012218-015231

Frone, M. R., Barnes, G. M., & Farrell, M. P. (1994). Relationship of work-family conflict to substance use among employed mothers: The role of negative affect. *Journal of Marriage and the Family, 56*(4), 1019–1030. https://doi.org/10.2307/353610

Frone, M. R., & Brown, A. L. (2010). Workplace substance-use norms as predictors of employee substance use and impairment: A survey of U.S. workers. *Journal of Studies on Alcohol and Drugs, 71*(4), 526–534. https://doi.org/10.15288/jsad.2010.71.526

Frone, M. R., Russell, M., & Cooper, M. L. (1995). Job stressors, job involvement, and employee health: A test of identity theory. *Journal of Occupational and Organizational Psychology, 68*(1), 1–11. https://doi.org/10.1111/j.2044-8325.1995.tb00684.x

Frone, M. R., Russell, M., & Cooper, M. L. (1997). Relation of work–family conflict to health outcomes: A four-year longitudinal study of employed parents. *Journal of Occupational and Organizational Psychology, 70*(4), 325–335. https://doi.org/10.1111/j.2044-8325.1997.tb00652.x

Frone, M. R., & Trinidad, J. R. (2012). Relation of supervisor social control to employee substance use: Considering the dimensionality of social control, temporal context of substance use, and substance legality. *Journal of Studies on Alcohol and Drugs, 73*(2), 303–310. https://doi.org/10.15288/jsad.2012.73.303

Frone, M. R., & Trinidad, J. R. (2014). Perceived physical availability of alcohol at work and workplace alcohol use and impairment: Testing a structural model. *Psychology of Addictive Behaviors, 28*(4), 1271–1277. https://doi.org/10.1037/a0037785

Golan, M., Bacharach, Y., & Bamberger, P. (2010). Peer assistance programs in the workplace. *Contemporary occupational health psychology: Global perspectives, 1*, 169–187.

Goplerud, E., Hodge, S., & Benham, T. (2017). A substance use cost calculator for US employers with an emphasis on prescription pain medication misuse. *Journal of Occupational and Environmental Medicine, 59*(11), 1063–1071. https://doi.org/10.1097/JOM.0000000000001157

Grandey, A. A., Frone, M. R., Malloy, B., & Sayre, G. M. (2019). When are fakers also drinkers? A self-control view of emotional labor and alcohol consumption among U.S. service workers. *Journal of Occupational Health Psychology, 24*(4), 482–497. https://doi.org/10.1037/ocp0000147

Greenberg, E. S., & Grunberg, L. (1995). Work alienation and problem alcohol behavior. *Journal of Health and Social Behavior, 36*(1), 83–102. https://doi.org/10.2307/2137289

Grunberg, L., Moore, S., Anderson-Connolly, R., & Greenberg, E. (1999). Work stress and self-reported alcohol use: The moderating role of escapist reasons for drinking. *Journal of Occupational Health Psychology, 4*(1), 29–36. https://doi.org/10.1037/1076-8998.4.1.29

Grunberg, L., Moore, S., & Greenberg, E. S. (1998). Work stress and problem alcohol behavior: A test of the spill-over model. *Journal of Organizational Behavior, 19*(5), 487–502. https://doi.org/10.1002/(SICI)1099-1379(199809)19:5<487::AID-JOB852>3.0.CO;2-Z

Harduar Morano, L., Steege, A. L., & Luckhaupt, S. E. (2018). Occupational patterns in unintentional and undetermined drug-involved and opioid-involved overdose deaths—United States, 2007–2012. *Morbidity and Mortality Weekly Report, 67*(33), 925–930. https://doi.org/10.15585/mmwr.mm6733a3

Hedegaard, H., Miniño, A. M., & Warner, M. (2020). *Drug overdose deaths in the United States, 1999–2019*. National Center for Health Statistics (Data Brief No. 394). Retrieved from https://www.cdc.gov/nchs/products/databriefs/db394.htm

Jacobson, J. M., Jones, A. L., & Bowers, N. (2011). Using existing employee assistance program case files to demonstrate outcomes. *Journal of Workplace Behavioral Health, 26*(1), 44–58. https://doi.org/10.1080/15555240.2011.540983

Joseph, B., Walker, A., & Fuller-Tyszkiewicz, M. (2018). Evaluating the effectiveness of employee assistance programmes: A systematic review. *European Journal of Work and Organizational Psychology, 27*(1), 1–15. https://doi.org/10.1080/1359432X.2017.1374245

Joseph Rowntree Foundation. (2004). *Drug testing in the workplace: The report of the independent inquiry into drug testing at work*.

Khantzian, E. J. (1997). The self-medication hypothesis of substance use disorders: A reconsideration and recent applications. *Harvard Review of Psychiatry, 4*(5), 231–244. https://doi.org/10.3109/10673229709030550

Kirkham, H. S., Clark, B. L., Bolas, C. A., Lewis, G. H., Jackson, A. S., Fisher, D., & Duncan, I. (2015). Which modifiable health risks are associated with changes in productivity costs? *Population Health Management, 18*(1), 30–38. https://doi.org/10.1089/pop.2014.0033

Kivimäki, M., Honkonen, T., Wahlbeck, K., Elovainio, M., Pentti, J., Klaukka, T., Virtanen, M., & Vahtera, J. (2007). Organisational downsizing and increased use of psychotropic drugs among employees who remain in employment. *Journal of Epidemiology and Community Health, 61*(2), 154–158. https://doi.org/10.1136/jech.2006.050955

Larimer, M. E., Dillworth, T. M., Neighbors, C., Lewis, M. A., Montoya, H. D., & Logan, D. E. (2012). Harm reduction for alcohol problems. In G. A. Marlatt, M. E. Larimer, & K. Witkiewitz (Eds.), *Harm reduction: Pragmatic strategies for managing high-risk behaviors* (pp. 63–106). The Guilford Press.

Li, P. Z., Sharar, D. A., Lennox, R., & Zhuang, W. (2015). Evaluating EAP counseling in the Chinese workplace: A study with a brief instrument. *Journal of Workplace Behavioral Health, 30*(1–2), 66–78. https://doi.org/10.1080/15555240.2015.1000143

Lim, D., Sanderson, K., & Andrews, G. (2000). Lost productivity among full-time workers with mental disorders. *The Journal of Mental Health Policy and Economics, 3*(3), 139–146. https://doi.org/10.1002/mhp.93

Liu, S., Wang, M., Bamberger, P., Shi, J., & Bacharach, S. B. (2015). The dark side of socialization: A longitudinal investigation of newcomer alcohol use. *Academy of Management Journal, 58*(2), 334–355. https://doi.org/10.5465/amj.2013.0239

Liu, S., Wang, M., Zhan, Y., & Shi, J. (2009). Daily work stress and alcohol use: Testing the cross-level moderation effects of neuroticism and job involvement. *Personnel Psychology, 62*(3), 575–597. https://doi.org/10.1111/j.1744-6570.2009.01149.x

Macdonald, S., Hall, W., Roman, P., Stockwell, T., Coghlan, M., & Nesvaag, S. (2010). Testing for cannabis in the work-place: A review of the evidence. *Addiction, 105*(3), 408–416. https://doi.org/10.1111/j.1360-0443.2009.02808.x

Macdonald, S., Wells, S., & Wild, T. C. (1999). Occupational risk factors associated with alcohol and drug problems. *The American Journal of Drug and Alcohol Abuse, 25*(2), 351–369. https://doi.org/10.1081/ADA-100101865

Madsen, I. E. H., Burr, H., Diderichsen, F., Pejtersen, J. H., Borritz, M., Bjorner, J. B., & Rugulies, R. (2011). Work-related violence and incident use of psychotropics. *American Journal of Epidemiology, 174*(12), 1354–1362. https://doi.org/10.1093/aje/kwr259

Maltby, L. (n.d.). *Impairment testing—does it work?* National Workrights Institute. https://www.workrights.org/nwi_drugTesting_impairmentTesting.html

Massachusetts Department of Public Health. (2018). *Opioid-related overdose deaths in Massachusetts by industry and occupation, 2011–2015.*

McCarthy, D. E., Curtin, J. J., Piper, M. E., & Baker, T. B. (2010). Negative reinforcement: Possible clinical implications of an integrative model. In J. D. Kassel (Ed.), *Substance abuse and emotion* (pp. 15–42). American Psychological Association. https://doi.org/10.1037/12067-001

Müller, C. P. (2020). Drug instrumentalization. *Behavioural Brain Research, 390,* 112672. https://doi.org/10.1016/j.bbr.2020.112672

National Drug Intelligence Center. (2011). *The economic impact of illicit drug use on American society.* United States Department of Justice.

Office of the Surgeon General. (2016). *Facing addiction in America: The surgeon general's report on alcohol, drugs, and health.* U.S. Department of Health and Human Services.

Osilla, K. C., dela Cruz, E., Miles, J. N., Zellmer, S., Watkins, K., Larimer, M. E., & Marlatt, G. A. (2010). Exploring productivity outcomes from a brief intervention for at-risk drinking in an employee assistance program. *Addictive Behaviors, 35*(3), 194–200. https://doi.org/10.1016/j.addbeh.2009.10.001

Osilla, K. C., Zellmer, S. P., Larimer, M. E., Neighbors, C., & Marlatt, G. A. (2008). A brief intervention for at-risk drinking in an employee assistance program. *Journal of Studies on Alcohol and Drugs, 69*(1), 14–20. https://doi.org/10.15288/jsad.2008.69.14

Pelfrene, E., Vlerick, P., Kittel, F., Mak, R. P., Kornitzer, M., & De Backer, G. (2002). Psychosocial work environment and psychological well-being: Assessment of the buffering effects in the job demand–control (–support) model in BELSTRESS. *Stress and Health, 18*(1), 43–56. https://doi.org/10.1002/smi.920

Pidd, K., & Roche, A. M. (2014). How effective is drug testing as a workplace safety strategy? A systematic review of the evidence. *Accident Analysis and Prevention, 71,* 154–165. https://doi.org/10.1016/j.aap.2014.05.012

PricewaterhouseCoopers. (2014). *Creating a mentally healthy workplace: Return on investment analysis.* Retrieved from https://apo.org.au/node/39705

Quest Diagnostics Inc. (2010). *The drug testing index.*

Quest Diagnostics Inc. (2022). *The drug testing index.*

Real Reporting Foundation. (2022, June 26). *Drug use testing related to employment.*

Richman, J. A., Shinsako, S. A., Rospenda, K. M., Flaherty, J. A., & Freels, S. (2002). Workplace harassment/abuse and alcohol-related outcomes: The mediating role of psychological distress. *Journal of Studies on Alcohol, 63*(4), 412–419. https://doi.org/10.15288/jsa.2002.63.412

Richmond, M. K., Shepherd, J. L., Pampel, F. C., Wood, R. C., Reimann, B., & Fischer, L. (2014). Associations between substance use, depression, and work outcomes: An evaluation study of screening and brief intervention in a large employee assistance program. *Journal of Workplace Behavioral Health, 29*(1), 1–18. https://doi.org/10.1080/15555240.2014.866470

Rotermann, M. (2021). Looking back from 2020, how cannabis use and related behaviours changed in Canada. *Health Reports, 32*(4), 3–14.

Sacks, J. J., Gonzales, K. R., Bouchery, E. E., Tomedi, L. E., & Brewer, R. D. (2015). 2010 national and state costs of excessive alcohol consumption. *American Journal of Preventive Medicine, 49*(5), e73–e79. https://doi.org/10.1016/j.amepre.2015.05.031

Sayette, M. A. (1999). Does drinking reduce stress? *Alcohol Research & Health, 23*(4), 250–255. https://www.ncbi.nlm.nih.gov/pmc/articles/PMC6760384/pdf/arh-23-4-250.pdf

Schou, L., & Moan, I. S. (2016). Alcohol use–sickness absence association and the moderating role of gender and socioeconomic status: A literature review. *Drug and Alcohol Review, 35*(2), 158–169. https://doi.org/10.1111/dar.12278

Sharar, D. A., & Lennox, R. (2014). The workplace effects of EAP use: Pooled results from 20 different EAPs with before and after WOS 5-item data. *EASNA Research Notes*, 4(1), 1–5. https://hdl.handle.net/10713/5139

Shi, Y., Sears, L. E., Coberley, C. R., & Pope, J. E. (2013). The association between modifiable well-being risks and productivity: A longitudinal study in pooled employer sample. *Journal of Occupational and Environmental Medicine*, 55(4), 353–364. https://doi.org/10.1097/JOM.0b013e3182851923

Sieck, C. J., & Heirich, M. (2010). Focusing attention on substance abuse in the workplace: A comparison of three workplace interventions. *Journal of Workplace Behavioral Health*, 25(1), 72–87. https://doi.org/10.1080/15555240903358744

Slaymaker, V. J., & Owen, P. L. (2006). Employed men and women substance abusers: Job troubles and treatment outcomes. *Journal of Substance Abuse Treatment*, 31(4), 347–354. https://doi.org/10.1016/j.jsat.2006.05.008

Snowden, C. B., Miller, T. R., Waehrer, G. M., & Spicer, R. S. (2007). Random alcohol testing reduced alcohol-involved fatal crashes of drivers of large trucks. *Journal of Studies on Alcohol and Drugs*, 68(5), 634–640. https://doi.org/10.15288/jsad.2007.68.634

Spetch, A., Howland, A., & Lowman, R. L. (2011). EAP utilization patterns and employee absenteeism: 3-year longitudinal study in a national Canadian retail corporation. *Consulting Psychology Journal*, 63(2), 110–128. https://doi.org/10.1037/a0024690

Steele, P. D. (1989). A history of job-based alcoholism programs: 1955–1972. *Journal of Drug Issues*, 19(4), 511–532. https://doi.org/10.1177/002204268901900406

Steele, P. D., & Trice, H. M. (1995). A history of job-based alcoholism programs: 1972–1980. *Journal of Drug Issues*, 25(2), 397–422. https://doi.org/10.1177/002204269502500211

Taylor, B., Irving, H. M., Kanteres, F., Room, R., Borges, G., Cherpitel, C., Greenfield, T., & Rehm, J. (2010). The more you drink, the harder you fall: A systematic review and meta-analysis of how acute alcohol consumption and injury or collision risk increase together. *Drug and Alcohol Dependence*, 110(1–2), 108–116. https://doi.org/10.1016/j.drugalcdep.2010.02.011

Van Hasselt, M., Keyes, V., Bray, J., & Miller, T. (2015). Prescription drug abuse and workplace absenteeism: Evidence from the 2008–2012 National Survey on Drug Use and Health. *Journal of Workplace Behavioral Health*, 30(4), 379–392. https://doi.org/10.1080/15555240.2015.1047499

Wadsworth, E. J. K., Moss, S. C., Simpson, S. A., & Smith, A. P. (2006). Cannabis use, cognitive performance and mood in a sample of workers. *Journal of Psychopharmacology*, 20(1), 14–23. https://doi.org/10.1177/0269881105056644

Walsh, J. M. (2008). New technology and new initiatives in U.S. workplace testing. *Forensic Science International*, 174(2–3), 120–124. https://doi.org/10.1016/j.forsciint.2007.03.011

Wang, M., Liu, S., Zhan, Y., & Shi, J. (2010). Daily work–family conflict and alcohol use: Testing the cross-level moderation effects of peer drinking norms and social support. *Journal of Applied Psychology*, 95(2), 377–386. https://doi.org/10.1037/a0018138

Weiss, P. A., Hitchcock, J. H., Weiss, W. U., Rostow, C., & Davis, R. (2008). The personality assessment inventory borderline, drug, and alcohol scales as predictors of overall performance in police officers: A series of exploratory analyses. *Policing and Society*, 18(3), 301–310. https://doi.org/10.1080/10439460802091708

Wolff, J. M., Rospenda, K. M., Richman, J. A., Liu, L., & Milner, L. A. (2013). Work-family conflict and alcohol use: Examination of a moderated mediation model. *Journal of Addictive Diseases*, 32(1), 85–98. https://doi.org/10.1080/10550887.2012.759856

Yu, J., Wang, S., & Yu, X. (2015). Health risk factors associated with presenteeism in a Chinese enterprise. *Occupational Medicine*, 65(9), 732–738. https://doi.org/10.1093/occmed/kqv115

19

Psychological Well-Being and Occupational Health

Caught in the Quicksand or Standing on a Firm Foundation?

Robert R. Sinclair, Thomas W. Britt, and Gwendolyn Paige Watson

Well-being continues to be a topic of broad interest in the social sciences and of specific interest in occupational health psychology (OHP). A recent literature search of three databases (Business Source Premier, Medline, and PsycInfo) on the terms *well-being* or *well being* or *wellbeing* with the terms *employee* or *staff* or *personnel* or *worker* revealed 9,317 citations in peer-reviewed academic journals between 2011 and 2021. This literature has been summarized in multiple reviews with a wide variety of personal, organizational, and contextual variables identified as antecedents and consequences of well-being (Bliese et al., 2017; Bowling et al., 2010; Danna & Griffin, 1999; Häusser et al., 2010; Loon et al., 2019; Nielsen et al., 2017; Warr, 2013). A full review of this literature lies well beyond the scope of this chapter. Rather, we set out to accomplish four aims.

First, we review the various usages of the term *well-being* in order to provide conceptual clarity on the nature of well-being. We present a typology based on two fundamental properties of well-being constructs: the extent to which they refer to well-being in a general sense or specific to one's work role, and the extent to which they emphasize the presence or absence of pleasure or self-actualization and the pursuit of meaning and purpose in one's life. Second, we provide a quantitative summary of the well-being literature from 2011 to 2020 with a focus on the various ways that researchers have conceptualized well-being. We also review several frameworks of well-being with the goal of highlighting the breadth of approaches to conceptualizing the term. Third, we discuss several developments in the literature related to

https://doi.org/10.1037/0000331-019
Handbook of Occupational Health Psychology, Third Edition, L. E. Tetrick, G. G. Fisher, M. T. Ford, and J. C. Quick (Editors)

well-being interventions. Finally, we discuss the need to consider the possible dark side to well-being.

CONCEPTUALIZATIONS OF WELL-BEING

Although it is beyond the scope of this chapter to exhaustively catalog the different definitions of well-being, it is necessary to highlight the breadth of viewpoints regarding well-being and to address the definitions that are used most often in OHP. Peter Warr (2013), who has conducted extensive research on work-related well-being, emphasized the importance of researchers' providing clear *conceptual* and *operational* definitions of well-being. Warr (2013) noted that in many cases the operationalization of well-being, in terms of the measure used, does not map onto the conceptual definition used by the researcher. Furthermore, researchers in OHP often use the term *well-being* when describing a measure or set of measures without supplying a conceptual definition of the construct. Unless researchers in the field of OHP are careful, well-being runs the risk of being what Connell and Nord (1996) referred to as a "quicksand term"—terms "that have so many conflicting definitions and connotations that they lead people into . . . 'conceptual quicksand' instead of to a sense of understanding" (p. 408). Nord and Connell (2011) further noted that quicksand terms may be used differently by those taking different perspectives on an issue, such as to gain rhetorical advantage in a debate. Quicksand terms therefore represent a potential obstacle to the advancement of occupational health science. To avoid conceptual quicksand, we will describe common elements in most researchers' definitions of well-being. We will also present a typology to categorize the differences in these definitions.

Common Elements in Researchers' Definitions

Most OHP researchers consider well-being as representing employees' subjective evaluations of their lived experience. Hesketh and Cooper (2019) emphasized well-being as involving subjective feelings regarding an individual's state of being. Similarly, Warr (2013) emphasized well-being as individuals perceiving an area of their life as beneficial. These conceptual definitions of well-being highlight the importance of subjectively experiencing some aspect of life in a positive manner. Furthermore, these definitions show that well-being does not simply reflect the absence of mental health symptoms but rather the presence of positive experiences in a particular domain. Defining well-being at work as something more than the absence of mental health symptoms was emphasized by Danna and Griffin (1999), who preferred the term *health* to address concerning physiological or psychological symptoms and the term *well-being* to address the perceived experience of the "whole person." Ryan and Deci (2001) further emphasized that "well-being is not the absence of mental illness" (p. 142). In a recent related post, Wilmar Schaufeli also noted, "We must be careful not to

confuse feelings of unwell-being with burnout" (https://www.linkedin.com/in/
schaufeli/detail/recent-activity/shares/).

A Typology of Well-Being Constructs

Figure 19.1 presents a 2 (hedonic vs. eudaimonic) × 2 (general or domain specific) typology to parsimoniously cover the breadth of well-being constructs
used by researchers in OHP. This typology contains examples of well-being
constructs falling under the four categories. The first dimension of well-being,
hedonic vs. eudaimonic, has been highlighted by researchers both within
OHP (Hesketh & Cooper, 2019) and outside the field (Ryff & Keyes, 1995).
Ryan and Deci (2001) pointed out that the hedonic approach focuses on the
experience of pleasure and the absence of pain, both physically and mentally
(e.g., participating in a desired activity). In contrast, the eudaimonic approach
highlights individuals living in accordance with their central values or their
"true self," emphasizing an experience of well-being resulting from being
engaged in activities that are perceived as authentic to the individual. The
other dimension highlighted in Figure 19.1 refers to whether the well-being
construct refers to the individual's general life experience at one end of the
continuum versus being contextualized within the work environment at the
other end.

Although OHP authors typically study indices of work-related well-being,
researchers will occasionally assess general measures of well-being. Briefly considering the more general conceptualizations of well-being, by far the most

FIGURE 19.1. A Typology of Well-Being Constructs

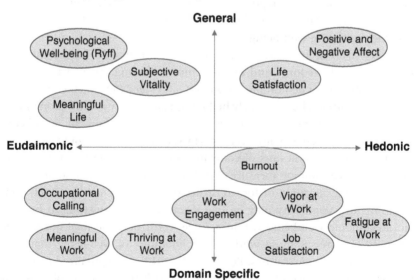

Note. With the exception of work engagement, location on the continuum is not meant
to imply relative standing on the dimensions.

popular hedonic approach was from Diener et al. (1999), who argued that the experience of *subjective well-being* was determined by high *life satisfaction*, high *positive affect*, low *negative affect*, and *satisfaction* in various life domains (i.e., roles). In contrast, there have been a wider variety of more general eudaimonic approaches to well-being. Ryan and Deci (2001) developed the construct of *subjective vitality* to emphasize feelings of aliveness and energy. Ryff and Keyes (1995) developed a multidimensional model of psychological well-being consisting of *autonomy, personal growth, self-acceptance, life purpose, mastery*, and *positive relatedness*. Whereas Ryff and Keyes argued these components were the defining features of psychological well-being, Ryan and Deci argued that these dimensions should be viewed as antecedents to well-being. The final eudaimonic approach to well-being identified in Figure 19.1 involves the *meaning in life* construct developed by Steger et al. (2006), highlighting an individual's experience of the presence of meaning in one's life.

Research on well-being within OHP typically includes measures that are contextualized to the work environment. Therefore, the bottom half of Figure 19.1 highlights a number of well-being constructs that are specific to the work domain and that vary along the hedonic–eudaimonic continuum. Considering the hedonic side of the continuum, the constructs of *job satisfaction* (Hackman & Lawler, 1971), *vigor at work* (Shirom, 2011), and *fatigue at work* (Frone & Tidwell, 2015) address either elements of satisfaction, the presence of positive affect, or the absence of negative affect. Although Figure 19.1 lists *burnout* as a hedonic and domain specific construct, some researchers have argued that burnout is better considered as a work-specific mental health problem (Schaufeli et al., 2009). Schonfeld and colleagues also have argued that measures of depression and the emotional exhaustion component of burnout are so highly related that burnout should be considered a measure of work-related depression (Bianchi et al., 2021). If burnout is classified as a work-related mental health problem, it should not be included as a construct indicating well-being.

The construct of *work engagement* is indicated in Figure 19.1 as having components of both hedonic and eudaimonic well-being, given the measure includes subscales of dedication, absorption, and vigor (Schaufeli et al., 2006). Vigor and absorption have a largely hedonic quality, whereas dedication implies an identity investment in work that is characteristic of eudaimonic well-being. Employee engagement has also been used by Gallup as an indicator of well-being linked to objective indicators of company performance (Harter et al., 2003). Engagement is a common measure of well-being in OHP, despite some controversy about the meaning of the construct (Macey & Schneider, 2008). One reason for this popularity may be that engagement addresses both hedonic and eudaimonic well-being within a single construct. The final quadrant in Figure 19.1 addresses those work-related indicators of well-being that have prominent eudaimonic features. Porath et al. (2012) conceptualized *thriving at work* as the experience of vitality combined with the reporting of continual learning and personal development. Thriving at work goes beyond vigor (a hedonic indicator of well-being) to emphasize the experience of a continued trajectory of growth at work. Another indicator of work-related eudaimonic well-being is the experience of being engaged in *meaningful work*. Rosso et al. (2010) discussed how employees experience meaning in their work, including doing work they perceive to be authentic, significant, or helping others (see also Allan et al., 2020; and Chapter 21, this volume). Martela and Pessi (2018) argued that meaningful work involves employees being engaged in significant activities that contribute to their own self-realization and/or a broader societal purpose. Related to meaningful work is the concept of fulfilling an *occupational calling* through work. Individuals with an occupational calling believe they were destined to do their work and that it is highly consistent with their identity (Dik & Duffy, 2009). Employees experiencing an occupational calling also believe they are pursuing work that betters themselves or others and experience a passion to do their work (Dobrow, 2013).

HOW HAS WELL-BEING BEEN CONCEPTUALIZED IN OHP RESEARCH?

Using Rigby and Traylor's (2020) text-mining application for the search terms *well-being, wellbeing,* and *well being,* we generated a list of articles published from 2011 to 2020 in the *Journal of Applied Psychology, Journal of Occupational Health Psychology,* and *Work & Stress*. The original list consisted of 239 articles on well-being. We removed 21 review and/or meta-analysis articles, resulting in our final list of 216 primary studies relevant to well-being. The remaining articles were randomly assigned to each author (72 articles per author) to be coded for the following information: publication journal, publication year, well-being variable(s) included in the study, and the well-being measure used for the variable(s). We removed an additional 40 articles after the coding process because they were review articles or did not specifically measure well-being, leaving 176 relevant articles to review.

Prior to discussing the results of this analysis, it is worth noting that authors differed in the extent to which they explicitly identified variables being examined as indicators of well-being. Although authors often specifically stated "indicators of well-being included," there were times when authors mentioned they were examining well-being in a given article, but then did not explicitly state that a given measure (e.g., emotional exhaustion) was an indicator of well-being. With that caveat in mind, there were 343 indicators of well-being present in the 176 articles that were coded. A summary of the indicators of well-being is provided in Exhibit 19.1.

As seen in the table, many indicators have been used to address well-being in OHP research. The most frequent indicator of well-being has been *burnout*, which includes burnout assessed through all three of its dimensions, as well as the dimensions being assessed separately. Of the 58 articles where burnout was assessed, the complete burnout construct was only assessed 15 times, whereas *emotional exhaustion* was assessed 40 times, and the remaining dimensions only assessed one time each. Therefore, emotional exhaustion is the

EXHIBIT 19.1. Broad Categories of Constructs Examined as Well-Being Indicators in 176 Journal Articles

Well-being indicator number of times assessed

Burnout 59

Mental health symptoms 38

Work engagement 36

Affect 28

Job satisfaction 27

Psychological well-being 19

Life satisfaction 17

Physical health 14

Fatigue 13

Stress 11

Positive psychology/meaningful work 10

Mood 10

Sleep 7

Psychological well-being/well-being 5

Cognitive functioning 5

Vitality 5

Psychological distress 4

Work–life balance 4

Ego depletion 2

Motivation 2

Psychophysiological 2

Withdrawal 2

Other single-mentioned indicators 27

Total indicators: 343

well-being measure most often included in the articles examined and represents the domain-specific and hedonic quadrant in Figure 19.1. The frequent use of burnout dimensions to address well-being has occurred despite the argument that burnout should not be viewed as an indicator of well-being (Schaufeli et al., 2009). Related to this point, the second most frequently used indicator of well-being in OHP research was *mental health symptoms* ($n = 38$). The most frequent mental health symptom indicators included *depression* ($n = 10$), *anxiety* ($n = 8$), and *general mental health symptoms* ($n = 8$). Mental health symptoms have been used as indicators of well-being despite the fact that mental health symptoms are better conceptualized as predictors of well-being as opposed to defining well-being (Danna & Griffin, 1999).

Representing a more positive approach to assessing well-being, *work engagement* emerged as the third most popular indicator of well-being. Of the 36 times work engagement was used as an indicator, the full work engagement construct was assessed 21 times, the subdimension of *vigor* was assessed 12 times, and the sub-dimension of *dedication* assessed 1 time. *Affect* and *job satisfaction* were the next most popular indicators of well-being. Affect was primarily conceptualized as either general negative ($n = 12$) or positive ($n = 8$), with only four studies using domain-specific job-related affect. Job satisfaction represents a straightforward indicator of a domain-specific indicator of hedonic well-being. *Psychological well-being*, an overall evaluation of psychological functioning (Goldberg & Hillier, 1979) representing a general and hedonic assessment of well-being, emerged as the next most popular indicator, followed by *life satisfaction*, another general indicator of hedonic well-being.

Rounding out the indicators that were used 10 or more times in OHP research, *physical health* includes overall ratings of physical health and specific physical symptoms, *fatigue* addresses reports primarily of physical exhaustion, and *stress* assesses general ratings of stress or strain. OHP researchers have also used assessed a variety of different *moods* as indicators of well-being, including anger, depressed mood, and irritation. Finally, a relatively small number of authors have used *eudaimonic indicators* of well-being. Examples of these indicators include flourishing, authenticity, and self-realization.

The content analysis also revealed that authors often used the term *well-being* within articles without providing a precise definition of the term and without justifying why specific indicators were used to assess well-being. In future research, authors should avoid the casual use of the term to refer to the presence of positive factors or the absence of negative factors. Instead, authors should be precise regarding the definition and why specific indicators were used to assess well-being within the context of the study being conducted. Authors also should explicitly identify whether hedonic or eudaimonic elements of well-being are being studied and provide a justification for why other variables examined in the study should be specifically related to either hedonic or eudaimonic well-being. Given the paucity of OHP research considering eudaimonic well-being, we also recommend that future research consider this type of well-being as both an outcome and a predictor.

MODELS OF WELL-BEING

Our content analysis clearly shows that there is no single model or approach to conceptualizing well-being. Most of the constructs we discussed have their own bodies of literature with nomological networks of antecedents and consequences developed to varying degrees. However, we judged four frameworks as worthy of discussion, in that each provides different approaches to integrate multiple components of well-being and/or the antecedents and consequences of well-being.

Warr's Vitamin Model

Warr's (1987) foundational work on job-related affective well-being described three continua representing dimensions of affective experiences as primary outcomes of interest: (a) anxious–comfortable, (b) depressed–actively pleased, and (c) discontented–contented. Whereas most OHP models then (and now) focus on linear relationships between measures of work characteristics and outcomes, Warr (1987) drew from the example of vitamins to propose that some work characteristics have linear relationships with outcomes, whereas others have nonlinear relationships. Some vitamins, such as vitamins C and E, have a "constant" effect such that taking them leads to health benefits up to a certain point, beyond which taking more leads to no additional benefits. Other vitamins, such as A and D, are beneficial but may have toxic effects when taken in very high doses.[1] Examples of job characteristics that follow the CE pattern include availability of money, physical security, valued social position, and supportive supervision. In contrast, characteristics such as job autonomy, skill variety, and task significance follow the AD pattern. The proposed AD pattern is especially noteworthy as it implies that researchers need to test nonlinear hypotheses about the effects of these characteristics on well-being. Although researchers continue to test the predictions of the model (e.g., De Jonge & Schaufeli, 1998; Stiglbauer & Kovacs, 2018), the vitamin model has received comparatively less attention than have other work stress–related models, and the general idea of nonlinear effects certainly requires more attention in occupational health psychology.

Job Demands–Resources Model

Initially conceived as a model of burnout, the job demands–resources (JD-R) model (Demerouti et al., 2001) has become one of the most widely used models in OHP (see also Chapter 3, this volume). In this model, job demands are conceptualized as any aspect of work that requires physical, emotional, or mental effort (e.g., high work pressure, job insecurity, irregular working hours). Chronic job demands lead to adverse health outcomes by creating work strain. A great deal of literature supports the link between job demands and poor health outcomes (cf. Bakker & Demerouti, 2017).

Job resources are the physical, psychological, social, or organizational aspects of the job that promote attainment of job-related goals, mitigate the demands-strain relationship, and/or enhance personal learning, development, and growth (Demerouti et al., 2001). Examples of job resources include social support, job control, and performance feedback as well as personal resources, such as self-esteem and self-efficacy (Xanthopoulou et al., 2007). Job resources are associated with higher employee motivation, reduced work strain, and positive outcomes such as job attitudes and employee engagement.

The JD-R model proposes that job demands and job resources initiate two underlying psychological processes, a health-impairment process and a motivational process, that explain the development of the demands-strain and resources-motivation relationships (Demerouti et al., 2001). The dual processes are referred to as the health-impairment process and the motivational process. The health-impairment process stems from job demands. Chronic job

---

[1]De Jonge and Schaufeli (1998) noted that vitamin overdose effects do not strictly follow the patterns described by Warr (1987).

demands expend employees' physical and psychological resources, leading employees to experience exhaustion and an increase in health problems. Burnout and engagement, the two most common indicators of well-being in the articles we reviewed, are commonly studied as proximal outcomes of the demands-strain and resource-motivation relationship.

Gallup–Sharecare Community Well-Being Index

Gallup and Sharecare have collaborated on the Sharecare Community Well-Being Index (CWBI; Sharecare.com, n.d.). The CWBI focuses on well-being in five domains: (a) physical, (b) community, (c) social, (d) purpose (also referred to as career well-being), and (e) financial. Although none of these directly reflect well-being as conceived in OHP, the purpose/career and financial dimensions reflect occupational health concerns, and the other dimensions highlight the importance of considering the relationship between well-being at work and in other life domains.

The CWBI is based on an impressive survey research program. Gallup interviews more than 500 U.S. adults 350 days per year to generate over 175,000 surveys each year, with over 2 million conducted since 2008 (Gallup.com, n.d.), and engages in international efforts to gather well-being data in over 120 countries (cf. Deaton, 2008). Although their approach has not been widely used in OHP, some Gallup publications have begun to focus on how organizations can improve employee well-being (e.g., Clifton & Harter, 2021). The CWBI research program offers important empirical data about well-being; the OHP research community would benefit from greater awareness of this work.

NIOSH Well-Being Model

The National Institute for Occupational Safety and Health (NIOSH) also has created a conceptual framework for worker well-being (Chari et al., 2018). Based on extensive literature review and expert panel input, this model consisted of five domains: (a) physical environment and safety climate; (b) workplace policies and culture; (c) health status; (d) work evaluation and experience; and (e) home, community, and society. This work integrates subjective and objective approaches to understanding well-being, with the subjective approach conceptualized as peoples' perceptions about the quality of their life and the objective approach reflecting whether people have sufficient access to resources needed to attain their desires, including physical health, material well-being, physical safety, social relationships, and spiritual harmony. As with the Gallup–Sharecare model, an important contribution of this approach is the recognition that workplace well-being is fundamentally related to well-being in other life domains. NIOSH also has developed the NIOSH Worker Well-Being Questionnaire (WellBQ; see NIOSH, n.d.) to capture the components of this model in a publicly available measure.

One direction for future research with models of psychological well-being is to consider the 2 × 2 framework of well-being constructs when examining the determinants of well-being. Researchers may find that eudaimonic indicators of well-being are uniquely predicted by typical determinants of well-being examined by OHP researchers (e.g., job resources such as developmental feedback). As one example, the work-related stressor of boredom has been examined as a predictor of depressive symptoms (van Hooff & van Hooft, 2016) but actually may be more strongly inversely related to eudaimonic indicators of well-being, such as dedication and authenticity at work.

PSYCHOLOGICAL WELL-BEING INTERVENTIONS AND INITIATIVES

Many organizations have engaged in efforts to promote the psychological well-being of their employees. The American Psychological Association (APA) developed a model of psychologically healthy workplaces with the goal of providing guidance to organizations about how to enhance employee well-being (Grawitch & Ballard, 2016; Grawitch et al., 2006). The APA framework categorized psychologically healthy workplace practices into five groups: (a) employee involvement, (b) work–life balance, (c) employee growth and development, (d) health and safety, and (e) employee recognition. OHP literature includes many interventions and initiatives that target the categories outlined by APA. We discuss examples of well-being interventions in each category, as well as two, mindfulness and job crafting, that do not clearly fall into the APA categories.

Employee Involvement

Employee involvement initiatives empower workers through increasing job autonomy and participative decision-making. Examples of employee involvement efforts include employee task forces, self-managed work teams, and employee suggestion forums (e.g., regular town halls, recommendation boxes). Nielsen and Randall (2012) demonstrated the benefits of an employee involvement intervention on well-being (e.g., affective well-being). They focused on creating self-managing teams and building a communicative climate with open discussions and group decision-making in eldercare centers. Prior to the intervention, employees primarily worked as one large, uncoordinated group that hindered the smooth transfer of information about clients and prevented collaboration on solutions for clients. The intervention involved creating smaller teams within the centers who were assigned to specific groups of clients and given the autonomy to allocate and execute tasks as the team deemed fit. Furthermore, the teams were encouraged to meet regularly to jointly discuss solutions for their clients. The procedures implemented through this intervention effectively increased employee well-being and perceived autonomy as well overall job satisfaction.

Work–Life Balance

Work–life balance programs intend to help employees manage their work demands and demands stemming from their roles and responsibilities outside of work (see Chapter 7, this volume). Examples of work–life balance interventions include flexible work arrangements (e.g., flextime, telecommuting), supervisor training interventions, childcare and eldercare assistance, extended benefits for family members, and flexible leave options beyond those legally required (e.g., the Family and Medical Leave Act in the United States).

A now sizable body of OHP literature offers a rich body of theory to explain the links between work–family concerns and health (Chapter 7, this volume) as well as empirically supported guidance for work–family interventions (Chapter 26, this volume). For example, using population survey data from Australia, Zheng et al. (2015) reported that perceived work–life balance was associated with better employee health and well-being (e.g., stress level). Work–life balance policies (e.g., flexible work arrangement, health and wellness programs, organizational understanding and support) positively influenced employee well-being in addition to health and perceived work–life balance. Interestingly, their findings highlighted that the availability of work–life balance programs—even when not used—improves employee well-being, suggesting that work–life balance initiatives signify the organization's concern for employees' well-being.

Employee Growth and Development

Employee growth and development opportunities focus on building employees' knowledge, skills, and abilities. Organizations may promote employee growth and development through educational programs (e.g., tuition reimbursement, continuing education courses), career development (e.g., mentoring, career counseling, promotions), and skills training. Employees with better perceptions of training and opportunities for career and skill development also experience greater well-being (Brunetto et al., 2012). Further, Huo and Boxall (2020) found that learning from supervisors, rather than coworkers, significantly mediated training and employee well-being. These results highlight that organizations should carefully design training programs to maximize their impact on well-being.

Health and Safety

Health and safety initiatives prevent, assess, and address potential health concerns to promote the physical and psychological health of workers (see Chapter 5, this volume). Organizations may introduce training and safeguards for workplace safety, offer healthy lifestyle interventions (e.g., stress management, wellness programs), make health resources more accessible (e.g., health insurance, health screenings, fitness memberships), and provide support for problems that may stem from outside of work (e.g., grief counseling, substance use programs, employee assistance programs). Research in this category closely aligns with the goals of government sponsored OHP programs such as *Total Worker Health®* (Schill & Chosewood, 2013). Anger et al. (2015) reviewed the effectiveness of *Total Worker Health* interventions on safety, health, and well-being and reported that the majority of intervention studies found significant improvements across a variety of well-being indicators (e.g., work stress, mental health, physical health). Pignata et al. (2016) found that employee awareness of health and safety initiatives improved employees' well-being (e.g., psychological strain, job satisfaction), regardless of whether they actually participated.

Employee Recognition

Employee recognition programs reward employees (individually or collectively) by acknowledging their work. Examples of rewards include competitive pay and benefits packages, performance-based bonuses, and acknowledgments of contributions and milestones through employee awards and/or recognition ceremonies. Although there has been considerably less focus on employee recognition interventions, the literature supports the expected positive influence of employee recognition programs on well-being. Khoreva and Wechtler (2018) found empirical support that motivation-enhancing human resource practices (e.g., competitive compensation, incentives and rewards, extensive benefits) increased employee psychological well-being (i.e., job satisfaction), ultimately improving performance. However, Grant et al. (2007) pointed out that these programs seem beneficial on the surface but may have weaker or even detrimental effects on well-being in certain contexts. For example, employee recognition programs may not be beneficial in competitive work environments, as employees' well-being may suffer when they compare their earnings to others or feel that they are constantly battling their coworkers for the promoted incentives.

Positive Psychology and Mindfulness

In recent years, researchers have bridged positive psychology and OHP to include positive psychology practices such as mindfulness (Jamieson & Tuckey, 2017; Pang & Ruch, 2019), gratitude (Winslow et al., 2017), and utility of character strengths interventions (Pang & Ruch, 2019). Mindfulness interventions have received the most attention of the positive psychology initiatives. *Mindfulness* involves "being attentive to and aware of what is taking place in the present" (Brown & Ryan, 2003, p. 822). A review of mindfulness interventions in the workplace by Jamieson and Tuckey (2017) found that 30 of the 40 studies (75%) in the review used some form of mindfulness-based stress reduction (MBSR) approach to the intervention, and almost all of these studies included health/well-being outcomes.

MBSR programs are traditionally administered in group settings over an 8-week period and train participants in stress-reducing activities such as meditation, yoga, and diaphragmatic breathing with the intention of improving their well-being through present-moment awareness. However, Jamieson and Tuckey (2017) noted that organizations sometimes modified the delivery, time frame, or content of the mindfulness intervention to better align with the organization's available resources and/or the specific work context. Some evidence also supports the effectiveness of virtual mindfulness training for improving employee well-being (e.g., perceived stress, resilience, and engagement; see Aikens et al., 2014).

Job Crafting

Although the bulk of the literature has focused on organization-initiated interventions, employees can also take a bottom-up approach to improving their well-being through job crafting. *Job crafting* involves employees altering their job characteristics such that they better align with how they want to perceive their work and who they are at work (Wrzesniewski & Dutton, 2001). Thus, rather than relying on programs provided by the organization, employees proactively improve their well-being through seeking social (e.g., requesting feedback, building support) and structural (e.g., seeking and utilizing autonomy) resources, seeking challenge demands (e.g., mentoring coworkers or subordinates, accepting training opportunities), and reducing hindrance demands such as creating clear boundaries between work and nonwork (Demerouti et al., 2019; Tims et al., 2012). Van Wingerden et al. (2017) provided a good example of a job crafting intervention in which they taught employees to create a personal crafting plan that would enable them to use job crafting strategies to match their personal strengths to their job duties. Their intervention group reported improvements over time in job crafting, basic need satisfaction, and work engagement as a result.

Future Interventions Research

As OHP scholars have shown a growing interest in well-being interventions (e.g., Beehr, 2019), there are some future research considerations to improve understanding and implementation of well-being interventions. For example, OHP researchers should take a more holistic approach in designing and empirically testing interventions by considering multiple avenues for creating a psychologically healthy workplace (i.e., employee involvement, work–life balance, employee growth and development, health and safety, and/or employee recognition) and devoting more efforts to promising areas (e.g., employee recognition) that are rarely tested in the literature. Conducting intervention research with pragmatic frameworks such as the APA categories in mind will contribute to bridging the scientist–practitioner gap by providing empirical support for the efficacy of well-being initiatives that can be practically implemented in organizations. Additionally, there is a need for more rigor in tests of interventions (e.g., randomized controlled trials, longitudinal designs that track the sustainability of the training). The gold standard of intervention implementation is to collect pre- and post-intervention measurement of well-being in a randomized controlled design to gauge the effectiveness of the intervention before using the resources to implement company-wide (Richardson & Rothstein, 2008). While many organizations do not have the necessary time, financial, or personnel resources to take this meticulous approach, where it is possible to implement, this design offers clearer indications of the causal effects of well-being interventions and reduces concerns about significant results occurring due to chance.

Finally, interventions to enhance well-being should also be considered in the context of the 2 × 2 framework of well-being offered in the present chapter. Some interventions may be more likely to affect some quadrants of well-being more than others. For example, interventions targeting the workplace may have stronger effects on work-specific aspects of well-being. On the other hand, interventions focused on multiple domains of an employee's life (e.g., work and family) have greater potential to affect general well-being. Further, some interventions may be more likely to affect eudaimonic indicators of well-being. For example, job crafting interventions may provide employees with a greater sense of purpose and authenticity, whereas interventions designed to reduce stressors may be primarily related to hedonic indicators of well-being.

THE DARK SIDE OF WELL-BEING

An important consideration for future well-being research is to examine possible deleterious outcomes associated with an intense organizational focus on well-being. Popular press articles have increasingly discussed the notion of "toxic positivity" at work. Torres (2020) described five scenarios reflecting toxic positivity: (a) workers' pressures to be positive in the face of legitimate concerns, (b) leaders' hesitance to acknowledge serious concerns, (c) refusing to acknowledge the impact of COVID-19, (d) employees being told to "look on the bright side" when experiencing job loss or other losses, and (e) minor efforts to address diversity and equity issues that ignore serious systemic concerns. The common theme across this and similar discussions is an emphasis on a hesitancy to acknowledge negative issues at work in order to focus on the positive. A heavy emphasis on well-being at work could produce some of these negative effects. However, to our knowledge, little or no empirical research has addressed this specific issue in terms of effects of managerial or other intervention strategies.

Some studies have begun to document potential negative effects associated with some "desirable" well-being constructs. For example, while mindfulness is generally regarded as desirable in terms of promoting adaptive responses to stressors, Walsh and Arnold (2020) showed that employees who scored higher on a measure of trait mindfulness reported lower vigor at work when exposed to higher levels of abusive leadership or lower levels of transformational leadership. They interpreted these effects as indicating that mindful employees may experience more difficulties disengaging from problems at work. Allan et al. (2020) found that people reported more adverse mental health consequences of meaningful work when they also were experiencing underemployment. Although it is important to note that this finding was not expected, they speculated that employees may be frustrated and disillusioned by meaningful work when they are prevented from fully utilizing their skills and abilities. Finally, Duffy et al. (2016) noted that having a calling at work may be associated with negative outcomes, particularly to the extent that people are unable to actually live out that calling at work. Each of these findings suggests that people have internal standards related to different aspects of well-being that may lead to negative health outcomes when not met.

Loon et al. (2019) discussed what they label as paradoxes in human resource management related to tensions between focusing on well-being and focusing on productivity. They noted that while focusing on employees' psychological well-being often leads to "win-win" outcomes that benefit both employees and their organization, it is possible that such efforts lead to unintended consequences. Examples they provided include the following: (a) increasing worker autonomy/discretion may reduce efficiencies gained through standardization; (b) flexible work arrangements that reduce work–family conflict could distract workers from their jobs; (c) providing more challenging jobs may be seen as exploitive, leading employees to reduce their citizenship behaviors; and (d) communication and information sharing may be undermined by performance-based pay systems. To avoid such tensions, Loon et al. suggested that managers and organizations attempt to reframe perceived tensions and acknowledge that while such tensions may not be able to be fully resolved, workarounds may be identified that minimize their negative impacts.

CONCLUSION

Employee well-being is a fundamental concept in OHP. Despite its importance, there is little consensus in the literature about how to conceptualize and operationalize the concept. This ambiguity represents an important potential barrier to the continued accumulation of knowledge about the nature of well-being at work but also represents an opportunity for researchers to offer empirically supported guidance about how to define and measure well-being. While researchers may be somewhat caught in the quicksand about the specific nature of well-being, a large body of empirical evidence supports the general importance of well-being, including several potential options for empirically supported interventions to actually improve employees' work lives. We look forward to continued developments in this literature so that occupational health science can better support employees' well-being at work.

REFERENCES

Aikens, K. A., Astin, J., Pelletier, K. R., Levanovich, K., Baase, C. M., Park, Y. Y., & Bodnar, C. M. (2014). Mindfulness goes to work: Impact of an online workplace intervention. *Journal of Occupational and Environmental Medicine*, 56(7), 721–731. https://doi.org/10.1097/JOM.0000000000000209

Allan, B. A., Rolniak, J. R., & Bouchard, L. (2020). Underemployment and well-being: Exploring the dark side of meaningful work. *Journal of Career Development*, 47(1), 111–125. https://doi.org/10.1177/0894845318819861

Anger, W. K., Elliot, D. L., Bodner, T., Olson, R., Rohlman, D. S., Truxillo, D. M., Kuehl, K. S., Hammer, L. B., & Montgomery, D. (2015). Effectiveness of Total Worker

Health interventions. *Journal of Occupational Health Psychology, 20*(2), 226–247. https://doi.org/10.1037/a0038340

Bakker, A. B., & Demerouti, E. (2017). Job demands–resources theory: Taking stock and looking forward. *Journal of Occupational Health Psychology, 22*(3), 273–285. https://doi.org/10.1037/ocp0000056

Beehr, T. A. (2019). Interventions in occupational health psychology. *Journal of Occupational Health Psychology, 24*(1), 1–3. https://doi.org/10.1037/ocp0000140

Bianchi, R., Verkuilen, J., Schonfeld, I. S., Hakanen, J. J., Jansson-Fröjmark, M., Manzano-García, G., Laurent, E., & Meier, L. L. (2021). Is burnout a depressive condition? A 14-sample meta-analytic and bifactor analytic study. *Clinical Psychological Science, 9*(4), 579–597. https://doi.org/10.1177/2167702620979597

Bliese, P. D., Edwards, J. R., & Sonnentag, S. (2017). Stress and well-being at work: A century of empirical trends reflecting theoretical and societal influences. *Journal of Applied Psychology, 102*(3), 389–402. https://doi.org/10.1037/apl0000109

Bowling, N., Eschleman, K. J., & Wang, Q. (2010). A meta-analytic examination of the relationship between job satisfaction and subjective well-being. *Journal of Occupational and Organizational Psychology, 83*(4), 915–934. https://doi.org/10.1348/096317909X478557

Brown, K. W., & Ryan, R. M. (2003). The benefits of being present: Mindfulness and its role in psychological well-being. *Journal of Personality and Social Psychology, 84*(4), 822–848. https://doi.org/10.1037/0022-3514.84.4.822

Brunetto, Y., Farr-Wharton, R., & Shacklock, K. (2012). Communication, training, well-being, and commitment across nurse generations. *Nursing Outlook, 60*(1), 7–15. https://doi.org/10.1016/j.outlook.2011.04.004

Chari, R., Chang, C.-C., Sauter, S. L., Petrun Sayers, E. L., Cerully, J. L., Schulte, P., Schill, A. L., & Uscher-Pines, L. (2018). Expanding the paradigm of occupational safety and health: A new framework for worker well-being. *Journal of Occupational and Environmental Medicine, 60*(7), 589–593. https://doi.org/10.1097/JOM.0000000000001330

Clifton, J., & Harter, J. (2021). *Well-being at work: How to build resilient and thriving teams.* The Gallup Press.

Connell, A. F., & Nord, W. R. (1996). The bloodless coup: The infiltration of organization science by uncertainty and values. *The Journal of Applied Behavioral Science, 32*(4), 407–427. https://doi.org/10.1177/0021886396324005

Danna, K., & Griffin, R. W. (1999). Health and well-being in the workplace: A review and synthesis of the literature. *Journal of Management, 25*(3), 357–384. https://doi.org/10.1177/014920639902500305

De Jonge, J., & Schaufeli, W. B. (1998). Job characteristics and employee well-being: A test of Warr's Vitamin Model in health care workers using structural equation modelling. *Journal of Organizational Behavior, 19*(4), 387–407. https://doi.org/10.1002/(SICI)1099-1379(199807)19:4<387::AID-JOB851>3.0.CO;2-9

Deaton, A. (2008). Income, health, and well-being around the world: Evidence from the Gallup World Poll. *The Journal of Economic Perspectives, 22*(2), 53–72. https://doi.org/10.1257/jep.22.2.53

Demerouti, E., Bakker, A. B., Nachreiner, F., & Schaufeli, W. B. (2001). The job demands-resources model of burnout. *Journal of Applied Psychology, 86*(3), 499–512. https://doi.org/10.1037/0021-9010.86.3.499

Demerouti, E., Peeters, M. C. W., & van den Heuvel, M. (2019). Job crafting interventions: Do they work and why? In E. E. van Zyl & S. Rothmann, Sr. (Eds.), *Positive psychological intervention design and protocols for multi-cultural contexts* (pp. 103–125). Springer Nature Switzerland AG. https://doi.org/10.1007/978-3-030-20020-6_5

Diener, E., Suh, E. M., Lucas, R. E., & Smith, H. L. (1999). Subjective well-being: Three decades of progress. *Psychological Bulletin, 125*(2), 276–302. https://doi.org/10.1037/0033-2909.125.2.276

Dik, B. J., & Duffy, R. D. (2009). Calling and vocation at work: Definitions and prospects for research and practice. *The Counseling Psychologist, 37*(3), 424–450. https://doi.org/10.1177/0011000008316430

Dobrow, S. R. (2013). Dynamics of calling: A longitudinal study of musicians. *Journal of Organizational Behavior, 34*(4), 431–452. https://doi.org/10.1002/job.1808

Duffy, R. D., Douglass, R. P., Autin, K. L., England, J., & Dik, B. J. (2016). Does the dark side of a calling exist? Examining potential negative effects. *The Journal of Positive Psychology, 11*(6), 634–646. https://doi.org/10.1080/17439760.2015.1137626

Frone, M. R., & Tidwell, M. O. (2015). The meaning and measurement of work fatigue: Development and evaluation of the Three-Dimensional Work Fatigue Inventory (3D-WFI). *Journal of Occupational Health Psychology, 20*(3), 273–288. https://psycnet.apa.org/doi/10.1037/a0038700

Gallup.com. (n.d.). *How does the Gallup-Sharecare Well-Being Index work?* https://www.gallup.com/175196/gallup-healthways-index-methodology.aspx

Goldberg, D. P., & Hillier, V. F. (1979). A scaled version of the General Health Questionnaire. *Psychological Medicine, 9*(1), 139–145. https://doi.org/10.1017/S0033291700021644

Grant, A. M., Christianson, M. K., & Price, R. H. (2007). Happiness, health, or relationships? Managerial practices and employee well-being tradeoffs. *The Academy of Management Perspectives, 21*(3), 51–63. https://doi.org/10.5465/amp.2007.26421238

Grawitch, M. J., & Ballard, D. W. (2016). Introduction: Building a psychologically healthy workplace. In M. J. Grawitch & D. W. Ballard (Eds.), *The psychologically healthy workplace: Building a win–win environment for organizations and employees* (pp. 3–11). American Psychological Association. https://doi.org/10.1037/14731-001

Grawitch, M. J., Gottschalk, M., & Munz, D. C. (2006). The path to a healthy workplace: A critical review linking healthy workplace practices, employee well-being, and organizational improvements. *Consulting Psychology Journal: Practice and Research, 58*(3), 129–147. https://doi.org/10.1037/1065-9293.58.3.129

Hackman, J. R., & Lawler, E. E. (1971). Employee reactions to job characteristics. *Journal of Applied Psychology, 55*(3), 259–286. https://doi.org/10.1037/h0031152

Harter, J. K., Schmidt, F. L., & Keyes, C. L. M. (2003). Well-being in the workplace and its relationship to business outcomes: A review of the Gallup studies. In C. L. M. Keyes & J. Haidt (Eds.), *Flourishing: Positive psychology and the life well-lived* (pp. 205–224). American Psychological Association. https://doi.org/10.1037/10594-009

Häusser, J. A., Mojzisch, A., Niesel, M., & Schulz-Hardt, S. (2010). Ten years on: A review of recent research on the Job Demand–Control (-Support) model and psychological well-being. *Work and Stress, 24*(1), 1–35. https://doi.org/10.1080/02678371003683747

Hesketh, I., & Cooper, C. L. (2019). *Wellbeing at work: How to design, implement, and evaluate an effective strategy.* Kogan Page Ltd.

Huo, M. L., & Boxall, P. (2020). Do workers respond differently to learning from supervisors and colleagues? A study of job resources, learning sources and employee wellbeing in China. *International Journal of Human Resource Management, 33*(4), 1–21.

Jamieson, S. D., & Tuckey, M. R. (2017). Mindfulness interventions in the workplace: A critique of the current state of the literature. *Journal of Occupational Health Psychology, 22*(2), 180–193. https://doi.org/10.1037/ocp0000048

Khoreva, V., & Wechtler, H. (2018). HR practices and employee performance: The mediating role of well-being. *Employee Relations, 40*(2), 227–243. https://doi.org/10.1108/ER-08-2017-0191

Loon, M., Otaye-Ebede, L., & Stewart, J. (2019). The paradox of employee psychological well-being practices: An integrative literature review and new directions for research. *International Journal of Human Resource Management, 30*(1), 156–187. https://doi.org/10.1080/09585192.2018.1479877

Macey, W. H., & Schneider, B. (2008). The meaning of employee engagement. *Industrial and Organizational Psychology: Perspectives on Science and Practice, 1*(1), 3–30. https://doi.org/10.1111/j.1754-9434.2007.0002.x

Martela, F., & Pessi, A. B. (2018). Significant work is about self-realization and broader purpose: Defining the key dimensions of meaningful work. *Frontiers in Psychology, 9,* 363. https://doi.org/10.3389/fpsyg.2018.00363

National Institute for Occupational Safety and Health. (n.d.). *The NIOSH Worker Well-Being Questionnaire (WellBQ).* https://www.cdc.gov/niosh/twh/wellbq/default.html

Nielsen, K., Nielsen, M., Ogbonnaya, C., Känsälä, M., Saari, E., & Isaksson, K. (2017). Workplace resources to improve both employee well-being and performance: A systematic review and meta-analysis. *Work and Stress, 31*(2), 101–120. https://doi.org/10.1080/02678373.2017.1304463

Nielsen, K., & Randall, R. (2012). The importance of employee participation and perceptions of changes in procedures in a teamworking intervention. *Work and Stress, 26*(2), 91–111. https://doi.org/10.1080/02678373.2012.682721

Nord, W. R., & Connell, A. F. (2011). *Organizational studies: A generative uncertainty perspective.* Routledge.

Pang, D., & Ruch, W. (2019). Fusing character strengths and mindfulness interventions: Benefits for job satisfaction and performance. *Journal of Occupational Health Psychology, 24*(1), 150–162. https://doi.org/10.1037/ocp0000144

Pignata, S., Boyd, C., Gillespie, N., Provis, C., & Winefield, A. H. (2016). Awareness of stress-reduction interventions: The impact on employees' well-being and organizational attitudes. *Stress and Health, 32*(3), 231–243. https://doi.org/10.1002/smi.2597

Porath, C., Spreitzer, G., Gibson, C., & Garnett, F. G. (2012). Thriving at work: Toward its measurement, construct validation, and theoretical refinement. *Journal of Organizational Behavior, 33*(2), 250–275. https://doi.org/10.1002/job.756

Richardson, K. M., & Rothstein, H. R. (2008). Effects of occupational stress management intervention programs: A meta-analysis. *Journal of Occupational Health Psychology, 13*(1), 69–93. https://doi.org/10.1037/1076-8998.13.1.69

Rigby, J., & Traylor, Z. (2020). Capturing trends in industrial-organizational psychology: A shiny web application. *Human Performance, 33*(4), 302–306. https://doi.org/10.1080/08959285.2020.1751165

Rosso, B. D., Dekas, K. H., & Wrzesniewski, A. (2010). On the meaning of work: A theoretical integration and review. *Research in Organizational Behavior, 30,* 91–127. https://doi.org/10.1016/j.riob.2010.09.001

Ryan, R. M., & Deci, E. L. (2001). On happiness and human potentials: A review of research on hedonic and eudaimonic well-being. *Annual Review of Psychology, 52*(1), 141–166. https://doi.org/10.1146/annurev.psych.52.1.141

Ryff, C. D., & Keyes, C. L. M. (1995). The structure of psychological well-being revisited. *Journal of Personality and Social Psychology, 69*(4), 719–727. https://doi.org/10.1037/0022-3514.69.4.719

Schaufeli, W. B., Bakker, A. B., & Salanova, M. (2006). The measurement of work engagement with a short questionnaire: A cross-national study. *Educational and Psychological Measurement, 66*(4), 701–716. https://doi.org/10.1177/0013164405282471

Schaufeli, W. B., Leiter, M. P., & Maslach, C. (2009). Burnout: 35 years of research and practice. *Career Development International, 14*(3), 204–220. https://doi.org/10.1108/13620430910966406

Schill, A. L., & Chosewood, L. C. (2013). The NIOSH Total Worker Health program: An overview. *Journal of Occupational and Environmental Medicine, 55*(Suppl. 12), S8–S11. https://doi.org/10.1097/JOM.0000000000000037

Sharecare.com. (n.d.). *What is the Sharecare Community Well-Being (CWBI) Index?* https://wellbeingindex.sharecare.com/

Shirom, A. (2011). Vigor as a positive affect at work: Conceptualizing vigor, its relations with related constructs, and its antecedents and consequences. *Review of General Psychology, 15*(1), 50–64. https://doi.org/10.1037/a0021853

Steger, M. F., Frazier, P., Oishi, S., & Kaler, M. (2006). The meaning in life questionnaire: Assessing the presence of and search for meaning in life. *Journal of Counseling Psychology, 53*(1), 80–93. https://doi.org/10.1037/0022-0167.53.1.80

Stiglbauer, B., & Kovacs, C. (2018). The more, the better? Curvilinear effects of job auto-nomy on well-being from vitamin model and PE-fit theory perspectives. *Journal of Occupational Health Psychology, 23*(4), 520–536. https://doi.org/10.1037/ocp0000107

Tims, M., Bakker, A. B., & Derks, D. (2012). Development and validation of the job crafting scale. *Journal of Vocational Behavior, 80*(1), 173–186. https://doi.org/10.1016/j.jvb.2011.05.009

Torres, M. (December 7, 2020). *Five signs you are experiencing toxic positivity at work.* Huffington Post. https://www.huffpost.com/entry/signs-experiencing-toxic-positivity-at-work_l_5fc7cedcc5b640945e52ce30

van Hooff, M. L. M., & van Hooft, E. A. J. (2016). Work-related boredom and depressed mood from a daily perspective: The moderating roles of work centrality and need satisfaction. *Work and Stress, 30*(3), 209–227. https://doi.org/10.1080/02678373.2016.1206151

van Wingerden, J., Bakker, A. B., & Derks, D. (2017). Fostering employee well-being via a job crafting intervention. *Journal of Vocational Behavior, 100,* 164–174. https://doi.org/10.1016/j.jvb.2017.03.008

Walsh, M. M., & Arnold, K. A. (2020). The bright and dark sides of employee mindful-ness: Leadership style and employee well-being. *Stress and Health, 36*(3), 287–298. https://doi.org/10.1002/smi.2926

Warr, P. (1987). *Work, unemployment, and mental health.* Oxford University Press.

Warr, P. (2013). How to think about and measure psychological well-being. In R. R. Sinclair, M. Wang, & L. E. Tetrick (Eds.), *Research methods in occupational health psy-chology: Measurement, design, and data analysis* (pp. 76–90). Routledge/Taylor & Francis Group.

Winslow, C. J., Kaplan, S. A., Bradley-Geist, J. C., Lindsey, A. P., Ahmad, A. S., & Hargrove, A. K. (2017). An examination of two positive organizational interventions: For whom do these interventions work? *Journal of Occupational Health Psychology, 22*(2), 129–137. https://doi.org/10.1037/ocp0000035

Wrzesniewski, A., & Dutton, J. E. (2001). Crafting a job: Revisioning employees as active crafters of their work. *Academy of Management Review, 26*(2), 179–201. https://doi.org/10.2307/259118

Xanthopoulou, D., Bakker, A. B., Demerouti, E., & Schaufeli, W. B. (2007). The role of personal resources in the job demands-resources model. *International Journal of Stress Management, 14*(2), 121–141. https://doi.org/10.1037/1072-5245.14.2.121

Zheng, C., Molineux, J., Mirshekary, S., & Scarparo, S. (2015). Developing individual and organisational work-life balance strategies to improve employee health and wellbeing. *Employee Relations, 37*(3), 354–379. https://doi.org/10.1108/ER-10-2013-0142

20

Psychological Recovery From Work Demands and Employee Well-Being

Charlotte Fritz

Understanding and facilitating employee well-being and performance capacity over time is a key factor in organizational success and sustainability. This is especially important considering the variety of work demands employees are exposed to and expected to deal with on a daily basis. Research over the past decade has pointed to the importance of psychological recovery from work demands for improving and maintaining positive employee and organizational outcomes. *Recovery from work* can be defined as "unwinding and restoration processes during which a person's strain level that has increased as a reaction to a stressor or any other demand returns to its prestressor level" (Sonnentag et al., 2017, p. 366). This chapter focuses on employee recovery during nonwork time (i.e., unwinding and restoration processes) and employee well-being (i.e., indicators of mental and physical health, job-related strain, and general well-being). The chapter starts out by describing several theoretical frameworks that have been used to examine psychological recovery from work. Next, the chapter elaborates on research findings regarding antecedents and outcomes of recovery from work. The chapter concludes with additional research considerations and practical implications.

THEORETICAL FRAMEWORKS

Research on recovery from work has built on a variety of theoretical frameworks, many of which stem from the field of work stress research. For example, early research on recovery from work built on the effort-recovery model

https://doi.org/10.1037/0000331-020
Handbook of Occupational Health Psychology, Third Edition, L. E. Tetrick, G. G. Fisher, M. T. Ford, and J. C. Quick (Editors)

(Meijman & Mulder, 1998), which suggests that effort expenditure at work is associated with "load reactions" that become visible in diminished well-being. In contrast, recovery is described as a process during which work demands and stressors are removed so that individual functional systems can return to their predemand levels (Meijman & Mulder, 1998). In turn, this is associated with a reduction in strain and an increase in well-being. Similarly, the cognitive activation theory of stress (Meurs & Perrewé, 2011; Ursin & Eriksen, 2010) suggests that sustained cognitive arousal (which is helpful for identifying and dealing with demands) is associated with decreased well-being. In the context of recovery from work, sustained cognitive activation during nonwork time due to work demands can hinder recovery processes, thereby further negatively impacting employee well-being. Similarly, the allostatic load model (Ganster & Rosen, 2013; Ganster et al., 2018; McEwen, 1998) proposes that extended exposure to demands in general is linked to a chronic overactivation of allostatic (e.g., cardiovascular, neuroendocrine) regulatory systems, which increases the probability of experiencing physical, psychological, or behavioral strain. Therefore, recovery from demands is crucial to help maintain employee well-being and health in the long term.

Another theoretical framework frequently used in research on recovery from work is the conservation of resources (COR) theory (Hobfoll, 1989; Hobfoll et al., 2018). According to COR theory, individuals generally strive to gain resources (i.e., valued objects, personal characteristics, conditions, and energies) and avoid the loss of resources. Halbesleben et al. (2014) expanded the concept of resources to suggest that resources include anything that helps an individual reach their goals. Nonwork time, a time during which work demands are reduced or removed, therefore provides the opportunity to replenish resources lost at work and to gain new resources.

Recent research has also built on self-determination theory (SDT; Ryan & Deci, 2000) as a framework to better understand recovery processes during nonwork time (e.g., Mojza et al., 2011; ten Brummelhuis & Trougakos, 2014). According to SDT, all humans have three basic human needs: autonomy, competence, and relatedness. Being able to fulfill these needs is associated with higher need satisfaction as well as well-being (Van den Broeck et al., 2016). In the context of recovery from work, nonwork time can provide the opportunity to fulfill these basic human needs. This is especially important if these needs cannot fully be satisfied at work.

A more direct description of links between recovery and well-being was suggested by Sonnentag and Fritz (2015) in their stressor-detachment model (SDM). Specifically, the SDM proposes that work demands are associated with lower psychological detachment (i.e., mental disengagement) from work during nonwork time, which in turn is linked to decreased employee well-being. Thus, detachment is expected to mediate the relationships between work demands and well-being. Furthermore, the model suggests that detachment can act as a moderator to alleviate the relationships between work demands and impaired well-being. In summary, central to the examination of recovery from work during nonwork time is the idea that taking breaks from the demands of work is crucial for the maintenance of employee short-term and long-term well-being.

RECOVERY ACTIVITIES, EXPERIENCES, AND STATES

Researchers suggest that it is beneficial to differentiate between recovery from work as a process and recovery from work as an outcome (Sonnentag & Geurts, 2009). The recovery process includes particular activities as well as specific experiences that are associated with an increase in well-being. Examining what people do (i.e., recovery activities) during nonwork time and their psychological experience of that time (i.e., recovery experiences) provides important insights into the reversal of the work strain process that often results from exposure to work demands. Recovery as an outcome refers to an employee's psychological or physiological state resulting from recovery processes during nonwork time.

Recovery Activities

When focusing on activities during nonwork time as indicators of the recovery process, research has examined different types of activities. With regard to types of activities, research has examined household and child care activities, physical activities, or social activities (e.g., Sonnentag, 2001). When examining nonwork activities, researchers have often categorized activities into those that support recovery (i.e., "low-duty activities" such as active or passive leisure activities) and those that may hinder recovery from work (i.e., "high-duty activities" such as household chores or work-related tasks; Sonnentag et al., 2017). Two nonwork activities that have received a great amount of research attention—although not necessarily always in the context of recovery from work—are sleep and physical activity (Calderwood et al., 2021; Litwiller et al., 2017). Some research has also examined the time spent on specific activities during nonwork time as well as the motivation and affect associated with these activities such as intentions (Payne et al., 2002), intrinsic motivation (ten Brummelhuis & Trougakos, 2014), or happiness during the activity (Oerlemans et al., 2014).

Recovery Experiences

Sonnentag and Fritz (2007) suggested that the experience associated with a nonwork activity may be more relevant for recovery from work than the activity itself. Therefore, they proposed four key recovery experiences during nonwork time: (a) psychological detachment, (b) relaxation, (c) mastery, and (d) control. *Psychological detachment* refers to mentally letting go of work during nonwork time. When employees are detaching from work during nonwork time, they are no longer engaged in work activities or work-related thoughts or feelings (Etzion et al., 1998; Sonnentag & Fritz, 2007). *Relaxation* during nonwork time includes the experience of ease and low effort and is often associated with nondemanding activities (Sonnentag & Fritz, 2007). *Mastery* experiences may require effort but provide opportunities for learning, growth, and broadening one's horizons (Sonnentag & Fritz, 2007). Finally, *control* during nonwork time refers to the extent to which employees experience that they are able to choose how to spend their nonwork time (Sonnentag & Fritz, 2007). Over the years, research on recovery has examined experiences beyond those four suggested by Sonnentag and Fritz (2007). For example, pleasure and enjoyment, positive and negative work reflection, meaning, and affiliation during nonwork time were examined as antecedents of employee well-being (Newman et al., 2014; Sonnentag et al., 2017).

Recovery as a State

Some research refers to recovery from work as a state that results from engagement in nonwork activities. For example, this research captures the "state of being recovered," which includes feeling full of energy, being mentally recovered, and feeling well rested (e.g., Binnewies et al., 2009; Sonnentag et al., 2012). The state of being recovered has also been considered an indicator of a successful recovery process (e.g., Binnewies et al., 2009).

RECOVERY SETTINGS

Recovery from work during nonwork time can occur during a variety of times. Accordingly, research has examined longer time frames such as sabbaticals or vacations as well as shorter time frames such as weekends or evenings (Fritz et al., 2013). In addition, research has examined recovery at work such as during lunch breaks (e.g., Trougakos et al., 2014) and "microbreaks" (e.g., Fritz et al., 2011). This chapter, however, focuses on recovery from work in the context of being outside of work only.

Sabbaticals—that is, a special case of extended respite from regular work—unfortunately, are only available to a small number of employees (e.g., university faculty). As a result, these work arrangements have received little research attention from organizational researchers so far (Davidson et al., 2010). Vacations include an extended time during which work demands are removed (or at least reduced) and therefore allow employees to spend more time engaging in activities and experiences that facilitate recovery from work. This extended time of low or removed work demands provides employees the opportunity to recover from short-term and accumulated or more chronic well-being impairments (e.g., burnout; Fritz & Sonnentag, 2006; Westman & Eden, 1997). While research shows improvements in employee well-being from before to directly after vacation, these positive effects seem to fade once the employee is exposed to work demands again (e.g., Fritz & Sonnentag, 2006; Horan et al., 2021). The weekend (i.e., one to three consecutive days of nonwork time) is another opportunity for employees to get a break from the demands of work and to replenish lost resources, resulting in higher well-being afterward (e.g., Fritz & Sonnentag, 2005). For example, weekends can provide better quality and quantity of sleep, which is associated with higher levels of vitality and lower levels of fatigue (Weigelt et al., 2021). Finally, non-work time in the evenings after work has received a great amount of research attention. For example, research has examined to what extent employee experiences (such as work demands or work resources) throughout the workday are associated with recovery during the evening. Furthermore, research has focused on possible links between recovery in the evening and increased well-being at bedtime or the following morning (see Sonnentag & Fritz, 2015, 2018; and Sonnentag et al., 2017, for reviews).

ANTECEDENTS OF PSYCHOLOGICAL RECOVERY FROM WORK

When considering antecedents of recovery from work, research so far has mostly focused on the role of work demands. There is, however, some research evidence for the role of nonwork demands, work and nonwork resources, as well as individual differences as antecedents of recovery from work during nonwork time.

Work and Nonwork Demands

Demands in work as well as in the nonwork domain require effort expenditure and are associated with negative activation (e.g., negative mood) that can impede psychological recovery during nonwork time. Furthermore, demands in either domain can limit the time available for recovery processes to occur. Considering the relationships between work, demands, recovery from work, and employee well-being, Sonnentag (2018) introduced the concept of a recovery paradox. Specifically, the recovery paradox builds on the vast amount of research indicating that work demands are linked to impaired short-term and long-term well-being and that recovery from work during nonwork time is associated with increased well-being. As a result, employees should especially engage in recovery activities and experiences when being exposed to high levels of work demands to counteract the commonly detrimental effects of these demands. Research, however, has pointed to the paradox that when experiencing high levels of work demands, employees are less likely (instead of more likely) to engage in recovery activities or experiences during nonwork time.

In a recent meta-analysis, Bennett et al. (2018) examined the relationships between work demands and the four recovery experiences introduced by Sonnentag and Fritz (psychological detachment, relaxation, mastery, and control). Findings indicated that challenge demands (such as time pressure) at work were negatively related to psychological detachment from work, relaxation, and control during nonwork time but were not related to mastery experiences. Furthermore, hindrance demands at work (such as role ambiguity or interpersonal conflict) were negatively associated with detachment and relaxation but were not related to control or mastery experiences during non-work time. Steed et al. (2021) conducted a more extensive meta-analysis on recovery from work to examine the links between a variety of work demands and employee recovery activities (i.e., low-duty vs. high-duty nonwork activities), recovery experiences, and the state of being recovered. Results generally indicated that work overload in addition to cognitive and emotional work demands were consistently negatively associated with recovery experiences and the state of being recovered (but neither with low-duty nor high-duty activities during nonwork time). Results for physical work demands were weaker and less consistent.

Research examining links between nonwork demands and psychological recovery from work has received little attention so far. This may be partially due to the assumption that activities and experiences during nonwork time—such as household chores or child care—could be described as part of recovery from work given that work demands are removed and employees are engaged in nonwork activities. These nonwork activities may be experienced as demanding and/or replenishing and as a result can be associated with lower or higher well-being, respectively. Some research on nonwork experiences has examined the role of nonwork hassles during vacations or weekends on employee well-being rather than directly on recovery activities or experiences (e.g., Fritz & Sonnentag, 2005, 2006; Fritz et al., 2010).

Research has also examined sleep as a specific activity that allows for the replenishment of physical and mental resources resulting in increased well-being. Cross-sectional and longitudinal research so far has suggested that work demands are associated with impaired sleep (see Sonnentag, 2018, for a summary). Again, these findings are in line with the recovery paradox indicating that employees may seek out recovery opportunities less (rather than more) when experiencing high levels of work demands. Meta-analytical research by Litwiller and colleagues (2017) indicates that workload was negatively related to employee sleep.

One nonwork activity that has received a large amount of research attention (although much of it outside the context of occupational health psychology) is physical activity (Calderwood et al., 2021; Fransson et al., 2012). For example, meta-analytical findings by Fransson et al. (2012) indicate that employees experiencing high levels of work demands and low levels of work control (i.e., high-strain jobs) report the highest levels of physical inactivity during nonwork time. Furthermore, initially physically active people became less active over time as a result of high-strain jobs or passive jobs (i.e., low work demands and low work control). These findings are in line with the recovery paradox suggested by Sonnentag (2018).

Work and Nonwork Resources

Research has indicated that work and nonwork resources can facilitate recovery from work. With regard to work resources, meta-analytical findings have shown that job autonomy was positively associated with three of the four recovery experiences introduced by Sonnentag and Fritz, namely, relaxation, mastery, and control during nonwork time (Bennett et al., 2018). Interestingly, job autonomy was not related to detachment from work (Bennett et al., 2018). Similarly, results from Litwiller et al.'s (2017) meta-analysis indicated that job autonomy was positively associated with employee sleep. Steed et al.'s (2021) more extensive meta-analysis on recovery from work expanded these findings. Overall, work resources such as social support were positively associated with recovery experiences and the state of being recovered but not with recovery activities (neither low-duty nor high-duty activities). The relationships between work resources and recovery experiences were stronger for mastery and control than for relaxation and detachment from work during nonwork time. It is important to consider that while some of the work resources linked to recovery during nonwork time may take place on the individual level, others may be on the team or organizational level. Accordingly, research shows that work team norms of segmenting work and nonwork life were linked to higher employee psychological detachment from work during nonwork time (Park et al., 2011). With regard to nonwork resources, meta-analytical evidence shows positive relationships such as spousal recovery support and recovery experiences (Steed et al., 2021). Again, the relationships were stronger for mastery and control than for relaxation and detachment during nonwork time. Due to lack of sufficient research, the relationships between nonwork resources and state of being recovered could not be meta-analytically calculated.

Individual Differences

Some research has also considered the role of individual differences in recovery from work. In their initial scale validation study of the four proposed recovery experiences, Sonnentag and Fritz (2007) found small or nonsignificant relationships between the Big Five personality factors and the four recovery experiences. However, individual differences related to the interface between work and nonwork life may be more relevant. For example, Park et al. (2011) found that the individual preference to separate work and nonwork life was associated with higher levels of psychological detachment from work. Similarly, Steed et al.'s (2021) findings indicate that personal resources (including more general as well as work- or nonwork-specific variables) were related to all four recovery experiences from work, and these relationships were stronger than those between work or nonwork resources and recovery experiences. Once again, relationships with activities and state of being recovered could not be meta-analytically calculated due to lack of research.

LINKS BETWEEN RECOVERY FROM WORK AND EMPLOYEE WELL-BEING

Recovery from work has been suggested as an important antecedent of employee well-being (Sonnentag & Fritz, 2007). Recovery from work can be linked to employee well-being in several specific ways (Steed et al., 2021).

For example, given that it includes the removal of or distancing from work demands, it facilitates the reduction of work-related strain and the improvement of well-being. Furthermore, specific nonwork experiences and activities allow employees to replenish individual resources invested at work, which becomes visible in increased well-being. During recovery from work, employees can explicitly enjoy their nonwork time and engage in activities that align with their personal goals and passions, resulting in decreased negative emotions and increased positive emotions (e.g., Fritz et al., 2010).

Accordingly, there is strong empirical evidence for links between recovery from work and employee well-being. In their meta-analysis, Bennett et al. (2018) examined associations between the four recovery experiences introduced by Sonnentag and Fritz (2007) and two indicators of employee well-being, namely vigor and fatigue. Findings indicated that all four recovery experiences were negatively associated with fatigue and positively associated with vigor, pointing to the important role of recovery from work for employee well-being. In their more extensive meta-analysis on recovery from work, Steed et al. (2021) examined relationships between recovery activities (i.e., low-duty and high-duty activities during nonwork time), recovery experiences, and the state of being recovered on one hand, and psychological (mental well-being, positive affect, negative affect, and life satisfaction) as well as psychosomatic well-being (fatigue, sleep, health) on the other hand. With regard to recovery activities, findings indicated that low-duty (but not high-duty) activities during nonwork time were associated with increased mental well-being.

In terms of recovery experiences, results suggested positive relationships with mental well-being. Furthermore, recovery experiences were consistently and positively related to positive affect and life satisfaction and negatively related to negative affect. In addition, recovery experiences were positively associated with psychosomatic well-being such as lower fatigue and improved sleep. Findings also pointed to positive relationships between the state of being recovered and psychological (mental well-being and positive affect) as well as psychosomatic (sleep and lower fatigue) well-being. Overall, recovery activities had the weakest and most inconsistent relationships with employee well-being. However, this may be due to the way in which recovery activities were categorized (e.g., high duty vs. low duty). That means that certain potentially demanding activities and experiences during nonwork time—such as household chores or child care—could be described as part of recovery from work given that work demands are removed and employees are engaged in nonwork activities. As mentioned previously, these nonwork activities may be experienced as demanding and/or replenishing and as a result can be associated with lower or higher well-being, respectively.

Physical activity can be considered as recovery activities during nonwork time that are especially beneficial for employee well-being and health. Accordingly, exercise has been linked to increased positive affect and decreased psychological distress immediately after the activity (see Calderwood et al., 2021, or Sonnentag, 2018, for a review). Furthermore, meta-analytical evidence suggests that regular exercise is associated with higher positive-activated affect

(Reed & Buck, 2009). Meta-analytical findings further indicate that exercise interventions are associated with reduced anxiety and reduced depressive symptoms (Conn, 2010a, 2010b). A recent multidisciplinary integrative review of research on employee physical activity (Calderwood et al., 2021) further suggests that acute and regular physical activity are both potentially linked to increased physical, affective, and cognitive resources (becoming visible in well-being indicators such as increased positive affect, better physical health, or mental resilience) that facilitate performance capacity at work.

Another crucial recovery activity outside of work is sleep. Numerous studies have shown that sleep is related to a wide variety of psychological and physical well-being indicators. Meta-analytical findings, for example, indicated that high sleep quality and quantity were both associated with lower anxiety, depressive symptoms, and fatigue (Litwiller et al., 2017). On the day level, research indicated that sleep quality the night before work is linked to fatigue, self-regulatory capacity, microbreaks, and work engagement during the workday (e.g., Kim et al., 2022). Overall, sleep as a nonwork activity seems to be a protective factor helping to reduce the risk of impaired well-being.

RECOVERY INTERVENTIONS

Given the amount of research indicating positive links between recovery from work and employee well-being and performance capacity, the development of interventions to facilitate employee recovery from work seems a fruitful endeavor. One approach would be to examine the potential impact of more general stress-reduction interventions on employee recovery from work. Accordingly, Michel et al. (2014) found that mindfulness training was associated with increased psychological detachment from work during nonwork time. Similarly, Ebert et al. (2016) reported that an internet-based stress management intervention focused on problem-solving and emotion regulation was associated with increased detachment from work. Another intervention approach would be to directly focus the intervention on the improvement of recovery from work. One such intervention study—conducted by Hahn et al. (2011)—focused on facilitating the four recovery experiences introduced by Sonnentag and Fritz (2007). Study findings showed that recovery experiences, recovery-related self-efficacy, and well-being increased as a result of the intervention.

Given that psychological detachment from work during nonwork time is the recovery experience most widely studied and often most strongly related to work demands and well-being, it has also received the most attention with regard to interventions. In a recent meta-analysis, Karabinski et al. (2021) examined the effectiveness of interventions designed to facilitate psychological detachment from work based on 30 studies (34 interventions, $N = 3,725$). Overall results indicated a positive effect of interventions on detachment from work. Furthermore, moderator analyses provided additional insights.

Interventions focused on reducing work demands or changing the primary (e.g., mindfulness) or secondary (e.g., increase in work resources) appraisal of work demands all were effective. Interventions focused on a change in primary appraisal, however, seemed most effective. In addition, longer interventions with higher dosage were more effective. In terms of participant characteristics, interventions were more effective for older employees and those with low levels of initial well-being or recovery. The authors suggest that essential components of detachment interventions should be strategies that help manage the boundaries between employees' work and nonwork domains, promote emotion regulation strategies, and improve sleep quality.

ADDITIONAL FINDINGS AND FURTHER CONSIDERATIONS

While a considerable amount of research has identified direct relationships between work characteristics and recovery as well as between recovery and well-being, additional research has suggested more complex relationships between these variables. For example, research also points to the role of recovery from work as a moderating or mediating factor in the relationships between work demands and employee well-being (e.g., Sonnentag & Fritz, 2015). In their qualitative review of the literature on psychological detachment from work, Sonnentag and Fritz (2015) were only able to find very few studies that examined detachment during nonwork time as a moderator or mediator in the relationship between work demands and well-being. Based on their review, the authors suggested an SDM in which detachment may act as a moderator as well as mediator. Furthermore, they suggested additional job and personal factors that may moderate the link between work demands and detachment (e.g., personal or job resources) in addition to the link between detachment and well-being (e.g., problem-focused coping). While research on recovery from work has clearly increased since that review, more research is needed examining recovery as a moderator or mediator in the relationships between work characteristics and employee well-being (Sonnentag & Fritz, 2015, 2018).

Similarly, other research has suggested that physical activity during nonwork time can help alleviate the relationships between work demands and impaired well-being (Puterman et al., 2017). Bennett et al. (2018) meta-analytically examined to what extent recovery experiences mediate the relationships between work characteristics (e.g., challenge and hindrance demands, work resources) and employee well-being (e.g., fatigue and vigor). Results indicated that challenge demands as well as resources at work were directly as well as indirectly (i.e., through recovery experiences) related to both fatigue and vigor. Hindrance demands were directly and indirectly associated with fatigue but only showed a direct (not an indirect) relationship with vigor. Furthermore, the authors examined the additional impact of recovery experiences during nonwork time on vigor and fatigue over and above the impact of work characteristics and found that there was a 26% increase in variance explained in fatigue and a 62% increase in variance explained in vigor through recovery experiences. Clearly, both job characteristics and recovery experiences impact employee well-being.

It is also important to consider the extent to which different aspects of recovery from work (activities, experiences, and the state of being recovered) may be related to each other. It is easy to assume that recovery activities and experiences are probably not independent from each other (Sonnentag, 2018). For example, exercise (especially certain forms) as a form of recovery activity during nonwork time may facilitate detachment from work, and detachment can facilitate sleep, another recovery activity (Hülsheger et al., 2014). Accordingly, Fritz and Crain (2016) suggested that a variety of activities (e.g., technology use, social interactions, exercise) and experiences (e.g., detachment from work, relaxation) during nonwork time were linked to employee sleep. Accordingly, findings indicated that cyber leisure (as a form of recovery activity) in the evening was negatively associated with sleep quantity and quality through bedtime procrastination (i.e., delaying sleep time) while cyber leisure was positively associated with sleep through psychological detachment.

In addition, recovery activities and experiences may interact with each other to predict short-term and/or long-term employee well-being (Bennett et al., 2016; Cho & Park, 2018). For example, Bennett et al. (2016) identified several profiles of recovery experiences (plus problem-solving pondering) that could be differentiated in their relationships with employee well-being (i.e., emotional exhaustion and work engagement). Similarly, Chawla et al. (2020) found that profiles of recovery experiences could be linked to different work demands and resources as well as employee well-being.

While most research on recovery from work and employee well-being has examined recovery as an antecedent of well-being, some research points to the possibility of reverse causality. Thus, in line with propositions based on COR theory, a lack of recovery from work after exposure to work demands may create a downward spiral in which well-being and recovery from work are increasingly impaired over time. In contrast, Sonnentag and Fritz (2018) have suggested that positive affective states—as an indicator of employee well-being—are not only an outcome of recovery from work but may also facilitate recovery. Intervention, in particular, or experimental studies will help shed more light on causal links between recovery from work and employee well-being. Thus, future research can contribute to the current knowledge on recovery from work by examining reciprocal, cyclical, or nonlinear processes of recovery from work (Sonnentag et al., 2022).

Related to the examination of reverse causality is also the deeper examination of relationships between work demands, recovery from work, and employee well-being over time. For example, it is important to understand how the short-term benefits of day-level recovery from work (e.g., during evenings after work) translate into longer term changes in employee physical and psychological well-being (Sonnentag et al., 2022). Relatedly, future research should also examine how long the benefits of different recovery activities, experiences, and time periods last (Sonnentag et al., 2022). Furthermore, by examining recovery processes using weekly or monthly assessments of recovery and well-being, research can expand the current knowledge based on day-level studies or longitudinal studies. This knowledge can provide further input into the development of specific strategies and interventions that help employees build the capacity for and implement successful recovery processes during nonwork time.

PRACTICAL IMPLICATIONS

Research findings regarding recovery from work provide considerable practical implications for work organizations. First, recovery during nonwork time is beneficial to employee well-being. This awareness can help organizations and their employees create opportunities for recovery during shorter (e.g., evenings) and longer (e.g., vacations) time periods outside of work. Research findings have suggested that work demands (especially work overload in addition to cognitive and emotional work demands) are negatively associated with recovery from work as well as employee well-being. Thus, whenever possible, organizations should reduce such demands on their employees. When work demands are reduced, less work-related strain is likely to occur, and recovery activities and experiences are less likely to be impaired. Given the link between recovery from work and employee well-being, organizations should also be aware that supporting employee recovery from work can potentially help reduce health care costs (Steed et al., 2021).

Beyond reducing work demands, organizations can facilitate employee recovery by providing increased job resources such as social support or greater autonomy and flexibility. Thus, by reducing work demands and increasing work resources, organizations may simultaneously reduce overall labor cost while improving employee well-being (Steed et al., 2021). Two job resources that may be especially important for employee recovery from work during nonwork time are workplace flexibility and supervisor support (Sonnentag & Fritz, 2018). Workplace flexibility can ease the burden associated with juggling work and nonwork demands and roles. For example, workplace flexibility strategies such as flexible start and end times each day, remote work, or shorter workweeks (e.g., four-day workweeks) increase employees' schedule control. The increased schedule control makes it easier for employees to take care of work and nonwork demands as needed and provides them with the opportunity to pursue recovery activities and experiences when most feasible and when needed most. With regard to supervisor support, a study by Bennett and colleagues (2016) indicated that supervisor support for recovery from work during nonwork time was positively related to employee recovery experiences.

Organizations may also explicitly facilitate employee recovery from work through minimizing expectations that employees engage in work activities (e.g., checking emails, answering work calls, finishing up work tasks) during nonwork time. Organizational leaders may also act as role models by, for example, not sending emails to employees after standard work hours. Accordingly, Koch and Binnewies (2015) found that employees with work–life friendly supervisors (i.e., supervisors that role model segmenting work from nonwork life) reported higher work–nonwork segmentation and lower burnout.

Organizations would also benefit from offering structured trainings to employees that help develop and expand employees' capacity to recover from work during nonwork time. Given that there is enough empirical evidence for the effectiveness of such trainings, it would be worth the organization's financial and time investment to provide such trainings to employees as an additional resource. As suggested by Karabinski et al. (2021), these trainings may be especially beneficial to older employees and those experiencing high levels of work-related strain or impaired recovery from work. It should be pointed out, however, that the opportunity for employees to participate in such trainings should not be a replacement for the reduction in work demands and the provision of work resources that can support employee recovery from work and facilitate well-being.

Given research findings pointing to the recovery paradox (especially including psychological detachment from work, physical activity, and sleep), organizations and employees should consider ways in which the paradox can be interrupted. Organizations may focus on reducing or eliminating work demands whenever possible. Employees may also be able to reduce the risk of the recovery paradox unfolding by approaching work in a more mindful way that helps alleviate the strain reactions resulting from work demands (Good et al., 2016; Sonnentag, 2018). Furthermore, employees may benefit from developing individual recovery habits that facilitate the engagement in recovery activities and experiences even (or especially) when work demands are high.

While organizations should be encouraged to facilitate employee recovery from work, so should employees themselves. As a first step, employees should be made aware of the potential negative impact that a lack of recovery may have for their well-being. As result, employees may be more motivated to engage in activities and experiences during nonwork time that support recovery from work. For example, employees may explicitly aim to detach from work and to seek out relaxation experiences. Given that organizations may not always be able to reduce employees' work demands or provide sufficient work resources, employees would benefit from proactively seeking out resources at work (e.g., requesting more scheduling flexibility) or outside of work (e.g., requesting spousal recovery support) as well as utilizing personal (e.g., increasing mindfulness through regular practice) resources that can facilitate their recovery from work.

It may also be helpful to employees to pursue recovery opportunities during different time frames so that unwinding effects can accumulate. For example, employees should consider that recovery activities and experiences are necessary and beneficial during shorter time frames (e.g., evenings after work) as well as longer time frames (e.g., weekends, vacations), and that one time period should not be considered as a replacement for another.

Employees would also benefit from developing strategies that help create boundaries between work and nonwork life that can facilitate recovery from work during nonwork time. For example, employees can set boundaries during vacations by not checking their emails and by setting up an automatic "out-of-office" email response that helps manage expectations regarding their response time. In addition, developing routines related to recovery from work to reduce the self-regulatory effort associated with recovery activities and experiences (Sonnentag & Fritz, 2018) could be helpful. For example, routines related to exercise, sleep, meditation, or socializing may help ensure that employees engage in these activities and experiences on a regular and frequent basis.

Employees may also draw on their social network outside of work for recovery support. Accordingly, Park and Fritz (2015) found that spousal recovery support was positively linked to employee recovery experiences and life satisfaction, which crossed over to the spouse's life satisfaction. Thus, employees should consider communicating their need for recovery to their spouse so that they can support each other in their pursuit of recovery from work and their well-being.

Steed et al. (2021) found that reports of recovery were relatively stable over time, suggesting that employees show substantial consistency in their state of being recovered as well as in their recovery experiences over time. Thus, some employees may be more likely to engage in recovery experiences (e.g., due to individual differences or routines) independent of contextual factors (e.g., demands, resources) at work or outside of work (Steed et al., 2021). The findings may also indicate that demands and resources are often stable over time. Thus, to create longer lasting positive changes in recovery, interventions or job design changes that facilitate changes in recovery processes and outcomes may be necessary.

CONCLUSION

When it comes to recovery from work, employees seem to face a dilemma: When facing high levels of (work and other) demands, recovery from work is particularly important; at the same time, during those time periods, recovery activities and experiences are often impaired (Sonnentag, 2018; Sonnentag et al., 2017). Recovery from work, however, is a crucial process through which well-being can be improved and maintained. While future research on recovery from work will provide additional insights, research over the past 20 years has provided empirical evidence for the important role of recovery from work in the field of occupational health psychology.

REFERENCES

Bennett, A. A., Bakker, A. B., & Field, J. G. (2018). Recovery from work-related effort: A meta-analysis. *Journal of Organizational Behavior, 39*(3), 262–275. https://doi.org/10.1002/job.2217

Bennett, A. A., Gabriel, A. S., Calderwood, C., Dahling, J. J., & Trougakos, J. P. (2016). Better together? Examining profiles of employee recovery experiences. *Journal of Applied Psychology, 101*(12), 1635–1654. https://doi.org/10.1037/apl0000157

Binnewies, C., Sonnentag, S., & Mojza, E. J. (2009). Daily performance at work: Feeling recovered in the morning as a predictor of day-level job performance. *Journal of Organizational Behavior, 30*(1), 67–93. https://doi.org/10.1002/job.541

Calderwood, C., ten Brummelhuis, L. L., Patel, A. S., Watkins, T., Gabriel, A. S., & Rosen, C. C. (2021). Employee physical activity: A multidisciplinary integrative review. *Journal of Management, 47*(1), 144–170. https://doi.org/10.1177/0149206320940413

Chawla, N., MacGowan, R. L., Gabriel, A. S., & Podsakoff, N. P. (2020). Unplugging or staying connected? Examining the nature, antecedents, and consequences of profiles of daily recovery experiences. *Journal of Applied Psychology, 105*(1), 19–39. https://doi.org/10.1037/apl0000423

Cho, S., & Park, Y. (2018). How to benefit from weekend physical activities: Moderating roles of psychological recovery experiences and sleep. *Stress and Health, 34*(5), 639–648. https://doi.org/10.1002/smi.2831

Conn, V. S. (2010a). Anxiety outcomes after physical activity interventions: Meta-analysis findings. *Nursing Research, 59*(3), 224–231. https://doi.org/10.1097/NNR.0b013e3181dbb2f8

Conn, V. S. (2010b). Depressive symptom outcomes of physical activity interventions: Meta-analysis findings. *Annals of Behavioral Medicine, 39*(2), 128–138. https://doi.org/10.1007/s12160-010-9172-x

Davidson, O. B., Eden, D., Westman, M., Cohen-Charash, Y., Hammer, L. B., Kluger, A. N., Krausz, M., Maslach, C., O'Driscoll, M., Perrewé, P. L., Quick, J. C., Rosenblatt, Z., & Spector, P. E. (2010). Sabbatical leave: Who gains and how much? *Journal of Applied Psychology, 95*(5), 953–964. https://doi.org/10.1037/a0020068

Ebert, D. D., Lehr, D., Heber, E., Riper, H., Cuijpers, P., & Berking, M. (2016). Internet- and mobile-based stress management for employees with adherence-focused guidance: Efficacy and mechanism of change. *Scandinavian Journal of Work, Environment & Health, 42*(5), 382–394. https://doi.org/10.5271/sjweh.3573

Etzion, D., Eden, D., & Lapidot, Y. (1998). Relief from job stressors and burnout: Reserve service as a respite. *Journal of Applied Psychology, 83*(4), 577–585. https://doi.org/10.1037/0021-9010.83.4.577

Fransson, E. I., Heikkilä, K., Nyberg, S. T., Zins, M., Westerlund, H., Westerholm, P., Väänänen, A., Virtanen, M., Vahtera, J., Theorell, T., Suominen, S., Singh-Manoux, A., Siegrist, J., Sabia, S., Rugulies, R., Pentti, J., Oksanen, T., Nordin, M., Nielsen, M. L., . . . Kivimäki, M. (2012). Job strain as a risk factor for leisure-time physical inactivity: An individual-participant meta-analysis of up to 170,000 men and women: The IPD-Work Consortium. *American Journal of Epidemiology, 176*(12), 1078–1089. https://doi.org/10.1093/aje/kws336

Fritz, C., & Crain, T. (2016). Recovery from work and employee sleep: Understanding the role of experiences and activities outside of work. In J. Barling, C. M. Barnes, D. T. Wagner, & E. L. Carleton (Eds.), *Sleep and work* (pp. 55–76). Oxford University Press. https://doi.org/10.1093/acprof:oso/9780190217662.003.0004

Fritz, C., Ellis, A. M., Demsky, C. A., Lin, B. C., & Guros, F. (2013). Embracing work breaks: Recovering from work stress. *Organizational Dynamics, 42*(4), 274–280. https://doi.org/10.1016/j.orgdyn.2013.07.005

Fritz, C., Lam, C. F., & Spreitzer, G. M. (2011). It's the little things that matter: An examination of knowledge workers' energy management. *The Academy of Management Perspectives, 25*(3), 28–39. https://doi.org/10.5465/amp.25.3.zol28

Fritz, C., & Sonnentag, S. (2005). Recovery, health, and job performance: Effects of weekend experiences. *Journal of Occupational Health Psychology, 10*(3), 187–199. https://doi.org/10.1037/1076-8998.10.3.187

Fritz, C., & Sonnentag, S. (2006). Recovery, well-being, and performance-related outcomes: The role of workload and vacation experiences. *Journal of Applied Psychology, 91*(4), 936–945. https://doi.org/10.1037/0021-9010.91.4.936

Fritz, C., Sonnentag, S., Spector, P. E., & McInroe, J. A. (2010). The weekend matters: Relationships between stress recovery and affective experiences. *Journal of Organizational Behavior, 31*(8), 1137–1162. https://doi.org/10.1002/job.672

Ganster, D. C., & Rosen, C. C. (2013). Work stress and employee health: A multidisciplinary review. *Journal of Management, 39*(5), 1085–1122. https://doi.org/10.1177/0149206313475815

Ganster, D. C., Rosen, C. C., & Fisher, G. G. (2018). Long working hours and well-being: What we know, what we do not know, and what we need to know. *Journal of Business and Psychology, 33*(1), 25–39. https://doi.org/10.1007/s10869-016-9478-1

Good, D. J., Lyddy, C. J., Glomb, T. M., Bono, J. E., Brown, K. W., Duffy, M. K., Baer, R. A., Brewer, J. A., & Lazar, S. W. (2016). Contemplating mindfulness at work: An integrative review. *Journal of Management, 42*(1), 114–142. https://doi.org/10.1177/0149206315617003

Hahn, V. C., Binnewies, C., Sonnentag, S., & Mojza, E. J. (2011). Learning how to recover from job stress: Effects of a recovery training program on recovery, recovery-related self-efficacy, and well-being. *Journal of Occupational Health Psychology, 16*(2), 202–216. https://doi.org/10.1037/a0022169

Halbesleben, J. R., Neveu, J. P., Paustian-Underdahl, S. C., & Westman, M. (2014). Getting to the "COR": Understanding the role of resources in conservation of resources theory. *Journal of Management, 40*(5), 1334–1364. https://doi.org/10.1177/0149206314527130

Hobfoll, S. E. (1989). Conservation of resources: A new attempt at conceptualizing stress. *American Psychologist, 44*(3), 513–524. https://doi.org/10.1037/0003-066X.44.3.513

Hobfoll, S. E., Halbesleben, J., Neveu, J. P., & Westman, M. (2018). Conservation of resources in the organizational context: The reality of resources and their consequences. *Annual Review of Organizational Psychology and Organizational Behavior, 5*(1), 103–128. https://doi.org/10.1146/annurev-orgpsych-032117-104640

Horan, S., Flaxman, P. E., & Stride, C. B. (2021). The perfect recovery? Interactive influence of perfectionism and spillover work tasks on changes in exhaustion and mood around a vacation. *Journal of Occupational Health Psychology, 26*(2), 86–107. https://doi.org/10.1037/ocp0000208

Hülsheger, U. R., Lang, J. W. B., Depenbrock, F., Fehrmann, C., Zijlstra, F. R. H., & Alberts, H. J. E. M. (2014). The power of presence: The role of mindfulness at work for daily levels and change trajectories of psychological detachment and sleep quality. *Journal of Applied Psychology, 99*(6), 1113–1128. https://doi.org/10.1037/a0037702

Karabinski, T., Haun, V. C., Nübold, A., Wendsche, J., & Wegge, J. (2021). Interventions for improving psychological detachment from work: A meta-analysis. *Journal of Occupational Health Psychology, 26*(3), 224–242. https://doi.org/10.1037/ocp0000280

Kim, S., Cho, S., & Park, Y. (2022). Daily microbreaks in a self-regulatory resources lens: Perceived health climate as a contextual moderator via microbreak autonomy. *Journal of Applied Psychology, 107*(1), 60–77. https://doi.org/10.1037/apl0000891

Koch, A. R., & Binnewies, C. (2015). Setting a good example: Supervisors as work-life-friendly role models within the context of boundary management. *Journal of Occupational Health Psychology, 20*(1), 82–92. https://doi.org/10.1037/a0037890

Litwiller, B., Snyder, L. A., Taylor, W. D., & Steele, L. M. (2017). The relationship between sleep and work: A meta-analysis. *Journal of Applied Psychology, 102*(4), 682–699. https://doi.org/10.1037/apl0000169

McEwen, B. S. (1998). Stress, adaptation, and disease: Allostasis and allostatic load. *Annals of the New York Academy of Sciences, 840*(1), 33–44. https://doi.org/10.1111/j.1749-6632.1998.tb09546.x

Meijman, T. F., & Mulder, G. (1998). Psychological aspects of workload. In P. J. D. Drenth, H. Thierry, & C. J. de Wolff (Eds.), *Handbook of work and organizational psychology: Work psychology* (pp. 5–33). Psychology Press/Erlbaum (UK) Taylor & Francis.

Meurs, J. A., & Perrewé, P. L. (2011). Cognitive activation theory of stress: An integrative theoretical approach to work stress. *Journal of Management, 37*(4), 1043–1068. https://doi.org/10.1177/0149206310387303

Michel, A., Bosch, C., & Rexroth, M. (2014). Mindfulness as a cognitive–emotional segmentation strategy: An intervention promoting work–life balance. *Journal of Occupational and Organizational Psychology, 87*(4), 733–754. https://doi.org/10.1111/joop.12072

Mojza, E. J., Sonnentag, S., & Bornemann, C. (2011). Volunteer work as a valuable leisure-time activity: A day-level study on volunteer work, non-work experiences, and well-being at work. *Journal of Occupational and Organizational Psychology, 84*(1), 123–152. https://doi.org/10.1348/096317910X485737

Newman, D. B., Tay, L., & Diener, E. (2014). Leisure and subjective well-being: A model of psychological mechanisms as mediating factors. *Journal of Happiness Studies: An Interdisciplinary Forum on Subjective Well-Being, 15*(3), 555–578. https://doi.org/10.1007/s10902-013-9435-x

Oerlemans, W. G. M., Bakker, A. B., & Demerouti, E. (2014). How feeling happy during off-job activities helps successful recovery from work: A day reconstruction study. *Work and Stress, 28*(2), 198–216. https://doi.org/10.1080/02678373.2014.901993

Park, Y., & Fritz, C. (2015). Spousal recovery support, recovery experiences, and life satisfaction crossover among dual-earner couples. *Journal of Applied Psychology, 100*(2), 557–566. https://doi.org/10.1037/a0037894

Park, Y., Fritz, C., & Jex, S. M. (2011). Relationships between work-home segmentation and psychological detachment from work: The role of communication technology use at home. *Journal of Occupational Health Psychology, 16*(4), 457–467. https://doi.org/10.1037/a0023594

Payne, N., Jones, F., & Harris, P. (2002). The impact of working life on health behavior: The effect of job strain on the cognitive predictors of exercise. *Journal of Occupational Health Psychology, 7*(4), 342–353. https://doi.org/10.1037/1076-8998.7.4.342

Puterman, E., Weiss, J., Beauchamp, M. R., Mogle, J., & Almeida, D. M. (2017). Physical activity and negative affective reactivity in daily life. *Health Psychology, 36*(12), 1186–1194. https://doi.org/10.1037/hea0000532

Reed, J., & Buck, S. (2009). The effect of regular aerobic exercise on positive-activated affect: A meta-analysis. *Psychology of Sport and Exercise, 10*(6), 581–594. https://doi.org/10.1016/j.psychsport.2009.05.009

Ryan, R. M., & Deci, E. L. (2000). Self-determination theory and the facilitation of intrinsic motivation, social development, and well-being. *American Psychologist, 55*(1), 68–78. https://doi.org/10.1037/0003-066X.55.1.68

Sonnentag, S. (2001). Work, recovery activities, and individual well-being: A diary study. *Journal of Occupational Health Psychology, 6*(3), 196–210. https://doi.org/10.1037/1076-8998.6.3.196

Sonnentag, S. (2018). The recovery paradox: Portraying the complex interplay between job stressors, lack of recovery, and poor well-being. *Research in Organizational Behavior, 38*, 169–185. https://doi.org/10.1016/j.riob.2018.11.002

Sonnentag, S., & Fritz, C. (2007). The Recovery Experience Questionnaire: Development and validation of a measure for assessing recuperation and unwinding from work. *Journal of Occupational Health Psychology, 12*(3), 204–221. https://doi.org/10.1037/1076-8998.12.3.204

Sonnentag, S., & Fritz, C. (2015). Recovery from job stress: The stressor-detachment model as an integrative framework. *Journal of Organizational Behavior, 36*(S1), 72–103. https://doi.org/10.1002/job.1924

Sonnentag, S., & Fritz, C. (2018). Recovery from work. In N. Anderson, D. S. Ones, H. K. Sinangil, & V. Chockalingam (Eds.), *The Sage handbook of industrial, work, & organizational psychology* (pp. 471–482). Sage. https://doi.org/10.4135/9781473914964.n21

Sonnentag, S., Cheng, B. H., & Parker, S. L. (2022). Recovery from work: Advancing the field toward the future. *Annual Review of Organizational Psychology and Behavior, 9*(1), 33–60. https://doi.org/10.1146/annurev-orgpsych-012420-091355

Sonnentag, S., & Geurts, S. (Ed.). (2009). Methodological issues in recovery research. In S. Sonnentag, P. L. Perrewé, & D. C. Ganster (Eds.), *Current perspectives on job-stress recovery* (Vol. 7, pp. 1–36). JAI Press/Emerald Group Publishing. https://doi.org/10.1108/S1479-3555(2009)0000007004

Sonnentag, S., Mojza, E. J., Demerouti, E., & Bakker, A. B. (2012). Reciprocal relations between recovery and work engagement: The moderating role of job stressors. *Journal of Applied Psychology, 97*(4), 842–853. https://doi.org/10.1037/a0028292

Sonnentag, S., Venz, L., & Casper, A. (2017). Advances in recovery research: What have we learned? What should be done next? *Journal of Occupational Health Psychology, 22*(3), 365–380. https://doi.org/10.1037/ocp0000079

Steed, L. B., Swider, B. W., Keem, S., & Liu, J. T. (2021). Leaving work at work: A meta-analysis on employee recovery from work. *Journal of Management, 47*(4), 867–897. https://doi.org/10.1177/0149206319864153

ten Brummelhuis, L. L., & Trougakos, J. P. (2014). The recovery potential of intrinsically versus extrinsically motivated off-job activities. *Journal of Occupational and Organizational Psychology, 87*(1), 177–199. https://doi.org/10.1111/joop.12050

Trougakos, J. P., Hideg, I., Cheng, B. H., & Beal, D. J. (2014). Lunch breaks unpacked: The role of autonomy as a moderator of recovery during lunch. *Academy of Management Journal, 57*(2), 405–421. https://doi.org/10.5465/amj.2011.1072

Ursin, H., & Eriksen, H. R. (2010). Cognitive activation theory of stress (CATS). *Neuroscience and Biobehavioral Reviews, 34*(6), 877–881. https://doi.org/10.1016/j.neubiorev.2009.03.001

Van den Broeck, A., Ferris, D. L., Chang, C.-H., & Rosen, C. C. (2016). A review of self-determination theory's basic psychological needs at work. *Journal of Management, 42*(5), 1195–1229. https://doi.org/10.1177/0149206316632058

Weigelt, O., Siestrup, K., & Prem, R. (2021). Continuity in transition: Combining recovery and day-of-week perspectives to understand changes in employee energy across the 7-day week. *Journal of Organizational Behavior, 42*(5), 567–586. https://doi.org/10.1002/job.2514

Westman, M., & Eden, D. (1997). Effects of a respite from work on burnout: Vacation relief and fade-out. *Journal of Applied Psychology, 82*(4), 516–527. https://doi.org/10.1037/0021-9010.82.4.516

Meaningful Work, Calling, and Occupational Health

Bryan J. Dik, Michael F. Steger, and Zachary A. Mercurio

Since the publication of the previous edition of this handbook, volatility, uncertainty, and change have continued to define the world of work. Beginning in 2020, the COVID-19 pandemic functioned as an accelerant of preexisting trends, such as a new labor contract in which workers trade security for flexibility, ubiquitous computing transforming more and more jobs into tech jobs, remote work arrangements inviting work into every minute and every space of people's lives, and the rise of automation causing anxiety about robots or artificial intelligence displacing human workers. A staggering proportion of workers apparently spent time during the pandemic reflecting on their current work or career trajectories and considering possible changes to them. In the United States, by the end of 2020 more than half of all workers in one national survey reported making plans to quit their jobs and explore new pathways, potentially triggering a "turnover tsunami" (Maurer, 2021). Similarly, more than two thirds of unemployed adults reported that they were considering changing occupations (Parker et al., 2021). Whether good or bad (or neither or both), such changes evoke feelings of uncertainty. In turn, uncertainty often spurs people to ask themselves existential questions about the world and their place in it. The process of seeking answers to such questions reflects what Frankl (2014) famously described as a "will to meaning"—people's instinctual desire to make sense of and derive purpose from their lives.

Within the career domain, early accounts of work's meaning date to religious teachings about the role of work in human life. The term *vocation*—derived from

https://doi.org/10.1037/0000331-021
Handbook of Occupational Health Psychology, Third Edition, L. E. Tetrick, G. G. Fisher, M. T. Ford, and J. C. Quick (Editors)

the Latin *vocare*, "to call"—reflects this tradition. For much of Western history, vocation was understood as God's call for certain people to live a monastic life. In time, Augustine, Aquinas, Benedict, and most notably the Protestant Reformers and Puritans began to develop the idea that any honest area of work could be pursued as a calling, provided that it glorified God and served the greater good. Modern perspectives on meaningful work retain some of these core assumptions, recognizing that humans live in communities that flourish when people engage in mutual service to address common needs. Within this framework, the work role is a life domain through which people have direct or indirect social impact (Hardy, 1990). The social and relational implications of work are in turn closely tied to people's experience of their work as meaningful.

The experience of meaningfulness (in life and in work) is a key component of eudaimonic well-being (Steger, 2016). *Eudaimonic well-being* focuses on personal growth, strengths, and meaningfulness and is usually contrasted with hedonic (pleasure-driven) well-being. Eudaimonic and hedonic well-being are related; meaningfulness, for example, has been found to buffer depression and anxiety and to positively predict various indicators of healthy psychological functioning (Steger et al., 2006). Meaningfulness has been described as a factor from which happiness arises (Lent, 2004) and also serves as a desirable end state. For these reasons, the aims of occupational health psychology (OHP)—that is, to "develop, maintain, and promote the health of employees directly and the health of their families" (Quick & Tetrick, 2011, p. 4)—are well aligned with contemporary research on, and practical implications of, meaningful work and calling. In our view, an important part of establishing safe, healthy working environments is ensuring that workers understand the point of their effort, can tie it to a broader sense of purpose in their lives, and can reap the personal benefits of their work's contributions to the greater good.

The purpose of this chapter is to introduce the most important concepts that consider meaningfulness in the context of work and OHP: calling and meaningful work. First, we explore the conceptual context by defining meaningful work and calling. Second, we provide an overview of meaningful work and calling theories. Third, we summarize the accumulating body of research on meaningful work and calling, highlighting linkages to safety, physical health, and psychological health and suggesting fruitful new directions to more directly tie this research to OHP objectives. Fourth, we explore the practical applications stemming from meaningful work research.

DEFINING MEANINGFUL WORK AND CALLING

Meaningful work may be considered a more general case than work as a calling, and it has usually been defined more loosely. The most facile definitions have posited that meaningful work is work that people judge to be meaningful to them. As a construct bridging multiple disciplines, meaningful work is viewed from multiple perspectives. Whereas early work in this area from industrial and organizational psychology, leadership, business, and management research regarded meaningful work as a characteristic of a person's job or as a motivating factor in how dedicated people might be to their work, more recent research has been influenced by the wider field of scholarship on meaning and purpose in life and by positive psychology more broadly. Each of these lines of inquiry may be seen in meaningful work scholarship with definitions mixing what motivates someone to work, and how meaningful and fulfilling the work seems to them. This blend of contributions to meaningful work distinguishes it from calling, which has deeper moral, ethical, and historical heritage. Thus, meaningful work is not simply whatever work is judged to be meaningful but also the expectation that in making that judgment, workers will appreciate elements of their job, find an outlet for their important motivations, and experience happiness and well-being because of their work. Therefore, we define *meaningful work* broadly as "work that is personally significant and worthwhile" (Lysova et al., 2019, p. 375).

Calling is usually understood as a particular expression of meaningful work. Definitions of calling have been explored in multiple conceptual and a few empirical papers. An early, seminal study by Wrzesniewski et al. (1997) popularized the idea that people view their work using one of three work orientations: job (i.e., motivated by extrinsic rewards), career (i.e., motivated by achievement and advancement), or calling (i.e., motivated by fulfilling, meaningful, socially salient work). However, most research has examined calling on its own rather than within this tripartite model, using one of at least 14 distinct formal definitions available in the literature (Thompson & Bunderson, 2019). One way of differentiating these conceptualizations is by placing them on a continuum anchored by the labels "neoclassical" and "modern." Neoclassical definitions broaden but build on historical and religious (i.e., classical) understandings of the term. As an example, Dik and Duffy (2009) framed calling as a "transcendent summons" toward prosocially oriented work that aligns with a person's broader sense of purpose. Modern approaches, in contrast, view calling as a secularized construct focused on self-actualization and self-fulfillment (e.g., "a consuming, meaningful passion . . . toward a domain"; Dobrow & Tosti-Kharas, 2011, p. 1005). Recently, Thompson and Bunderson (2019) reoriented the neoclassical/modern distinction by proposing that callings reflect both the "inner requiredness" described by modern views and the "outer requiredness" described by neoclassical views. Callings characterized by high inner and outer requiredness, they suggested, are "transcendent callings." The notion of transcendence has been identified as the most unique element of the calling construct (Brown & Lent, 2016), but scholars have also suggested that diverse calling definitions are linked by a common core—a sense of purpose. Evidence from cluster (Hirschi, 2011) and taxometric analyses (Shimizu et al., 2019) supports this perspective, revealing that people's sense of calling differs in degree rather than kind. This is likely why studies investigating correlates of calling, despite their diverse measures reflecting diverse (but overlapping) conceptualizations, find remarkably consistent results. Given this, we follow the integrative approach taken by Duffy et al. (2018) and refer to *calling* as "an approach to work that reflects seeking a sense of overall purpose and meaning and is used to help others or contribute to the common good, motivated by an external or internal summons" (p. 426).

MEANINGFUL WORK AND CALLING THEORY

Theoretical advancement in meaningful work scholarship has come in fits and starts but appears to be building some momentum with a range of approaches that anticipate the tenor, qualities, and types of work people judge to be meaningful. Following a time when it was common to use ad hoc measures and definitions of meaningful work or to conflate meaningful work and calling, several conceptual models were proposed that set the stage for more rigorous and focused research. Four models showcase different approaches and provide a useful range of perspectives for understanding meaningful work. Research on calling has taken a parallel path, growing exponentially without the guidance of a unifying theory—until recently, when the inductively built work as a calling theory (WCT; Duffy et al., 2018) emerged.

The next section provides brief summaries of Hackman and Oldham's job characteristics theory (JCT; Hackman & Oldham, 1975), Rosso and colleagues' (2010) model of major pathways to meaningful work, Steger and colleagues' (2012) three-part model of meaningful work, and Lips-Wiersma and Wright's (2012) comprehensive meaningful work model, before shifting focus to calling and WCT.

Job Characteristics Theory

The first effort to integrate meaningful work into models of work adjustment and performance was developed by Hackman and Oldham (1975) as part of their influential JCT. The theory emphasized how work could be described and then designed in such a way as to yield important psychological and performance outcomes from workers. Critical job characteristics included the variety of skills workers need to use to complete work tasks, how well workers can see the entirety of the completed project to which they contribute, the potential significance or impact that one's work can have on others, the degree to which employees have discretion or autonomy in doing their work, and access to feedback concerning work outcomes. These characteristics purportedly led to three critical psychological mediators: (a) autonomy to create accountability and responsibility for work outcomes, (b) feedback to create knowledge of one's work outcomes, and (c) the other three characteristics to create the variable of central focus here: work meaningfulness. These psychological states were in turn proposed to enhance the important outcomes of motivation, satisfaction, and performance. Thus, perceived work meaningfulness in the JCT was positioned as one of several drivers of greater satisfaction and performance.

It may be difficult from a contemporary perspective to understand why work meaningfulness is viewed as causally upstream from other similarly "psychological" work attitudes, such as motivation and satisfaction. Work meaningfulness in the JCT was defined as the "degree to which the employee experiences the job as one which is generally meaningful, valuable, and worthwhile" (Hackman & Oldham, 1975, p. 162). Using that definition as a basis, many scholars were inspired to upgrade meaningful work from a means for achieving other outcomes to an outcome of value in its own right. There is a measurement instrument available (described elsewhere in this chapter) to assess elements of the JCT, including work meaningfulness, which spurred significant research interest. Despite the large volume of JCT-related research, very little of it has focused specifically on meaningful work, but the model did lay the groundwork for later research that more intently probed what meaningful work is, how it benefits people and their occupational functioning, and where it might come from.

Pathways to Meaningful Work

Rosso et al. (2010) proposed that meaningful work could be achieved in a variety of ways, depending on where people direct their intended impact and what their basic motivations are. In both cases, issues of independence versus communion created the impact and motivation poles. Some workers focus their work efforts on their own outcomes whereas others focus on other people as the intended recipients of their efforts, creating a self–other axis. When it comes to motivation, some workers are more motivated to distinguish themselves as individuals whereas some are more motivated to connect with others (including higher powers) and form communities. Thus, layered on top of the self–other axis is an agency–communion axis. This 2 × 2 space creates four quadrants that illustrate archetypal paths to meaningful work: (a) individuation, (b) self-connection, (c) contribution, and (d) unification. Thus, meaningful work may be experienced as a drive for self-understanding and the development of one's potential for people in the self-connection quadrant as well as a desire to join with others to make important positive contributions to the greater good for people in the contribution quadrant.

Three Dimensions of Meaningful Work

The idea of contributing to the greater good has emerged as a connective tissue of sorts in meaningful work theories. Like Rosso et al. (2010), Steger and colleagues (e.g., Steger & Dik, 2009, 2010; Steger et al., 2012) looked to previous research to develop the themes in their model. They drew primarily on previous research on meaningful work, the psychological literature on meaning and purpose in life, and studies on the positive role work plays in people's lives (often referred to as the "meaning of work" as distinguished from meaningfulness in work; e.g., Harpaz & Fu, 2002). Meaning and purpose in life theory emphasizes the value of making sense of one's experience and of being motivated to work toward identifiable outcomes (e.g., Steger et al., 2006), which, when translated into the workplace, develop into three dimensions: *positive meaning* emphasizes the sense and purpose people find in their work and careers, *meaning making* emphasizes the contributions work makes to individual personal growth and life beyond the workplace, and *greater good motivations* capture the most salient positive role of work in people's lives: the drive to benefit some greater good beyond oneself. Each of these dimensions were conceived to be additive. That is, the more positive meaning, meaning making, and greater good motivations people had, the more meaningful their work would be. The Work and Meaning Inventory (WAMI; Steger et al., 2012) was developed to assess these three dimensions of meaningful work and propel research to understand meaningful work predictors, correlates, and outcomes.

Comprehensive Meaningful Work

Unlike the previous models discussed, all of which were based on published theory and research, the *comprehensive meaningful work* model was developed by Lips-Wiersma and Wright (2012) on the basis of qualitative interviews with working adults in New Zealand. This model paid particular attention to some of the tensions in pursuing meaningful work that emerged from the interviews. These addressed some of the balances that need to be struck between internal reflective practices and the drive to act, the desire to help others and also to develop the self, as well as the wide distance that sometimes exists between inspiration and reality. Alongside these new insights, there are some familiar themes that resonate with previous scholarship, particularly the pathways to meaningful work developed by Rosso and colleagues (2010). As with the work of Steger et al. (2012), the intention behind developing this model was to create a measurement instrument. Thus, the resulting scale sought to reflect meaningful work through these dimensions: unity with others, serving others, expressing one's full potential, developing oneself, reality, inspiration, and balancing tensions. Although the JCT scale and the WAMI purport to measure meaningful work, the comprehensive meaningful work scale appears more rooted in the ways that people discover meaningful work, which is more in line with a pathways to meaningful work approach (cf. Rosso et al., 2010).

Work as a Calling Theory

Work as a calling theory (WCT) was developed by Duffy et al. (2018) to pull together converging patterns of results from calling research into an integrative model while also proposing novel directions for research. The theory builds on a key distinction in the calling literature between perceiving a calling and living one out. This distinction forms the basis of WCT's primary mediation hypothesis, in which perceiving a calling is a predictor of work outcomes (both positive and in some circumstances negative) and living a calling is the key mediating variable. Several secondary mediation and moderation hypotheses are proposed within WCT to further explicate the linkages between perceiving a calling, living a calling, and positive (job satisfaction, job performance) and negative (workaholism, burnout, exploitation) outcomes. For example, according to the theory, the link between perceiving a calling and living a calling is itself mediated by person–environment fit and also by the experience of meaningful work and career commitment. Access to opportunity also serves as a predictor in the model, recognizing the role that privilege and work volition play in facilitating one's ability to live out a calling.

The link between perceiving a calling and positive outcomes such as job satisfaction, mediated by living a calling, is well-established. Less clearly understood is how living a calling can serve as a vulnerability, leading to workaholism, burnout, and exploitation. WCT proposes that factors related to a person's personality and the psychological climate of the organization can create conditions in which calling's "dark side" emerges. For example, workers who are living out a calling and also have potentially maladaptive personality traits (e.g., high neuroticism, perfectionism, and need for achievement; low agreeableness, conscientiousness, and self-esteem) may be inclined to rationalize an unhealthy overinvestment in their work, leading to workaholism, burnout, and possibly exploitation at the hands of unscrupulous employers. When such workers operate in work environments with toxic psychological climates (marked by role stress, high demands and low control, poor leadership), these vulnerabilities for negative outcomes are, theoretically, all the more salient.

RESEARCH ON MEANINGFUL WORK AND CALLING

During the 2010s, the pace of meaningful work and calling publications accelerated dramatically, to the extent that the first scholarly handbook on meaningful work was published in 2019 (Yeoman et al., 2019) and a wide-ranging review was able to address notable research findings across multiple levels (e.g., individual, job, organizational, and societal; Lysova et al., 2019). Within this rich body of research are numerous studies that highlight the potential benefits of meaningful work and calling for workplace safety, health, and well-being.

Safety

One approach to understanding how matters of safety dovetail with meaningful work and calling comes from research on *decent work*, which is defined as work that provides safe working conditions; work schedules that enable free time and rest; and workplace culture that is compatible with family and social values, adequate financial compensation, and access to health care (Duffy et al., 2016). Meaningful work was most strongly correlated with compensation and compatibility among work culture and family/social values (Duffy et al., 2016), but other research has shown significant ties between psychological safety and meaningful work as well (e.g., May et al., 2004).

Unfortunately, safety, and particularly physical safety at work, has not been a common research topic in the meaningful work and calling literatures, leaving scholars mainly to bootstrap from theories that suggest workers need to feel respected or participate in decent work in order to find it meaningful (e.g., Duffy et al., 2016; Steger, 2016).

Physical Health

From the perspective that meaningful work is a well-being asset, it should have a similar pattern of relations with other correlates of well-being, including physical health. This area of research has received somewhat more attention than safety, with a consistent stream of studies finding positive links between meaningful work and reports of better subjective general health (e.g., Arnold & Walsh, 2015, Soane et al., 2013), as well as reports of better health behaviors (e.g., Lease et al., 2019). Much of this research has looked specifically at ways meaningful work can protect people from psychologically noxious elements of their jobs, such as customer incivility (Arnold & Walsh, 2015). For example, a large study of 1,658 Finnish teachers found that workplace stressors were associated with worse self-reported general health, whereas meaningful work was associated with better health as well as with a buffering of the impact of stress on health (Minkkinen et al., 2020). Thus, meaningful work shows potential to be a buffer for work-related stressors and a positive health asset. Research examining calling and physical health is sparse by comparison but has yielded similar results. For example, Wrzesniewski et al. (1997) reported positive associations between calling and both self-rated health and health satisfaction. A more recent study found that U.S. academics with unanswered callings (e.g., a sense of calling they are not currently living out) reported significantly worse physical health symptoms than those with answered callings or no calling at all (Gazica & Spector, 2015). However, a replication with a stratified national sample of American workers found that those with answered callings reported better health than those with no calling at all, but neither group significantly differed from those with unanswered callings (Marsh et al., 2020).

Certainly, more research is needed, particularly given the reliance on self-report measures. One interesting extension of this line of research examined whether meaningful work was protective of health among 181 working adults in Denmark who also were engaged in taking care of a family member (Dich et al., 2019). Rather than use self-reported general health, this study used a composite health score calculated from a range of biomarkers for cardiovascular, metabolic, and immune health, such as blood pressure, cholesterol, and inflammatory cytokine levels. Using a community sample with diverse employment and physical health markers provides a conservative test of the hypothesis that meaningful work is related to health. Dich et al. (2019) found that while meaningful work was associated with better mental health, its relationship with physical health was surprising; there was no relationship between meaningful work and biomarkers of health among men, and the relationship trended in the opposite direction than expected for women. That is, women who were taking care of a family member and also felt their work was meaningful had worse biomarkers of health. Clearly this is a research result that needs replication given the nature of the sample, but it is provocative nonetheless and highlights the need to advance methods beyond self-report surveys alone.

Psychological Health and Well-Being

In contrast to research on safety and physical health, there is an abundance of research supporting positive associations between meaningful work and psychological health and well-being. A meta-analysis concluded that there were medium-to-large relations between meaningful work and leading well-being indicators such as life satisfaction, meaning in life, and negative affect (Allan, Batz-Barbarich, et al., 2019). Beyond these indicators, researchers have reported inverse relations between meaningful work and hostility and depression (Lease et al., 2019; Steger et al., 2012), and between meaningful work and stress and burnout (e.g., Lease et al., 2019; Minkkinen et al., 2020). Research on calling has yielded similar results, with numerous studies establishing a positive, moderate-to-strong association between a sense of calling and meaning in life, zest, lower emotional exhaustion, greater psychological adjustment, and greater affective well-being. Despite a heavy reliance upon cross-sectional designs, accumulating longitudinal research suggests that the causal arrows likely go in both directions, such that a sense of calling and well-being are mutually reinforcing (for reviews, see Dik et al., 2020, and Duffy et al., 2018).

An important new direction for this line of inquiry will be in assessing the toll taken by essential workers during the pandemic. One early report on a convenience sample of Portuguese doctors and nurses found that among doctors, meaningful work was inversely related to disengagement, while unrelated to either workload or burnout, whereas among nurses meaningful work was inversely related to both disengagement and burnout (Correia & Almeida, 2020). Another interesting finding from this study was that meaningful work was unrelated to workload.

Calling's "Dark Side"

Despite the evidence that meaningfulness and calling are consistently linked to positive outcomes, some workers in some circumstances may find the opposite—that a sense of calling can foster vulnerabilities for negative outcomes. Some evidence supports this. For example, studies of health care workers (e.g., Vinje & Mittelmark, 2007) found that a sense of calling was linked to elevated burnout. Relatedly, Clinton et al. (2017) found that a sense of calling was associated with working longer hours. Keller et al. (2016) also reported a link between calling and working more hours, and added that having a calling was weakly but significantly linked to workaholism. Several qualitative studies have described calling as a "double-edged sword," with participants describing both joy and difficult sacrifices (e.g., Bunderson & Thompson, 2009). Some workers may also find themselves taken advantage of by employers given their high levels of intrinsic motivation, a finding first reported in Bunderson and Thompson's (2009) classic study of zookeepers and later found in a study of animal shelter workers (Schabram & Maitlis, 2017). More research, beginning with tests of the moderators proposed by WCT, is needed to better elucidate the conditions in which an ordinarily positive approach to work can provoke negative consequences—including identifying a possible "tipping point."

PRACTICAL APPLICATIONS

Given the linkages usually found between meaningful work, calling, and positive outcomes, a natural question is how individuals and organizations might intervene to help people derive meaning from their work and maintain their well-being. This section discusses applications for experiencing meaningful work and living a calling, along with relevant cautions and considerations.

Experiencing Meaningful Work: Individual Applications

Research concurs that people's propensity for experiencing meaning and discerning a calling can be amplified by at least three practices: (a) fostering self-knowledge and activating personal strengths and values; (b) developing a positive and prosocial approach to work; and (c) initiating changes to perceptions, tasks, and relationships in work. These practices can increase self-knowledge. They can also enable personal agency, activating the mechanisms for experiencing meaningful work theorized by Rosso et al. (2010): individuation and self-connection.

Using Strengths and Clarifying Values

Because factors rooted in individual differences predispose people to experience meaningful work (Lysova et al., 2019), facilitating ongoing opportunities for people to explore and develop a full, accurate understanding of themselves within the context of their work environment is foundational. One personal characteristic found to enhance experiences of meaningful work is the use of strengths. Using unique strengths in work situations has consistently correlated with increased perceptions of meaningfulness (Littman-Ovadia & Steger, 2010), a sense of calling (Harzer & Ruch, 2012), and psychological well-being (Dik et al., 2015). One practice-tested instrument for helping people discover and use their strengths is the Values in Action character strengths survey (Peterson & Seligman, 2004), which conceptualizes strengths as critical parts of people's overall character that impact how they think, feel, and behave. A second is the CliftonStrengths assessment (Clifton et al., 2006), which conceptualizes strengths as talents. Being able to identify and deploy signature strengths in either approach is associated with experiences of meaningful work (Littman-Ovadia & Steger, 2010).

Evidence also suggests that using character strengths can reduce burnout by increasing experiences of meaningful work. For example, in a study of counselors, Allan, Owens, and Douglass (2019) found that activating greater levels of certain character strengths (i.e., zest, perspective, self-regulation) predicted higher perceptions of meaningful work and less burnout, which is consistent with previous findings that meaningful work is negatively related to burnout and positively moderated by using character strengths (e.g., Tei et al., 2015). Therefore, we advocate for strengths-based supervision approaches, where supervisors help workers continually identify and implement strengths in job situations (e.g., Thompson et al., 2011).

Beyond strengths, evidence suggests that clarifying personal values and aligning those values to work roles and tasks may also increase people's perceptions of meaningfulness (Lysova et al., 2019). For example, prosocial and self-actualization values are associated with meaningful work (Fairlie, 2011). Furthermore, when people self-select into certain occupations based on their values, they report increased feelings of meaningfulness (Rosso et al., 2010). Research also shows that self-concept and job fit—the fit between a person's perceived values and the job—positively predicts meaningful work (Scroggins, 2008). Several practical applications can illuminate values and help people connect their values to their work activities. First, using assessments to help people evaluate the fit between their values and their current work environment can be fruitful. Second, identifying new work activities people could undertake to more fully realize their values can help them pursue "unused opportunities for meaningful work" (Fairlie, 2011, p. 518).

Developing Positive and Prosocial Approaches Toward Work

Developing a positive and prosocial approach to work also is linked to experiences of meaningful work (Lysova et al., 2019; Rosso et al., 2010), and studies indicate that people can adjust both motives *to* work and dispositions *toward* work to discern and experience more positive meaning (e.g., Lips-Wiersma et al., 2015). When people adopt a greater good motivation in work and when they can live a calling in their work, studies show increased experiences of meaningfulness and well-being (Dik et al., 2015). One experimental study by Allan et al. (2018) demonstrated that working to help others can increase people's perceptions of meaningful work. Specifically, researchers asked participants to hit alternating numbers on a keyboard as fast as possible. Participants who were instructed to do the task to earn money "for a charity" versus for themselves experienced more meaningfulness. Practically, this study reveals that the pleasantness or unpleasantness of a task may have less to do with experienced meaningfulness than does the motive for the task. Therefore, engaging in active reflection and discussion on how everyday tasks ultimately benefit others may increase perceptions of meaningfulness.

Another way to enact a personal prosocial approach to work is to discern, develop, and live a calling (Dik & Duffy, 2014). The practice of discerning a calling often entails a lengthy exploration process to identify a "summons" to do particular work that manifests through continual reflection on how unique personal strengths fit and contribute to certain environments and help other people. One practice for discerning a calling is connecting with a mentor or guide to help facilitate one's understanding of how unique gifts best meet human needs. Leaders and supervisors can also help with this process by continually showing people how their personal strengths make a positive difference in the workplace and by providing space for people to continually reflect on how their work impacts the greater good (Dik et al., 2015). Recognizing that a sense of calling can have a "dark side" is important as well. Efforts to prevent such vulnerabilities are best framed in a proactive manner. For example, coaching individuals to pursue goals in diverse life domains, including those outside of work (e.g., "Spend two hours of quality time with my children each night this week"), are likely more effective at thwarting workaholism than are negatively framed goals (e.g., "Just don't get overcommitted at work").

Job Crafting

Another practice-tested application for increasing meaningfulness is empowering and equipping individuals to introduce changes to their perceptions of tasks, relationships at work, and the nature of tasks themselves. This process of active shaping one's work is known as *job crafting*. Research demonstrates that job crafting can increase meaningfulness, resilience, and performance and contribute to a positive self-image (Berg, Dutton, & Wrzesniewski, 2013). Individuals can change perceptions of their tasks, called *cognitive crafting*, in three ways: expanding, focusing, and linking perceptions. Individuals can expand perceptions by thinking about how their jobs relate to a larger whole and how their jobs impact other people. For example, in a study on how building cleaners experience meaningful work (Mercurio, 2019), a janitor described experiencing more positive meaning when she thought about the unpleasant task of cleaning dormitory bathrooms as helping prevent illness among students. Second, individuals can focus their perceptions by thinking more about the parts of their jobs they find valuable. Third, individuals can link perceptions by cognitively connecting parts of their work with parts of their own identity that are meaningful to them. Berg, Dutton, and Wrzesniewski (2013) described the example of a customer service representative making a link between telling jokes with colleagues with the personal hobby of performing stand-up comedy.

Employees can also craft the relationships they have in work by building, reframing, and adapting relationships. Building relationships with those who provide positive interpersonal cues that reaffirm self-worth and dignity is found to increase meaningfulness (Wrzesniewski et al., 2013). Individuals can also reframe relationships by conceptualizing them as serving a different purpose (i.e., thinking of supervision as "supporting" others vs. "managing" others) or adapting relationships by taking a different role in the relationship, like helping or encouraging. Finally, people can craft the tasks themselves by adding tasks that are meaningful to them, emphasizing tasks they already complete that they find positive and significant, or redesigning tasks by changing aspects (i.e., time, quantity, location) of the task to incite more meaningfulness. Berg, Dutton, and Wrzesniewski's (2013) Job Crafting Exercise is a workbook designed to facilitate the job crafting process and has been tested in practice (Berg, Dutton, Wrzesniewski, & Baker, 2013).

Facilitating Meaningful Work: Organizational Applications

Although individuals can create meaningfulness for themselves, organizations play an important role in designing environments that facilitate or thwart meaningful work. At their best, organizations foster the mechanisms of meaningful work that are other-centered: contribution and unification (Rosso et al., 2010). In this section, four evidence-based organizational applications for facilitating meaningful work are reviewed: job design, leadership, culture, and organizational practices and policies (Bailey et al., 2019; Lysova et al., 2019). However, to mitigate one potential "dark side" of meaningful work (e.g., Allan et al., 2020), it is important for organizations to ensure access to *decent work* that provides physical and emotional safety, predictable and livable work schedules, living wages, and access to adequate health care (Duffy et al., 2016). Similarly, organizations can ensure people who already experience meaningful work have adequate opportunities to fully use their strengths and pursue objectives that are important for maintaining and enhancing their well-being (Allan et al., 2020).

Job Design

Most existing organizational practices to facilitate meaningfulness are derived from Hackman and Oldham's (1976) JCT (e.g., Kahn, 1990; Lysova et al., 2019; May et al., 2004; Rosso et al., 2010). Whereas job crafting is a bottom-up, individual approach to creating meaningfulness, job design using the JCT can be conceptualized as the top-down, organizational shaper of meaningfulness (Berg, Dutton, & Wrzesniewski, 2013). Two elements of the JCT, task identity and task significance, are found to be significantly connected to the experience of meaningful work. *Task identity* is best defined as "the degree to which the job requires completion of a 'whole' and identifiable piece of work—that is, doing a job from beginning to end with a visible outcome" (Hackman & Oldham, 1976 p. 161). Ensuring work is structured to allow employees to see the end outcome of their work, especially along the way, can increase the experience of meaningful work (e.g., May et al., 2004). For example, in an archival study of NASA's management approach during the effort to land astronauts on the moon, Carton (2018) uncovered that some supervisors frequently referenced a "ladder to the moon," by which employees could tangibly connect how their tasks enabled measurable objectives that would ultimately put a person on the moon by the end of the 1960s.

Organizations can also create a clear line of sight between employee's work and the impact on beneficiaries of the work or the organization's higher purpose. *Task significance* describes the degree to which the job or task has an objective or perceived "substantial impact" on the lives of other people (Hackman & Oldham, 1976). One evidence-based practice to increase a sense of task significance is to ensure frequent contact with the work's beneficiaries (Allan et al., 2018). Collecting and regularly sharing real stories of the work's impact on others is another way to enhance the experience of meaningful work.

Leadership

While causal links are yet to be empirically established, leaders may be able to create the conditions that allow for employees to experience meaningfulness (e.g., Carton, 2018; Lysova et al., 2019; Steger, 2016). Leadership approaches associated with employee experiences of meaningful work include transformational leadership, empowering leadership, and ethical leadership (Lysova et al., 2019). Studies on each of these leadership approaches indicate that, in general, leadership behaviors that facilitate employees' self-awareness and personal development, give autonomy, provide meaningful recognition, create a sense of unity, and connect everyday work to a larger other-centered purpose can create the conditions for meaningful work (Lysova et al., 2019; Frémeaux & Pavageau, 2020; Lips-Wiersma & Morris, 2009). Also, a leader's integrity or "moral correctness" (as evidenced by espousing and enacting values like justice, fairness, equity, and dignity) can create a socio-moral climate which is linked to employee experiences of meaningful work (Demirtas et al., 2017).

Finally, as theorized by Steger and Dik (2010) and echoed in Frémeaux and Pavageu's (2020) qualitative study of 42 leaders, another important way leaders can contribute to creating cultures that foster meaningfulness is to develop their own experiences of meaningful work. By developing self-awareness, demonstrating their commitment to the greater good, and ensuring their behaviors are aligned with prosocial belief systems and values, leaders can mitigate the risk of meaningful work applications being perceived as inauthentic (Bailey et al., 2017).

Organizational Culture

Organizational culture is another key component for sustaining employee experiences of meaningful work (Lysova et al., 2019; Pratt & Ashforth, 2003). Practices theorized to craft cultures that cultivate meaningfulness include imbuing a shared sense of a higher other-centered purpose (Quinn & Thakor, 2014); fostering high-quality connections and relationships (Lips-Wiersma & Morris, 2009); creating mattering (Flett, 2018); and norming the enactment of humane values such as support, care, and compassion (e.g., Cardador & Rupp, 2011; Lips-Wiersma et al., 2015). "Learning cultures" that foster innovation and entrepreneurial thinking through encouraging ideas, feedback, and demonstrating openness to new ideas are also theorized to create more meaningfulness as they may allow people to fully deploy their strengths to make a difference (Cardador & Rupp, 2011).

Although more research is needed on how the social context of work affects meaningfulness, the quality of relationships and interactions in work are also theorized to be important shapers of positive meaning (Wrzesniewski et al., 2003). Because research suggests individuals may look to others for "cues" about the meaningfulness of their work (Wrzesniewski et al., 2003), organizations can help employees maintain meaningfulness by supporting and modeling relationships that reinforce others' significance, are respectful, and focus on assisting, mentoring, and caring for others (Colbert et al., 2016; Lysova et al., 2019).

Organizational Practices and Policies

Organizational policies and practices can also create the scaffolding to maintain experiences of meaningfulness. Because meaningfulness is amplified by one's self-understanding of unique strengths and values, strengths-based and values-based learning and development pathways can reinforce meaningfulness (Bailey et al., 2019). Further, organizations that adopt corporate social responsibility or volunteer programs are found to associate with meaningfulness by creating a mechanism for greater good motivations (Rodell, 2013). Research also demonstrates that organizational practices like recruitment, selection, and socialization that reinforce personal values, foster personal development, and prompt others to develop a prosocial motivation to work may contribute to experiences of meaningful work (Pratt & Ashforth, 2003; Pratt et al., 2013; Rosso et al., 2010). These practices may reinforce desired work orientations, the subjective valuations of what makes the work worth doing. Studies on work orientations have uncovered three factors that relate to meaningful work: kinship (doing with), serving (doing good), and craftsmanship (doing well; Pratt et al., 2013). Organizational practices can serve as the context in which these work orientations are primed, maintained, and reinforced (Pratt et al., 2013). Individual and organizational applications intended to increase experiences of meaningful work should be sensitive to two emerging considerations. First, some workers may more readily experience meaningful work than others (Bailey et al., 2019; Lips-Wiersma et al., 2015; Lysova et al., 2019). Second, some jobs simply offer more volition, dignity, autonomy, and freedom than others (Blustein, 2011). Therefore, when considering the reviewed meaningful work applications,we recommend an approach sensitive to the unique needs of individuals, employee groups, and occupational contexts. In addition, where workers already experience meaninglessness, Bailey et al. (2017) cautioned that organizational applications for increasing meaningfulness are susceptible to employee perceptions of inauthenticity or manipulation. Ensuring that authenticity and trust are established through the consistent enactment of values that prioritize meaningful work is important to reduce a gap between rhetoric and employees' lived experiences.

FUTURE RESEARCH PRIORITIES

Collectively, the body of research that has emerged around OHP topics is international (including data from Denmark, Finland, Portugal, South Africa, and the United States, just in the articles cited in this chapter) and diverse in terms of the occupations sampled (e.g., teachers, nurses, call center workers). Yet, significant gaps need to be addressed in both basic and applied research. First, given the vast range of occupations, worker protections, working conditions, and economic factors around the world, a priority should be set to initiate or support studies within occupations or countries that are not well represented in meaningful work research. For example, we know little about how well theoretical models developed in Western, industrialized countries (often using white-collar jobs as the template) pertain to work in developing countries, or in occupations where safety, stability, or employee benefits are less emphasized.

Second, there is not enough research on occupational safety practices and meaningful work. One might hypothesize that where worker health is visibly prioritized through safety practices, workers would feel more valued and view their work as more meaningful. However, the opposite sequence of relations also is plausible. Workers who see meaning in what they do may be more likely to engage in formal and informal behaviors that protect each other (e.g., organizational citizenship behavior is positively related to meaningful work; Steger et al., 2012) and may be more likely to adhere to existing safety practices.

Third, research on occupational health to date is overly reliant on self-report measures. Interestingly, the exception to the seemingly beneficial role played by meaningful work is from a study that looked at biomarkers of health (Dich et al., 2019). More research is needed to understand why workers in most contexts who say their work is meaningful also say they experience less stress and are healthier despite scant evidence that they are physically healthier. Feeling good is arguably as important as having biomarker values in a range indicating good health, but it will be difficult to develop convincing theoretical models without data to better understand the mechanisms and the limitations of meaningful work's potential impact on health.

Fourth, more intervention and experimental research on meaningful work are needed (Steger, 2016). Many of the practical applications discussed here are related to other well-being variables that are connected to meaningful work, yet intervention research that directly investigates meaningful work in diverse occupational contexts is lacking. To develop a fuller picture of the individual process of experiencing meaningful work, it will be important to continue to explore how certain qualities of individual, occupational, organizational, and societal forces relate to the process of constructing work as meaningful.

CONCLUSION

Research on the nature, benefits, and facilitators of meaningful work and calling has accelerated dramatically in recent years, with wide-ranging implications for occupational health. We have provided an overview of some of the research showing that meaningful work and having a calling appear to support greater health, safety, and well-being at work, and we pointed toward some of the steps that individuals and organizations can take to foster these benefits. As a closing note, we express significant optimism concerning the pace of advances in this field. Yet we also acknowledge some concerns that meaningful work and calling, like so many human-centered and promising concepts before them, will fall prey to oversimplification and lip service in the name of profit and corporate bottom lines. It would be tragic if such richly textured, personal, and existential ideas were reduced to platitudes about meaningful work cultures or corporate purpose statements meant to inspire workers without tangibly influencing the structures in which they operate. On the whole, research identifying meaningful work and calling as strong contributors to people's workplace health, well-being, and performance captures their genuine efforts to cultivate meaning in their work lives. It is worth seeking ways to preserve the authenticity at the heart of such personal journeys to meaningful work and calling.

REFERENCES

Allan, B. A., Batz-Barbarich, C., Sterling, H. M., & Tay, L. (2019). Outcomes of meaningful work: A meta-analysis. *Journal of Management Studies, 56*(3), 500–528. https://doi.org/10.1111/joms.12406

Allan, B. A., Duffy, R. D., & Collisson, B. (2018). Helping others increases meaningful work: Evidence from three experiments. *Journal of Counseling Psychology, 65*(2), 155–165. https://doi.org/10.1037/cou0000228

Allan, B. A., Owens, R. L., & Douglass, R. P. (2019). Character strengths in counselors: Relations with meaningful work and burnout. *Journal of Career Assessment, 27*(1), 151–166. https://doi.org/10.1177/1069072717748666

Allan, B. A., Rolniak, J. R., & Bouchard, L. (2020). Underemployment and well-being: Exploring the dark side of meaningful work. *Journal of Career Development, 47*(1), 111–125. https://doi.org/10.1177/0894845318819861

Arnold, K. A., & Walsh, M. M. (2015). Customer incivility and employee well-being: Testing the moderating effects of meaning, perspective taking and transformational leadership. *Work and Stress, 29*(4), 362–378. https://doi.org/10.1080/02678373.2015.1075234

Bailey, C., Madden, A., Alfes, K., Shantz, A., & Soane, E. (2017). The mismanaged soul: Existential labor and the erosion of meaningful work. *Human Resource Management Review, 27*(3), 416–430. https://doi.org/10.1016/j.hrmr.2016.11.001

Bailey, C., Yeoman, R., Madden, A., Thompson, M., & Kerridge, G. (2019). A review of the empirical literature on meaningful work: Progress and research agenda. *Human Resource Development Review, 18*(1), 83–113. https://doi.org/10.1177/1534484318804653

Berg, J. M., Dutton, J. E., & Wrzesniewski, A. (2013). Job crafting and meaningful work. In B. J. Dik, Z. S. Byrne, & M. F. Steger (Eds.), *Purpose and meaning in the workplace* (pp. 81–104). American Psychological Association. https://doi.org/10.1037/14183-005

Berg, J. M., Dutton, J. E., Wrzesniewski, A., & Baker, W. E. (2013). *Job crafting exercise.* University of Michigan.

Blustein, D. L. (2011). A relational theory of working. *Journal of Vocational Behavior, 79*(1), 1–17. https://doi.org/10.1016/j.jvb.2010.10.004

Brown, S. D., & Lent, R. W. (2016). Vocational psychology: Agency, equity, and well-being. *Annual Review of Psychology, 67*(1), 541–565. https://doi.org/10.1146/annurev-psych-122414-033237

Bunderson, J. S., & Thompson, J. A. (2009). The call of the wild: Zookeepers, callings, and the double-edged sword of deeply meaningful work. *Administrative Science Quarterly, 54*(1), 32–57. https://doi.org/10.2189/asqu.2009.54.1.32

Cardador, M. T., & Rupp, D. E. (2011). Organizational culture, multiple needs, and the meaningfulness of work. In N. M. Ashkanasy, C. P. M. Wilderom, & M. F. Peterson (Eds.), *Handbook of organizational culture and climate* (2nd ed., pp. 158–180). Sage.

Carton, A. M. (2018). "I'm not mopping the floors, I'm putting a man on the moon": How NASA leaders enhanced the meaningfulness of work by changing the meaning of work. *Administrative Science Quarterly, 63*(2), 323–369. https://doi.org/10.1177/0001839217713748

Clifton, D. O., Anderson, E. C., & Schreiner, L. A. (2006). *StrengthsQuest: Discover and develop your strengths in academics, career, and beyond.* Gallup.

Clinton, M. E., Conway, N., & Sturges, J. (2017). "It's tough hanging-up a call": The relationships between calling and work hours, psychological detachment, sleep quality, and morning vigor. *Journal of Occupational Health Psychology, 22*(1), 28–39. https://doi.org/10.1037/ocp0000025

Colbert, A. E., Bono, J. E., & Purvanova, R. K. (2016). Flourishing via workplace relationships: Moving beyond instrumental support. *Academy of Management Journal, 59*(4), 1199–1223. https://doi.org/10.5465/amj.2014.0506

Correia, I., & Almeida, A. E. (2020). Organizational justice, professional identification, empathy, and meaningful work during COVID-19 pandemic: Are they burnout protectors in physicians and nurses? *Frontiers in Psychology, 11*, 566139. https://doi.org/10.3389/fpsyg.2020.566139

Demirtas, O., Hannah, S. T., Gok, K., Arslan, A., & Capar, N. (2017). The moderated influence of ethical leadership, via meaningful work, on followers' engagement, organizational identification, and envy. *Journal of Business Ethics, 145*(1), 183–199. https://doi.org/10.1007/s10551-015-2907-7

Dich, N., Lund, R., Hansen, Å. M., & Rod, N. H. (2019). Mental and physical health effects of meaningful work and rewarding family responsibilities. *PLOS ONE, 14*(4), e0214916. https://doi.org/10.1371/journal.pone.0214916

Dik, B. J., & Duffy, R. D. (2009). Calling and vocation at work: Definitions and prospects for research and practice. *The Counseling Psychologist, 37*(3), 424–450. https://doi.org/10.1177/0011000008316430

Dik, B. J., & Duffy, R. D. (2014). Best practices in promoting calling and vocation in career counseling. In M. Pope, L. Flores, & P. Rottinghaus (Eds.), *The role of values in careers* (pp. 167–177). Information Age Publishing.

Dik, B. J., Duffy, R. D., Allan, B. A., O'Donnell, M. B., Shim, Y., & Steger, M. F. (2015). Purpose and meaning in career development applications. *The Counseling Psychologist, 43*(4), 558–585. https://doi.org/10.1177/0011000014546872

Dik, B. J., Steger, M. F., & Autin, K. (2020). Calling, meaning, and volition: Emerging perspectives. In S. Brown & R. Lent (Eds.), *Career development and counseling: Putting theory and research to work* (3rd ed., pp. 237–270). Wiley.

Dobrow, S. R., & Tosti-Kharas, J. (2011). Calling: The development of a scale measure. *Personnel Psychology, 64*(4), 1001–1049. https://doi.org/10.1111/j.1744-6570.2011.01234.x

Duffy, R. D., Blustein, D. L., Diemer, M. A., & Autin, K. L. (2016). The psychology of working theory. *Journal of Counseling Psychology, 63*(2), 127–148. https://doi.org/10.1037/cou0000140

Duffy, R. D., Dik, B. J., Douglass, R. P., England, J. W., & Velez, B. L. (2018). Work as a calling: A theoretical model. *Journal of Counseling Psychology, 65*(4), 423–439. https://doi.org/10.1037/cou0000276

Fairlie, P. (2011). Meaningful work, employee engagement, and other key employee outcomes: Implications for human resource development. *Advances in Developing Human Resources, 13*(4), 508–525. https://doi.org/10.1177/1523422311431679

Flett, G. (2018). *The psychology of mattering: Understanding the human need to be significant.* Academic Press.

Frankl, V. E. (2014). *The will to meaning: Foundations and applications of logotherapy.* Penguin.

Frémeaux, S., & Pavageau, B. (2020). Meaningful leadership: How can leaders contribute to meaningful work? *Journal of Management Inquiry, 31*(1), 54–66. https://doi.org/10.1177/1056492619897126

Gazica, M. W., & Spector, P. E. (2015). A comparison of individuals with unanswered callings to those with no calling at all. *Journal of Vocational Behavior, 91*(1), 1–10. https://doi.org/10.1016/j.jvb.2015.08.008

Hackman, J. R., & Oldham, G. R. (1975). Development of the job diagnostic survey. *Journal of Applied Psychology, 60*(2), 159–170. https://doi.org/10.1037/h0076546

Hackman, J. R., & Oldham, G. R. (1976). Motivation through the design of work: Test of a theory. *Organizational Behavior and Human Performance, 16*(2), 250–279. https://doi.org/10.1016/0030-5073(76)90016-7

Hardy, L. (1990). *The fabric of this world: Inquiries into calling, career choice, and the design of human work*. William B. Eerdmans Publishing.

Harpaz, I., & Fu, X. (2002). The structure of the meaning of work: A relative stability amidst change. *Human Relations, 55*(6), 639–667. https://doi.org/10.1177/0018726702556002

Harzer, C., & Ruch, W. (2012). When the job is a calling: The role of applying one's signature strengths at work. *The Journal of Positive Psychology, 7*(5), 362–371. https://doi.org/10.1080/17439760.2012.702784

Hirschi, A. (2011). Callings in career: A typological approach to essential and optional components. *Journal of Vocational Behavior, 79*(1), 60–73. https://doi.org/10.1016/j.jvb.2010.11.002

Kahn, W. A. (1990). Psychological conditions of personal engagement and disengagement at work. *Academy of Management Journal, 33*(4), 692–724. https://doi.org/10.5465/256287

Keller, A. C., Spurk, D., Baumeler, F., & Hirschi, A. (2016). Competitive climate and workaholism: Negative sides of future orientation and calling. *Personality and Individual Differences, 96*(1), 122–126. https://doi.org/10.1016/j.paid.2016.02.061

Lease, S. H., Ingram, C. L., & Brown, E. L. (2019). Stress and health outcomes: Do meaningful work and physical activity help? *Journal of Career Development, 46*(3), 251–264. https://doi.org/10.1177/0894845317741370

Lent, R. W. (2004). Toward a unifying theoretical and practical perspective on well-being and psychosocial adjustment. *Journal of Counseling Psychology, 51*(4), 482–509. https://doi.org/10.1037/0022-0167.51.4.482

Lips-Wiersma, M., & Morris, L. (2009). Discriminating between 'meaningful work' and the 'management of meaning.' *Journal of Business Ethics, 88*(3), 491–511. https://doi.org/10.1007/s10551-009-0118-9

Lips-Wiersma, M., Souter, A., & Wright, S. (2015). The lived experience of meaningful work. *New Zealand Journal of Human Resources Management, 15*, 134–150.

Lips-Wiersma, M., & Wright, S. (2012). Measuring the meaning of meaningful work: Development and validation of the Comprehensive Meaningful Work Scale (CMWS). *Group & Organization Management, 37*(5), 655–685. https://doi.org/10.1177/1059601112461578

Littman-Ovadia, H., & Steger, M. (2010). Character strengths and well-being among volunteers and employees: Toward an integrative model. *The Journal of Positive Psychology, 5*(6), 419–430. https://doi.org/10.1080/17439760.2010.516765

Lysova, E. I., Allan, B. A., Dik, B. J., Duffy, R. D., & Steger, M. F. (2019). Fostering meaningful work in organizations: A multi-level review and integration. *Journal of Vocational Behavior, 110*(A1–A2), 374–389. https://doi.org/10.1016/j.jvb.2018.07.004

Marsh, D. R., Alayan, A. J., & Dik, B. J. (2020). Answered callings, unanswered callings, or no calling: Examining a nationally representative sample. *The Career Development Quarterly, 68*(4), 374–380. https://doi.org/10.1002/cdq.12243

Maurer, R. (2021, March 12). *Turnover 'tsunami' expected once pandemic ends*. Society for Human Resource Management. https://www.shrm.org/resourcesandtools/hr-topics/talent-acquisition/pages/turnover-tsunami-expected-once-pandemic-ends.aspx

May, D. R., Gilson, R. L., & Harter, L. M. (2004). The psychological conditions of mean-ingfulness, safety and availability and the engagement of the human spirit at work. *Journal of Occupational and Organizational Psychology, 77*(1), 11–37. https://doi.org/10.1348/096317904322915892

Mercurio, Z. A. (2019). *The lived experience of meaningful work in a stigmatized occupation: A descriptive phenomenological inquiry* [Doctoral dissertation, Colorado State University]. ProQuest Dissertations. https://www.proquest.com/openview/f2400a7a4a06a9cbe7cb988a8fb8cbde/1?pq-origsite=gscholar&cbl=18750&diss=y

Minkkinen, J., Auvinen, E., & Mauno, S. (2020). Meaningful work protects teachers' self-rated health under stressors. *Journal of Positive School Psychology, 4*(2), 140–152. https://jyx.jyu.fi/handle/123456789/72095

Parker, K., Igielnik, R., & Kochhar, R. (2021, February 10). *Unemployed Americans are feeling the emotional strain of job loss; most have considered changing occupations.* Pew Research Center. https://www.pewresearch.org/fact-tank/2021/02/10/unemployed-americans-are-feeling-the-emotional-strain-of-job-loss-most-have-considered-changing-occupations/

Peterson, C., & Seligman, M. E. (2004). *Character strengths and virtues: A handbook and classification.* Oxford University Press.

Pratt, M. G., & Ashforth, B. E. (2003). Fostering meaningfulness in working and at work. In K. Cameron, J. Dutton, & R. Quinn (Eds.), *Positive organizational scholarship: Foundations of a new discipline* (pp. 309–327). Berrett-Koehler.

Pratt, M. G., Pradies, C., & Lepisto, D. A. (2013). Doing well, doing good, and doing with: Organizational practices for effectively cultivating meaningful work. In B. Dik, Z. Byrne, & M. Steger (Eds.), *Purpose and meaning in the workplace* (pp. 173–196). American Psychological Association. https://doi.org/10.1037/14183-009

Quick, J. C., & Tetrick, L. E. (2011). *Handbook of occupational health psychology* (2nd ed.). American Psychological Association.

Quinn, R. E., & Thakor, A. V. (2014). Imbue the organization with a higher purpose. In J. E. Dutton & G. M. Spreitzer (Eds.), *How to be a positive leader: Small actions, big impact* (pp. 100–112). Berrett-Koehler.

Rodell, J. B. (2013). Finding meaning through volunteering: Why do employees volunteer and what does it mean for their jobs? *Academy of Management Journal, 56*(5), 1274–1294. https://doi.org/10.5465/amj.2012.0611

Rosso, B. D., Dekas, K. H., & Wrzesniewski, A. (2010). On the meaning of work: A theo-retical integration and review. *Research in Organizational Behavior, 30*(1), 91–127. https://doi.org/10.1016/j.riob.2010.09.001

Schabram, K., & Maitlis, S. (2017). Negotiating the challenges of a calling: Emotion and enacted sensemaking in animal shelter work. *Academy of Management Journal, 60*(2), 584–609. https://doi.org/10.5465/amj.2013.0665

Scroggins, W. A. (2008). Antecedents and outcomes of experienced meaningful work: A person job fit perspective. *Journal of Business Inquiry, 7*(1), 68–78. https://journals.uvu.edu/index.php/jbi/article/view/167

Shimizu, A. B., Dik, B. J., & Conner, B. T. (2019). Conceptualizing calling: Cluster and taxometric analyses. *Journal of Vocational Behavior, 114*(1), 7–18. https://doi.org/10.1016/j.jvb.2018.07.006

Soane, E., Shantz, A., Alfes, K., Truss, C., Rees, C., & Gatenby, M. (2013). The associa-tion of meaningfulness, well-being, and engagement with absenteeism: A moder-ated mediation model. *Human Resource Management, 52*(3), 441–456. https://doi.org/10.1002/hrm.21534

Steger, M. F. (2016). Hedonia, eudaimonia, and meaning: Me versus us; fleeting versus enduring. In J. Vitters\u00f6 (Ed.), *Handbook of eudaimonic well-being* (pp. 175–182). Springer. https://doi.org/10.1007/978-3-319-42445-3_11

Steger, M. F., & Dik, B. J. (2009). If one is looking for meaning in life, does it help to find meaning in work? *Applied Psychology. Health and Well-Being, 1*(3), 303–320. https://doi.org/10.1111/j.1758-0854.2009.01018.x

Steger, M. F., & Dik, B. J. (2010). Work as meaning: Individual and organizational benefits of engaging in meaningful work. In P. A. Linley, S. Harrington, & N. Page (Eds.), *Handbook of positive psychology and work* (pp. 131–142). Oxford University Press.

Steger, M. F., Dik, B. J., & Duffy, R. D. (2012). Measuring meaningful work: The Work and Meaning Inventory (WAMI). *Journal of Career Assessment, 20*(3), 322–337. https://doi.org/10.1177/1069072711436160

Steger, M. F., Frazier, P., Oishi, S., & Kaler, M. (2006). The meaning in life questionnaire: Assessing the presence of and search for meaning in life. *Journal of Counseling Psychology, 53*(1), 80–93. https://doi.org/10.1037/0022-0167.53.1.80

Tei, S., Becker, C., Sugihara, G., Kawada, R., Fujino, J., Sozu, T., Murai, T., & Takahashi, H. (2015). Sense of meaning in work and risk of burnout among medical professionals. *Psychiatry and Clinical Neurosciences, 69*(2), 123–124. https://doi.org/10.1111/pcn.12217

Thompson, E. H., Frick, M. H., & Trice-Black, S. (2011). Counselor-in-training perceptions of supervision practices related to self-care and burnout. *The Professional Counselor, 1*(3), 152–162. https://doi.org/10.15241/eht.1.3.152

Thompson, J. A., & Bunderson, J. S. (2019). Research on work as a calling . . . and how to make it matter. *Annual Review of Organizational Psychology and Organizational Behavior, 6*(1), 421–443. https://doi.org/10.1146/annurev-orgpsych-012218-015140

Vinje, H. F., & Mittelmark, M. B. (2007). Job engagement's paradoxical role in nurse burnout. *Nursing & Health Sciences, 9*(2), 107–111. https://doi.org/10.1111/j.1442-2018.2007.00310.x

Wrzesniewski, A., Dutton, J. E., & Debebe, G. (2003). Interpersonal sensemaking and the meaning of work. *Research in Organizational Behavior, 25*, 93–135. https://doi.org/10.1016/S0191-3085(03)25003-6

Wrzesniewski, A., LoBuglio, N., Dutton, J. E., & Berg, J. M. (2013). Job crafting and cultivating positive meaning and identity in work. In A. B. Bakker (Ed.), *Advances in positive organizational psychology* (Vol. 1, pp. 281–302). Emerald Group Publishing Limited.

Wrzesniewski, A., McCauley, C., Rozin, P., & Schwartz, B. (1997). Jobs, careers, and callings: People's relations to their work. *Journal of Research in Personality, 31*(1), 21–33. https://doi.org/10.1006/jrpe.1997.2162

Yeoman, R., Bailey, C., Madden, A., & Thompson, M. (Eds.). (2019). *The Oxford handbook of meaningful work*. Oxford University Press. https://doi.org/10.1093/oxfordhb/9780198788232.001.0001

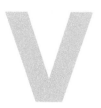

INTERVENTIONS AND TREATMENT

INTRODUCTION: INTERVENTIONS AND TREATMENT

Part V of this handbook covers methods of intervening to prevent and treat occupational stress, illness, and conflicts between work and family roles. Chapter 22 focuses on participatory organizational interventions, reviewing the key principles of communication, participation, management support, and intervention-organization fit. Chapter 22 also delves into five phases of participatory interventions, explaining how attention to the entire lifetime of the intervention is critical to success. Chapter 23 discusses different targets for change at the individual and organizational levels, taking a holistic, social ecological, and systems science perspective. Chapter 24 focuses on employee assistance programs, which provide counseling and assistance to workers to address personal and work-related problems. Chapter 25 discusses the role of leadership in occupational health and safety, identifying and reviewing research on key leadership constructs such as supervisor support and destructive leadership. Finally, Chapter 26 reviews work–family policies such as flexible work arrangements, along with interventions such as those focused on family supportive supervisor behavior. We encourage the readers to consider primary, secondary, and tertiary interventions across these various chapters— all of which have their place in occupational health—while also recognizing particular benefits to primary prevention approaches.

The purpose of Part V is to focus on targets and methods for intervention to help prevent illness and promote health in the workforce. Content in Part V overlaps with some other chapters, particularly from Parts II and III. For example, Chapters 22 and 23 discuss some of the stressors and stress processes initially described in Chapters 3 and 4. Chapter 26 describes practices on the work–family interface, whereas Chapter 7 discusses theory on this topic. Chapter 25 explores leadership constructs that also come up in Chapter 14 on mistreatment in organizations. However, despite these similarities, Part V has a specific focus on targets and methods of intervention among individuals, leaders, and organizations at large.

22

Improving Employee Well-Being Through Improving Working Conditions

A Review on How We Can Make Participatory Organizational Interventions Work

Karina Nielsen

articipatory organizational interventions can be defined as "planned, behavioral, theory-based actions that aim to improve employee well-being through changing the way work is organized, designed and managed" (Nielsen, 2013, p. 1030). Central to such interventions is the focus on changing work practices, policies, and procedures (Sorensen et al., 2019). Participatory organizational interventions are recommended by key international bodies (European Trade Union Confederation, 2004; International Labor Office, 2001) because they address the causes of poor well-being, rather than the symptoms. Despite being the recommended method, systematic reviews reveal that participatory organizational interventions show inconsistent results in their ability to improve working conditions and employee well-being (Richardson & Rothstein, 2008). In the wake of these findings, a growing body of research has started to explore why such interventions may succeed or fail (Havermans et al., 2016; Nielsen & Abildgaard, 2013; Nielsen & Randall, 2013) and how we can make such interventions work in order to successfully improve employee well-being (Nielsen & Noblet, 2018; Nielsen, Randall, et al., 2010).

Well-being in this context is seen as a broad outcome of interventions covering life and nonwork satisfactions (e.g., with social/family life, spirituality), work and job-related satisfactions (e.g., with pay, promotion opportunities, the job itself, coworkers), as well as general health (e.g., mental/psychological indicators such as affect, frustration, and anxiety; stress and

https://doi.org/10.1037/0000331-022
Handbook of Occupational Health Psychology, Third Edition, L. E. Tetrick, G. G. Fisher, M. T. Ford, and J. C. Quick (Editors)

FIGURE 22.1. Organizational Intervention Implementation Model

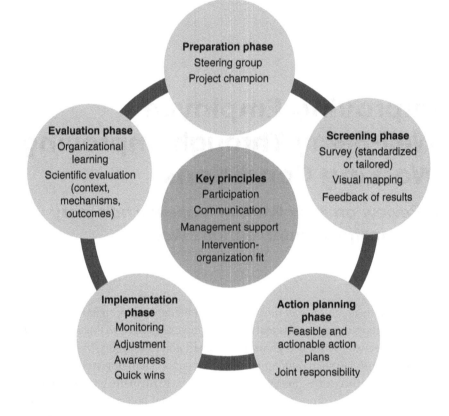

physical/physiological indicators such as blood pressure, heart condition, and general physical health; Danna & Griffin, 1999).

In this chapter, I review the literature on how to make interventions work such that they achieve their intended outcomes. I first briefly outline participatory organizational interventions, then detail four key principles of such interventions—namely, communication, participation, management support, and intervention fit. Finally, I discuss the key elements of each of the five intervention phases, as detailed in Figure 22.1, reviewing the evidence that supports these phases.

PARTICIPATORY ORGANIZATIONAL INTERVENTIONS

Work stress and well-being theories underpin participatory organizational interventions (Nielsen, Taris, & Cox, 2010). These theories all suggest that the work environment has an impact on employee well-being. The job demand–control theory (Karasek & Theorell, 1990) suggests that jobs designed to be demanding but that also offer employees a high level of control in their job can be considered active jobs. Such jobs result in positive employee well-being. Conversely, jobs characterized by high demands and low control are considered high-strain jobs that result in poor employee well-being. In their job demands–resources model (JD-R), Demerouti et al. (2001) extended this line of thinking in the job demand–control model and suggested a broader view on the working conditions, which may influence employee well-being. According to the JD-R model, working conditions can be classified as demands and resources. *Demands* are defined as the physical, social, and organizational aspects of the job that require physical or mental effort and thus may lead to poor employee well-being. *Resources* are defined as the working conditions that may help employees achieve their goals—that is, maintain or improve their well-being (Halbesleben, 2010). Importantly, in an intervention context, resources may buffer adverse job demands that cannot be eliminated or reduced (Vignoli et al., 2017).

Nielsen et al. (2017) and Day and Nielsen (2017) suggested that demands and resources can be classified into four levels in the Individual-Group-Leader-Organization (IGLO) model. At the individual level, demands and resources inherent within the individual may influence employee well-being. Examples of inherent demands that employees put on themselves are their expectations of their performance levels and career aspirations. Examples of inherent resources may be employees' ability to successfully manage the challenges they face at work (i.e., self-efficacy; Bandura, 1986) and their ability to craft a job that enables them to thrive and develop (Nielsen & Abildgaard, 2012). At the group level, examples of demands may be group conflict and incivility, and examples of resources may be a positive team climate and social support. At the leader level, examples of demands may be laissez-faire leadership or abusive leadership with leaders either not supporting their employees or bullying their employees (Mackey et al., 2020; Schyns & Schilling, 2013). Examples of leaders' resources may be a positive relationship between the leader and their employees, leader–member exchange, or transformational leadership—that is, leaders who provide a vision for their employees, stimulate their workers, and demonstrate an understanding of individual workers' needs (Harms et al., 2017; Inceoglu et al., 2018). Finally, demands at the organizational level may be a heavy workload or role conflict, whereas examples of job resources include autonomy or human resources (HR) policies, such as flexible working hours and high-performance work practices that motivate employees through rewards, give them opportunities to participate in decision making, and enable them to use their abilities (Bailey, 1993). Participatory organizational interventions can focus on reducing or eliminating demands and enhancing resources at any or all of these four levels (Nielsen & Christensen, 2021d).

Participatory organizational interventions employ a problem-solving cycle approach whereby problems in the working conditions are identified and action plans are developed to address these problems and evaluate their effectiveness (Nielsen, Randall, et al., 2010). Using this approach, such interventions go through a systematic, structured process of setting up the intervention, screening of the demands and resources that need to change, feedback of results, developing and prioritizing actions to minimize or eliminate adverse demands and increase or maintain resources, implementation of action plans, evaluating the effects of action plans, extracting learning about the barriers and facilitators to a successful process, and integrating this learning into future interventions.

FOUR KEY PRINCIPLES OF THE PARTICIPATORY ORGANIZATIONAL INTERVENTION PROCESS

The intervention process is key to participatory organizational interventions achieving their intended outcomes of improving working conditions and employee well-being (Havermans et al., 2016). The intervention process has been defined as the "individual, collective and management perceptions and actions in implementing any intervention and their influence on the overall result of the intervention" (Nytrø et al., 2000, p. 214). Four key elements of the intervention process are crucial for the participatory organizational intervention to be successfully implemented, running throughout the phases of the intervention (Schelvis et al., 2016; Sorensen et al., 2019). These four elements are communication, participation, management support, and context-intervention fit (i.e., integration of the intervention into the organizational context; Nielsen & Noblet, 2018; Schelvis et al., 2016; Sorensen et al., 2019).

Communication

In all phases of the participatory organizational intervention, *communication* is an important vehicle for driving the participatory process (Nielsen & Randall, 2013; Sorensen et al., 2019). The content, the process, and the quality of communication may influence the intervention's outcomes (Bakhuys Roozeboom et al., 2020; Havermans et al., 2016). The specifics of the intervention need to be communicated. Communication needs to focus on how the intervention will be implemented, including details about, for instance, who is on the steering group, what the methods are, a survey to identify demands and resources and interactive workshops to develop action plans, and how the intervention will be integrated into existing practices and procedures. The overall goals and objectives of the intervention, as well as the benefits that employees and line managers can gain from engaging with the intervention, need to be communicated. Key activities and phases of the intervention and when these will happen also need to be discussed. It is important to continually communicate about progress and what activities will happen next. The targets of information—the participants in the intervention but also who is responsible for communication (e.g., management, union, and safety representatives)—also must be decided. The channels of communication (e.g., posters, emails, intranet, meetings) need to be confirmed (Nielsen et al., 2013).

The advantages of communication are at least twofold: Communication facilitates employees' sensemaking of the intervention and ensures their commitment to the intervention, as expectations of them are clarified (Bakhuys Roozeboom et al., 2020; Schelvis et al., 2016). Previous research has found that employees who felt they lacked sufficient information about their roles and responsibilities worked in groups where the intervention was not implemented according to plan (Augustsson et al., 2015). Bakhuys Roozeboom et al. (2020) found that communication helps build the organizational resource of autonomy and increased job satisfaction.

Participation

In the context of participatory organizational interventions, *participation* has been defined as employees' involvement in the design and implementation of the intervention or the process (Hurrell, 2005) and the content of the intervention (i.e., the changes made to policies, procedures, and practices; Abildgaard et al., 2016). The participatory intervention process may help successful implementation in multiple ways. First, it ensures the use of employees' firsthand knowledge of which changes to policies, practices, and procedures are needed and feasible (Rosskam, 2009). Second, as employees have a say in which changes to make, they are more likely to feel a sense of ownership over action plans developed and will proactively work to implement these, thus ensuring a smooth integration of action plans into existing policies, practices, and procedures (Daltuva et al., 2009; Nielsen et al., 2014). Nielsen et al. (2007) found that employees who reported that they had been provided the opportunity to influence the intervention process were more likely to engage in intervention activities. Augustsson et al. (2015) saw that the intervention was implemented according to plan in groups where employees felt they had an opportunity to participate in the intervention process.

There is evidence that the participatory intervention process has had a direct impact on the intervention's outcomes (Tafvelin et al., 2019). Like the content of the intervention (i.e., action plans can address demands and resources at the four IGLO levels), the participatory intervention process itself may develop resources at the four levels, thus explaining how the process influences the outcomes. First, engagement in the participatory process may enhance employees' and managers' sensemaking process. Participants actively generate meaning about the intervention process as they take action through engaging in the process (Ashmos & Nathan, 2002).

Second, group-level resources may also be developed as a result of the participatory process. Abildgaard et al. (2020) found that collective efficacy increased in some departments undergoing a participatory organizational intervention. Collective efficacy concerns the team or work group's beliefs that they can collectively implement action plans successfully and overcome any challenges they may face as they implement action plans (Abildgaard et al., 2020). Furthermore, social support has also been found to increase as a result of participatory interventions (Nielsen & Randall, 2012). The collaborative problem-solving dialogue that is key to the participatory process makes employees feel supported and increases their shared understanding of the challenges and changes to policies, practices, and procedures (Nielsen, Antino, et al., 2021). As employees engage in a colearning process, they feel a strengthened working relationship with their colleagues (Landsbergis & Vivona-Vaughan, 1995). Comparing employees' sensemaking of the participatory process as an individual phenomenon or a collective phenomenon, Nielsen, Antino, et al. (2021) found that the intervention had a more powerful impact on employee well-being when employees felt that they as a team had exerted influence over the process and the content of the intervention. Ipsen et al. (2015) found that across three small enterprises, the participatory process was the second most important factor ensuring a successful intervention implementation.

Third, at the leader level, the participatory process may develop leaders' behaviors. Leaders or line managers are often responsible for implementing the intervention at the team and departmental levels (Nielsen, 2017). One change-focused leadership style is that of transformational leadership (Carter et al., 2013). Transformational leaders' formulation of a vision for the intervention and their involvement of employees in the participatory process, thus enhancing employees' identification with the intervention, lead to a successful intervention outcome (Abildgaard et al., 2020; Lundmark et al., 2017).

At the organizational level, the participatory intervention process may enhance employees' job control. Key to the participatory intervention process is that managers and employees are colearners in an empowerment process as they agree on the process and the content of the intervention (Mikkelsen, 2005). Bond and Bunce (2001) found support in a participatory organizational intervention that indicated that job control did lead to successful intervention outcomes. The combination of a high level of control over which changes to make and the co-learning process may result in active jobs, as formulated by the JD-R model (Karasek & Theorell, 1990).

Management Support

Management support of the intervention at all levels is important throughout all five phases (Nielsen, 2017). The advantages of management support are multiple. It helps ensure there are sufficient resources to implement changes to policies, work practices, and procedures; creates accountability; and puts well-being on the agenda (Ipsen et al., 2015; Sorensen et al., 2019). The line manager plays a significant role in communicating about the intervention, creating a vision for the intervention, involving employees in the intervention process, and driving and prioritizing intervention activities (Nielsen, 2017; Niks et al., 2018). Augustsson et al. (2015) found that in groups where line managers encouraged the use of intervention tools and were positive about integrating them into existing practices and procedures, the intervention was more likely to be implemented; there was no such effect of senior managers' activities as they were perceived to be too distant from the work of the groups. Line managers' active support of and involvement in the intervention has been found to lead to a successful intervention outcome (Lundmark et al., 2017; Nielsen & Randall, 2009).

Senior managers play an important role in demonstrating their commitment to the intervention. First, they must allocate the necessary resources for the intervention activities to be developed and implemented (Ipsen et al., 2015; Schelvis et al., 2016). Second, they must communicate effectively with line management levels and employee representatives to ensure a smooth implementation of the intervention (Schelvis et al., 2016) and acknowledge sensitive results (Jenny et al., 2015). It is crucial to involve senior managers in all phases of the project to ensure their support. Ramos et al. (2020) noted that after a group identified and developed actions plans for addressing adverse working conditions, a senior manager closed down the intervention as he did not approve of the content of the action plans that had been developed.

Intervention-Organization Fit

Crucial to successful intervention implementation is tailoring the intervention process and content to the organizational context (Nielsen, Axtell, & Sorensen, 2021). The perspective of *intervention-organizational fit* has its roots in person–environment fit theory (Kristof-Brown & Guay, 2011). There are five key elements to intervention-organization fit. First, the intervention needs to be aligned with the organization's objectives and core business. If the intervention contrasts with central organizational objectives, participants are unlikely to buy into and support the intervention, as it may prevent them from delivering on their key performance indicators (Randall et al., 2005). Second, the intervention needs to address the demands and resources that participants feel need addressing (von Thiele Schwarz et al., 2021). If employees do not feel positively about the intervention, they are more likely to be resistant as they do not feel it will be beneficial to them (Aust et al., 2010). Third, changes brought about by the intervention need to be integrated into existing work practices, procedures, and policies (Sørensen & Holman, 2014. If the changes are not integrated, they are unlikely to be sustained in the long term and may be abandoned once the intervention project has finished (Randall et al., 2005). Fourth, the intervention processes need to be integrated into existing structures (von Thiele Schwarz et al., 2017). Making use of and extending the purpose of existing management systems to also consider well-being issues facilitates the alignment to organizational objectives and ensures that well-being considerations become part of daily business. It may also take the pressure off participants by reducing the number of additional activities they have to engage in (Andersen & Westgaard, 2013; Poulsen et al., 2015). Finally, intervention processes need to consider existing levels of maturity—for example, the abilities of participants to engage in problem-solving processes. Nielsen et al. (2006) found that employees in industrial canteens struggled to implement action plans as they had little experience engaging in problem-solving processes, and Augustsson et al. (2015) saw that action plans were more likely to be implemented in groups where employees had previous experience in using the Kaizen tools used as part of the intervention.

FIVE PHASES OF PARTICIPATORY ORGANIZATIONAL INTERVENTIONS

The four key principles run through the five phases of participatory organizational interventions. In the following sections, I outline each of the five phases and the supporting evidence from the research.

Preparation Phase

At the first step, the *preparation phase*, a steering group should be implemented (Nielsen & Noblet, 2018). The steering group has a dual purpose. At the operational level, it should oversee the day-to-day progress of project activities, including developing a communication plan for the intervention, designing and approving the screening tool, solidifying the feedback strategy, developing the action planning strategy, and monitoring the action plan implementation (Nielsen et al., 2013). At the strategic level, the steering group should identify groups at risk, ensure that the intervention aligns with organizational objectives, ensure sufficient resources throughout the intervention, and reflect on how learning from the intervention can be integrated into HR and occupational health management structures. The steering group should represent all who have an interest in well-being issues (i.e., senior and line management, occupational health and HR, and employee representatives; Nielsen et al., 2013). Dahler-Larsen et al. (2020) found that when key stakeholders were involved in the intervention process, more actions were taken to improve psychosocial working conditions.

An important member of the steering group is the project champion who can act as the driver of change (Nielsen et al., 2013). This individual's responsibility is to manage the process, facilitate meetings and workshops, and keep up momentum (Nielsen et al., 2013). Project champions can be employees (Nielsen, Dawson, et al., 2021), line managers (Ipsen et al., 2015), senior managers (Schelvis et al., 2016), or consultants (Nielsen, Antino, et al., 2021; von Thiele Schwarz et al., 2017). Although project champions are key to drive the implementation, it is important that the project is embedded in the organization through the steering group to ensure shared responsibility. Ipsen et al. (2015) found that facilitators were the single biggest factor facilitating intervention implementation. Too much emphasis on one person makes the intervention vulnerable to stagnation if that person leaves the role or the organization (Schelvis et al., 2016). The representatives on the steering group and the power balance need to be considered. Schelvis et al. (2016) found that in an organization where management was overrepresented in the steering group, employees felt they had few opportunities for participation; conversely, in an organization with a smaller steering group, employees reported they had greater opportunities for participation.

Screening Phase

Key to participatory organizational interventions is that changes to work policies, practices, and procedures are not predetermined but are developed based on participants' prioritization of what demands and resources need to be addressed. A thorough screening is needed in order to ensure that changes target the most prominent issues (Nielsen et al., 2013). Most often, standardized questionnaires and a number of validated questionnaires are used—for example, the Management Standards HSE Indicator tool, which captures six resources: demands, control, support, relationships, roles, and change (Cousins et al., 2004), or the Copenhagen Psychosocial Questionnaire (Kristensen et al., 2005), which addresses more than 35 demands and resources. These questionnaires measure a fixed set of psychosocial working conditions. One limitation of the HSE Indicator tool is that it does not measure any well-being outcomes, making it impossible to determine whether any of the psychosocial working conditions evaluated influence employee outcomes (Nielsen et al., 2021d). Standardized questionnaires often rest on the assumption that a restricted set of working conditions are important to all occupation groups and that there is a cut-off point above which a working condition is harmful, much like chemical risks (Cousins et al., 2004). Benchmarks are often calculated assuming that if an intervention group scores lower than the national or occupational average, this is an indication of a necessary change. This assumption is problematic for at least three reasons. First, in some occupations, specific working conditions may play a particular role; for example, in health care occupations, emotional demands from patients and their families are inherent to the job (Dewe & Trenberth, 2012). It has therefore been argued that questionnaires should capture the conditions most relevant to the occupation in question (Di Tecco et al., 2020). Second, cognitive appraisals play a key role in determining the effect of working conditions (Lazarus & Folkman, 1992); people in the same job do not perceive their job in the same way (Persson et al., 2012). Third, benchmarks may not be relevant to all groups—certain occupational groups, such as postal workers, for example, may not expect high levels of autonomy (Nielsen et al., 2014).

An alternative strategy has therefore been explored where tailored questionnaires are developed to capture the demands and resources specific to the intervention group. Tailored questionnaires may capture the appraisals of participants by asking whether a working condition is a positive or negative aspect of the work, and subsequently calculating the percentage of participants who feel that the working condition is a problem (Nielsen et al., 2014). In one study, participants in a participatory organizational intervention felt that the tailored questionnaire provided them with more precise information about key policies, practices, and procedures that needed to change and facilitated the development of the feasible and appropriate action plans (Nielsen et al., 2014), however, the authors emphasized that the method required high levels of expertise and time.

Questionnaires may not be suitable in smaller organizations; methods such as visual mapping (using sticky notes to map out working conditions) or focus groups may be more suitable for these groups (Gupta et al., 2018). Using these methods, groups of workers engage in dialogue workshops to identify which demands and resources need addressing. Gupta et al. (2018) found that visual mapping was a useful technique to identify both demands and resources. An advantage of such methods is that they overcome the translation process from abstract concepts such as "social support" and "autonomy" (Gupta et al., 2018). The steering group plays a key role in determining which screening process is appropriate in a given organization (Nielsen, Randall, et al., 2010).

Once screening has taken place, the results should be fed back to participants to enable them to prioritize which actions to take. Providing survey feedback in an anonymized form has been found to lead to more actions taken to improve psychosocial working conditions (Dahler-Larsen et al., 2020).

Action Planning Phase

In the *action planning phase*, the results of the screening process are translated into changes to work practices, policies, and procedures (Nielsen & Noblet, 2018). Informed action is key, and action planning needs to be based on the results of the screening. It is important that these action plans are developed to be feasible and actionable (Nielsen & Noblet, 2018). Identifying quick wins and action plans that can easily be implemented may build employee confidence (Schelvis et al., 2016).

It is important that the action planning is seen as a joint responsibility between managers and employees. Schelvis et al. (2016) found that employees viewed action plans positively when they had been given the opportunity to participate. Furthermore, the translation of screening results into action plans needs to be clearly communicated in order for employees to understand the link between the two. In one organization where participation was perceived to be high, action plans were mostly seen as appropriate, whereas in another organization where employees felt participation was low, they were unable to understand how survey results had resulted in the actions that had been decided upon (Schelvis et al., 2016). This study also revealed that in the organization where employees felt they had few opportunities for participation in the overall process, participation was also low in the action planning phase; however, employees still felt responsible for the content of the action plan. Similarly, Gupta et al. (2018) reported a high level of participation in screening and action planning workshops and saw that more than four out of five participants felt that action plans targeted the most relevant problems.

Implementation Phase

Implementation of action plans requires careful monitoring and adjustment (von Thiele Schwarz et al., 2021). In Gupta et al.'s (2018) study, 75% of employees reported having continuously revisited the action plans, and 79% reported having implemented the planned plans.

A number of key factors drive the implementation of action plans. First, it is crucial that responsibilities to implement action plans are taken seriously. Those employees who have been allocated responsibility for implementing action plans need to be proactive in driving change (Sørensen & Holman, 2014). Second, awareness of action plans leads to more actions being taken; if employees are not aware of which changes to work polices, practices, and procedures are planned, they cannot be expected to implement these changes (Dahler-Larsen et al., 2020). Schelvis et al. (2016) found that despite low participation in the previous phases of the intervention and despite feeling poorly informed about progress, employees still felt responsible for the implementation of action plans. Furthermore, in groups where action plans were implemented, managers and employees in working groups ensured all participants were informed about progress (e.g., through producing posters and leaflets; Sørensen & Holman, 2014). Communication about progress is key, and celebrating the implementation of quick wins helps create a positive perception of the intervention. It is important to strike a balance and ensure that real change is occurring (Schelvis et al., 2016); if not, there is a risk that improvements are seen as negligible (Schelvis et al., 2016). Third, line managers need to support the implementation of changes. Dahler-Larsen et al. (2020) reported that line manager support led to more actions being taken to improve psychosocial working conditions. Fourth, it is crucial that the implementation of action plans is prioritized (Ipsen et al., 2015) and integrated into existing procedures (e.g., integration into HR and strategy procedures; Dahler-Larsen et al., 2020; von Thiele Schwarz et al., 2017).

Evaluation Phase

In the final phase, the intervention should be evaluated. *Evaluation* should take place at two levels: organizational and scientific (von Thiele Schwarz et al., 2021).

The objective of organizational evaluation is to promote the organization's learning capability (von Thiele Schwarz et al., 2021. Organization members utilize organizational evaluation to reflect on their ability to implement changes successfully and determine whether implemented action plans achieved their intended outcomes, whether the tools and methods used were appropriate in the organizational context, and whether processes were implemented according to plan and were successful (i.e., whether communication reached the intended audience and the messages were successfully transmitted). These reflections will enable organizations to evaluate what worked well and what did not work well and integrate these findings into future interventions within the organization (Nielsen & Abildgaard, 2013). Organizational evaluation is crucial to ensure organizational learning and sustainable change (Nielsen & Abildgaard, 2013). One method to perform organizational evaluation is chronicle workshops (Poulsen et al., 2015), in which organizational members reflect on the intervention, enabling them to understand the outcomes and influencing factors. Chronicle workshops help create a shared story about the intervention process, detailing what happened when and why, using visual materials such as sticky notes (Poulsen et al., 2015).

The objective of scientific evaluation is to explicate the effects of the intervention and the extent to which it was successful in improving working conditions and promoting employee well-being. As participatory organizational interventions are complex with emergent and reverse causality (Rogers, 2008), scientific evaluation calls for sophisticated evaluation methods. Realist evaluation (Pawson & Tilley, 1997) enables researchers to answer the questions of what works for whom in which circumstances. Central to realist evaluation is the formulation and testing of context-mechanism-outcomes configurations, the exploration of whether the mechanisms bring about the intended outcomes in terms of improved working conditions and employee well-being. Mechanisms are what make the intervention work (e.g., line manager support, effective communication about the intervention, or active participation in the intervention design and implementation; Nielsen & Miraglia, 2017). Whether mechanisms are triggered or activated depends on whether the context supports these mechanisms (i.e., that there is a certain level of trust within the organization enabling participants to engage in the participatory process; Nielsen & Miraglia, 2017). Central to scientific evaluation are the quantitative before-and-after measurements of outcomes to determine whether improvements in outcomes can be detected; however, contextual factors and mechanisms can be captured using both qualitative (Abildgaard et al., 2020) and quantitative methods (von Thiele Schwarz et al., 2017).

Regardless of the level of evaluation, it is crucial to evaluate the impact of the different phases and understand how one phase influences subsequent phases (Nielsen & Abildgaard, 2013). Schelvis et al. (2016) found that already in the early phases of an intervention, process issues around participation were a challenge and therefore the intervention failed to achieve its outcomes. Sørensen and Holman (2014) observed that only in the implementation phase did variations in the intervention process influence outcomes differentially across intervention groups.

DISCUSSION

In this chapter, I discussed the "how to" of participatory organizational interventions. I outlined the key principles of participation, management support, intervention fit, and communication that need to be considered throughout the intervention process as well as the considerations at each of the five phases of intervention. One limitation of the chapter is that the intervention process may come across as a fairly linear process and that the four process principles operate separately from each other; this is not the case. One process factor influences the others (Schelvis et al., 2016). Schelvis and colleagues found that when managers took too much ownership over the process, employees did not feel they had the opportunity to engage with the intervention. Another study found that preexisting levels of participation predicted the engagement of line managers and employee job satisfaction in the early phases of an intervention (Tafvelin et al., 2019). Likewise, line manager support at the early stages ensured participation in the implementation phase (Tafvelin et al., 2019) and a good intervention fit (Lundmark et al., 2018).

It is important to be aware that what happens at one phase of the intervention influences the subsequent phases. Nielsen et al. (2007) found that information about intervention activities influenced the extent to which employees were involved in designing the intervention and its activities, which in turn predicted whether they participated in the activities. Those who had participated in intervention activities had a positive attitude toward the intervention, which was related to improvements in employee well-being. Schelvis et al. (2016) found that dissatisfaction with the feedback report could partly explain disappointing intervention outcomes; in particular, senior management's dissatisfaction with issues identified could partly explain their lack of support in later phases.

Although organizational interventions are the recommended method due to their potential to address the causes of poor well-being (International Labor Office, 2001), it is important to note that they require high levels of investment. The intervention process itself may build resources (Nielsen & Christensen, 2021), but the intervention processes may also be perceived as a strain. Bakhuys Roozeboom et al. (2020) noted that in organizations where the dialogue about stress had improved, workers reported less of a decrease in job demands, possibly because the dialogue was related to increased activities to strengthen this dialogue, e.g., participation in workshops.

A cautionary word should be raised about intervention fit. Although the intervention needs to be integrated into organizational practices, it also needs its own identity. Schelvis et al. (2016) found that when action plans were integrated into overall performance indicators, this reduced an opportunity for employees to be involved in the implementation, and employees were unaware of progress. It is important to maintain momentum in the later phases to avoid cynicism and waning levels of engagement (Schelvis et al., 2016).

CONCLUSION

Participatory organizational interventions hold great promise for improving working conditions and employee well-being; however, they are not easy to implement. The process is as essential as the content of the intervention, and careful attention needs to be paid throughout the entire lifetime of an intervention to ensure that it is implemented according to plan and succeeds in developing organizational learning to promote sustainable results.

REFERENCES

Abildgaard, J. S., Nielsen, K., Wåhlin-Jacobsen, C. D., Maltesen, T., Christensen, K. B., & Holtermann, A. (2020). 'Same, but different': A mixed-methods realist evaluation of a cluster-randomized controlled participatory organizational intervention. *Human Relations, 73*(10), 1339–1365. https://doi.org/10.1177/0018726719866896

Abildgaard, J. S., Saksvik, P. Ø., & Nielsen, K. (2016). How to measure the intervention process? An assessment of qualitative and quantitative approaches to data collection in the process evaluation of organizational interventions. *Frontiers in Psychology, 7*, 1380. https://doi.org/10.3389/fpsyg.2016.01380

Andersen, G. R., & Westgaard, R. H. (2013). Understanding significant processes during work environment interventions to alleviate time pressure and associated sick leave of home care workers—A case study. *BMC Health Services Research, 13*(1), 477. https://doi.org/10.1186/1472-6963-13-477

Ashmos, D. P., & Nathan, M. L. (2002). Team sense-making: A mental model for navigating uncharted territories. *Journal of Managerial Issues, 14*(2), 198–217. https://www.jstor.org/stable/40604384

Augustsson, H., von Thiele Schwarz, U., Stenfors-Hayes, T., & Hasson, H. (2015). Investigating variations in implementation fidelity of an organizational-level occupational health intervention. *International Journal of Behavioral Medicine, 22*(3), 345–355. https://doi.org/10.1007/s12529-014-9420-8

Aust, B., Rugulies, R., Finken, A., & Jensen, C. (2010). When workplace interventions lead to negative effects: Learning from failures. *Scandinavian Journal of Public Health, 38*(3, Suppl.), 106–119. https://doi.org/10.1177/1403494809354362

Bailey, T. R. (1993). *Discretionary effort and the organization of work: Employee participation and work reform since Hawthorne.* Teachers College and Conservation of Human Resources, Columbia University.

Bakhuys Roozeboom, M. C., Schelvis, R. M. C., Houtman, I. L. D., Wiezer, N. M., & Bongers, P. M. (2020). Decreasing employees' work stress by a participatory, organizational level work stress prevention approach: A multiple-case study in primary education. *BMC Public Health, 20*(1), 676. https://doi.org/10.1186/s12889-020-08698-2

Bandura, A. (1986). The explanatory and predictive scope of self-efficacy theory. *Journal of Social and Clinical Psychology, 4*(3), 359–373. https://doi.org/10.1521/jscp.1986.4.3.359

Bond, F. W., & Bunce, D. (2001). Job control mediates change in a work reorganization intervention for stress reduction. *Journal of Occupational Health Psychology, 6*(4), 290–302. https://doi.org/10.1037/1076-8998.6.4.290

Carter, M. Z., Armenakis, A. A., Feild, H. S., & Mossholder, K. W. (2013). Transformational leadership, relationship quality, and employee performance during continuous incremental organizational change. *Journal of Organizational Behavior, 34*(7), 942–958. https://doi.org/10.1002/job.1824

Cousins, R., Mackay, C. J., Clarke, S. D., Kelly, C., Kelly, P. J., & McCaig, R. H. (2004). 'Management standards' work-related stress in the UK: Practical development. *Work and Stress, 18*(2), 113–136. https://doi.org/10.1080/02678370410001734322

Dahler-Larsen, P., Sundby, A., & Boodhoo, A. (2020). Can occupational health and safety management systems address psychosocial risk factors? An empirical study. *Safety Science, 130,* 104878. https://doi.org/10.1016/j.ssci.2020.104878

Daltuva, J. A., King, K. R., Williams, M. K., & Robins, T. G. (2009). Building a strong foundation for occupational health and safety: Action research in the workplace. *American Journal of Industrial Medicine, 52*(8), 614–624. https://doi.org/10.1002/ajim.20711

Danna, K., & Griffin, R. W. (1999). Health and well-being in the workplace: A review and synthesis of the literature. *Journal of Management, 25*(3), 357–384. https://doi.org/10.1177/014920639902500305

Day, A., & Nielsen, K. (2017). What does our organization do to help our well-being? Creating healthy workplaces and workers. In N. Chmiel, F. Fraccoroli, & M. Sverke (Eds.), *An introduction of work and organizational psychology* (pp. 295–314). Wiley Blackwell. https://doi.org/10.1002/9781119168058.ch16

Demerouti, E., Bakker, A. B., Nachreiner, F., & Schaufeli, W. B. (2001). The job demands-resources model of burnout. *Journal of Applied Psychology, 86*(3), 499–512. https://doi.org/10.1037/0021-9010.86.3.499

Dewe, P., & Trenberth, L. (2012). Exploring the relationships between appraisals of stressful encounters and the associated emotions in a work setting. *Work and Stress, 26*(2), 161–174. https://doi.org/10.1080/02678373.2012.687042

Di Tecco, C., Nielsen, K., Ghelli, M., Ronchetti, M., Marzocchi, I., Persechino, B., & Iavicoli, S. (2020). Improving working conditions and job satisfaction in healthcare: A study concept design on a participatory organizational level intervention in psychosocial risks management. *International Journal of Environmental Research and Public Health, 17*(10), 3677. https://doi.org/10.3390/ijerph17103677

European Trade Union Confederation. (2004). *Framework agreement on work-related stress.*

Gupta, N., Wåhlin-Jacobsen, C. D., Abildgaard, J. S., Henriksen, L. N., Nielsen, K., & Holtermann, A. (2018). Effectiveness of a participatory physical and psychosocial intervention to balance the demands and resources of industrial workers: A cluster-randomized controlled trial. *Scandinavian Journal of Work, Environment & Health, 44*(1), 58–68. https://doi.org/10.5271/sjweh.3689

Halbesleben, J. R. (2010). A meta-analysis of work engagement: Relationships with burnout, demands, resources, and consequences. In A. Bakker & M. Leiter (Eds.), *Work engagement: A handbook of essential theory and research* (pp. 102–117). Psychology Press.

Harms, P. D., Credé, M., Tynan, M., Leon, M., & Jeung, W. (2017). Leadership and stress: A meta-analytic review. *The Leadership Quarterly, 28*(1), 178–194. https://doi.org/10.1016/j.leaqua.2016.10.006

Havermans, B. M., Schelvis, R. M. C., Boot, C. R. L., Brouwers, E. P. M., Anema, J. R., & van der Beek, A. J. (2016). Process variables in organizational stress management intervention evaluation research: A systematic review. *Scandinavian Journal of Work, Environment & Health, 42*(5), 371–381. https://doi.org/10.5271/sjweh.3570

Hurrell, J. (2005). Organizational stress intervention. In J. Barling, E. K. Kelloway, & M. R. Frone (Eds.), *Handbook of work stress* (pp. 623–646). Sage. https://doi.org/10.4135/9781412975995.n27

Inceoglu, I., Thomas, G., Chu, C., Plans, D., & Gerbasi, A. (2018). Leadership behavior and employee well-being: An integrated review and a future research agenda. *The Leadership Quarterly, 29*(1), 179–202. https://doi.org/10.1016/j.leaqua.2017.12.006

International Labor Office. (2001). *Guidelines on occupational safety and health management systems.*

Ipsen, C., Gish, L., & Poulsen, S. (2015). Organizational-level interventions in small and medium-sized enterprises: Enabling and inhibiting factors in the PoWRS program. *Safety Science, 71*, 264–274. https://doi.org/10.1016/j.ssci.2014.07.017

Jenny, G. J., Brauchli, R., Inauen, A., Füllemann, D., Fridrich, A., & Bauer, G. F. (2015). Process and outcome evaluation of an organizational-level stress management intervention in Switzerland. *Health Promotion International, 30*(3), 573–585. https://doi.org/10.1093/heapro/dat091

Karasek, R. A., & Theorell, T. (1990). *Healthy work: Stress, productivity and the reconstruction of working life.* Basic Books.

Kristensen, T. S., Hannerz, H., Høgh, A., & Borg, V. (2005). The Copenhagen Psychosocial Questionnaire—A tool for the assessment and improvement of the psychosocial work environment. *Scandinavian Journal of Work, Environment & Health, 31*(6), 438–449. https://doi.org/10.5271/sjweh.948

Kristof-Brown, A., & Guay, R. P. (2011). Person–environment fit. In S. Zedeck (Ed.), *APA handbook of industrial and organizational psychology: Vol. 3. Maintaining, expanding, and contracting the organization* (pp. 3–50). American Psychological Association. https://doi.org/10.1037/12171-001

Landsbergis, P., & Vivona-Vaughan, E. (1995). Evaluation of an occupational stress intervention in a public agency. *Journal of Organizational Behavior, 16*(1), 29–48. https://doi.org/10.1002/job.4030160106

Lazarus, R., & Folkman, S. (1992). *Stress, appraisal and coping.* Springer Publications.

Lundmark, R., Hasson, H., von Thiele Schwarz, U., Hasson, D., & Tafvelin, S. (2017). Leading for change: Line managers' influence on the outcomes of an occupational health intervention. *Work and Stress, 31*(3), 276–296. https://doi.org/10.1080/02678373.2017.1308446

Lundmark, R., von Thiele Schwarz, U., Hasson, H., Stenling, A., & Tafvelin, S. (2018). Making it fit: Associations of line managers' behaviours with the outcomes of an organizational-level intervention. *Stress and Health, 34*(1), 163–174. https://doi.org/10.1002/smi.2770

Mackey, J. D., Huang, L., & He, W. (2020). You abuse and I criticize: An ego depletion and leader–member exchange examination of abusive supervision and destructive voice. *Journal of Business Ethics, 164*, 579–591. https://doi.org/10.1007/s10551-018-4024-x

Mikkelsen, A. (2005). Methodological challenges in the study of organizational interventions in flexible organizations. In A. M. Fuglseth & I. A. Kleppe (Eds.), *Anthology for Kjell Grønhaug in celebration of his 70th birthday* (pp. 150–178). Fagbokforlaget.

Nielsen, K. (2013). How can we make organizational interventions work? Employees and line managers as actively crafting interventions. *Human Relations, 66*(8), 1029–1050. https://doi.org/10.1177/0018726713477164

Nielsen, K. (2017). Leaders can make or break an intervention—but are they the villains of the play? In K. Kelloway, K. Nielsen, & J. Dimoff (Eds.), *Leading to occupational health and safety: How leadership behaviours impact organizational safety and well-being* (pp. 197–210). Wiley.

Nielsen, K., & Abildgaard, J. S. (2012). The development and validation of a job crafting measure for use with blue-collar workers. *Work and Stress, 26*(4), 365–384. https://doi.org/10.1080/02678373.2012.733543

Nielsen, K., & Abildgaard, J. S. (2013). Organizational interventions: A research-based framework for the evaluation of both process and effects. *Work and Stress, 27*(3), 278–297. https://doi.org/10.1080/02678373.2013.812358

Nielsen, K., Abildgaard, J. S., & Daniels, K. (2014). Putting context into organizational intervention design: Using tailored questionnaires to measure initiatives for worker well-being. *Human Relations, 67*(12), 1537–1560. https://doi.org/10.1177/0018726714525974

Nielsen, K., Antino, M., Rodríguez-Muñoz, A., & Sanz-Vergel, A. (2021). Is it me or us? The impact of individual and collective participation on work engagement and burnout in a cluster-randomized organisational intervention. *Work and Stress, 35*(4), 374–397. https://doi.org/10.1080/02678373.2021.1889072

Nielsen, K., Axtell, C., & Sorensen, G. (2021). Organizational interventions—fitting the intervention to the context to ensure the participatory process. In E. K. Kelloway & C. Cooper (Eds.), *A research agenda for workplace stress and wellbeing* (pp. 191–200). Edward Elgar Publishing.

Nielsen, K., Axtell, C., & Taylor, S. (2021). National approaches to wellbeing interventions: The UK management standards as an example. In T. Wall, C. Cooper, & X. P. Brough (Eds.), *The SAGE handbook of organizational wellbeing* (pp. 368–382).

Nielsen, K., & Christensen, M. (2021). Positive participatory organizational interventions: A multilevel approach for creating healthy workplaces. *Frontiers in Psychology: Positive Psychology.* https://doi.org/10.3389/fpsyg.2021.696245

Nielsen, K., Dawson, J., Hasson, H., & von Thiel Schwarz, U. (2021). What about me? The impact of employee change agents' person-role fit on their job satisfaction during organisational change. *Work and Stress, 35*(1), 57–73. https://doi.org/10.1080/02678373.2020.1730481

Nielsen, K., Fredslund, H., Christensen, K. B., & Albertsen, K. (2006). Success or failure? Interpreting and understanding the impact of interventions in four similar worksites. *Work and Stress, 20*(3), 272–287. https://doi.org/10.1080/02678370601022688

Nielsen, K., & Miraglia, M. (2017). What works for whom in which circumstances? On the need to move beyond the 'what works?' question in organizational intervention research. *Human Relations, 70*(1), 40–62. https://doi.org/10.1177/0018726716670226

Nielsen, K., Nielsen, M. B., Ogbonnaya, C., Känsälä, M., Saari, E., & Isaksson, K. (2017). Workplace resources to improve both employee well-being and performance: A systematic review and meta-analysis. *Work and Stress, 31*(2), 101–120. https://doi.org/10.1080/02678373.2017.1304463

Nielsen, K., & Noblet, A. (2018). Introduction: Organizational interventions: Where we are, where we go from here? In K. Nielsen & A. Noblet (Eds.), *Organizational interventions for health and well-being: A handbook for evidence-based practice* (pp. 1–23). Routledge. https://doi.org/10.4324/9781315410494-1

Nielsen, K., & Randall, R. (2009). Managers' active support when implementing teams: The impact on employee well-being. *Applied Psychology. Health and Well-Being, 1*(3), 374–390. https://doi.org/10.1111/j.1758-0854.2009.01016.x

Nielsen, K., & Randall, R. (2012). The importance of employee participation and perceptions of changes in procedures in a teamworking intervention. *Work and Stress, 26*(2), 91–111. https://doi.org/10.1080/02678373.2012.682721

Nielsen, K., & Randall, R. (2013). Opening the black box: Presenting a model for evaluating organizational-level interventions. *European Journal of Work and Organizational Psychology, 22*(5), 601–617. https://doi.org/10.1080/1359432X.2012.690556

Nielsen, K., Randall, R., & Albertsen, K. (2007). Participants' appraisals of process issues and the effects of stress management interventions. *Journal of Organizational Behavior, 28*(6), 793–810. https://doi.org/10.1002/job.450

Nielsen, K., Randall, R., Holten, A. L., & González, E. R. (2010). Conducting organizational-level occupational health interventions: What works? *Work and Stress, 24*(3), 234–259. https://doi.org/10.1080/02678373.2010.515393

Nielsen, K., Stage, M., Abildgaard, J. S., & Brauer, C. V. (2013). Participatory intervention from and organizational perspective: Employees as active agents in creating a healthy work environment. In G. Bauer & G. Jenny (Eds.), *Concepts of salutogenic organizations and change: The concepts behind organizational health intervention research* (pp. 327–350). Springer Publications. https://doi.org/10.1007/978-94-007-6470-5_18

Nielsen, K., Taris, T. W., & Cox, T. (2010). The future of organizational interventions: Addressing the challenges of today's organizations. *Work and Stress, 24*(3), 219–233. https://doi.org/10.1080/02678373.2010.519176

Niks, I., de Jonge, J., Gevers, J., & Houtman, I. (2018). Work stress interventions in hospital care: Effectiveness of the *DISCovery* method. *International Journal of Environmental Research and Public Health, 15*(2), 332. https://doi.org/10.3390/ijerph15020332

Nytrø, K., Saksvik, P. Ø., Mikkelsen, A., Bohle, P., & Quinlan, M. (2000). An appraisal of key factors in the implementation of occupational stress interventions. *Work and Stress, 14*(3), 213–225. https://doi.org/10.1080/02678370010024749

Pawson, R., & Tilley, N. (1997). *Realistic evaluation*. Sage.

Persson, R., Hansen, Å. M., Garde, A. H., Kristiansen, J., Nordander, C., Balogh, I., Ohlsson, K., Ostergren, P. O., & Ørbæk, P. (2012). Can the job content questionnaire be used to assess structural and organizational properties of the work environment? *International Archives of Occupational and Environmental Health, 85*(1), 45–55. https://doi.org/10.1007/s00420-011-0647-2

Poulsen, S., Ipsen, C., & Gish, L. (2015). Applying the chronicle workshop as a method for evaluating participatory interventions. *International Journal Human Factors and Ergonomics, 3*(3/4), 271–290. https://doi.org/10.1504/IJHFE.2015.073002

Ramos, S., Costa, P., Passos, A. M., Silva, S. A., & Sacadura-Leite, E. (2020). Intervening on burnout in complex organizations—The incomplete process of an action research in the hospital. *Frontiers in Psychology, 11*, 2203. https://doi.org/10.3389/fpsyg.2020.02203

Randall, R., Griffiths, A., & Cox, T. (2005). Evaluating organizational stress-management interventions using adapted study designs. *European Journal of Work and Organizational Psychology, 14*(1), 23–41. https://doi.org/10.1080/13594320444000209

Richardson, K. M., & Rothstein, H. R. (2008). Effects of occupational stress management intervention programs: A meta-analysis. *Journal of Occupational Health Psychology, 13*(1), 69–93. https://doi.org/10.1037/1076-8998.13.1.69

Rogers, P. J. (2008). Using programme theory to evaluate complicated and complex aspects of interventions. *Evaluation, 14*(1), 29–48. https://doi.org/10.1177/1356389007084674

Rosskam, E. (2009). Using participatory action research methodology to improve worker health. In P. Schnall, M. Dobson, & E. Rosskam (Eds.), *Unhealthy work: Causes, consequences, cures* (pp. 211–229). Baywood Publishing Company.

Schelvis, R. M., Wiezer, N. M., Blatter, B. M., van Genabeek, J. A., Oude Hengel, K. M., Bohlmeijer, E. T., & van der Beek, A. J. (2016). Evaluating the implementation process of a participatory organizational level occupational health intervention in schools. *BMC Public Health, 16*(1), 1212. https://doi.org/10.1186/s12889-016-3869-0

Schyns, B., & Schilling, J. (2013). How bad are the effects of bad leaders? A meta-analysis of destructive leadership and its outcomes. *The Leadership Quarterly, 24*(1), 138–158. https://doi.org/10.1016/j.leaqua.2012.09.001

Sorensen, G., Peters, S., Nielsen, K., Nagler, E., Karapanos, M., Wallace, L., Burke, L., Dennerlein, J. T., & Wagner, G. R. (2019). Improving working conditions to promote worker safety, health, and wellbeing for low-wage workers: The workplace organizational health study. *International Journal of Environmental Research and Public Health, 16*(8), 1449. https://doi.org/10.3390/ijerph16081449

Sørensen, O. H., & Holman, D. (2014). A participative intervention to improve employee well-being in knowledge work jobs: A mixed-methods evaluation study. *Work and Stress, 28*(1), 67–86. https://doi.org/10.1080/02678373.2013.876124

Tafvelin, S., von Thiele Schwarz, U., Nielsen, K., & Hasson, H. (2019). Employees' and line managers' active involvement in participatory organizational interventions: Examining direct, reversed, and reciprocal effects on well-being. *Stress and Health, 35*(1), 69–80. https://doi.org/10.1002/smi.2841

Vignoli, M., Nielsen, K., Guglielmi, D., Tabanelli, M. C., & Violante, F. S. (2017). The importance of context in screening in occupational health interventions in organizations: A mixed methods study. *Frontiers in Psychology, 8*, 1347. https://doi.org/10.3389/fpsyg.2017.01347

von Thiele Schwarz, U., Nielsen, K. M., Stenfors-Hayes, T., & Hasson, H. (2017). Using kaizen to improve employee well-being: Results from two organizational intervention studies. *Human Relations, 70*(8), 966–993. https://doi.org/10.1177/0018726716677071

von Thiele Schwarz, U., Nielsen, K., Edwards, K., Hasson, H., Ipsen, C., Savage, C., Abildgaard, J. S., Richter, A., Lornudd, C., Mazzocato, P., & Reed, J. E. (2021). How to design, implement and evaluate organizational interventions for maximum impact: The Sigtuna Principles. *European Journal of Work and Organizational Psychology, 30*(3), 415–427. https://doi.org/10.1080/1359432X.2020.1803960

23

Promoting Worker Health and Well-Being: Targets for Change and Strategies for Attaining Them

Catherine A. Heaney

Much has changed in the worlds of work and health since the last edition of this handbook, and the rate of change is accelerating as the world recovers from the global coronavirus pandemic. More workers are self-employed or involved in informal or contingent work, are working remotely from home, and are changing jobs more often. The nature of work also continues to change, with a growing proportion of the workforce involved in the technical or service sectors as opposed to the agricultural or manufacturing sectors (Bureau of Labor Statistics, 2021). These changes have sparked modifications in the expectations and preferences of both employers and workers. In the world of health, there has been a growing commitment to the definition of health originally put forth in the preamble to the constitution of the World Health Organization: "Health is a state of complete physical, mental and social well-being and not merely the absence of disease or infirmity" (1946, bullet 1).

What does this mean for the arena of worker health interventions? This chapter identifies current challenges to mounting effective worker health interventions and suggests strategies for overcoming these challenges. More specifically, we discuss the various outcomes that worker health interventions attempt to bring about, a social ecological approach to identifying targets of change, and the strategies for attaining the desired changes.

https://doi.org/10.1037/0000331-023
Handbook of Occupational Health Psychology, Third Edition, L. E. Tetrick, G. G. Fisher, M. T. Ford, and J. C. Quick (Editors)

DESIRED OUTCOMES OF WORKER HEALTH INTERVENTIONS

Occupational safety and health (OSH) professionals have long had the mission of protecting workers from physical and chemical hazards in the workplace. With the growth of the service sector in the United States and our enhanced understanding of how psychosocial stress can contribute to poor health, OSH broadened its mission to include psychosocial hazards such as job stress, job insecurity, unpredictability and lack of control, lack of fairness, and poor social relationships at work. At the same time, there was a growing call to integrate efforts to protect workers from hazards with health promotion efforts that focused on improving workers' personal health behaviors (e.g., smoking, physical activity, and nutrition; Sorensen et al., 2013).

Most recently, there has been a movement to further broaden the purview of worker health programs to include the promotion of positive experiences, positive emotions, and other assets that are important constituents of well-being (Chari et al., 2018). This movement has had several catalysts. The advancement of the field of positive psychology, with its emphasis on the processes of thriving and flourishing, provided some of the initial theories and research (Seligman, 2018). While the study of well-being has a long intellectual history across several academic disciplines (e.g., philosophy, economics, psychology), more recent research has linked well-being to longevity and to prevention of disease (Zaninotto & Steptoe, 2019). These studies have helped bring the pursuit of well-being into the biomedical arena.

Figure 23.1 presents the broad array of outcomes that worker health interventions can address. Adapted from the field of mental health intervention (National Research Council and Institute of Medicine, 2009), the figure presents four overarching categories of interventions: promotion, protection and prevention, treatment, and maintenance. Of course, all worker health interventions have the ultimate goal of enhancing worker health and well-being. However, they approach this ultimate goal through different proximal goals. The promotion category stems from the newfound commitment to emphasizing the positive aspects of well-being. For example, these interventions may have the goal of making work more meaningful or more engaging for workers. The protection and prevention interventions have the goal of reducing workers' risks for illness and/or injuries. These risks include both those found in the work environment and workers' personal risk behaviors. Sometimes these interventions are labeled "universal," meaning that they address a need (or risk) relevant to all workers. Selective interventions target a group of employees perceived to be at higher risk than others (e.g., the risk of pulmonary disease among coal miners), and indicated prevention interventions attempt to reduce the risk of individuals at high personal risk of ill health (e.g., coal miners who smoke). Occupational medicine addresses the diagnosis and treatment of work-related disorders. Maintenance interventions attempt to sustain positive changes at both the individual and organizational levels. The sustainability of organizational change (Buchanan et al., 2005) and individual behavior change

FIGURE 23.1. Spectrum of Worker Health Interventions

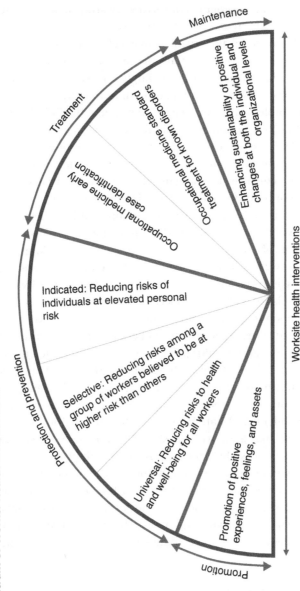

(Fjeldsoe et al., 2011) is a burgeoning area of investigation given the high rates of program collapse and worker relapse.

There are several implications of the wide array of desired proximal outcomes presented in Figure 23.1. First, in any given employment sector or workplace, any or all of these four intervention categories might be necessary. Thus, needs assessments should provide information relevant to each of the categories. Second, in order to address a wide array of desired outcomes, multidisciplinary teams are needed. Psychologists are needed to examine and help modify both individual and organizational behaviors. Communication specialists are needed to convey important messages about worker health and well-being to all relevant stakeholders. Engineers are needed to discover and implement strategies for removing or minimizing physical and chemical hazards. Health professionals are needed to examine the links between risks and ill health, to diagnose and treat health problems, and to measure biomedical outcomes. And given that any worker health intervention needs to be mounted in as cost-effective a manner as possible and with the opportunity to provide an adequate return on investment, economists are needed to develop and evaluate these concepts. Third, many different outcomes need to have valid and reliable measures in order to assess intervention effectiveness: positive aspects of work; risks for ill health including aspects of work organization, work content, physical and social environments at work, and personal risk behaviors; as well as incidence and prevalence of disease and injury. Special attention needs to be paid to the time course and sustainability of any changes.

The recognition of universal, selective, and indicated prevention and protection interventions raises some important issues. The universal designation alerts us to the need to examine which workers (if any) are not being adequately addressed. For example, OSH professionals have struggled mightily to bring worker health interventions to those who work in small businesses (Ingram et al., 2021). A more nascent struggle is that of providing adequate protection and prevention to contingent and self-employed workers who do not benefit from many federal and state labor protection regulations. Indeed, some evidence suggests that these workers should be the targets of selective interventions because of possible higher exposure to both physical and psychosocial hazards and weaker government protections, in addition to the inherent precariousness of such work arrangements (Benach et al., 2016). Recognizing these three types of interventions also raises the possibility that there are distinct challenges inherent in each type, and thus perhaps differences in how each of the three categories of interventions should be developed and implemented.

TARGETS FOR CHANGE

No matter what category of worker health intervention is mounted, there are strong benefits to using a social ecological approach to identifying potential targets for change. Such an approach identifies varying levels of influence on worker health. For example, Figure 23.2 shows that public policy,

FIGURE 23.2. Targets for Change With Intervention Examples

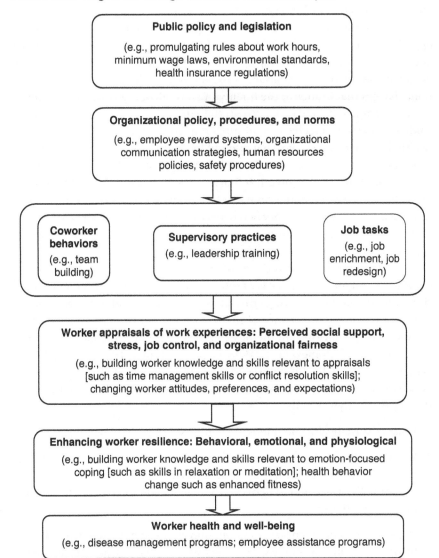

organizational policy and procedures, job tasks, and the behaviors of supervisors and coworkers all contribute to the experience of work. Thus, interventions at any of these levels may influence worker appraisals of stress,
social support, job control, and other work characteristics. The descending
flow (indicated by the arrows in Figure 23.2) suggests that higher level targets for change may constrain or otherwise influence lower level targets.
For example, minimum wage laws constrain organizational employee compensation policies. These policies, in turn, influence how supervisors conduct
performance reviews of employees. All of these factors may influence the
extent to which employees perceive that they are fairly compensated for

their work. Of course, employee expectations and attitudes also influence employee appraisals of fairness.

Historically, much research has investigated the link between employee appraisals of their work experiences and worker health, with little research addressing the linkages among specific organizational factors, supervisory behaviors, and worker appraisals. However, interest in identifying organizational factors that influence the quality of work life has grown tremendously (see, for example, Scholl et al., 2018). Nonetheless, there are still many more studies that assess perceived social support at work and its relation to worker health than there are studies that attempt to identify the organizational structures and policies or the supervisory behaviors that lead to worker perceptions of social support (Gilbreath & Benson, 2004; Härenstam, 2008). Because of the limited research in this arena, at this point, the extent to which organizational factors and supervisory behaviors that contribute to worker appraisals of social support or job control are specific to local context versus widely applicable across worksites is not known.

Several planning frameworks in public health intervention development suggest that targets for change for protection and prevention interventions be chosen based on the following criteria: (a) importance and prevalence of the health problem, (b) prevalence of the risk factors, (c) strength of association between the risk factors and the health problem, and (d) modifiability of the risk factors (Bartholomew et al., 1998; Green & Kreuter, 1999; Jeffery, 1989). When these public health criteria are applied to the development of worker health interventions, they translate into the following questions (adapted from Heaney & van Ryn, 1990):

1. What adverse health conditions are being experienced by workers?

2. What are the various physical, social, and organizational conditions that are potentially contributing to these adverse health conditions? What is the strength of association between these work conditions and the adverse health conditions?

3. Who is experiencing these conditions and appraising them as being harmful or potentially harmful (e.g., a few idiosyncratic individuals, an identifiable subgroup, or all workers)?

4. How modifiable are these conditions?

5. If exposure to these conditions cannot be reduced, what individual and social resources are effective buffers against the adverse effects of these conditions?

The questions that guide promotion interventions are somewhat different, focusing on the identification of positive conditions and experiences at work that contribute to worker well-being. However, the logic of identifying the assets, exploring which workers and how many workers are experiencing them, estimating the magnitude of their effect on well-being, and assessing their modifiability is the same as the logic of the traditional public health intervention frameworks. These procedures are not yet as well developed as those for identifying hazards and risks.

However, these questions are rarely systematically asked and answered during the planning of worker health interventions. Instead, the choice of what worker health interventions attempt to change has typically been determined more by philosophy, disciplinary assumptions, and perceived feasibility rather than critical assessment of empirical criteria. For example, occupational health and safety practitioners who are trained as engineers or safety science specialists tend to give priority to reducing exposure to hazards by engineering them out of the work process (Goldenhar & Schulte, 1994). Interventions addressing stress-related health problems have tended to emphasize enhancing worker resilience or changing worker appraisals (Murphy & Sauter, 2004). Interestingly, when asked about their preferences or expectations for intervention, workers seem to prefer interventions that target employee knowledge and skills or that target employee health behaviors more generally (Elo et al., 2008; Saksvik et al., 2002). These beliefs are very much aligned with the "fundamental attribution error" in social psychology (Ross & Nisbett, 1991) and the "context minimization error" in community psychology (Shinn & Toohey, 2003), which describe the tendency of observers to overestimate the importance of individual characteristics and underestimate the importance of situational or contextual factors when describing the causes of phenomena. Such information-processing biases may contribute to the continued overemphasis on individual-level targets for change in worker health interventions.

A social ecological perspective emphasizes the dynamic interplay among the parts of a system and suggests that sole reliance on any one target or level of intervention is unlikely to yield optimal results (Sallis et al., 2015). This perspective reminds us that the effectiveness of change at one level is likely to be dependent on the extent to which factors at the other levels are aligned with or facilitative of that change. For example, the quality of a supervisor's relationship with their boss has been shown to influence the extent to which the supervisor is able to have a positive impact on their employees' attitudes toward work (Tangirala et al., 2007). Indeed, managers have expressed reservations about engaging in worksite health interventions if they perceive that upper management is not willing to support or reward the effort (Härenstam et al., 2022). Thus, an intervention that plans for integrated change across numerous targets at multiple levels (e.g., employee, supervisor, work team, organization) will be most likely to effectively reduce health problems.

In addition, a social ecological perspective suggests that effective change at one level is likely to bring about changes at other levels. Sometimes, such changes are unintended, unexpected, and, in a worst-case scenario, unwanted. For example, it has been suggested that the implementation of autonomous work groups may result in changes in coworker relationships that undermine the availability of coworker support (Semmer, 2006). In addition, there is some evidence that worksite programs addressing personal health behaviors may increase stigma and discrimination against workers who do not enact the healthy behaviors (Powroznik, 2017).

A social ecological perspective also suggests the importance of identifying "high impact leverage points" (Stokols, 1996, p. 290) as targets for change. These leverage points are people, behaviors, roles, and environmental conditions that exert a disproportionately large influence on worker health and well-being. For example, Rasmussen et al. (2006) found that the elected safety representatives in a Danish manufacturing facility were tremendously central to the success of an intervention intended to reduce the incidence of eczema and traumatic injuries among workers. By involving these safety representatives in the planning of any production system changes and encouraging them to seek input from a broader base of employees, the intervention was successful at improving the safety climate in the facility and reducing the incidence of injuries and illness. Front-line supervisors can also be an important leverage point. If front-line supervisors increase their supportive exchanges with coworkers and subordinates, many employees stand to benefit in terms of enhanced well-being (Stein et al., 2020). Finally, opinion leaders may serve as high-impact leverage points because of their ability to bring about changes in others' attitudes and behaviors, and thus the identification and inclusion of opinion leaders is often a part of frameworks supporting worker health (see, for example, Safeer et al., 2021).

STRATEGIES FOR CHANGE

Although the model in Figure 23.2 shows a variety of potential targets for change, it provides little guidance in terms of identifying strategies for change. *Strategies for change* are the activities that change agents engage in or implement to bring about the desired intervention outcomes. Once a target for change has been identified, how does one go about effecting that change in as timely, appropriate, and cost-effective a manner as possible? What tactics should be used to reduce the likelihood of undesirable outcomes while optimizing desired change?

Most planning frameworks suggest that social science theories, intervention effectiveness research, program evaluation results, and knowledge gained from local needs and resource assessments should inform choices of tactics and strategies (Green & Kreuter, 1999; Kok et al., 2016). However, these criteria are not without controversy. For example, several systematic reviews of behavior change interventions that claim to be guided by behavior change theories have not concluded that these interventions are any more effective than interventions that are not guided by theory (see, for example, Cahill et al., 2010), and relevant scholars are publicly debating the usefulness of theory (Hagger & Weed, 2019). A growing literature addresses this issue by focusing on how theories are translated into intervention development and implementation (Michie et al., 2018), claiming that theory-based interventions have not been rigorously tested in part because they have not been rigorously developed. Through the development of integrated syntheses of various behavior change theories (Cane et al., 2012; Fishbein, 2009) and explicit linking of behavior change theory to mechanisms of action, intervention developers have better guidance for ensuring that their interventions are theory based and not just theory inspired (Michie et al., 2018).

Another controversy centers on the extent to which any particular intervention research study can inform subsequent interventions targeting different workers in various worksites. This has long been an issue in the organizational change literature, which often emphasizes the influence of the organizational context on the change process (Molinsky, 1999). Such contextualizing limits the ability of the intervention developer to apply the findings from one organization to another and strongly suggests that "off the shelf" programs are not likely to be effective if adopted without modification (Argyris, 1993; Colarelli, 1998). Perhaps because of the contextual nature of this work, organizational change research tends to be more idiographic than nomothetic (Quick, 1997).

The need to consider characteristics of workers in the development of interventions has a storied intellectual history in the person–environment fit literature (see, for example, Caplan, 1987). Recently, investigators have turned significant attention to the notion of fit between an intervention and the organization in which it is being developed and implemented (Nielsen & Randall, 2015). Using an array of qualitative research methods, strategies for better matching an intervention with the work culture and preferences of workers have been identified (see, for example, Peters et al., 2020).

Both of these controversies about the usefulness of theory and single-organization intervention research studies are likely to be settled through using both theory and intervention research results at an appropriate level of abstraction and accompanied by strategies for ensuring fit with both worker characteristics and preferences, as well as employer norms and worksite culture. In the following discussion, strategies for change are categorized as follows: (a) individual-level change strategies that focus on changing employees' beliefs, attitudes, and behaviors; and (b) organizational-level change strategies that focus on changing organizational structures, policies, priorities, and procedures.

Individual-Level Change

When attempting to change employee beliefs, attitudes, and behaviors, theories of social influence and social learning have been used to guide intervention development. The most commonly used theories include social cognitive theory (Bandura, 1986), the transtheoretical model of change (Prochaska et al., 2015), fear arousal theories (Tannenbaum et al., 2015), and the theory of reasoned action (Ajzen et al., 2007); as previously mentioned, there are several models for integrating these various theories. Although these theories place differing amounts of emphasis on cognitive, affective, and behavioral processes, they all aid in identifying the major explanatory factors that influence the target of change, and in some cases they also identify strategies for modifying the explanatory factors. For example, social cognitive theory (Bandura, 1986) places great emphasis on efficacy expectations (beliefs regarding one's ability to successfully carry out a course of action or perform a behavior) and outcome expectations (beliefs that the performance of a behavior will have desired effects or consequences) as explanatory factors for behavior. The theory further posits that both types of expectations can be influenced through observational and experiential learning (Bandura, 1986). Thus, to increase health care employees' compliance with universal precautions, an intervention might incorporate learning activities that allow employees to hear about or observe others' successful use of the desired procedures and to practice the procedures themselves in order to develop confidence in their ability to carry them out. Theories that have undergone rigorous testing and that have been applied in many different settings and with various target populations are the most useful for developing intervention strategies (Glanz et al., 2015).

Although psychological theories of learning and social influence have not been well integrated into a preponderance of worker health interventions, a few studies serve as useful examples of how worker health intervention strategies that are attempting individual-level change can be well guided by theory. For example, Pedersen et al. (2018) applied self-determination theory to an intervention to improve physical activity and related cardiovascular health indicators among postal workers. As another example, Greene et al. (2005) used concepts from social cognitive theory to guide the development and evaluation of an ergonomics training program for computer users. And Wright et al. (2019) used fear arousal theory to enhance compliance with the use of personal protective equipment among wastewater management workers.

Organizational-Level Change

Work and health researchers and practitioners have made less use of organizational change theory and its associated body of research than they have of theories describing individual-level change. Several factors may inhibit application of organizational change theory and research to worksite health programs. The idiographic nature of organizational change has already been mentioned. Methodologies focus on case studies and include more ethnographic approaches rather than experimental or epidemiological methods. Thus, the application of the findings in the literature tends to be in terms of "lessons learned" from diverse cases rather than empirically derived generalizations about effective change processes. Although these lessons can be instructive, they may be less compelling to intervention developers who have been steeped in positivist, experimental research traditions.

Another factor that hinders the use of the organizational change literature among worker health intervention developers is that the outcomes of interest for many published organizational change interventions revolve around the health of the organization (productivity, efficiency, profits) rather than the health of the employee. And although several conceptualizations of healthy organizations include the well-being of employees (DiFabio, 2017; Lawler et al., 1995; Pfeffer, 1998), much of the research does not examine health outcomes. Thus, the process of translating results from the organizational change literature to the field of worksite health is not straightforward.

In spite of these complexities and inconsistencies, various organizational change scholars have suggested strategies for maximizing the success of planned change efforts (Boonstra, 2004; Kotter, 1996), and several health policy investigators have contributed to this literature (Weiner, 2009; Weiner et al., 2008). There are striking similarities among the guidelines put forth by different authors. Their intellectual roots are firmly entrenched in Lewin's influential model for conceptualizing change (Lewin, 1951), which posited three stages to the change process: unfreezing the old behavior, moving to a new behavior, and then refreezing or stabilizing the new behavior. Building on this framework, organizational change theorists linked the stages to action steps that change agents should take to facilitate progress through the stages.

The *unfreezing stage* involves creating a readiness for change among members of the organization. This stage needs to address employee beliefs about the need for change, perhaps by disconfirming current conceptions of and stimulating dissatisfaction with the status quo (Cummings & Worley, 2001). Employee beliefs about the likelihood that change can be successfully accomplished should also be addressed in order to build a shared sense of collective capacity. According to Lewin's original theory, this stage involves conducting a "force field analysis" that identifies the major forces that both facilitate and hinder change. This process encourages organization members to think about why change has not already occurred and how the change process should be crafted in order to be optimally successful. Cummings and Worley (2001) suggested that this involves creating a vision for the planned change.

The *moving stage* centers on the development and implementation of an action plan to bring about the desired change. Such a plan should include developing political support for the change among the relevant stakeholders, identifying and accessing the needed resources, providing leadership and assigning responsibility for the change, modifying organizational structures and policies to support the change effort, and providing training and problem-solving assistance (Cummings, 2004; Kotter, 1996).

The *refreezing stage* involves sustaining the momentum of the change effort and institutionalizing the change. This is a particularly important stage if the change effort has been initiated or managed by researchers or experts from outside the organization who will leave once the change effort has been implemented. Strategies associated with this stage include reinforcing changes by making rewards contingent on compliance with them, socializing newcomers into the organizational culture that informed the change effort, and disseminating the change more broadly throughout the organization in order to normalize it (Cummings, 2004).

CONCLUSION

The social ecological perspective (Sallis et al., 2015) and the systems science approach (Green, 2006) strongly suggest that worksite interventions incorporate multiple targets of change at various levels of influence. Multilevel studies across multiple organizations will help identify organizational structures and practices that consistently influence employee perceptions of stress, social support, control, organizational justice, and organizational commitment to employees' health and well-being. In addition, well-documented local efforts are needed to ascertain these linkages within specific organizations. Such activity will support the inclusion of a broader array of targets for change for worksite health programs.

Thus, it is important to move past an either/or framing of the choice of targets for change. Worksite health interventions that incorporate change at multiple levels provide the opportunity for organizational structures and processes to reinforce adaptive employee norms and facilitate healthy behaviors, as well as for individual behaviors to support and augment the effects of the implementation and institutionalization of organizational processes that increase exposure to positive aspects of work, reduce exposure to hazards, and enhance healthy decision making.

The *Total Worker Health®* program at the National Institute for Occupational Safety and Health in the United States is an exemplar of an effort to take a holistic view of worker health, integrating disciplinary perspectives in the service of optimizing the effectiveness of worker health interventions. Not only does the *Total Worker Health* program recognize the importance of and integrate efforts to improve workplace physical and chemical conditions, psychosocial aspects of work, and personal health behaviors, but it also broadens the focus of worker health to include aspects of the home and community (Punnett et al., 2020). This is an important innovation as the interface between work and nonwork becomes more porous due to technology and nontraditional work arrangements. There is growing recognition of the potential interplay between worksites and the communities in which they are located, as well as the communities in which workers reside (Baron et al., 2019).

With a few notable exceptions, the worker health intervention literature continues to provide minimal attention to issues of strategy. Published accounts of interventions rarely provide detailed descriptions of the program activities and change processes, nor do they explicate the basis for decisions about strategies for change. It is even more rare for intervention research to formally compare the effectiveness of various strategies for bringing about targeted changes. For example, no published studies have compared the implementation and effectiveness of worksite health interventions that incorporate employee participation in the change process with interventions that are guided solely by outside experts. Such studies would be difficult to design and implement, but they could potentially provide some definitive answers to long-standing questions about how to optimize worker health interventions.

Only with more systematic attention to the development and implementation phases of intervention research (Goldenhar et al., 2001) will we be able to maximize the effectiveness of worker health interventions. The NIOSH (2020) *Total Worker Health* program suggests that this can be accomplished through "policies, programs, and practices that integrate protection from work-related safety and health hazards with promotion of injury and illness prevention efforts to advance worker well-being."

REFERENCES

Ajzen, I., Albarracin, D., & Hornik, R. (Eds.). (2007). *Prediction and change of health behavior: Applying the reasoned action approach*. Erlbaum. https://doi.org/10.4324/9780203937082

Argyris, C. (1993). *Knowledge for action: A guide to overcoming barriers to organizational change*. Jossey-Bass.

Bandura, A. (1986). *Social foundations of thought and action*. Prentice Hall.

Baron, S., Tsui, E. K., Cuervo, I., & Islam, N. (2019). Community health programs: Promising practices and opportunities for expanding Total Worker Health®. In H. L. Hudson, J. A. S. Nigam, S. L. Sauter, L. C. Chosewood, A. L. Schill, & J. Howard (Eds.), *Total Worker Health* (pp. 193–208). American Psychological Association. https://doi.org/10.1037/0000149-012

Bartholomew, L. K., Parcel, G. S., & Kok, G. (1998). Intervention mapping: A process for developing theory and evidence-based health education programs. *Health Education & Behavior, 25*(5), 545–563. https://doi.org/10.1177/109019819802500502

Benach, J., Vives, A., Tarafa, G., Delclos, C., & Muntaner, C. (2016). What should we know about precarious employment and health in 2025? Framing the agenda for the next decade of research. *International Journal of Epidemiology, 45*(1), 232–238. https://doi.org/10.1093/ije/dyv342

Boonstra, J. J. (Ed.). (2004). *Dynamics of organizational change and learning*. John Wiley & Sons. https://doi.org/10.1002/9780470753408

Buchanan, D., Fitzgerald, L., Ketley, D., Gollop, R., Jones, J. L., Lamont, S. S., Neath, A., & Whitby, E. (2005). No going back: A review of the literature on sustaining organizational change. *International Journal of Management Reviews, 7*(3), 189–205. https://doi.org/10.1111/j.1468-2370.2005.00111.x

Bureau of Labor Statistics. (2021) *Labor force statistics from the Current Population Survey*. U.S. Department of Labor. https://www.bls.gov/cps/lfcharacteristics.htm

Cahill, K., Lancaster, T., & Green, N. (2010). Stage-based interventions for smoking cessation. *Cochrane Database of Systematic Reviews, 11*(11), CD004492. https://doi.org/10.1002/14651858.CD004492.pub4

Cane, J., O'Connor, D., & Michie, S. (2012). Validation of the theoretical domains framework for use in behaviour change and implementation research. *Implementation Science, 7*(1), 37. https://doi.org/10.1186/1748-5908-7-37

Caplan, R. (1987). Person–environment fit theory and organizations: Commensurate dimensions, time perspectives, and mechanisms. *Journal of Vocational Behavior, 31*(3), 248–267. https://doi.org/10.1016/0001-8791(87)90042-X

Chari, R., Chang, C. C., Sauter, S. L., Petrun Sayers, E. L., Cerully, J. L., Schulte, P., Schill, A. L., & Uscher-Pines, L. (2018). Expanding the paradigm of occupational safety and health: A new framework for worker well-being. *Journal of Occupational and Environmental Medicine, 60*(7), 589–593. https://doi.org/10.1097/JOM.0000000000001330

Colarelli, S. M. (1998). Psychological interventions in organizations: An evolutionary perspective. *American Psychologist, 53*(9), 1044–1056. https://doi.org/10.1037/0003-066X.53.9.1044

Cummings, T. (2004). Organizational development and change: Foundations and applications. In J. J. Boonstra (Ed.), *Dynamics of organizational change and learning* (pp. 25–42). John Wiley & Sons. https://doi.org/10.1002/9780470753408.ch2

Cummings, T., & Worley, C. (2001). *Organizational development and change* (7th ed.). Southwestern College Publishing.

Di Fabio, A. (2017). Positive healthy organizations: Promoting well-being, meaningfulness, and sustainability in organizations. *Frontiers in Psychology, 8*, 1938. https://doi.org/10.3389/fpsyg.2017.01938

Elo, A.-L., Ervasti, J., Kuosma, E., & Mattila, P. (2008). Evaluation of an organizational stress management program in a municipal public works organization. *Journal of Occupational Health Psychology, 13*(1), 10–23. https://doi.org/10.1037/1076-8998.13.1.10

Fishbein, M. (2009). An integrative model for behavioral prediction and its application to health promotion. In R. J. DiClemente, R. A. Crosby, & M. C. Kegler (Eds.), *Emerging theories in health promotion practice and research* (pp. 215–234). Jossey-Bass/Wiley.

Fjeldsoe, B., Neuhaus, M., Winkler, E., & Eakin, E. (2011). Systematic review of maintenance of behavior change following physical activity and dietary interventions. *Health Psychology, 30*(1), 99–109. https://doi.org/10.1037/a0021974

Gilbreath, B., & Benson, P. G. (2004). The contribution of supervisor behaviour to employee psychological well-being. *Work and Stress, 18*(3), 255–266. https://doi.org/10.1080/02678370412331317499

Glanz, K., Rimer, B. K., & Viswanath, K. (Eds.). (2015). *Health behavior: Theory, research, and practice* (5th ed.). Jossey-Bass.

Goldenhar, L. M., LaMontagne, A. D., Katz, T., Heaney, C. A., & Landsbergis, P. (2001). The intervention research process in occupational safety and health: An overview from the National Occupational Research Agenda Intervention Effectiveness Research team. *Journal of Occupational and Environmental Medicine, 43*, 616–622. https://doi.org/10.1097/00043764-200107000-00008

Goldenhar, L. M., & Schulte, P. A. (1994). Intervention research in occupational health and safety. *Journal of Occupational Medicine, 36*(7), 763–775. https://pubmed.ncbi.nlm.nih.gov/7931743/

Green, L. W. (2006). Public health asks of systems science: To advance our evidence-based practice, can you help us get more practice-based evidence? *American Journal of Public Health, 96*(3), 406–409. https://doi.org/10.2105/AJPH.2005.066035

Green, L. W., & Kreuter, M. W. (1999). *Health promotion planning: An educational and ecological approach* (3rd ed.). Mayfield.

Greene, B. L., DeJoy, D. M., & Olejnik, S. (2005). Effects of an active ergonomics training program on risk exposure, worker beliefs, and symptoms in computer users. *Work, 24*(1), 41–52. https://pubmed.ncbi.nlm.nih.gov/15706071/

Hagger, M. S., & Weed, M. (2019). Debate: Do interventions based on behavioral theory work in the real world? *International Journal of Behavioral Nutrition and Physical Activity 16*(1), 36. https://doi.org/10.1186/s12966-019-0795-4

Härenstam, A. (2008). Organizational approach to studies of job demands, control and health. *Scandinavian Journal of Work, Environment and Health*, (Suppl. 6), 144–149. https://www.researchgate.net/publication/41464069_Organizational_approach_to_studies_of_job_demands_control_and_health

Härenstam, A., Pousette, A., & Berntson, E. (2022). Improving organizational and working conditions for managers in the Swedish public sector: A conceptual model and evaluation of interventions. *Economic and Industrial Democracy, 43*(1), 72–97. https://doi.org/10.1177/0143831X19883017

Heaney, C. A., & van Ryn, M. (1990). Broadening the scope of worksite stress programs: A guiding framework. *American Journal of Health Promotion, 4*(6), 413–420. https://doi.org/10.4278/0890-1171-4.6.413

Ingram, M., Wolf, A. M. A., Lopez-Galvez, N. I., Griffin, S. C, & Beamer, P. I. (2021). Proposing a social ecological approach to address disparities in occupational exposures and health for low-wage and minority workers employed in small businesses. *Journal of Exposure Science & Environmental Epidemiology, 31*(3), 404–411. https://doi.org/ 10.1038/s41370-021-00317-5.

Jeffery, R. W. (1989). Risk behaviors and health: Contrasting individual and population perspectives. *American Psychologist, 44*(9), 1194–1202. https://doi.org/10.1037/ 0003-066X.44.9.1194

Kok, G., Gottlieb, N. H., Peters, G.-J. Y., Mullen, P. D., Parcel, G. S., Ruiter, R. A. C., Fernández, M. E., Markham, C., & Bartholomew, L. K. (2016). A taxonomy of behavior change methods: An intervention mapping approach. *Health Psychology Review, 10*(3), 297–312. https://doi.org/10.1080/17437199.2015.1077155

Kotter, J. P. (1996). *Leading change.* Harvard Business School Press.

Lawler, E. E., Mohrman, S. A., & Ledford, G. E., Jr. (1995). *Creating high performance organizations.* Jossey-Bass.

Lewin, K. (1951). Field theory and learning. In D. Cartwright (Ed.), *Field theory in social science: Select theoretical papers* (pp. 60–86). Harper-Collins.

Michie, S., Carey, R. N., Johnston, M., Rothman, A. J., de Bruin, M., Kelly, M. P., & Connell, L. E. (2018). From theory-inspired to theory-based interventions: A protocol for developing and testing a methodology for linking behaviour change techniques to theoretical mechanisms of action. *Annals of Behavioral Medicine, 52*(6), 501–512. https://doi.org/10.1007/s12160-016-9816-6

Molinsky, A. L. (1999). Sanding down the edges: Paradoxical impediments to organizational change. *The Journal of Applied Behavioral Science, 35*(1), 8–24. https://doi.org/ 10.1177/0021886399351002

Murphy, L., & Sauter, S. (2004). Work organization interventions: State of knowledge and future directions. *Sozial- und Präventivmedizin, 49,* 79–86. https://doi.org/ 10.1007/s00038-004-3085-z

National Institute of Occupational Safety and Health. (2020). NIOSH *Total Worker Health® program.* Centers for Disease Control and Prevention. https://www.cdc.gov/ NIOSH/twh/

National Research Council and Institute of Medicine. (2009). Preventing mental, emotional, and behavioral disorders among young people: Progress and possibilities. Committee on the Prevention of Mental Disorders and Substance Abuse Among Children, Youth, and Young Adults: Research Advances and Promising Interventions. In M. E. O'Connell, T. Boat, & K. E. Warner (Eds.), *Board on Children, Youth, and Families, Division of Behavioral and Social Sciences and Education.* The National Academies Press.

Nielsen, K., & Randall, R. (2015). Assessing and addressing the fit of planned interventions to the organizational context. In M. Karanika-Murray & C. Biron (Eds.), *Derailed organizational interventions for stress and well-being* (107–113). Springer Dordrecht. https://doi.org/10.1007/978-94-017-9867-9_12

Pedersen, C., Halvari, H., & Williams, G. C. (2018). Worksite intervention effects on motivation, physical activity, and health: A cluster randomized controlled trial. *Psychology of Sport and Exercise, 35,* 171–180. https://doi.org/10.1016/j.psychsport.2017.11.004

Peters, S. E., Nielsen, K. M., Nagler, E. M., Revette, A. C., Madden, J., & Sorensen, G. (2020). Ensuring organization-intervention fit for a participatory organizational intervention to improve food service workers' health and wellbeing: Workplace organizational health study. *Journal of Occupational and Environmental Medicine, 62*(2), e33–e45. https://doi.org/10.1097/JOM.0000000000001792

Pfeffer, J. (1998). *The human equation: Building profits by putting people first.* Harvard Business School Press.

Powroznik, K. M. (2017). Healthism and weight-based discrimination: The unintended consequences of health promotion in the workplace. *Work and Occupations, 44*(2), 139–170. https://doi.org/10.1177/0730888416682576

Prochaska, J. O., Redding, C. A., & Evers, K. E. (2015). The transtheoretical model and stages of change. In K. Glanz, B. K. Rimer, & K. Viswanath (Eds.), *Health behavior: Theory, research and practice* (5th ed., pp. 125–148). Jossey-Bass.

Punnett, L., Cavallari, J. M., Henning, R. A., Nobrega, S., Dugan, A. G., & Cherniack, M. G. (2020). Defining 'integration' for Total Worker Health®: A new proposal. *Annals of Work Exposures and Health, 64*(3), 223–235. https://doi.org/10.1093/annweh/wxaa003

Quick, J. C. (1997). Idiographic research in organizational behavior. In C. L. Cooper (Ed.), *Creating tomorrow's organizations: A handbook for future research in organizational behavior* (pp. 475–492). John Wiley & Sons.

Rasmussen, K., Glasscock, D. J., Hansen, O. N., Carstensen, O., Jepsen, J. F., & Nielsen, K. J. (2006). Worker participation in change processes in a Danish industrial setting. *American Journal of Industrial Medicine, 49*(9), 767–779. https://doi.org/10.1002/ajim.20350

Ross, L., & Nisbett, R. (1991). *The person and the situation: Perspectives in social psychology*. McGraw Hill.

Safeer, R. S., Lucik, M. M., & Christel, K. C. (2021). Using the CDC Worksite Health Scorecard to promote organizational change. *American Journal of Health Promotion, 35*(7), 997–1001. https://doi.org/10.1177/08901171211012948

Saksvik, P. O., Nytrø, K., Dahl-Jørgensen, C., & Mikkelsen, A. (2002). A process evaluation of individual and organizational occupational stress and health interventions. *Work and Stress, 16*(1), 37–57. https://doi.org/10.1080/02678370110118744

Sallis, J. F., Owen, N., & Fisher, E. B. (2015). Ecological models of health behavior. In K. Glanz, B. K. Rimer, & K. Viswanath (Eds.), *Health behavior: Theory, research and practice* (5th ed., pp. 443–464). Jossey-Bass.

Sauter, S. L., & Murphy, L. R. (2004). Work organization interventions: State of knowledge and future directions. *Sozial- und Präventivmedizin, 49*(2), 79–86. https://doi.org/10.1007/s00038-004-3085-z

Scholl, I., LaRussa, A., Hahlweg, P., Kobrin, S., & Elwyn, G. (2018). Organizational- and system-level characteristics that influence implementation of shared decision-making and strategies to address them—A scoping review. *Implementation Science, 13*(1), 40. Advance online publication. https://doi.org/10.1186/s13012-018-0731-z

Seligman, M. (2018). PERMA and the building blocks of well-being. *The Journal of Positive Psychology, 13*(4), 333–335. https://doi.org/10.1080/17439760.2018.1437466

Semmer, N. K. (2006). Job stress interventions and the organization of work. *Scandinavian Journal of Work, Environment & Health, 32*(6), 515–527. https://doi.org/10.5271/sjweh.1056

Shinn, M., & Toohey, S. M. (2003). Community contexts of human welfare. *Annual Review of Psychology, 54*(1), 427–459. https://doi.org/10.1146/annurev.psych.54.101601.145052

Sorensen, G., McLellan, D., Dennerlein, J. T., Pronk, N. P., Allen, J. D., Boden, L. I., Okechukwu, C. A., Hashimoto, D., Stoddard, A., & Wagner, G. R. (2013). Integration of health protection and health promotion: Rationale, indicators, and metrics. *Journal of Occupational and Environmental Medicine, 55*(Suppl. 12), S12–S18. https://doi.org/10.1097/JOM.0000000000000032

Stein, M., Vincent-Höper, S., & Gregersen, S. (2020). Why busy leaders may have exhausted followers: A multilevel perspective on supportive leadership. *Leadership and Organization Development Journal, 41*(6), 829–845. https://doi.org/10.1108/LODJ-11-2019-0477

Stokols, D. (1996). Translating social ecological theory into guidelines for community health promotion. *American Journal of Health Promotion, 10*(4), 282–298. https://doi.org/10.4278/0890-1171-10.4.282

Tangirala, S., Green, S. G., & Ramanujam, R. (2007). In the shadow of the boss's boss: Effects of supervisors' upward exchange relationships on employees. *Journal of Applied Psychology, 92*(2), 309–320. https://doi.org/10.1037/0021-9010.92.2.309

Tannenbaum, M. B., Hepler, J., Zimmerman, R. S., Saul, L., Jacobs, S., Wilson, K., & Albarracín, D. (2015). Appealing to fear: A meta-analysis of fear appeal effectiveness and theories. *Psychological Bulletin, 141*(6), 1178–1204. https://doi.org/10.1037/a0039729

Weiner, B. J. (2009). A theory of organizational readiness for change. *Implementation Science, 4*(1), 67. https://doi.org/10.1186/1748-5908-4-67

Weiner, B. J., Lewis, M. A., & Linnan, L. A. (2008). Using organization theory to understand the determinants of effective implementation of worksite health promotion programs. *Health Education Research, 24*(2), 292–305. https://doi.org/10.1093/her/cyn019

World Health Organization. (1946). *Constitution.* Retrieved January 5, 2023, from https://www.who.int/about/governance/constitution

Wright, T., Adhikari, A., Yin, J., Vogel, R., Smallwood, S., & Shah, G. (2019). Issue of compliance with use of personal protective equipment among wastewater workers across the southeast region of the United States. *International Journal of Environmental Research and Public Health, 16*(11), 2009. https://doi.org/10.3390/ijerph16112009

Zaninotto, P., & Steptoe, A. (2019). Association between subjective well-being and living longer without disability or illness. *JAMA Network Open, 2*(7), e196870. https://doi.org/10.1001/jamanetworkopen.2019.6870

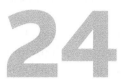

Employee Assistance Programs

Strengths, Challenges, and Future Roles

Zofia Bajorek, Andrew Kinder, and Cary L. Cooper

This chapter discusses organization-wide approaches to support employees and reviews these from a U.K. point of view, especially as there have been some noteworthy developments within this geographical area. Over the last 2 decades, there has been an increase in organizational research and policy about the role of "well-being" and the implications that workplace well-being can have on employee and organizational outcomes. This research is outlined in this chapter prior to introducing the important role of employee assistance programs (EAPs). EAPs are designed to help the employer assist employees in terms of work performance issues as well as personal problems that may occur, including emotional, practical, or familial issues. Winwood and Beer (2008) provided some history on how EAPs have developed, as well as the different types that occur. More recently, EAPs have expanded significantly in their digital offerings, which have increased their potential for accessibility in addition to their coverage and reach.

Sickness absence rates have been increasing, and we do not yet understand the true impact that the pandemic has had on the health and well-being of the working age population and organizational sickness absence levels. Although some sickness absence from work is unavoidable, it is generally agreed that creating the right conditions at work can improve employee health and well-being and improve sickness absence levels. When sickness absence becomes unduly prolonged, it becomes more difficult for employees to return to work;

https://doi.org/10.1037/0000331-024
Handbook of Occupational Health Psychology, Third Edition, L. E. Tetrick, G. G. Fisher, M. T. Ford, and J. C. Quick (Editors)

it can also become damaging to the employee, the organization, and to the wider society.

As a result, policy makers in the field have taken steps to make workplace health and well-being a priority and encourage employers to optimize the health of their workforce. In 2008, Black wrote a seminal report in which evidence clearly demonstrated the link between good employee health and positive business outcomes and showed that improving employee health and well-being could generate both organizational and government cost savings. It is now not contentious to assert that a healthy workforce is more innovative, resourceful, and productive than an unhealthy one. The Black report also recognized the need for more robust business models that could effectively measure and analyze the benefits of any well-being interventions that were integrated so that business cases could be made for implementing further practices in the future. This was echoed by Bajorek et al. (2014), who argued that despite an increase in the understanding about the importance of health and well-being in the workplace, organizations still face a number of barriers when introducing health and well-being programs, which do need to be overcome if any initiatives are to have their intended outcomes.

Taylor et al. (2017) put workplace well-being into the policy and public agenda once again. The report emphasized the findings of the Waddell and Burton (2006) review: that "good quality work" has positive implications for both organizational productivity and health outcomes, but employers still had to take a number of steps to reach fair and decent work, including further progress in the health and well-being agenda. The Taylor review found that "we need to develop a more proactive approach to workplace health" (p. 9) and that "better quality work is healthier work" (p. 98).

But what is the evidence that organizations are putting this knowledge into practice? A report by Farmer and Stevenson (2017), which focused specifically on mental health in the workplace, suggested that organizations still need to "pull their socks up" when it comes to mental health, and more work needs to be done to further prioritize this issue. The report found that around 15% of people at work have some symptoms of existing mental health conditions, and there was evidence to suggest that having a mental health condition could hamper upward progression in the workplace. The report noted that people living with mental health conditions at work were more likely to lose their jobs, with 300,000 people with long-term health conditions leaving the workplace each year—much higher than those who work with physical impairments. Mental health stigma is still an obstacle to disclosure and seeking support, with only 11% of surveyed employees feeling comfortable with discussing a recent mental health problem with their line manager.

The report found that the cost of poor mental health at work for employers was estimated to be between £33 billion and £42 billion. Over half of these costs resulted from presenteeism, with additional costs coming from turnover and sickness absence. Farmer and Stevenson (2017) made a number of practical recommendations to help outline changes to mental health management at work and set a vision about the future of mental health and well-being in the workplace. The authors suggested required workplace modifications, including employees in all types of occupations having access to good quality work, and all employees having the knowledge of and the confidence to use the tools available to support their mental health at work and the mental health of those around them. Importantly, organizations should provide tools to (a) prevent employees' mental ill-health caused or worsened by work, (b) make employees aware of how they can access timely help in an attempt to reduce sickness absence caused by mental ill-health, and (c) support individuals to help them thrive at work.

Employee mental health has been a frequent topic of discussion, especially as a result of the COVID-19 pandemic and resultant lockdowns. Alongside any logistical and operational challenges that the pandemic presented for organizations and employees, workers also had to adjust to a number of changes, including balancing work and home lives (which may have involved homeschooling and/or elder caring responsibilities), isolation from work colleagues, and becoming acclimated to new working conditions and communication channels with the need to remain productive amid all this uncertainty and the fear of becoming ill. These challenges posed a risk to individuals' physical and emotional well-being.

Bajorek et al. (2020) undertook a survey to understand the initial lockdowns' effects on employee health and well-being. A large majority of survey respondents had begun working from home as a result of the pandemic (71%), and those new to working from home reported significantly poorer emotional health compared with individuals who had been working from home regularly pre-pandemic. This could have been because working from home was enforced and not a choice. Employees may have struggled to adjust to their new working conditions, for example, a lack of routine, coping mechanisms, and communication channels necessary to work from home effectively. The level of social isolation that employees experienced was one of the main issues reported. Employees who had increased weekly contact with organizational colleagues reported higher levels of organizational commitment and job satisfaction, indicating how important social connectedness at work is for mental health and well-being. Managers and employers should be aware of these changes in emotional well-being; especially as the future of the workplace and employees' return to the workplace continues to be uncertain, organization leaders should consider how any health and well-being policies and practices may need to be adapted in the future. The widescale issue is how mental health and well-being at work can be effectively managed now and in the post-pandemic environment.

LEVELS OF INTERVENTION

By helping employees cope with stress and mental and physical well-being in the work environment, organizations also hope to reduce absenteeism, improve staff morale, and consequently boost overall organizational productivity (Highley & Cooper, 1994). Investment in early prevention and pointing to sources or services of help has been found to make good business sense. Dewe (1994) described an explosion of interest in well-being services and noted that these interventions could be introduced at a number of levels.

These levels can be understood by grouping them from primary through to secondary and then tertiary. *Primary prevention* is concerned with taking action to reduce or eliminate stressors (i.e., sources of stress) and to promote a supportive and healthy work environment. *Secondary prevention* is concerned with the prompt detection and management of mental concerns such as depression and anxiety by increasing individual and collective awareness of stress and improving stress-management skills. *Tertiary prevention* involves the rehabilitation and recovery process of those individuals who have suffered, or are suffering from, mental or physical ill-health as a result of stress.

Primary Prevention

The most effective way of tackling stress and improving well-being is to eliminate it at its source. This may involve changes in personnel policies, such as improving communications systems, redesigning jobs, or allowing more decision making and autonomy at lower levels. Primary prevention is a main factor of "good work." Waddell and Burton (2006) concluded that "work is generally good for physical and mental health and wellbeing . . . the provisos are that account must be taken for the nature and the quality of work and its social context; jobs should be safe and accommodating" (p. ix). Parker and Bevan (2011) identified other elements that make the workplace inherently "good," including (a) balance between the effort expended at work and the rewards gained; (b) management support and the extent to which any decisions made are fair and just; (c) employees having a "voice" at work; (d) employees' level of social support and social interaction at work; (e) having control, autonomy, and discretion in work roles; (f) skill development and skill utilization; and (g) job security.

Secondary Prevention

Initiatives that fall into the category of secondary prevention generally focus on training and education and involve awareness-raising activities and skills training programs (Biron et al., 2009), which serve a useful function in helping individuals as well as their line managers to recognize the symptoms of mental ill-health in themselves and others and to extend or develop their coping skills. The form and content of this kind of training can vary immensely but often includes simple relaxation techniques, lifestyle advice and planning, as well as basic training in time management, assertiveness, and problem-solving skills.

Tertiary Prevention

One of the main aspects of tertiary prevention that organizations can consider in assisting with the recovery and rehabilitation of mental ill-health and well-being is workplace counseling. In this approach, organizations provide access to confidential professional counseling services for employees who are experiencing problems in the workplace or in personal settings. An EAP is a development of workplace-based professional counseling. EAPs can be in-house or (more commonly) delivered through an expert external agency or contractor. An EAP provides counseling, information, and/or referral to appropriate internal or external counseling treatment and support services for employees.

DEFINING AND DESCRIBING AN EAP

EAP history has been associated with attempts during the 19th and 20th centuries to deal with alcohol abuse in U.S. workplaces. However, EAPs have since evolved to help employees adjust to a range of personal and psychological situations that are caused by or worsened by work, to benefit organizational productivity. Berridge et al. (1997) defined an EAP as a systematic, organized, and ongoing provision of counseling, advice, and assistance, provided or funded by the employer, designed to help employees and (in most cases) their families with problems arising from work-related and external sources.

The U.K. Employee Assistance Professionals Association (EAPA; 2012) defined EAPs as

> a set of professional services specifically designed to improve and/or maintain the productivity and healthy functioning of the workplace, and to address a work organisation's particular business needs through the application of specialised knowledge and expertise about human behaviour and mental health. More specifically, as EAP is a workplace programme designed to assist: (1) work organisations in addressing productivity issues, and (2) "employee clients" in identifying and resolving personal concerns, including health, marital, family, financial, alcohol, drug, legal, emotional stress, or other personal issues that may affect job performance. (p. 6)

In Britain and Europe more widely, EAPs tend to have two primary objectives: (a) to help the employees distracted by a range of personal concerns, including (but not limited to) emotional, stress, relationship, family, alcohol, drug, financial, legal, and other problems to cope with such concerns and learn to control the stresses produced; and (b) to assist the organization in the identification and amelioration of productivity issues in employees whose job performance is adversely affected by such personal concerns (UK EAPA, 2012). An EAP can also generate benefits at the organizational level because "being more or less deeply embedded into the organizational processes of the firm, it becomes part of organizational discourse, it reflects and nourishes the organizational culture, and it becomes part of the organizational learning, problem-solving and adaptation mechanisms" (Berridge & Cooper, 1994, p. 5). EAPs can keep organizations operating efficiently and competitively by helping employees tackle complex issues and retain high levels of performance. Carchietta (2015) reported that at any given time, 20% of employees can have personal problems that may influence their work role. If employees are encouraged or choose to access an EAP before a problem worsens, then organizations may be able to mitigate any costs of any long-term or short-term sickness absence.

Others have defined EAPs as an organizational risk management tool (Compton & McManus, 2015). Through providing an early counseling intervention to employees who may have mental ill-health, there is then a greater chance that problems experienced by employees can be avoided or reduced. Kirk and Brown (2003) highlighted that EAPs are now frequently offered to employees as an "employee benefit" and regarded as evidence of organizations' duty of care.

The essential components of an EAP should reflect the provider's and the employer's preferred methods of implementing assistance, the resources available to the organization, the needs of its employees, as well as the size and the configuration of the organization (Davis & Gibson, 1994; Lee & Gray, 1994). Berridge et al. (1997) provided the following list featuring many of the essential elements that distinguish the EAP by its integrated approach and its systematic design, meshing with the administrative and social systems of the organization and its environment:

- a systematic survey of the organization to determine the nature, causes, and extent of problems perceived by individuals, also taking into account the viewpoints of all stakeholders and functional specialists in the organization;

- a continuing commitment on the part of the employing organization at the top level to provide counseling, advisory, and assistance services to "troubled" employees on a no-blame and no-cost, totally confidential basis;

- an effective program of promotion and publicity of the EAP to all employees as potential clients, emphasizing in particular its confidentiality, access, and scope in issues covered;

- a linked program of education and training on the goals and methods of the EAP for all staff members in terms of the definition of "troubled employees"; the individual's responsibility for well-being; the roles of managers, supervisors, and shop stewards within the design and implementation of the EAP; and the duties and capabilities of counselors, including any limitations on their activities;

- a procedure for contact with the EAP and referral to counseling, details of procedures for self-referral, and (if appropriate) managerial referral;

- a definition of problem-assessment procedures, including diagnosis routes, confidentiality guarantees, timeliness, scope of counselors' training, as well as their accreditation, competencies, and organizational knowledge;

- a protocol outlining the extent of short-term counseling and longer-term treatment and assistance;

- a statement of the macro- and micro-linkages with other services in the community, or with specialist resources or support mechanisms;

- a procedure for the follow-up and monitoring of employees subsequent to their use of the EAP service, with the necessary provisions for their appropriate use and deployment;

- an administrative channel for the feedback of aggregated statistics on the age and short- and longer-term outcomes of the EAP, provided by the contractor; and

- an evaluation procedure of individual and corporate benefits of the EAP on the most impartial basis that is practical.

EAPs can also vary in scope: Some cover an employee's family and a broader range of issues (including those extrinsic to work, including financial well-being, legal concerns, bereavement, retirement, domestic violence), while others focus solely on issues that have an effect on work performance (e.g., mental ill-health, unacceptable/bullying behaviors at work). Some may also provide trauma counseling, and specialized training for line managers. EAPs may also vary in terms of whether an organization decides on internal or external service provision. According to Newton et al. (2005), some advantages of an internal EAP could include a recognition and understanding of organizational needs. The service can also be monitored to ensure that maximum provisions are being offered to employees. However, external EAPs may portray greater confidentiality and independence of service provision. Due to the increase in EAP providers, Cekiso and Terblanche (2015) commented that any EAP service must now be seen as flexible in complex and changing environments, and must be refined or tailored to meet an organization's demands.

Trauma therapy is an important component of an EAP for those organizations where posttraumatic stress disorder is a potential hazard that needs to be mitigated. Ørner (2012) charted how psychological trauma has been managed within organizations, tracing its origins to World War II. This approach was then adapted to organizations involved in law enforcement and emergency services where first responders deal with psychological trauma on a daily basis. Mitchell (1983) was an early proponent of psychological debriefing, and there has been a long debate about the effectiveness of such early interventions ever since (see Rick & Briner, 2012; Rick et al., 2006; Rose & Bisson, 1998; Wessley, 2001). Within the United Kingdom, the National Institute for Health and Care Excellence concluded that psychological debriefing should not be carried out, but instead called for active monitoring and trained peer supporters to be involved in the aftermath of a trauma within an organization (NICE, 2018).

Organizations have responded to this in different ways; for instance, the U.K. College of Policing outlined a culturally tailored posttrauma intervention called the Emergency Services Trauma Intervention Programme (College of Policing, 2018), and within workplaces where there is a high potential risk of traumatic incidents occurring, Trauma Risk Management (TRiM) has been implemented (Brooks et al., 2019). Active monitoring (sometimes referred to as "watchful waiting") of those employees continues to be an important aspect of any trauma response, and for those individuals who are not recovering over the active monitoring period and may have chronic or complex post-traumatic stress symptoms, the EAP must have available effective treatments, such as trauma-focused cognitive behavior therapy and eye-movement desensitization and reprocessing (Wilson et al., 2018). Regardless of the direction of this debate, it is clear that EAPs need to have a clear evidence-based approach to psychological trauma within organizations so that employers can inform, educate, and effectively plan effective interventions with their clients.

ASSESSMENT OF THE EFFECTIVENESS OF EAPs

EAPs are being introduced more frequently into organizations as a health and well-being staff benefit and also with the hope of improving employee productivity. Consequently, their effectiveness should be explored more fully: what evidence is there in terms of their effectiveness, and what do these effectiveness studies actually measure?

Kirk and Brown (2003) argued that a clear and decided definition of EAPs is nonexistent and a plethora of intervention types have been subsumed under this label. This makes it extremely difficult, if not impossible, to rigorously evaluate the effectiveness of EAPs because the form and content of interventions can vary dramatically. Kirk and Brown observed that it is common for evaluations to report high levels of employee satisfaction with EAP services. Although this is important information, it is of limited use in terms of any objective assessment of their value.

Effectiveness studies frequently include satisfaction as a criterion variable (Arthur, 2000). Typically, employee satisfaction with EAP interventions has been found to be quite high, and counselor satisfaction is (perhaps not surprisingly) also high (Harlow, 1998). For example, Macdonald and his colleagues reported that over 90% of employees at a Canadian transportation company indicated high levels of satisfaction with the EAP services provided, and 69% said that these services had a positive effect on their overall quality of life. With respect to job performance, 46% of employees reported some or great improvement in their own job performance. Reports from counselors in the program also suggested a favorable reaction to the outcomes of the program (Macdonald et al., 1997, 2000).

A literature review of the impact of EAPS on workplace behavior and client satisfaction also reported that 90% of EAP clients in studies indicated that they were happy with the services they received (McLeod, 2001). McLeod updated this literature in 2008, reporting that clients would use the service again and recommend it to their colleagues. However, these measures tend to reflect how professionally the service was delivered rather than the overall quality of the services and their implications for employee health and well-being and organizational productivity (McLeod, 2008). The updated review did try to ameliorate this, providing evidence to suggest that those who had received workplace counseling experienced improvements in their reported stress and well-being, including a positive effect on depression, but the review of the literature could not claim that EAPs had an enduring impact on psychological difficulties, or whether the service merely helped clients deal with current symptoms. With regard to outcomes such as job attitudes, satisfaction, motivation, and organizational commitment, EAPs did seemingly appear to lead to positive changes in work attitudes, but some of the data also suggested that there was not a sufficient level of "work dysfunction" for there to be clear and measurable changes in work outcomes, and so concluded that on these measures the outcomes still remained uncertain. In terms of work behavior (with a special focus on sickness absence), studies in the report mentioned that the use of EAPs had resulted in reduced sickness absence (between 20% and 60% were reported in the range of studies included, and some of these also reported a longitudinal positive effect), but there was a caveat that even after using EAPs, client sickness absence was still higher than organizational averages.

Mellor-Clark et al. (2013) measured the effectiveness of EAP service provision in comparison with the U.K. National Health Service primary care and U.K. education CORE systems benchmark. This analysis showed EAPs to be an effective intervention for those who experience common mental health problems (e.g., anxiety, depression, stress), as clients reported improved well-being outcomes after receiving between four and six counseling sessions. Another positive of EAPs was the quick access to counseling provision, with mean waiting times between the referral and assessment to therapy being just under 9 days. A state of the market study into EAP provision and use was undertaken using a survey of HR managers followed up by qualitative interviews (Bajorek, 2016). The survey reported that EAPs were most commonly used for issues related to work-related stress, depression, and family conflicts. A number of other workplace issues were also reported, including concerns with line management, workplace restructuring, and bullying. Human resources (HR) managers often reported EAPs to be an "invaluable service" even though confidentiality could make evaluations difficult.

More recent measures have been developed to understand EAP effectiveness for workplace outcomes. The Workplace Outcomes Suite (WOS) measures five key aspects of the workplace that can be seen as proxy measures for well-being, including (a) presenteeism, (b) absenteeism, (c) workplace distress, (d) work engagement, and (e) life satisfaction (Chestnut Global Partners, 2017). Pre-EAP and post-EAP data (post-EAP data were collected 3 months after EAP use) showed improvements on each of the WOS measures, although they did differ substantially in terms of the relative change seen. For example, measures of life satisfaction and presenteeism reported greater improvements in comparison to work distress, work engagement, and absenteeism. It was also reported that through the reduction of presenteeism, EAPs could also have positive implications for organizational productivity.

Other measures of EAP evaluation have been reported. For example, Winwood and Beer (2008) outlined what makes a good EAP, identifying what they believe to be the "core technology" of EAPs, including (a) collaboration on the training and development of those managing troubled employees,

(b) timely and confidential provision of problem identification and assessment opportunities, (c) the use of constructive techniques that address in the immediate short-term job performance problems, (d) the referral of employees for treatment and assistance, (e) the establishment and maintenance of service provision and consultation in relation to other services that may be required, and (f) program evaluation at both the organizational and individual levels as well as in terms of identifiable performance outcome measures.

In contrast to these positive evaluations of EAPs, some studies have reported little or no systematic advantages over other forms of treatment or counseling. Whatmore et al. (1999) found that most of the gains that had been observed at 3 months postintervention had virtually dissipated by 6 months following completion of the intervention, suggesting that positive benefits may not be sustained, particularly if there is no systematic follow-up. De Groot and Kiker (2003) concluded that EAPs were most useful when clients approached them with a specific outcome to be focused on and when EAPs were approached voluntarily; however, the programs also seemed to have little or no effect on job satisfaction or turnover levels.

Overall, it would appear that EAPs can and often do yield positive benefits for individual employee well-being, but these programs' relation to productivity and other organizationally relevant outcomes is far from clear. The literature has also shown that organizational choices and decisions to use EAPs can also depend on economic factors (Berridge & Cooper, 1994). In 2013, a report by the U.K. EAPA highlighted that costs of EAPs have fallen, and this could present a challenge for EAPs to remain competitive and profitable while still providing a quality service. Measuring the economic benefits of EAPs has also been a focus of research, but care has to be given regarding on the type of economic benefits that are being measured. A cost–benefit analysis compares the money spent on providing services with the monetary values produced by the change. This is in comparison to a cost–effectiveness that focuses on more unspecified outcomes (e.g., well-being), aiming to establish which organizational interventions implemented achieve the best therapeutic results. Finally, there is the return on investment (ROI), which is an important finding as organizations often have to justify the costs of interventions to see if they provide enough business value to cover their costs.

Some of the literature discusses economic data with regard to EAP use. Dainas and Marks (2000) reported a favorable 2:1 cost savings of an organizational EAP, as employees and their family members who had access to the service also had reduced medical and health care costs. Bajorek (2016) found that only 9% of surveyed HR managers conducted ROIs of EAPs, with interview data reporting that senior managers did not ask for proof of cost–effectiveness of EAPs as they were often viewed as the right thing to have in organizations. For other managers, the logistics in undertaking ROIs, including the development of robust methodologies were a barrier, and the usage information provided by EAPs themselves does not provide the relevant information to undertake ROIs, although some assumptions could be made. More recently, Bevan and Bajorek (2019) developed a tool with U.K. EAPA that HR professionals could use to capture workplace data to estimate the ROIs of EAPs. The initial first wave of data collected and used in the tool reported that the ROI of EAPs is very positive, even in the case of low sickness absence and low utility figures.

However, much of the EAP research also reveals a number of methodological issues when undertaking evaluations. Confidentiality is a concern in terms of client confidentiality (Highley & Cooper, 1994), leading to difficulties in obtaining organizational data that could help with undertaking evaluations, and making longitudinal research difficult. Some EAPs do ask clients to provide feedback about the service, but there are differences in how reliably clients answer these questions, as well as resistance on the part of EAPs toward having their efforts evaluated (Davis & Gibson, 1994).

How the utilization of EAPs is measured can also differ, with Bajorek (2016) arguing that a standardized definition is needed to aid future evaluations. Csiernik (2003) had previously found that organizations used 19 different formulae for collating EAP utilization reports, and consequently reports may not be comparing like-for-like. Masi (2011) concluded that "true" measures of utilization will always be difficult because EAPs want to remain competitive and profitable; a common measuring tool to gauge performance may therefore be difficult.

Highley and Cooper (1994) commented that evaluations can be difficult because EAPs frequently have multiple goals, including enhancing employee morale and motivation, promoting an image of the organization as caring for the welfare of its employees, improving productivity (e.g., by reducing absenteeism and tardiness, as well as through more direct effects on job performance), and reducing disciplinary problems. Given the range of intended benefits and given that achieving significant improvements in all of these areas is unlikely, the assessment of whether a particular intervention has been effective poses considerable challenges for the evaluator (Noblet & Lamontagne, 2009).

Alongside the different goals of EAPs are different research designs that EAP evaluations use. The simplest form of evaluation is the pre- and postcounseling comparison, which aims to show that change has occurred as a result of the intervention. But as Bajorek (2016) reported, EAPs are usually one of a number of interventions that employers implement to improve employee health and well-being; thus, it is important to develop more robust methodologies to determine the influence of EAPs, but it can be difficult to implement these in organizational settings.

In summary, this brief overview of EAP evaluations illustrates that findings on the outcomes of EAPs are mixed (e.g., Arthur, 2000) and that it is simply not possible to draw general conclusions about the effectiveness of these interventions. One reason for this lack of conclusiveness lies in the design of EAP evaluations, which are often suboptimal and do not include longitudinal pre- and postintervention assessments, data comparative with other forms of intervention, multiple sources of information (e.g., managers and organizational clients as well as counselors and employees), and the variety of types of information needed to ensure that benefits are not limited to self-reports of satisfaction levels or financial outcomes. An additional problem is that the term

EAP encompasses a wide variety of types and foci of intervention, ranging from substance abuse programs to stress-management training and even more global wellness programs. The multidimensionality of EAPs means that it may not be possible to derive general conclusions that reflect all intervention types and formats. Rather, it may be more appropriate to examine the specific goals of a particular program and the extent to which those goals have been achieved. Nevertheless, it is evident that evaluations of EAPs need to be more systematic and rigorous than has often been the case until now, and they must examine a range of outcomes that demonstrate benefits to a variety of stakeholders.

FUTURE ROLE OF EAPs

The COVID-19 pandemic has once again highlighted the importance of employee health and well-being and the role that organizations have in supporting staff. However, it is important that the management of health and well-being does not become a mere tick-box exercise and that organizations implement interventions that will be of benefit to employees. So, what does this mean for the future of EAPs?

Given the levels of uncertainty and inconsistency around current EAP research findings, further research and education is required regarding the benefits of EAPs and how they can be effectively implemented in organizations. Bajorek and Bevan (2020) reported that what makes high quality counselling and EAPs needs to be determined. To achieve this, developing methodologies for organizations to fully evaluate outcomes (both well-being and financial outcomes) needs to be a key priority, as well as developing a standardized measure of utilization to improve the accuracy of recording across providers and organizations. This will also help with the identification of baseline measures to make comparisons within and between organizations to see if or when changes in service use occur, and how this impacts organizational outcomes measured. Alongside this, greater understanding is needed about how organizations actually use EAPs, and consequently service providers could match the services they offer to organizational needs.

These evaluations could be enhanced by including a range of stakeholder perspectives that are typically involved in implementing, promoting, using, and evaluating EAPs. For example, as line managers have been viewed as important in employee health and well-being, it may be valuable to understand what they think of the service, whether they promote the service (and how), and what benefits they recognize. Senior managers should also be engaged as they are critical in service implementation, in determining how the service is evaluated, and in reviewing whether cost benefits of the service are an important evaluative criteria (or whether health and well-being is the most important outcome). As these various stakeholders may have differing views regarding the value of EAPs and how they should be evaluated, it is important that these views are captured.

Further research into the client experience of EAPs is also needed. Current research into the client experience has often been filtered through the questions asked, the purpose of the research, or the theoretical lens of the researcher. For example, questions usually focus on clients' satisfaction with the service or whether they would recommend the service to others. However, more focus could and should be placed on measurements of changes in well-being, what clients would like to see from EAPs, and how services could be further improved.

Bajorek (2016) reported that one of the factors that has made workplace counseling and EAP evaluations notoriously difficult is that service providers typically have had little or no engagement in evaluations because they are, rightly, concerned about sharing what could be commercially sensitive data, having implications for provider competition. Where EAP providers have shared data, the amount of missing data made any significant research evaluation difficult (with providers mentioning that data were unavailable, records may not be up-to-date, or the data being requested could not be calculated from their records). The limited nature of provider engagement does have an impact on understanding the extent and level of EAP service use. The future of EAP use and development could be enhanced by engaging with service providers so that there is an increased understanding in their role in service promotion and evaluation. It is thus necessary to uncover this reticence in engaging with evaluative research and determine how this challenge can be overcome.

Bajorek and Bevan (2020) argued that one aspect of provider reticence could be related to the future funding of EAPs with respect to any increase in future utilization. In a consultation with service providers, Bajorek and Bevan saw that service providers were questioning what organizations hoped to receive from EAPs when they paid on average £5 per employee per year (in the United Kingdom). If the demand for EAPs does increase (as seen during the COVID-19 pandemic), but the number of suppliers remains similar, then a crisis could emerge in relation to the price of the service and the quality of the counseling provided. Individuals are not only seeking mental well-being counseling; they are also seeking counseling for financial well-being and legal advice. If more (and a wider range of) counselors are needed to meet this demand, EAP services may be at risk of outpricing themselves.

In relation to concerns about prospective service provision, there have also been discussions about the future training and accreditation of counselors. Counselors require supervision and need to receive ongoing training to keep up with new and continual developments in counseling methodologies; there are concerns that if this ongoing training is not maintained, the future of the profession could be at risk. Although counseling is a popular profession, extra development is needed to undertake workplace counseling as provided by EAPs to understand the specific needs of employees and how their mental ill-health could be worsened by work. Developing an accredited course based on core competencies and modules could be a method to improve and shape the future of workplace counseling.

The effects of COVID-19 on the implementation and promotion of EAPs could also be reviewed. Many EAPs already provide their services across a range of digital interfaces; however, promotional activities typically still occur via posters, word of mouth, or through organizational well-being days. If the COVID-19 pandemic does result in the increase in hybrid working or the use of more digital technologies, including delivering remote therapies via video or telephone, organizations and EAP service providers may need to become more creative in how their service is implemented and promoted for maximum employee and organizational benefits.

Finally, for employee health and well-being to be maintained at work, organizations must take on a preventative role, whereas traditional EAP provision is still in essence reactive. More still could be done to understand where EAPs can fit into the "good work" agenda, focusing on the quality of work as well as how it is done and managed, so that EAPs can have a more meaningful contribution to employee well-being in the future.

REFERENCES

Arthur, A. R. (2000). Employee assistance programmes: The emperor's new clothes of stress management? *British Journal of Guidance & Counselling, 28*(4), 549–559. https://doi.org/10.1080/03069880020004749

Bajorek, Z. (2016). *Employee assistance programmes (EAPs): Supporting good work for UK employers?* The Work Foundation.

Bajorek, Z., & Bevan, S. (2020). *Demonstrating the effectiveness of workplace counselling.* Institute for Employment Studies.

Bajorek, Z., Mason, B., & Bevan, S. (2020). Wellbeing under lockdown: Results of a survey of British homeworkers. *Occupational Health at Work, 17*(2), 29–34. https://www.atworkpartnership.co.uk/journal/issue/17_2/contents/wellbeing-under-lockdown

Bajorek, Z., Shreeve, V., Bevan, S., & Taskila, T. (2014). *The way forward: Policy options for improving workforce health in the UK.* The Work Foundation. https://www.bl.uk/collection-items/way-forward-policy-options-for-improving-workforce-health-in-the-uk

Berridge, J., & Cooper, C. L. (1994). The employee assistance programme: Its role in organizational coping and excellence. *Personnel Review, 23*(7), 4–20. https://doi.org/10.1108/00483489410072190

Berridge, J., Cooper, C., & Highley-Marchington, C. (1997). *Employee assistance programmes and workplace counselling.* Wiley.

Bevan, S., & Bajorek, Z. (2019). *Designing and testing a return-on-investment tool for EAPs.* Institute for Employment Studies.

Biron, C., Cooper, C. L., & Bond, F. (2009). Mediators and moderators of organizational stress interventions to prevent occupational stress. In S. Cartwright & C. L. Cooper (Eds.), *The Oxford handbook of organizational well-being* (pp. 441–465). Oxford University Press.

Black, C. (2008, March 17). *Working for a healthier tomorrow: Review of the health of Britain's working age population.* Presentation to the Secretary of State for Health and the Secretary of State for Works and Pensions. London, England: The Stationery Office.

Brooks, S. K., Rubin, G. J., & Greenberg, N. (2019). Traumatic stress within disaster-exposed occupations: Overview of the literature and suggestions for the management of traumatic stress in the workplace. *British Medical Bulletin, 129*(1), 25–34. https://doi.org/10.1093/bmb/ldy040

Carchietta, G. A. (2015). Five steps to increasing utilization of your employee assistance program. *Workplace Health & Safety, 63*(3), 132. https://doi.org/10.1177/2165079915585054

Cekiso, N. A., & Terblanche, L. S. (2015). Pricing models of employee assistance programs: Experiences of corporate clients serviced by a leading employee assistance program service provider in South Africa. *Journal of Workplace Behavioral Health*, *30*(1–2), 154–178. https://doi.org/10.1080/15555240.2015.1000162

Chestnut Global Partners. (2017). *Comparing improvement after EAP counselling for different outcomes.* Workplace Outcome Suite (WOS) Annual Report 2017. https://www.eapassn.org/Portals/11/Docs/WOS/WOS_AnnualReportFinal2017.pdf?ver=2017-09-15-173501-900

College of Policing. (2018). *Responding to trauma in policing: A practical guide.*

Compton, R.-L., & McManus, J. G. (2015). Employee assistance programs in Australia: Evaluating success. *Journal of Workplace Behavioral Health*, *30*(1–2), 32–45. https://doi.org/10.1080/15555240.2015.998971

Cooper, C. L., & Cartwright, S. (1994). Healthy mind; Healthy organization—A proactive approach to occupational stress. *Human Relations*, *47*(4), 455–471. https://doi.org/10.1177/001872679404700405

Csiernik, R. (2003). Employee assistance programme utilization: Developing a comprehensive scorecard. *Employee Assistance Quarterly*, *18*, 45–60. https://doi.org/10.1300/J022v18n03_04

Dainas, C., & Marks, D. (2000). Evidence of an EAP cost offset. *Behavioural Health Management.* July/August.

Davis, A., & Gibson, L. (1994). Designing employee welfare provision. *Personnel Review*, *23*(7), 33–45. https://doi.org/10.1108/00483489410072208

De Groot, T., & Kiker, D. S. (2003). A meta-analysis of the non-monetary effects of employee health management programs. *Human Resource Management*, *42*(1), 53–69. https://doi.org/10.1002/hrm.10064

Dewe, P. J. (1994). EAPs and stress management: From theory to practice to comprehensiveness. *Personnel Review*, *23*(7), 21–32. https://doi.org/10.1108/00483489410072217

Employee Assistance Professionals Association. (1997). *U.K. EAPA guidelines for the audit and evaluation of workplace counselling programmes.*

Farmer, P., & Stevenson, D. (2017). *Thriving at work. The Stevenson/Farmer review of mental health and employers.* https://assets.publishing.service.gov.uk/government/uploads/system/uploads/attachment_data/file/658145/thriving-at-work-stevenson-farmer-review.pdf

Harlow, K. (1998). Employee attitudes toward an internal employee assistance program. *Journal of Employment Counseling*, *35*(3), 141–150. https://doi.org/10.1002/j.2161-1920.1998.tb00995.x

Highley, J. C., & Cooper, C. L. (1994). Evaluating EAPs. *Personnel Review*, *23*(7), 46–59. https://doi.org/10.1108/00483489410072226

Kirk, A. K., & Brown, D. F. (2003). Employee assistance programs: A review of the management of stress and well-being through workplace counselling and consulting. *Australian Psychologist*, *38*(2), 138–143. https://doi.org/10.1080/00050060310001707137

Lee, C., & Gray, J. A. (1994). The role of employee assistance programmes. In C. L. Cooper & S. Williams (Eds.), *Creating healthy work organizations* (pp. 215–242). Wiley.

Macdonald, S., Lothian, S., & Wells, S. (1997). Evaluation of an employee assistance program at a transportation company. *Evaluation and Program Planning*, *20*(4), 495–505. https://doi.org/10.1016/S0149-7189(97)00028-1

Macdonald, S., Wells, S., Lothian, S., & Shain, M. (2000). Absenteeism and other workplace indicators of employee assistance program clients and matched controls. *Employee Assistance Quarterly*, *15*(3), 41–57. https://doi.org/10.1300/J022v15n03_04

Masi, D. A. (2011). Redefining the EAP field. *Journal of Workplace Behavioral Health*, *26*(1), 1–9. https://doi.org/10.1080/15555240.2011.540971

McLeod, J. (2001). *Counselling in the workplace: The facts.* British Association for Counselling and Psychotherapy.

McLeod, J. (2008). *Counselling in the workplace: A comprehensive review of the research evidence* (2nd ed.). British Association for Counselling and Psychotherapy.

Mellor-Clark, J., Twigg, E., Farrell, E., & Kinder, A. (2013). Benchmarking key service quality indicators in UK Employee Assistance Programme Counselling: A CORE system data profile. *Counselling & Psychotherapy Research, 13*(1), 14–23. https://doi.org/10.1080/14733145.2012.728235

Mitchell, J. T. (1983). When disaster strikes . . . the critical incident stress debriefing process. *JEMS: A Journal of Emergency Medical Services, 8*(1), 36–39.

National Institute for Health and Care Excellence (NICE). (2018). Recommendations. *Post-traumatic stress disorder: NICE Guidelines [NG116].* https://www.nice.org.uk/guidance/ng116/chapter/Recommendations

Newton, L., Hayday, S., & Barkworth, R. (2005). *Employee assistance programmes.* Institute for Employment Studies.

Noblet, A. J., & Lamontagne, A. D. (2009). The challenges of developing, implementing, and evaluating interventions. In S. Cartwright & C. L. Cooper (Eds.), *The Oxford handbook of organizational well-being* (pp. 466–496). Oxford University Press.

Ørner, F. J. (2012). The evolution of models of early intervention for adults: From inspired help giving toward evidence-based pragmatism. In R. Hughes, A. Kinder, & C. L. Cooper (Eds.), *International handbook of workplace trauma support.* Wiley-Blackwell. https://doi.org/10.1002/9781119943242.ch1

Parker, L., & Bevan, S. (2011). *Good work and our times: Report of the Good Work Commission.* The Work Foundation.

Rick, J., & Briner, R. B. (2012). Evidence-based trauma management for organizations: Developments and prospects. In R. Hughes, A. Kinder, & C. L. Cooper (Eds.), *International handbook of workplace trauma support.* Wiley-Blackwell. https://doi.org/10.1002/9781119943242.ch2

Rick, J., O'Regan, S., & Kinder, A. (2006). *Early Intervention Following Trauma: A Controlled Longitudinal Study at Royal Mail Group* [Report 435]. Institute for Employment Studies.

Rose, S., & Bisson, J. (1998). Brief early psychological interventions following trauma: A systematic review of the literature. *Journal of Traumatic Stress, 11*(4), 697–710. https://doi.org/10.1023/A:1024441315913

Taylor, M., Marsh, G., Nicol, D., & Broadbent, P. (2017). *Good work: The Taylor review of modern working practices.* RSA.

UK Employee Assistance Professionals Association. (2012). *EAP Guidelines.*

Waddell, G., & Burton, A. K. (2006). *Is work good for your health and well-being?* The Stationery Office.

Wessley, S. (2001). Psychological injury: Fact and fiction. In A. Braidwood (Ed.), *Psychological injury: Understanding and supporting* (pp. 34–44). Department of Social Security. The Stationery Officer.

Whatmore, L., Cartwright, S., & Cooper, C. (1999). United Kingdom: Evaluation of a stress management programme in the public sector. In M. Kompier & C. Cooper (Eds.), *Preventing stress, improving productivity: European case studies in the workplace* (pp. 149–174). Routledge.

Wilson, G., Farrell, D., Barron, I., Hutchins, J., Whybrow, D., & Kiernan, M. D. (2018) The use of eye-movement desensitization reprocessing (EMDR) therapy in treating post-traumatic stress disorder—A systematic narrative review. *Frontiers in Psychology, 6*(9). https://doi.org/10.3389/fpsyg.2018.00923

Winwood, M. A., & Beer, S. (2008). What makes a good employee assistance programme? In A. Kinder, R. Hughes, & C. Cooper (Eds.), *Employee well-being support: A workplace resource* (pp. 183–200). Wiley. https://doi.org/10.1002/9780470773246.ch16

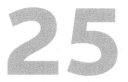

Occupational Health and Safety Leadership

Jane Mullen, Tabatha Thibault, and E. Kevin Kelloway

There is widespread acknowledgment in occupational health research that organizational leadership influences employee health and safety (Barling, 2014). Indeed, virtually every variable of interest in occupational health psychology (OHP) has been linked to leadership (Mullen & Kelloway, 2011). A great deal of research has demonstrated that effective—and in particular, transformational—leadership is associated with a variety of positive employee health and safety outcomes (Arnold, 2017; Mullen & Kelloway, 2011; Nielsen & Taris, 2019). Poor leadership (i.e., abusive, laissez-faire) is undeniably harmful to employees (Harms et al., 2017; Montano et al., 2017). Leaders use a range of high-quality leadership behaviors (Clarke & Taylor, 2018), and displaying them consistently (Mullen et al., 2011) leads to better employee health and safety-related outcomes within workplaces. In this chapter, we review the literature on leadership as a mechanism for enhancing employee health and safety in organizations. We begin with a review of the most widely researched leadership styles and their associations with various health and safety-related outcomes, followed by an examination of destructive forms of leadership. We conclude with a discussion of topics for future research.

LEADERSHIP FOR CREATING HEALTHY AND SAFE WORKPLACES

Transformational and transactional styles of leadership, and their unique effects on employee health and safety-related outcomes, continue to receive considerable attention from researchers in the OHP literature (Kelloway &

https://doi.org/10.1037/0000331-025
Handbook of Occupational Health Psychology, Third Edition, L. E. Tetrick, G. G. Fisher, M. T. Ford, and J. C. Quick (Editors)

Barling, 2010; Mullen & Kelloway, 2011). *Transformational leadership* comprises idealized influence, intellectual stimulation, inspirational leadership, and individualized consideration (Bass, 1990). Leaders exhibiting idealized influence act as a role model for their subordinates. *Inspirational motivation* involves setting high yet attainable goals and challenging subordinates. Leaders who engage in intellectual stimulation encourage creativity and solicit input from their subordinates. Finally, *individualized consideration* means that leaders attend to each of their subordinates' needs (Hildenbrand et al., 2018; Judge & Piccolo, 2004). Simply put, transformational leadership involves behaviors that go beyond basic transactions to result in higher levels of performance.

Transactional leadership, on the other hand, focuses on exchanges between leaders and their subordinates and what behaviors the leaders engage in as a response to subordinate behavior (Judge & Piccolo, 2004). Contingent reward is the most positive type of transactional leadership. Leaders exhibiting *contingent reward* clarify their expectations of their subordinates, set concrete goals, provide rewards for those who meet those goals or expectations, and provide immediate and contingent feedback for subordinates (Judge & Piccolo, 2004).

Meta-analyses have found positive associations between transformational leadership and employee health and safety outcomes (e.g., Montano et al., 2017). For example, meta-analytic evidence demonstrates that both transformational leadership and contingent reward uniquely predict employee job satisfaction and follower satisfaction with their leader (Judge & Piccolo, 2004). According to a recent meta-analysis, transformational leadership is positively related to employee psychological well-being and psychological functioning, and negatively related to affective symptoms (including anger, anxiety, frustration, and fear), burnout (measured as general burnout and emotional exhaustion), stress, and health complaints (e.g., fatigue; Montano et al., 2017). Clarke's (2013) meta-analysis found that transformational leadership is positively linked to employee safety compliance (i.e., safety-related behaviors required by the organization) and participation (i.e., voluntary behaviors that do not contribute to personal safety but support organizational safety), in addition to safety climate (i.e., perceptions of safety in the organization based on policies, procedures, and practices). Studies have also examined potential mediators for the relationship between transformational leadership and employee mental health, including trust in one's leader (Kelloway et al., 2012; Liu et al., 2010), job demands (Hentrich et al., 2017), self-efficacy (Hentrich et al., 2017; Liu et al., 2010), meaningful work (i.e., finding a purpose in work; Arnold et al., 2007; Nielsen et al., 2008), and involvement (Nielsen et al., 2008).

Positive leader behaviors can be taught and increased through intervention (Duygulu & Kublay, 2011; Kelloway & Barling, 2010). Leadership interventions can include classroom-based training, individual coaching, and/or feedback sessions, all of which can be effective (Kelloway et al., 2000). By increasing effective leadership types such as transformational leadership, these interventions can improve subordinate health and safety outcomes (Mullen & Kelloway, 2009). Increased transformational leadership through leadership interventions have been found to increase employee engagement (Biggs et al.,

2014), job satisfaction (Biggs et al., 2014), and employee-rated safety climate (von Thiele Schwarz et al., 2016). Furthermore, Mullen and Kelloway (2009) found that safety-specific transformational leadership training enhanced safety attitudes, self-efficacy, and intent to promote safety, which then led to improved safety climate perceptions and safety participation from employees, and reduced safety-related events and injuries 3 months after training compared with control groups.

In addition to exploring general leadership styles that encompass a wide range of behaviors, researchers suggest a need to examine specific leader behaviors and their unique effects on health and safety outcomes (Griffin & Hu, 2013; Nielsen & Taris, 2019; Wong et al., 2015). Studies examining the effectiveness of leadership development programs provide insight into what leaders can do and the specific behaviors that lead to improved health and safety (for a review, see Wong et al., 2016). For example, frequently speaking about safety is an important leadership behavior (Wong et al., 2015) that serves as a mechanism through which leaders communicate organizational values, priorities, and expectations for safety (Halbesleben et al., 2013; Zohar, 2002; Zohar & Luria, 2003). Leaders enhance their communication skills by incorporating health and safety-related topics into their verbal communication with employees, which in turn leads to improved health and safety outcomes at the employee level (Kines et al., 2010).

Leadership theories also suggest that supervisors are important role models of desired behavior in organizations; thus, researchers are interested in examining role modeling as a mechanism for influencing employee health and safety-related behavior. For example, transformational leaders are "role models for followers to emulate . . . and display high standards of ethical and moral conduct" (Avolio, 1999, p. 43). In a survey study of leaders and employees from 54 organizations, Tucker et al. (2016) found that frontline employee injuries were related to the collective safety actions of leaders at various levels of an organization. Through the trickle-down effect of leader actions, CEOs, managers, and supervisors shape the organizational safety climate, which in turn influences employee perceptions of their supervisors' support for safety. When employees perceived higher levels of supervisor support for safety (i.e., supervisor sets a good safety example by "walking the talk"), they reported fewer work-related injuries. Similarly, Halbesleben et al. (2013) examined leader safety behavioral integrity, defined as the alignment of actions for improving espoused safety expectations, and found that safety behavioral integrity was associated with psychological safety toward one's supervisor and employee safety compliance, which in turn predicted employee self-reports of injury severity. Researchers have also examined leader safety hypocrisy, defined as the misalignment of leaders' demonstrated safety actions and speaking about safety (Kelloway et al., 2018), and found that the positive effects of speaking about safety on employee safety behavior were significant only when leaders also modeled safety behaviors.

Kranabetter and Niessen (2017) saw that the negative relationship between employee ratings of transformational leadership and exhaustion was stronger when leaders reported higher levels of health awareness (i.e., knowing when they require a break for recovery; awareness of personal health limits) and positive health behaviors (i.e., taking regular breaks, caring about healthy lifestyle, following safety rules under pressure). Similarly, Koch and Binnewies (2015) found that employees with positive work–life-friendly supervisory role models (i.e., supervisor demonstrates positive work–life balance behaviors) reported lower levels of exhaustion and disengagement. However, leaders may also serve as negative role models of health and safety in organizations. In a three-wave survey study of employees and their direct supervisors, Dietz et al. (2020) examined the long-term effects of leader presenteeism behavior on employee health outcomes and found that employees reported higher presenteeism days and longer sick leave when their leaders reported working frequently while being ill. Hammer et al. (2015) evaluated a safety and health program designed to improve family-supportive supervisor behavior (i.e., family-supportive role modeling, creative work–family management) and supervisor safety behavior (i.e., safety communication, safety role modeling). Results of the intervention were mixed, with no significant increases in employee safety behaviors or general health; however, there were significant reductions in employee blood pressure at 12 months postintervention. Hammer et al. (2015) suggested that although the findings were promising, further research needs to examine the unique effects of each training component (i.e., supervisor versus team component of the training program). Furthermore, it would be useful to examine the unique effects of each leadership behavior (i.e., role modeling versus communication) on employee health outcomes and safety behaviors.

The results from studies examining specific leadership behaviors suggest that leading by example and talking about health and safety may uniquely and effectively strengthen health and safety outcomes in organizations. Combined, these studies suggest that managers should be aware of the significant impacts of their health and safety-related actions and communication, as well as how these factors may influence others within the work environment.

SUPERVISOR SUPPORT

Researchers are increasingly interested in exploring the relationships between social support from supervisors and employee health and safety outcomes. Two types of *supervisor support* commonly examined in the literature are instrumental support (i.e., flexibility in work schedules) and emotional support (i.e., showing employees care and concern; Cohen & Wills, 1985). Research suggests that perceived supervisor support generally results in better employee health and safety outcomes. For example, McIlroy and colleagues' (2021) quasi-experimental field study showed that unanswered support from supervisors (i.e., when an employee actively requests support from their supervisor and it is not received) indirectly affected employee emotional exhaustion through a lower need satisfaction. In a study of health care workers from 52 organizations, supervisor support emerged as a stronger predictor of employee safety behavior than other job resources, including social support from coworkers and job autonomy (Bronkhorst, 2015).

Resource theories (i.e., conservation of resources theory, job demands–resources model) classify support from leaders as an important job resource that serves to mitigate the negative impact of stressors on employee health outcomes. Both forms of supervisor support are strongly interrelated and buffer the negative effects of a broad range of job stressors on employee attitudes, behaviors, and health-related outcomes (Mathieu et al., 2019). For example, Van de Ven et al. (2013) found that emotional job demands resulted in lower levels of emotional exhaustion when employees experienced high levels of emotional support from supervisors. Witnessing bullying in the workplace was associated with increased anxiety and depression 6 months later, but only when employees reported low levels of supervisor support (Sprigg et al., 2019). Similarly, supervisor support was shown to temper the negative effects of family-to-work conflict (FWC) among employees with caregiving responsibilities such that employees who experienced high levels of FWC were more likely to report increased depression, but only when they reported low supervisor support. Combined, these findings are consistent with the literature suggesting that the absence of effective leadership behavior (i.e., lack of support) is associated with negative consequences for employee health and safety as opposed to having a null effect (Kelloway et al., 2006).

A growing body of research explores specific forms of support and suggests that family-supportive supervisor behavior (FSSB; i.e., expressing care and concern for an employee's nonwork life; providing resources to assist employees with managing work and nonwork life) is associated with a broad range of employee psychological and physical health outcomes (for a review, see Crain & Stevens, 2018). Studies suggest that supportive supervisory behaviors can be developed through leadership training interventions and serve as a means to effectively enhance employees' positive emotions (e.g., calm, quiet, happy), reduce negative emotions, and protect against declines in employee safety compliance and citizenship behaviors (i.e., behaviors that are above and beyond the defined role and benefit the organization and its members; Hammer et al., 2016; Mohr et al., 2021).

DESTRUCTIVE LEADERSHIP

To further our understanding of the link between leadership and employee health and safety, researchers have studied destructive styles of leadership (i.e., abusive supervision, passive leadership styles; see Kelloway et al., 2005; Martinko et al., 2013; Skogstad et al., 2017). *Abusive supervision* is a commonly used construct to describe destructive leadership and is defined as "the sustained display of hostile verbal and nonverbal behaviors, excluding physical contact" (Tepper, 2000, p. 178). Organizations should be aware of the research highlighting the severity and type of effects that abusive supervision has on employee health and safety-related outcomes (Montano et al., 2017; Mullen et al., 2018; Schyns & Schilling, 2013). Employees who experience abusive supervisory behavior report higher levels of psychological distress, emotional exhaustion and burnout (Harms et al., 2017; Martinko et al., 2013), as well as increased psychosomatic symptoms (e.g., headaches, sleep problems, backaches; Velez & Neves, 2016). Additionally, abusive supervision is negatively associated with employee safety behavior, including compliance with safety protocols and voluntary participation in safety programs (Mullen et al., 2018). Abusive supervisory behavior undermines employee safety behavior by weakening an employee's sense of belonging to the workgroup and can be more harmful to some employees than others (e.g., when employees report higher uncertainty of their social standing; Yang et al., 2020).

Researchers are increasingly interested in examining strategies that will alleviate the damaging effects of abusive supervision on employee health and safety. One stream of research is focused on job and personal resources as a buffer against abusive supervision on employee health outcomes (Rafferty et al., 2010; Skogstad et al., 2017). For example, Velez and Neves (2016) found that job autonomy attenuated the positive association between abusive supervision and employee psychosomatic symptoms, but the positive relationship was significant only when employee job autonomy was low. Li et al. (2016) found that a leader's psychological distress, through their abusive behavior, affected team members' levels of psychological distress. Furthermore, the positive relationship between abusive supervision and employees' psychological distress was stronger when employees' psychological capital (i.e., employees' positive psychological state, including self-efficacy, optimism, hope, and resilience) was lower. This research suggests that increasing personal and job resources may help employees cope with their abusive leaders.

Other research focuses on preventing or reducing the occurrence of abusive supervisory behavior, as opposed to mitigating the negative outcomes, as a strategy for improving employee health. For example, Gonzalez-Morales et al. (2018) conducted a quasi-experimental field study to evaluate a training intervention designed to displace abusive behavior with supportive supervisory strategies (i.e., benevolence, fairness, sincerity, and mindfulness). Employees whose supervisors received the training reported less abusive supervision and higher levels of supervisor support compared to employees in the no-training condition. Although intervention studies aimed at displacing abusive supervisory behavior are rare, there is a growing body of literature that supports the effectiveness of leadership development as a strategy for positively influencing employee health and safety outcomes (for a review, see Kelloway & Barling, 2010).

Passive leadership (Avolio, 1999) appears to be just as harmful to employees as abusive supervision and other destructive leadership styles (Skogstad et al., 2017). For example, *laissez-faire leadership*, characterized by the avoidance of leadership responsibilities (Bass, 1985), is negatively associated with employee safety climate and employee safety behavior (Mullen et al., 2011; Smith et al., 2016) and mental health (Montano et al., 2017), and positively associated with depressive symptoms (Barling & Frone, 2017), burnout, and physical symptoms (Che et al., 2017). However, studies have shown mixed results, depending on the length of time between data collection periods. For example, the association between laissez-faire leadership and employee state anxiety was found to be nonsignificant in a study with a 6-month time lag between Time 1 and 2 data collection (Nielsen, Skogstad, et al., 2019), whereas other studies have suggested that the appropriate length of time to detect the negative effects of passive leadership may require a relatively long period (i.e., 2-year period; Skogstad et al., 2014). In a 30-day diary study that examined daily fluctuations in employee safety compliance behavior, Olsen et al. (2021) found that an increase in perceived daily passive leadership was associated with increased daily safety noncompliance beyond the variance accounted for by transformational leadership. The results showed that even very short periods of perceived passive leadership may negatively influence employee safety behavior. Again, the results suggested that the absence of effective leadership is of equal importance to the presence of effective leadership for employee health and safety. Managers undermine safety systems in organizations and weaken the positive impact of effective leadership when they avoid their leadership responsibilities (Mullen et al., 2011, 2017).

FUTURE RESEARCH

Despite the considerable amount of research that has improved our understanding of leadership and occupational health and safety, there remain many unanswered questions and opportunities to expand our knowledge on the topic. We conclude with several suggestions for future research. These suggestions are not intended to provide a comprehensive research agenda but rather to highlight several key issues that have emerged in the literature.

Longitudinal studies that assess the underlying mediating and moderating processes in the relationships between leadership behaviors, employee health, and safety-related outcomes are essential for advancing research on this topic and for providing empirical evidence that will guide organizational leadership training. For example, Inceoglu et al. (2018) identified 384 studies of leadership and well-being and noted that only 71 of those studies examined a mediation model. On the basis of their review, the authors concluded that "very few studies provided well-developed theoretical justifications for why the chosen well-being construct(s) were examined in relation to one or several leadership behaviors . . . very few studies attempted to conceptually align leadership behavior predictors and well-being criteria, let alone mediators" (p. 185).

Researchers have also called for more studies that examine the positive and negative crossover effects of leaders' and employees' mental health (Harms et al., 2017; Nielsen & Taris, 2019). Although emerging data provide support for crossover effects of leaders' mental health on employees' health (Li et al., 2016), the health-related antecedents of leadership behavior represent a developing area of research (for a review of this literature, see Barling & Cloutier, 2017) along with the nature and direction of health crossover effects. For example, drawing on resource theories (e.g., Hobfoll's, 1989, conservation of resources theory), researchers suggest that leaders' well-being is a resource that is positively associated with effective leadership behavior (i.e., transformational), and depleted leader resources (i.e., poor mental health) are associated with destructive and abusive leader behavior (Byrne et al., 2014). Indeed, recent meta-analytic studies show that effective leadership styles are positively associated with leader well-being, and destructive leadership is negatively associated with leader well-being (Harms et al., 2017; Kaluza et al., 2020). Similarly, there is evidence supporting the link between leader well-being and employee health outcomes (Li et al., 2016). However, the findings reported in the literature are based on a small number of correlation studies, which limits conclusions about causality and the underlying theoretical frameworks used to explain the mediation/moderation processes linking leader and employee health and safety.

To advance our knowledge of the mediating and moderating processes, researchers call for studies that adopt a true longitudinal design (i.e., evaluation of the same variables at three or more time points) to allow for an evaluation of complex theoretical models, changes in variables over time, and tests of causality (for a review of longitudinal designs, see Kelloway & Francis, 2013). Much of the extant research relies on cross-sectional or two-wave designs with variables assessed at one time point. Additionally, when research is time-lagged, researchers often report that there is a lack of theoretical justification for the appropriate length of time between data collection points or the appropriate amount of time required to assess the immediate and longer term effects of different leadership behaviors or to capture fluctuations in leader behaviors. Thus, future longitudinal studies should measure variables repeatedly over varying time periods (e.g., daily, weekly, monthly, yearly), and incorporate personal and situational antecedents of leaders' behavior (i.e., Barling & Cloutier, 2017) into models linking leadership and employee health and safety outcomes.

There is also a need to explore the harmful effects of a broader range of leadership behaviors rather than focusing primarily on destructive styles (i.e., passive, abusive behavior). Emerging research suggests that effective leadership behaviors (e.g., transformational leadership, supervisor support) may also result in negative unintended health-related consequences for both the leader and their employees (Breevaart & Bakker, 2018). For example, Nielsen and Daniels (2016) found that transformational leadership positively predicted employee absenteeism a year later. Furthermore, employee presenteeism moderated the relationship between transformational leadership and employee absenteeism 2 years later (Nielsen & Daniels, 2016). Specifically, the relationship between transformational leadership and absenteeism was positive at high levels of employee presenteeism but negative at low levels of employee presenteeism (Nielsen & Daniels, 2016). Perhaps employees need more time to recover their resources from the pressure their leader is putting on them, and/or those with a transformational leader feel pushed to make an extra effort (Nielsen & Daniels, 2016).

In one of their two samples, Franke and Felfe (2011) saw that the idealized influence component of transformational leadership positively predicted employee strain. While having a leader who has high standards may be motivating for some, it may inadvertently be putting added pressure on other employees (Franke & Felfe, 2011). Somewhat similarly, intellectual stimulation negatively predicted employee well-being in a faculty sample (both staff and academics within the same faculty; Zineldin & Hytter, 2012). Zineldin and Hytter (2012) posited that a leader who ranks highly in terms of intellectual stimulation would be a demanding leader and could be challenging for subordinates. These findings indicate that contextual factors may impact the influence of individual transformational leadership dimensions on employee health.

Research also suggests that social support from supervisors is not always helpful and can exacerbate employee strain outcomes (i.e., reverse buffering effect). Meta-analytic evidence demonstrates that the beneficial/harmful moderation effects of supervisor support are equally common (Mathieu et al., 2019). Harmful effects may occur if the specific leadership behaviors are perceived by an employee as unhelpful or if the support is unwanted (Beehr et al., 2010; Gray et al., 2020). For example, in a qualitative study on employees' return to work after experiencing the loss of an immediate family member, Gilbert et al. (2021) found that employees experienced both positive and negative psychological and behavioral strain in response to the support they received from their leader. They suggested that support from leaders may worsen employees' experience of grief if it is unwanted, draws more attention to the stressor, or is perceived as unhelpful or insincere. This study points to the need to consider the types of leadership behaviors that are most important depending on the situational context (Clarke, 2013), and under what conditions the behavior will alleviate or worsen the effects of stressors on employee outcomes.

There remains a concern about the influence of common method variance (CMV) as ratings of leadership and employee health and safety variables are typically obtained from the same source (i.e., employee ratings). Future studies should focus on gathering data from multiple sources (e.g., supervisors, managers, employees) to mitigate the concern of CMV effects (Podsakoff et al., 2003). Furthermore, researchers should include a combination of self-ratings with objective measures of health and safety variables (e.g., injury/accident/ claim records, blood pressure, cortisol levels, sleep). For example, Wong and Kelloway (2016) measured employee systolic blood pressure and self-reports of perceived interactions with their supervisor throughout the day and found that perceived negative supervisory interactions are associated with adverse employee health outcomes (e.g., heightened blood pressure at work and delayed recovery after work). Diebig et al. (2016) measured hair cortisol levels in their study of the relationship between full-range leadership behaviors (e.g., transformational, transactional, and laissez-faire leadership) and employee stress. Future studies will benefit from multiple sources of data and a combination of subjective ratings as well as objective measures of health and safety-related variables.

Finally, longitudinal and intervention research that focuses on the effectiveness of leadership styles for enhancing distributed worker health and safety is also warranted. *Distributed work* includes a variety of flexible work arrangements that allow people to work autonomously away from the central organizational location (Bélanger & Collins, 1998). Since the outbreak of the COVID-19 pandemic (WHO, 2020), telecommuting, a well-known form of distributed work, has increased significantly, and many organizations are opting for permanent full-time telecommuting arrangements for their employees (McLean, 2020). Pre-pandemic data suggest that telecommuting is negatively associated with role stress, work–family conflict, and turnover intentions, and positively associated with job satisfaction, performance, and autonomy (Gajendran & Harrison, 2007). However, there remains a need for further research that examines the complexity of the links between telecommuting and employee psychological, physical, and behavioral health-related outcomes such as injuries associated with physical workstations, physical activity, sleep, exhaustion, and other health behaviors (Allen et al., 2015; Moen et al., 2011). Furthermore, much of the extant research on leadership and occupational health and safety has been conducted within organizational settings where leaders and their employees have in-person interactions. Leading remotely creates unique challenges as there is limited face-to-face interaction, employees work in various locations, and there is reduced access to organizational health and safety information (Nielsen, Daniels, et al., 2019). Emerging cross-sectional survey studies are promising and suggest that leaders' safety leadership is positively associated with distributed workers' safety behaviors and performance (for a review, see Nayani et al., 2018). However, there remain many future research opportunities to explore the aforementioned theoretical and methodological issues.

CONCLUSION

Transformational leadership and other forms of positive leadership tend to lead to positive employee health and safety outcomes, whereas negative leadership styles (e.g., abusive) tend to lead to negative employee health and safety outcomes. Leadership interventions such as transformational leadership training can aid in improving health and safety. While there is ample evidence for the positive impacts of leadership, more research is still warranted. For example, using multisource data, examining multiple leadership styles at once, and analyzing the impact of leadership in atypical work settings (e.g., the growing use of the remote work environment) would advance the literature on leadership.

REFERENCES

Allen, T. D., Golden, T. D., & Shockley, K. M. (2015). How effective is telecommuting? Assessing the status of our scientific findings. *Psychological Science in the Public Interest, 16*(2), 40–68. https://doi.org/10.1177/1529100615593273

Arnold, K. A. (2017). Transformational leadership and employee psychological well-being: A review and directions for future research. *Journal of Occupational Health Psychology, 22*(3), 381–393. https://doi.org/10.1037/ocp0000062

Arnold, K. A., Turner, N., Barling, J., Kelloway, E. K., & McKee, M. C. (2007). Transformational leadership and psychological well-being: The mediating role of meaningful work. *Journal of Occupational Health Psychology, 12*(3), 193–203. https://doi.org/10.1037/1076-8998.12.3.193

Avolio, B. J. (1999). *Full leadership development: Building the vital forces in organizations.* Sage.

Barling, J. (2014). *The science of leadership: Lessons from research for organizational leaders.* Oxford University Press. https://doi.org/10.1093/acprof:oso/9780199757015.001.0001

Barling, J., & Cloutier, A. (2017). Leaders' mental health at work: Empirical, methodological, and policy directions. *Journal of Occupational Health Psychology, 22*(3), 394–406. https://doi.org/10.1037/ocp0000055

Barling, J., & Frone, M. R. (2017). If only my leader would just do *something*! Passive leadership undermines employee well-being through role stressors and psychological resource depletion. *Stress and Health, 33*(3), 211–222. https://doi.org/10.1002/smi.2697

Bass, B. M. (1985). *Leadership and performance beyond expectations.* Free Press.

Bass, B. M. (1990). From transactional to transformational leadership: Learning to share the vision. *Organizational Dynamics, 18*(3), 19–31. https://doi.org/10.1016/0090-2616(90)90061-S

Beehr, T. A., Bowling, N. A., & Bennett, M. M. (2010). Occupational stress and failures of social support: When helping hurts. *Journal of Occupational Health Psychology, 15*(1), 45–59. https://doi.org/10.1037/a0018234

Belanger, F., & Collins, R. W. (1998). Distributed work arrangements: A research framework. *The Information Society, 14*(2), 137–152. https://doi.org/10.1080/019722498128935

Biggs, A., Brough, P., & Barbour, J. P. (2014). Enhancing work-related attitudes and work engagement: A quasi-experimental study of the impact of an organizational intervention. *International Journal of Stress Management, 21*(1), 43–68. https://doi.org/10.1037/a0034508

Breevaart, K., & Bakker, A. B. (2018). Daily job demands and employee work engagement: The role of daily transformational leadership behavior. *Journal of Occupational Health Psychology, 23*(3), 338–349. https://doi.org/10.1037/ocp0000082

Bronkhorst, B. (2015). Behaving safely under pressure: The effects of job demands, resources, and safety climate on employee physical and psychosocial safety behavior. *Journal of Safety Research, 55*, 63–72. https://doi.org/10.1016/j.jsr.2015.09.002

Byrne, A., Dionisi, A., Barling, J., Akers, A., Robertson, J., Lys, R., & Dupré, K. (2014). The depleted leader: The influence of leaders' diminished psychological resources on leadership behaviors. *The Leadership Quarterly, 25*(2), 344–357. https://doi.org/10.1016/j.leaqua.2013.09.003

Che, X. X., Zhou, Z. E., Kessler, S. R., & Spector, P. E. (2017). Stressors beget stressors: The effect of passive leadership on employee health through workload and work–family conflict. *Work and Stress, 31*(4), 338–354. https://doi.org/10.1080/02678373.2017.1317881

Clarke, S. (2013). Safety leadership: A meta-analytic review of transformational and transactional leadership styles as antecedents of safety behaviours. *Journal of Occupational and Organizational Psychology, 86*(1), 22–49. https://doi.org/10.1111/j.2044-8325.2012.02064.x

Clarke, S., & Taylor, I. (2018). Reducing workplace accidents through the use of leadership interventions: A quasi-experimental field study. *Accident Analysis and Prevention, 121*, 314–320. https://doi.org/10.1016/j.aap.2018.05.010

Cohen, S., & Wills, T. A. (1985). Stress, social support, and the buffering hypothesis. *Psychological Bulletin, 98*(2), 310–357. https://doi.org/10.1037/0033-2909.98.2.310

Crain, T. L., & Stevens, S. C. (2018). Family-supportive supervisor behaviors: A review and recommendations for research and practice. *Journal of Organizational Behavior, 39*(7), 869–888. https://doi.org/10.1002/job.2320

Diebig, M., Bormann, K. C., & Rowold, J. (2016). A double-edged sword: Relationship between full-range leadership behaviors and followers' hair cortisol level. *The Leadership Quarterly, 27*(4), 684–696. https://doi.org/10.1016/j.leaqua.2016.04.001

Dietz, C., Zacher, H., Scheel, T., Otto, K., & Rigotti, T. (2020). Leaders as role models: Effects of leader presenteeism on employee presenteeism and sick leave. *Work and Stress, 34*(3), 300–322. https://doi.org/10.1080/02678373.2020.1728420

Duygulu, S., & Kublay, G. (2011). Transformational leadership training programme for charge nurses. *Journal of Advanced Nursing, 67*(3), 633–642. https://doi.org/10.1111/j.1365-2648.2010.05507.x

Franke, F., & Felfe, J. (2011). How does transformational leadership impact employees' psychological strain?: Examining differentiated effects and the moderating role of affective organizational commitment. *Leadership, 7*(3), 295–316. https://doi.org/10.1177/1742715011407387

Gajendran, R. S., & Harrison, D. A. (2007). The good, the bad, and the unknown about telecommuting: Meta-analysis of psychological mediators and individual consequences. *Journal of Applied Psychology, 92*(6), 1524–1541. https://doi.org/10.1037/0021-9010.92.6.1524

Gilbert, S., Mullen, J., Kelloway, E. K., Dimoff, J., Teed, M., & McPhee, T. (2021). The CARE model of employee bereavement support. *Journal of Occupational Health Psychology, 26*(5), 405–420. https://doi.org/10.1037/ocp0000287

Gonzalez-Morales, M. G., Kernan, M. C., Becker, T. E., & Eisenberger, R. (2018). Defeating abusive supervision: Training supervisors to support subordinates. *Journal of Occupational Health Psychology, 23*(2), 151–162. https://doi.org/10.1037/ocp0000061

Gray, C., Spector, P., Lacey, K., Young, B., Jacobsen, S., & Taylor, M. (2020). Helping may be harming: Unintended negative consequences of providing social support. *Work and Stress, 34*(4), 359–385. https://doi.org/10.1080/02678373.2019.1695294

Griffin, M. A., & Hu, X. (2013). How leaders differentially motivate safety compliance and safety participation: The role of monitoring, inspiring, and learning. *Safety Science, 60*, 196–202. https://doi.org/10.1016/j.ssci.2013.07.019

Halbesleben, J. R. B., Leroy, H., Dierynck, B., Simons, T., Savage, G. T., McCaughey, D., & Leon, M. R. (2013). Living up to safety values in health care: The effect of leader behavioral integrity on occupational safety. *Journal of Occupational Health Psychology, 18*(4), 395–405. https://doi.org/10.1037/a0034086

Hammer, L. B., Johnson, R. C., Crain, T. L., Bodner, T., Kossek, E. E., Davis, K. D., Kelly, E. L., Buxton, O. M., Karuntzos, G., Chosewood, L. C., & Berkman, L. (2016). Intervention effects on safety compliance and citizenship behaviors: Evidence from the Work, Family, and Health Study. *Journal of Applied Psychology, 101*(2), 190–208. https://doi.org/10.1037/apl0000047

Hammer, L. B., Truxillo, D. M., Bodner, T., Rineer, J., Pytlovany, A. C., & Richman, A. (2015). Effects of a workplace intervention targeting psychosocial risk factors on safety and health outcomes. *BioMed Research International, 2015*, 1–12. https://doi.org/10.1155/2015/836967

Harms, P. D., Credé, M., Tynan, M., Leon, M., & Jeung, W. (2017). Leadership and stress: A meta-analytic review. *The Leadership Quarterly, 28*(1), 178–194. https://doi.org/10.1016/j.leaqua.2016.10.006

Hentrich, S., Zimber, A., Garbade, S. F., Gregersen, S., Nienhaus, A., & Petermann, F. (2017). Relationships between transformational leadership and health: The mediating role of perceived job demands and occupational self-efficacy. *International Journal of Stress Management, 24*(1), 34–61. https://doi.org/10.1037/str0000027

Hildenbrand, K., Sacramento, C. A., & Binnewies, C. (2018). Transformational leadership and burnout: The role of thriving and followers' openness to experience. *Journal of Occupational Health Psychology, 23*(1), 31–43. https://doi.org/10.1037/ocp0000051

Hobfoll, S. E. (1989). Conservation of resources: A new attempt at conceptualizing stress. *American Psychologist, 44*(3), 513–524. https://doi.org/10.1037/0003-066X.44.3.513

Inceoglu, I., Thomas, G., Chu, C., Plans, D., & Gerbasi, A. (2018). Leadership behavior and employee well-being: An integrated review and a future research agenda. *The Leadership Quarterly, 29*(1), 179–202. https://doi.org/10.1016/j.leaqua.2017.12.006

Judge, T. A., & Piccolo, R. F. (2004). Transformational and transactional leadership: A meta-analytic test of their relative validity. *Journal of Applied Psychology, 89*(5), 755–768. https://doi.org/10.1037/0021-9010.89.5.755

Kaluza, A. J., Boer, D., Buengeler, C., & van Dick, R. (2020). Leadership behaviour and leader self-reported well-being: A review, integration and meta-analytic examination. *Work and Stress, 34*(1), 34–56. https://doi.org/10.1080/02678373.2019.1617369

Kelloway, E. K., & Barling, J. (2010). Leadership development as an intervention in occupational health psychology. *Work and Stress, 24*(3), 260–279. https://doi.org/10.1080/02678373.2010.518441

Kelloway, E. K., Barling, J., & Helleur, J. (2000). Enhancing transformational leadership: The roles of training and feedback. *Leadership and Organization Development Journal, 21*(3), 145–149. https://doi.org/10.1108/01437730010325022

Kelloway, E. K., & Francis, L. (2013). Longitudinal research and data analysis. In R. R. Sinclair, M. Wang, & L. E. Tetrick (Eds.), *Research methods in occupational health psychology: Measurement, design and data analysis* (pp. 374–394). Routledge.

Kelloway, E. K., Mullen, J., & Francis, L. (2006). Divergent effects of transformational and passive leadership on employee safety. *Journal of Occupational Health Psychology, 11*(1), 76–86. https://doi.org/10.1037/1076-8998.11.1.76

Kelloway, E. K., Mullen, J., Ozblizir, T., & Wong, J. (2018, September 16). *The definition and effects of leaders' safety hypocrisy* [Paper presentation]. The European Association of Occupational Health Psychology Conference, Lisbon, Portugal.

Kelloway, E. K., Sivanathan, N., & Francis, L. (2005). Poor leadership. In J. Barling, E. K. Kelloway, & M. Frone (Eds.), *Handbook of workplace stress* (pp. 89–112). Sage. https://doi.org/10.4135/9781412975995.n5

Kelloway, E. K., Turner, N., Barling, J., & Loughlin, C. (2012). Transformational leadership and employee psychological well-being: The mediating role of employee trust in leadership. *Work and Stress, 26*(1), 39–55. https://doi.org/10.1080/02678373.2012.660774

Kines, P., Andersen, L. P., Spangenberg, S., Mikkelsen, K. L., Dyreborg, J., & Zohar, D. (2010). Improving construction site safety through leader-based verbal safety communication. *Journal of Safety Research, 41*(5), 399–406. https://doi.org/10.1016/j.jsr.2010.06.005

Koch, A. R., & Binnewies, C. (2015). Setting a good example: Supervisors as work-life-friendly role models within the context of boundary management. *Journal of Occupational Health Psychology, 20*(1), 82–92. https://doi.org/10.1037/a0037890

Kranabetter, C., & Niessen, C. (2017). Managers as role models for health: Moderators of the relationship of transformational leadership with employee exhaustion and cynicism. *Journal of Occupational Health Psychology, 22*(4), 492–502. https://doi.org/10.1037/ocp0000044

Li, Y., Wang, Z., Yang, L.-Q., & Liu, S. (2016). The crossover of psychological distress from leaders to subordinates in teams: The role of abusive supervision, psychological capital, and team performance. *Journal of Occupational Health Psychology, 21*(2), 142–153. https://doi.org/10.1037/a0039960

Liu, J., Siu, O., & Shi, K. (2010). Transformational leadership and employee well-being: The mediating role of trust in the leader and self-efficacy. *Applied Psychology, 59*(3), 454–479. https://doi.org/10.1111/j.1464-0597.2009.00407.x

Martinko, M. J., Harvey, P., Brees, J. R., & Mackey, J. (2013). A review of abusive supervision research. *Journal of Organizational Behavior, 34*(S1), S120–S137. https://doi.org/10.1002/job.1888

Mathieu, M., Eschleman, K. J., & Cheng, D. (2019). Meta-analytic and multiwave comparison of emotional support and instrumental support in the workplace. *Journal of Occupational Health Psychology, 24*(3), 387–409. https://doi.org/10.1037/ocp0000135

McIlroy, T. D., Parker, S. L., & McKimmie, B. M. (2021). The effects of unanswered supervisor support on employees' well-being, performance, and relational outcomes.

Journal of Occupational Health Psychology, 26(1), 49–68. https://doi.org/10.1037/ocp0000270

McLean, R. (2020). *These companies plan to make working from home the new normal. As in forever.* CNN. https://www.cnn.com/2020/05/22/tech/work-from-home-companies/index.html

Moen, P., Kelly, E. L., Tranby, E., & Huang, Q. (2011). Changing work, changing health: Can real work-time flexibility promote health behaviors and well-being? *Journal of Health and Social Behavior, 52*(4), 404–429. https://doi.org/10.1177/0022146511418979

Mohr, C. D., Hammer, L. B., Brady, J. M., Perry, M. L., & Bodner, T. (2021). Can supervisor support improve daily employee well-being? Evidence of supervisor training effectiveness in a study of veteran employee emotions. *Journal of Occupational and Organizational Psychology, 94*(2), 400–426. https://doi.org/10.1111/joop.12342

Montano, D., Reeske, A., Franke, F., & Hüffmeier, J. (2017). Leadership, followers' mental health and job performance in organizations: A comprehensive meta-analysis from an occupational health perspective. *Journal of Organizational Behavior, 38*(3), 327–350. https://doi.org/10.1002/job.2124

Mullen, J., Fiset, J., & Rhéaume, A. (2018). Destructive forms of leadership: The effects of abusive supervision and incivility on employee health and safety. *Leadership & Organization Development Journal, 39*(8), 946–961. https://doi.org/10.1108/LODJ-06-2018-0203

Mullen, J., & Kelloway, E. K. (2011). Occupational health and safety leadership. In J. C. Quick & L. E. Tetrick (Eds.), *Handbook of occupational health psychology* (2nd ed., pp. 357–372). American Psychological Association.

Mullen, J., Kelloway, E. K., & Teed, M. (2011). Inconsistent style of leadership as a predictor of safety behaviour. *Work and Stress, 25*(1), 41–54. https://doi.org/10.1080/02678373.2011.569200

Mullen, J., Kelloway, E. K., & Teed, M. (2017). Employer safety obligations, transformational leadership and their interactive effects on employee safety performance. *Safety Science, 91*, 405–412. https://doi.org/10.1016/j.ssci.2016.09.007

Mullen, J. E., & Kelloway, E. K. (2009). Safety leadership: A longitudinal study of the effects of transformational leadership on safety outcomes. *Journal of Occupational and Organizational Psychology, 82*(2), 253–272. https://doi.org/10.1348/096317908X325313

Nayani, R. J., Nielsen, K., Daniels, K., Donaldson-Feilder, E. J., & Lewis, R. C. (2018). Out of sight and out of mind? A literature review of occupational safety and health leadership and management of distributed workers. *Work and Stress, 32*(2), 124–146. https://doi.org/10.1080/02678373.2017.1390797

Nielsen, K., & Daniels, K. (2016). The relationship between transformational leadership and follower sickness absences: The role of presenteeism. *Work and Stress, 30*(2), 193–208. https://doi.org/10.1080/02678373.2016.1170736

Nielsen, K., Daniels, K., Nayani, R., Donaldson-Feilder, E., & Lewis, R. (2019). Out of mind, out of sight? Leading distributed workers to ensure health and safety. *Work and Stress, 33*(2), 173–191. https://doi.org/10.1080/02678373.2018.1509402

Nielsen, K., & Taris T. W. (2019). Leading well: Challenges to researching leadership in occupational health psychology–and some ways forward. *Work and Stress, 33*(2), 107–118. https://doi.org/10.1080/02678373.2019.1592263

Nielsen, K., Yarker, J., Brenner, S. O., Randall, R., & Borg, V. (2008). The importance of transformational leadership style for the well-being of employees working with older people. *Journal of Advanced Nursing, 63*(5), 465–475. https://doi.org/10.1111/j.1365-2648.2008.04701.x

Nielsen, M. B., Skogstad, A., Gjerstad, J., & Einarsen, S. V. (2019). Are transformational and laissez-faire leadership related to state anxiety among subordinates? A two-wave prospective study of forward and reverse associations. *Work and Stress, 33*(2), 137–155. https://doi.org/10.1080/02678373.2018.1528307

Olsen, O. K., Hetland, J., Berge Matthiesen, S., Løvik Hoprekstad, Ø., Espevik, R., & Bakker, A. B. (2021). Passive avoidant leadership and safety non-compliance:

A 30 days diary study among naval cadets. *Safety Science, 138,* Article 105100. https://doi.org/10.1016/j.ssci.2020.105100

Podsakoff, P. M., MacKenzie, S. B., Lee, J. Y., & Podsakoff, N. P. (2003). Common method biases in behavioral research: A critical review of the literature and recommended remedies. *Journal of Applied Psychology, 88*(5), 879–903. https://doi.org/10.1037/0021-9010.88.5.879

Rafferty, A., Restubog, S. L., & Jimmieson, N. (2010). Losing sleep: Examining the cascading effects of supervisors' experience of injustice on subordinates' psychological health. *Work and Stress, 24*(1), 36–55. https://doi.org/10.1080/02678371003715135

Schyns, B., & Schilling, J. (2013). How bad are the effects of bad leaders? A meta-analysis of destructive leadership and its outcomes. *The Leadership Quarterly, 24*(1), 138–158. https://doi.org/10.1016/j.leaqua.2012.09.001

Skogstad, A., Hetland, J., Glasø, L., & Einarsen, S. (2014). Is avoidant leadership a root cause of subordinate stress? Longitudinal relationships between laissez-faire leadership and role ambiguity. *Work and Stress, 28*(4), 323–341. https://doi.org/10.1080/02678373.2014.957362

Skogstad, A., Nielsen, M. B., & Einarsen, S. (2017). Destructive forms of leadership and their relationships with employee well-being. In E. K. Kelloway, K. Nielsen, & J. K. Dimoff (Eds.), *Leading to occupational health and safety* (pp. 163–195). Wiley.

Smith, T. D., Eldridge, F., & DeJoy, D. M. (2016). Safety-specific transformational and passive leadership influences on firefighter safety climate perceptions and safety behavior outcomes. *Safety Science, 86,* 92–97. https://doi.org/10.1016/j.ssci.2016.02.019

Sprigg, C. A., Niven, K., Dawson, J., Farley, S., & Armitage, C. J. (2019). Witnessing workplace bullying and employee well-being: A two-wave field study. *Journal of Occupational Health Psychology, 24*(2), 286–296. https://doi.org/10.1037/ocp0000137

Tepper, B. J. (2000). Consequences of abusive supervision. *Academy of Management Journal, 43*(2), 178–190. https://doi.org/10.2307/1556375

Tucker, S., Ogunfowora, B., & Ehr, D. (2016). Safety in the C-suite: How chief executive officers influence organizational safety climate and employee injuries. *Journal of Applied Psychology, 101*(9), 1228–1239. https://doi.org/10.1037/apl0000116

Van de Ven, B., van den Tooren, M., & Vlerick, P. (2013). Emotional job resources and emotional support seeking as moderators of the relation between emotional job demands and emotional exhaustion: A two-wave panel study. *Journal of Occupational Health Psychology, 18*(1), 1–8. https://doi.org/10.1037/a0030656

Velez, M. J., & Neves, P. (2016). Abusive supervision, psychosomatic symptoms, and deviance: Can job autonomy make a difference? *Journal of Occupational Health Psychology, 21*(3), 322–333. https://doi.org/10.1037/a0039959

von Thiele Schwarz, U., Hasson, H., & Tafvelin, S. (2016). Leadership training as an occupational health intervention: Improved safety and sustained productivity. *Safety Science, 81,* 35–45. https://doi.org/10.1016/j.ssci.2015.07.020

Wong, J., Ozbilir, T., & Mullen, J. (2016). Developing safety leadership. In E. K. Kelloway, K. Neilsen, & J. Dimoff (Eds.), *Leading to occupational health and safety* (pp. 49–68). Wiley.

Wong, J. H. K., & Kelloway, E. K. (2016). What happens at work stays at work? Workplace supervisory social interactions and blood pressure outcomes. *Journal of Occupational Health Psychology, 21*(2), 133–141. https://doi.org/10.1037/a0039900

Wong, J. H. K., Kelloway, E. K., & Makhan, D. W. (2015). Safety leadership. In S. Clarke, T. M. Probst, F. Guldenmund, & J. Passmore (Eds.), *The Wiley Blackwell handbook of the psychology of occupational safety and workplace health* (pp. 83–110). Wiley-Blackwell. https://doi.org/10.1002/9781118979013.ch5

World Health Organization (WHO). (2020). *WHO Director-General's opening remarks at the media briefing on COVID-19—11 March 2020.* https://www.who.int/director-general/speeches/detail/who-director-general-s-opening-remarks-at-the-media-briefing-on-covid-19---11-march-2020

Yang, L.-Q., Zheng, X., Liu, X., Lu, C. Q., & Schaubroeck, J. M. (2020). Abusive supervision, thwarted belongingness, and workplace safety: A group engagement perspective. *Journal of Applied Psychology, 105*(3), 230–244. https://doi.org/10.1037/apl0000436

Zineldin, M., & Hytter, A. (2012). Leaders' negative emotions and leadership styles influencing subordinates' well-being. *International Journal of Human Resource Management, 23*(4), 748–758. https://doi.org/10.1080/09585192.2011.606114

Zohar, D. (2002). Modifying supervisory practices to improve subunit safety: A leadership-based intervention model. *Journal of Applied Psychology, 87*(1), 156–163. https://doi.org/10.1037/0021-9010.87.1.156

Zohar, D., & Luria, G. (2003). The use of supervisory practices as leverage to improve safety behavior: A cross-level intervention model. *Journal of Safety Research, 34*(5), 567–577. https://doi.org/10.1016/j.jsr.2003.05.006

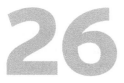

The Work–Nonwork Interface

Policy and Practice

Leslie B. Hammer and Tori L. Crain

Occupational health psychology (OHP) has traditionally been based at the intersection of the organization, the individual, and the work–nonwork interface (Quick, 1999). Thus, a new chapter in this edition of the handbook is devoted to work–nonwork policies and practices. Focusing on the organization of work and the workplace environment as the primary lever for reducing employee work–nonwork stress, in addition to improving health, safety, and well-being, such workplace policies and practices are critical to achieving positive employee outcomes. Furthermore, such organizational approaches as policies and practices are seen as primary prevention strategies for changing the workplace environment to achieve improvements in employee well-being. While a review of employee stress and well-being is covered in prior chapters of this volume, and specifically in Chapter 19, the present chapter focuses on the workplace policies and practices that have shown promise in preventing and reducing work–nonwork stress, ultimately improving employee health, safety, and well-being.

Occupational stress has contributed up to $190 billion in annual U.S. health care costs, with one of the largest contributing factors being work–nonwork stress, costing up to $24 billion (Goh et al., 2015). Work–nonwork stress is identified as an occupational hazard that should be given the same attention as other workplace environmental hazards (Hammer & Sauter, 2013). Work–nonwork stress impacts numerous health and well-being outcomes, as well as work and family outcomes, and is consistently named as one of the most

https://doi.org/10.1037/0000331-026
Handbook of Occupational Health Psychology, Third Edition, L. E. Tetrick, G. G. Fisher, M. T. Ford, and J. C. Quick (Editors)

significant stressors affecting today's workforce (American Psychological Association [APA], 2016, 2020).

Additionally, the focus on employee well-being has never been so important, as reports reveal extreme levels of psychological distress among the general population in relation to the COVID-19 pandemic (e.g., APA, 2020). Much of this stress has been reported by younger workers, working parents, and single parents more specifically. Given the increased attention to the work–nonwork interface, and the more recent recognition by workplaces of the importance of employee well-being in light of the COVID-19 pandemic, the focus of this chapter is timely. While the pandemic has brought the topic of work–nonwork balance to the forefront of workplace policies and practice, especially related to gendered patterns in child care and the newly revised flexible and hybrid work schedules, the importance of worker well-being was more formally recognized at the national level before the pandemic (Hammer & Brady, 2021). For example, in 2019 the U.S. Surgeon General reported that the National Academy of Medicine and the Occupational Safety and Health Administration had identified worker well-being as a "nationally important health issue" and that working conditions (including workplace policies and practices), in particular, can improve or damage individual well-being (Adams, 2019, p. 583). Furthermore, critical efforts are underway to advance a much-needed U.S. national paid family and medical leave policy, greatly enhancing the Family and Medical Leave Act of 1993 by guaranteeing *paid* leave; unfortunately, only 21% of the U.S. workforce currently has access to paid family and medical leave through their employer (Scalia & Beach, 2020).

Given these high levels of work–nonwork stress, an increasing need to support employees' family life as a result of the COVID-19 pandemic, and a lack of federal legislation that supports working families, in this chapter we explore work–nonwork policies and practices in hopes of facilitating future research and applied work.

When using the term *work–nonwork policies*, we are referring broadly to any formal standards, rules, or guidelines put forward by organizations, that address the intersection between work and nonwork and are fairly permanent, until there is a proposed policy change. *Work–nonwork practices*, on the other hand, involve less formal initiatives, interventions, and programs provided by the organization or implemented by supervisors/managers that aim to improve employee experiences of the work–nonwork interface. Such policies and practices include, but are not limited to, human resource policies (e.g., hybrid work, flexible work arrangements, reduced work hours) and leadership trainings and interventions (e.g., family-supportive supervisor behavior training) that can impact the work–nonwork interface. In other work, these policies and practices have fallen under the umbrella term of *work–family supports*; Masterson et al. (2021) referred to discretionary and formal work–family supports in their review, and French and Shockley (2020) differentiated between formal supports provided by the organization and informal support provided by other individuals through their behaviors. Similarly, Hammer et al. (2005) identified formal work–family supports that included "policies (e.g., flexible work arrangements), services (e.g., resource and referral information about dependent care options), and benefits (e.g., child care subsidies)" (p. 799).

It is the expectation that such work–family supports—in the form of policies, practices, services, and benefits—provide workers with resources, leading to a reduction in occupational stressors such as work–family stress (i.e., physical and psychological reactions that result from engaging in one role that in turn interferes with engaging in the other role). However, the rest of this chapter focuses primarily on policies and practices within workplaces, and less on services and benefits related to the work–nonwork interface. Furthermore, we abstain from discussing national family policy in depth, although our future directions section does mention it, given that excellent resources exist elsewhere (e.g., Ferragina, 2020; Nieuwenhuis & Van Lancker, 2020; Ooms, 2019). We next describe theories that have informed this work, review existing research on workplace work–nonwork policies and practices, and conclude the chapter by discussing future directions for research.

THEORETICAL FOUNDATIONS FOR WORK-NONWORK POLICY AND PRACTICE

As described in Chapter 7 of this volume, environmental and personal resources and demands impact work–nonwork balance through work–family conflict and work–family enrichment perceptions. The present chapter focuses on resources and demands associated with workplace policies and practices, drawing on the *Total Worker Health*® approach to worker safety, health, and well-being, as well as the conservation of resources theory (Hobfoll, 1989).

The *Total Worker Health* (TWH) Approach

Launched by the National Institute for Occupational Safety and Health (NIOSH) in 2011 (Schill & Chosewood, 2013), TWH is defined as policies, programs, and practices that integrate protection from work-related safety and health hazards with promotion of injury and illness prevention efforts to advance worker well-being (Tamers et al., 2019). TWH approaches recognize the importance of workplace risk factors, as well as broader societal and economic risk factors, impacting worker health, safety, and well-being. Workplace hazard reduction is the first step in any TWH approach, and work–nonwork stress is an important occupational hazard (Hammer & Sauter, 2013). Furthermore, the *Total Worker Health* Agenda (2016–2026) identifies work–nonwork issues as a crucial area of national research (Department of Health and Human Services, Centers for Disease Control and Prevention, & National Institute for Occupational Safety and Health, 2016). Thus, given the significant impact of work–nonwork stress and conflict on worker health and well-being, many have argued that the work–nonwork interface is an ideal focus for TWH interventions (Hammer & Perry, 2019).

Conservation of Resources Theory

Conservation of resources (COR) *theory* suggests that individuals strive to obtain, maintain, and protect resources. COR assumes that a number of resources are universally valued across all individuals, including family, health, self-esteem, and a sense of purpose in life, and thus a threat to these resources is particularly stressful (Hobfoll et al., 2018). However, in addition to these common and universal resources, individuals also appraise certain resources as being more or less important to them personally. *Resources* can be broadly characterized as objects, personal characteristics, conditions, or energies of value to the individual or that serve to help the individual gain more resources; anything an individual perceives that helps them attain goals (Halbesleben et al., 2014). Indeed, a strength of the COR framework is that it acknowledges the potential for a multitude of resources, which is complemented by other theoretical frameworks that are more specific in nature (Hobfoll et al., 2018). However, given the central role of family as a universal motivator within the COR framework, work–nonwork policy and practice is necessarily concerned with how organizations can develop systems for ensuring that employees have access to resources that sustain family and nonwork life. Work–nonwork stress can occur when individuals experience loss of resources, threat of loss, or failure to gain expected resources (Hobfoll, 1989, 2002). One key resource often targeted within work–family policies and practices is social support in the workplace, which can serve as a buffer of work–nonwork stress, as well as a resource, impacting health and well-being outcomes for workers (Bakker & Demerouti, 2007; Cohen & Wills, 1985; Karasek, 1979).

Together, the TWH approach and COR are foundations for the development of policies and practices aimed at improving the work–nonwork interface. Such approaches that are designed to increase employees' perceived existing and available resources, and decrease perceptions of loss and threat to resources, are expected to decrease strain and lead to further resource gains, having a beneficial effect on the work–nonwork interface. Similarly, a recent review by Bakker and de Vries (2021) suggests that human resources practices, such as remote working policies, healthy leadership practices, and associated leadership social support training, all increase individual resources and are related to increased self-regulation. This increased self-regulation is suggested as an important mechanism through which we see improvements in well-being outcomes, such as decreased burnout and work–nonwork conflict. Thus, both frameworks offer a unique lens in terms of understanding policies, practices, resources, and demands associated with the work and nonwork interface.

HUMAN RESOURCES POLICIES AND PRACTICES AND THE WORK–NONWORK INTERFACE

Human resources policies and practices related to the work–nonwork interface have needed to evolve over the past 35 years, as workforce demographics have changed. The workplace is increasingly needing to support a diversity of families, with more single-parent employees, greater gender integration in organizations, increased ethnically and racially diverse workplaces, more varied cultural and religious representation across the workforce, greater visibility among members of the LGBTQ+ community within organizations, as well as greater diversity in age and disability status among workers. Such policies include, but are not limited to, flexible work arrangements, newly developing hybrid work policies, telecommuting policies, and family leave policies, as well as dependent support programs and educational assistance programs, to name a few.

In addition, organizational policies and practices aimed at supporting families were developed in response to greater numbers of women entering the workforce in the 1980s and 1990s, resulting in organizations being motivated to retain women in particular. Simultaneously, the Reagan administration implemented tax legislation limiting government social service expenditures by encouraging employers to create their own human service programs such as child care (Goodstein, 1994). More recently, these policies and practices are fueled by the recognition that employee health and well-being is intimately tied to support for work and nonwork. Thus, while employee attraction, retention, and organizational performance were traditionally important factors affecting organizational adoption of work–nonwork integration policies, worker health and well-being have recently advanced as critical strategic outcomes of such policies. As corporate policies and practices continue to develop around wellness and well-being, workplaces are motivated to cut health care costs and spending, and are becoming more interested in putting people first. This is consistent with societal trends over the past few decades, as scholarly research in the work–nonwork field has highlighted the critical need to support working families as both a community and corporate responsibility.

Much of this progression toward support for work and nonwork has also proven necessary due to virtually nonexistent national policies supporting families. Thus, the advancement of human resource policies and practices that support work and nonwork has occurred despite a lack of national leadership in the provision of federal supports for working families and, quite frankly, in response to the failure of the United States to prioritize working families' needs. An area in which this has become evident is during the COVID-19 pandemic, when work-from-home policies were mandated in many U.S. workplaces; despite no national leave policies being in place to support such arrangements and with a lack of nationally mandated guidelines regarding workplace flexibility, workers were still expected to continue at full pace. The impact was particularly felt among working families with young, school-aged children, as U.S. workers were expected to continue working while also caring for their children without missing a beat.

Utilization and Availability of Work Policies

Reviews and empirical research have demonstrated mixed findings on flexible work schedule policy effectiveness (e.g., Butts et al., 2013; Hammer et al., 2005; Masterson et al., 2021), suggesting that the effects of availability and use are not always consistent. For example, in a meta-analysis examining the relationship between work–family support initiatives and employee attitudes, Butts et al. (2013) found significant, positive associations between work–family policy availability and use with job satisfaction, affective commitment, and intentions to stay with the organization, and a negative relationship with work–family conflict. Alternatively, a recent meta-analysis on the relationship between flexible work arrangements and health demonstrated stronger positive relationships for availability of flexible work schedules, as compared with utilization of flexible work arrangements (Shifrin & Michel, 2021). Possible explanations for these inconsistencies include the challenges associated with actual utilization, which tends to be dependent on a supportive culture enabling such use (e.g., Shifrin & Michel, 2021); lack of cross-level analyses, as suggested by Masterson et al. (2021); lack of information on occupational differences and the possibility that those who were in most need, while they may be most likely to use the supports when available (Hammer et al., 2011), also may be least likely to have such supports available (e.g., people in lower wage occupations; Kossek & Lautsch, 2018). Additionally, reviews indicate that different types of employees experience the benefits of different work–family policies to different degrees; gender, marital status, and life stage associated with parenting can determine whether or not employees are able to reap the benefits of these policies (e.g., Allen et al., 2013; Masterson et al., 2021). Finally, while some of these policies and practices are less formal and can be implemented at the discretion of the manager or supervisor, others are more formalized within the workplace and available to all workers.

Work–Nonwork Policies and Occupational Level

Research shows that simply having a policy available impacts employee perceptions of organizational support. Unfortunately, such policies tend to be available only to certain occupational groups, and thus occupational status and flexibility practices vary and lead to work–nonwork inequality, as demonstrated by Kossek and Lautsch (2018). Many people in hourly, lower level jobs are unable to access policies or practices, which tend to benefit those who occupy middle- and upper-level positions. This showed up in a review of U.S. Census data demonstrating that unionized workers had less access to flexibility than other workers (Golden, 2009), and Kossek and Distelberg (2009) similarly showed that white-collar workers had greater access to flexibility.

Unfortunately, work–nonwork policies and practices are most often available to employees in professional-level jobs and those employed by larger organizations, thereby limiting access to employees in low-wage, hourly positions, who are most in need of such policies. Kossek and Lautsch (2018) demonstrated occupational differences in the location of work, with professionals and managers having more control over location. This sharp inequality was most recently seen in the treatment, health, and safety policies for "essential" and "nonessential" workers during the pandemic (Kossek & Lee, 2020), with a negative disparate impact on racially and ethnically diverse workers. However, much of the existing research has not been able to adequately account for such occupational differences due to the lack of a clear flexibility policy and lack of comparative information on occupational levels (Kossek & Lautsch, 2018). In general, what the research and practice related to work–nonwork policies and practices reveal is that both formal human resources policies and less formalized flexibility practices around where, when, and how people work generally lead to improvements in employee engagement at work, reductions in work–nonwork conflict, and improved overall well-being for employees, their families, and for the organizations in which they work (e.g., Kelly & Moen, 2007); however, differences exist in terms of who benefits based on the type of occupation and job level.

WORK–NONWORK HUMAN RESOURCE POLICIES DURING THE COVID-19 PANDEMIC

During the coronavirus pandemic, there has been an exponential increase in remote work policies, and the effects are appearing to be significant in terms of the work–nonwork interface. For example, in their qualitative study of dual-earner couples with young children during the COVID-19 pandemic, Shockley et al. (2021) found that while some families had very gendered approaches to the pandemic and remote work practices, with women taking on a majority of the child care responsibilities, even more families seemed to work out what was referred to as a more egalitarian approach to work and child care, which appeared to be more positively related to well-being. Such egalitarian approaches potentially required some additional informal flexibility from employers due to each member of the couple needing to split shifts and/or alternate working times to enable them to achieve work and care for their young children. Furthermore, in a study of boundary management among employees who switched to remote work during the pandemic, Allen et al. (2021) found that, contrary to their expectations, boundary management preferences for segmentation were related to higher levels of work–nonwork balance among the remote workers, and not surprisingly, this relationship was stronger for those who had a dedicated home office working space. The authors suggested that while most of these employees had traditionally worked in an office setting pre-COVID and thus may have been more oriented toward segmentation boundary management styles, perhaps the lack of a commute helped increase their nonwork time, thereby improving their work–nonwork balance.

Another critical issue to consider is the distinction between work–nonwork flexibility and work–nonwork flexible work schedule policies. The former is related to flexibility in where, when, and how one works, and as can be seen by the effects of the pandemic, people are much more effective and trustworthy than managers and supervisors previously gave them credit for being. Many people have worked more effectively without the added burden and time that is involved with commuting to and from work. Thus, providing workplace flexibility in where, when, and how people work can significantly affect employee well-being. At the same time, many people have been constrained due to limited or no workspace at home, coworking partners, and school-aged and younger children or older dependents at home needing assistance and attention during the workday.

Finally, it is clear that there is more need for compassion, support, and flexibility on the part of managers and supervisors to enable employees to work effectively during the pandemic and beyond (e.g., Sinclair et al., 2020; Vaziri et al., 2020). There also appears to be a greater move away from a focus on location of work to a focus on the results of work, similar to arguments in line with the results-only work environment approach that have demonstrated positive effects on work–nonwork outcomes (e.g., Kelly et al., 2011).

WORK–NONWORK POLICIES AND PRACTICES AND THE ROLE OF LEADERSHIP TRAININGS

Few work–nonwork policies or practices have been systematically evaluated using experimental designs and theoretically driven targets allowing for strong scientific conclusions about their effectiveness. One exception is those practices focused on leadership trainings (Hammer et al., 2016; Hammer & Perry, 2019). Because leaders, and especially supervisors and managers, work directly with employees daily as nonwork issues arise and act as gatekeepers and translators of organizational policies that can aid families, they have received special focus in the work–nonwork literature. Three key practices identified as impacting the work–nonwork interface are increasing control over work, increasing social support, and decreasing job demands, consistent with TWH, COR, as well as the job demand–control theory (Karasek, 1979). Control over where, when, and how one works, also referred to as workplace flexibility, was addressed earlier in the chapter, and thus we focus here on practices that aim to increase social support and decrease demands.

Family-Supportive Supervisor Behavior Training

Family-supportive supervisor behaviors (FSSBs; Hammer et al., 2009), in addition to organizational support for work and family, have been shown to be more strongly related to reduced work–family conflict than general nonspecific workplace supports (see Kossek et al., 2011). FSSBs consist of enacting four types of behaviors related to emotional support, instrumental support, role modeling, and creative work–family management. *Emotional support* refers to behaviors demonstrating a worker is cared for, and their feelings are being considered, especially with respect to their family and nonwork lives (e.g., having face-to-face contact with employees, asking how employees are doing, or communicating genuine concern about employees' work–life challenges). *Instrumental support* involves behaviors such as helping workers manage schedules and working with employees to solve schedule conflicts (e.g., helping an employee find a replacement, if absent). *Role modeling* refers to behaviors that demonstrate how a supervisor is taking care of their own work/nonwork challenges (e.g., discussing taking time out to attend a child's school activities and talking about one's own family, leaving work at reasonable hours, or showing that managers value involvement in nonwork life). *Creative work–family management* has to do with behaviors aimed at redesigning work to support conflicting employee work–nonwork demands in a manner that is mutually beneficial for both employees and employers (e.g., promoting cross-training and giving employees the ability to trade shifts to enable schedule flexibility and work coverage).

FSSB training was effectively evaluated as part of the Work, Family, and Health Network (WFHN) randomized study in the information technology and health care industries, the most extensive evaluation of a work–nonwork intervention to date. As part of the initial research, the beneficial effects of FSSB training were found on worker job satisfaction, turnover intentions, and reports of physical health among those employees with high work–family conflict at baseline (Hammer et al., 2011). The work–nonwork practices evaluated included increasing control over work and increasing supervisor support for work and family (i.e., FSSB). The WFHN study focused on training supervisors to be more supportive of employees who were managing work and family demands and also involved facilitated sessions prompting employees to discuss where and when they work in the information technology and health care industry sectors. Researchers found that together the practices led to an increase in employees' perceived schedule control and significantly increased employee perceptions of their supervisor eliciting supervisor support for family and personal life, as well as decreased work–family conflict (Kelly et al., 2014). Likewise, Moen et al. (2016) found that the WFHN intervention (made up of supervisor FSSB training and practices to increase control over work) had significant effects on reduced burnout, perceived stress, and psychological distress, and increased job satisfaction among information technology workers. Kossek et al. (2019) evaluated the effects of the WFHN intervention among health care workers and found that it decreased psychological distress for employees with elder care responsibilities. Thus, this leader intervention, with primary components focused on improving social support and increasing flexibility provided by managers and supervisors, demonstrated having significant effects on employee psychological health outcomes, hence improving well-being. A number of additional studies have demonstrated the beneficial impact of the WFHN workplace intervention on worker health, safety, and well-being as well as child well-being and organizational outcomes (e.g., Crain et al., 2019; Davis et al., 2015; Hammer et al., 2016; Hurtado et al., 2016; Kelly et al., 2014; McHale et al., 2015; Olson et al., 2015; see https://workfamilyhealthnetwork.org/).

Hammer and colleagues, as part of the Oregon Healthy Workforce Center (OHWC), a TWH center of excellence, developed and evaluated the implementation of the Safety and Health Improvement Program (SHIP) based on the integration of FSSB training, and supervisor support for safety, in combination with a team-based approach called Team Effectiveness Process developed by Work Family Directions (Hammer et al., 2015; Hammer, Truxillo, et al., 2019). While no effects of the work–life stress reduction practices were found for safety outcomes, the program did reduce blood pressure at the 12-month follow-up as well as increased reports of employee work–life effectiveness (see the Oregon Healthy Workforce Center website for SHIP and other evidence-based TWH intervention materials [https://www.yourworkpath.com/ship]).

Veteran supportive supervisor training was designed to improve workplace resources and support for reintegrated veterans in the general workforce across industries. It teaches supervisors and managers to appreciate and foster the unique skills, leadership experience, and dedication that veterans bring to the workplace, and improves veterans' work–nonwork balance, health, and well-being. This program was originally developed and evaluated through the Study for Employment Retention of Veterans (https://www.servestudy.org). Training produced significant improvements in employee stress (among those whose supervisors' attitudes toward veterans improved), physical health and sleep quality, marital relationship quality and parenting behaviors, and job outcomes (e.g., Brady et al., 2021; Hammer et al., 2015; Hammer, Wan, et al., 2019; Mohr et al., 2021).

FUTURE RESEARCH AND PRACTICAL SUGGESTIONS

Although extensive research to date has evaluated work–nonwork policies and practices, we provide suggestions in the next section to further improve our understanding of the availability, use, and effectiveness of these supports. A unique characteristic of this topic is that a number of key stakeholders at different levels are involved with the design, implementation, utilization, and evaluation of policies and practices, both within organizations (i.e., employees, supervisors, executive-level decision makers, human resources departments) and outside of organizations (i.e., employees' families, legislators). Thus, many of our recommendations for future directions involve interactions between these stakeholders across levels and contexts. As a general recommendation, we suggest that future research move beyond just employee experiences and capture the effects of policies and practices within family systems, while also considering how the employee is embedded within multilevel organizational hierarchies as well as national and local contexts.

THE ROLE OF PUBLIC AND PRIVATE WORK–FAMILY POLICY

The United States lags far behind other industrialized countries in terms of public family policies. Despite the Family and Medical Leave Act of 1993 providing eligible workers, albeit approximately less than 60%, with unpaid caregiving leave, organizations are not required by federal law to provide employees with paid leave (Williams, 2021). Currently, nine states (i.e., Washington, Oregon, California, Colorado, New York, Massachusetts, Rhode Island, Connecticut, New Jersey) and the District of Columbia have enacted paid family and medical leave policies, with Hawaii providing paid medical leave in the form of temporary disability insurance. Furthermore, research indicates that of those individuals who do take leave, they frequently take less time off than they believe is necessary for their situation (Stepler, 2017). Although President Biden released the American Families Plan in 2021 that will be put before Congress, other countries have progressed much farther in their support of working families. For example, Estonia provides 86 weeks of paid leave to new parents, with a number of other countries offering more than a full year (e.g., Japan, Norway, Bulgaria; Livingston & Thomas, 2019). Yet, as described by Hammer and Brady (2021), certain groups in the United States are likely to face more challenges in accessing leave of any type (e.g., fathers, parents with eldercare responsibilities, and LGBTQ+ individuals and families). Other findings from the Stepler (2017) indicate that Black and Latinx workers, individuals without a college education, and employees making less than $30,000 per year were less likely to be able to take the amount of family and/or medical leave needed.

Although an increase in rigorous methods to evaluate national policy effectiveness has recently been implemented (e.g., better survey data, program evaluation, randomized controlled trials), one noted obstacle and critique of family policy research is that few policy analysts and academics collaborate to understand the effectiveness of policy initiatives and their impact on individual workers (Ooms, 2019). Furthermore, decisions on how to spend money related to policy is often not informed by rigorous scientific evidence (Baron, 2018). Thus, there is a major need for policy reform in the United States to improve the lives of working families, interdisciplinary collaborations are necessary for future evaluation, and scientific evidence should be better used to inform future policy use.

Interestingly, research across all parts of the globe has often failed to evaluate the interaction between public work–family policy at national and state levels (e.g., paid parental leave, flexible work schedules, universal child care, vacation and sick time, cash allowances to parents) and workplace family policy and practices (Wiß & Greve, 2020). While some countries provide work–family policies as a common social benefit (e.g., Australia), other countries consider work–family support to be up to the discretion of each individual employer and even, in some cases, a benefit to attract highly qualified employees (e.g., the United States). Notably, some countries have adopted generous public family policies (e.g., Denmark), and organizations have also followed suit, likely due to the presence of effective and widespread union representation (Wiß & Greve, 2020) in addition to cultural beliefs about family and gender ideologies (Budig et al., 2016; Haney, 2010). In the United States, we must rely on workplace interventions for reducing work–nonwork stress because there is little support at the national level (Hammer & Brady, 2021). As

French and Shockley (2020) suggested, there is a need for future research that integrates an understanding of public policy at both the national and state levels, with organizations' provisions of policies to employees. For example, an examination of how the effectiveness of a work–nonwork policy provided by the organization is either strengthened or weakened in certain national or local contexts, and how this in turn affects both the employee and family, could be particularly valuable for future policy adoption and funding decisions. Understanding how and why organizational decision makers implement work–nonwork policies and practices in differing state and national contexts could provide beneficial insight into future intervention effectiveness.

AN EXPANDED UNDERSTANDING OF LEADERSHIP TRAINING

A growing and rigorous randomized controlled trial literature now shows that FSSB interventions are effective (Crain & Stevens, 2018). We encourage researchers to expand their focus to better encompass research questions that are of practical importance, namely, that of how FSSB can be promoted, encouraged, fostered, and sustained in actual workplaces. These studies might also answer the question of for whom FSSB training is the least and most effective. Although some research has found these interventions to be most effective for individuals with the highest levels of work–family conflict (Hammer et al., 2011), in teams with poor leadership relations and low cohesion (Hammer, Truxillo, et al., 2019), and among those with greater elder caregiving demands (Kossek et al., 2019), other recent work also suggests that implementation of some work–nonwork policies and practices can result in negative attitudes, emotions, and behaviors (i.e., "work–family backlash") for certain groups—for example, when a certain policy benefits one group more than others, resulting in perceptions of inequity (Perrigino et al., 2018). As such, there is a need for continued rigorous evaluation of these practices across occupational groups and employees with different demands. Yet it is also critical to target groups who are most in need of resources, while still improving the quality of life for the overall workforce.

An additional future direction addresses what organizations can do prior to training to establish a climate ripe for supervisor support. In a new line of research, Ellis et al. (2021) evaluated the extent to which supervisors who have not received FSSB training believed that FSSB was an expected part of their job duties. Interestingly, 9% of their sample disagreed or strongly disagreed that FSSB was an expected part of their job, while 54% reported that they agreed or strongly agreed that it was an expected part of their job, and 37% reported they were unsure of whether FSSB was an expected part of their job. The more supervisors believed FSSB to be a part of their job role, the more likely they were to actually engage in FSSB. Organizations hoping to foster a family-supportive culture need to make this expectation of supervisors clearer through documentation, communications from leadership, and throughout the performance review process.

DIVERSE FAMILIES IN WORK–FAMILY RESEARCH ON POLICY AND PRACTICE

As work–nonwork scholars have increasingly noted, both the workforce and families are growing increasingly diverse. However, recent research indicates that although gender and work–nonwork experiences have been well-addressed, race and class have often been left out of the conversation (Perry-Jenkins & Gerstel, 2020), and the research to date has largely ignored intersectional approaches to studying working families. For example, much of the FSSB intervention research to date has not evaluated whether there are differing intervention effects based on income and/or race/ethnicity, and how discrimination and inequity may be present in the availability and encouragement of policy utilization. Some research has begun to explore the experiences of immigrant workers, finding that work–family support from coworkers, as opposed to that from supervisors or the organization, is most beneficial (Robles-Saenz et al., 2021). Thus, different forms of support targeted in future interventions may be more helpful for certain groups. Additionally, as Murphy et al. (2021) suggested, the majority of research on work–nonwork experiences in general has been centered on the heteronormative couple and largely ignored the challenges and obstacles faced by LGBTQ+ employees and families. Future research in this vein could explore the unique experiences of LGBTQ+ employees requesting and receiving access to work–nonwork policies in the workplace, the necessity of having to disclose sexual or gender identities in the workplace in order to access work–nonwork benefits, and the potential for discrimination.

While much of the work–nonwork policy investigation so far has centered on workplace schedules and leaves, in addition to child care, little research to date has examined how economic inequity between families creates very different work–nonwork experiences and access to supports. Other research indicates, as previously mentioned, that individuals who are the most under resourced and most in need of work–nonwork support are the least likely to have access (Kossek & Lautsch, 2018). To complicate matters, new hires— especially in professional-level positions—are increasingly negotiating with employers for idiosyncratic deals (i-deals), which are defined as "voluntary, personalized agreements of a nonstandard nature negotiated between individual employees and their employers regarding terms that benefit each party" (Rousseau et al., 2006, p. 978). These proactive attempts to customize work arrangements (e.g., a flexible schedule, reduced work hours) are likely creating more inequity between certain groups of individuals, especially when hires from majority groups tend to hold greater negotiation power.

Understanding these informal practices, as opposed to more formal policies that are implemented broadly, is an important point of exploration related to equity.

CONCLUSION

Overall, human resources policies and practices are critical to the work–nonwork interface, due to the lack of public policies in the United States, and rigorous studies have demonstrated the key role that supervisor support training has on employee safety, health, well-being, and family-related outcomes. Addressing the stress that results from the integration of work and nonwork through the implementation of workplace policies and practices is consistent with suggestions that OHP interventions focus on primary prevention (Tetrick & Quick, 2011). The importance of this chapter is further amplified by the stress that the COVID-19 pandemic has brought to the work–nonwork interface. We have identified the important effects of policies and practices related to both formal and informal workplace flexibility on employees, the need for leader support, and the recognition that such policies and practices can have differential impacts on employees based on their occupational and income level, gender, race, identity, and family diversity—all factors that need to be considered in future research on work–nonwork policies and practices.

REFERENCES

Adams, J. M. (2019). The value of worker well-being. *Public Health Reports, 134*(6), 583–586. https://doi.org/10.1177/0033354919878434

Allen, T. D., Johnson, R. C., Kiburz, K. M., & Shockley, K. M. (2013). Work–family conflict and flexible work arrangements: Deconstructing flexibility. *Personnel Psychology, 66*(2), 345–376. https://doi.org/10.1111/peps.12012

Allen, T. D., Merlo, K., Lawrence, R. C., Slutsky, J., & Gray, C. E. (2021). Boundary management and work-nonwork balance while working from home. *Applied Psychology, 70*(1), 60–84. https://doi.org/10.1111/apps.12300

American Psychological Association. (2016). *Stress in America: The impact of discrimination.* Stress in America™ survey. https://www.apa.org/news/press/releases/stress/2015/impact-of-discrimination.pdf

American Psychological Association. (2020). *Stress in America™ 2020: A national mental health crisis.* https://www.apa.org/news/press/releases/stress/2020/report-october

Bakker, A. B., & de Vries, J. D. (2021). Job demands–resources theory and self-regulation: New explanations and remedies for job burnout. *Anxiety, Stress, and Coping, 34*(1), 1–21. https://doi.org/10.1080/10615806.2020.1797695

Bakker, A. B., & Demerouti, E. (2007). The job demands-resources model: State of the art. *Journal of Managerial Psychology, 22*(3), 309–328. https://doi.org/10.1108/02683940710733115

Baron, J. (2018). A brief history of evidence-based policy. *The Annals of the American Academy of Political and Social Science, 678*(1), 40–50. https://doi.org/10.1177/0002716218763128

Brady, J. M., Hammer, L. B., Mohr, C. D., & Bodner, T. E. (2021). Supportive supervisor training improves family relationships among employee and spouse dyads. *Journal of Occupational Health Psychology, 26*(1), 31–48. https://doi.org/10.1037/ocp0000264

Budig, M. J., Misra, J., & Boeckmann, I. (2016). Work–family policy trade-offs for mothers? Unpacking the cross-national variation in motherhood earnings penalties. *Work and Occupations, 43*(2), 119–177. https://doi.org/10.1177/0730888415615385

Butts, M. M., Casper, W. J., & Yang, T. S. (2013). How important are work–family support policies? A meta-analytic investigation of their effects on employee outcomes. *Journal of Applied Psychology, 98*(1), 1–25. https://doi.org/10.1037/a0030389

Cohen, S., & Wills, T. A. (1985). Stress, social support, and the buffering hypothesis. *Psychological Bulletin, 98*(2), 310–357. https://doi.org/10.1037/0033-2909.98.2.310

Crain, T. L., Hammer, L. B., Bodner, T., Olson, R., Kossek, E. E., Moen, P., & Buxton, O. M. (2019). Sustaining sleep: Results from the randomized controlled work, family, and health study. *Journal of Occupational Health Psychology, 24*(1), 180–197. https://doi.org/10.1037/ocp0000122

Crain, T. L., & Stevens, S. C. (2018). Family-supportive supervisor behaviors: A review and recommendations for research and practice. *Journal of Organizational Behavior, 39*(7), 869–888. https://doi.org/10.1002/job.2320

Davis, K. D., Lawson, K. M., Almeida, D. M., Kelly, E. L., King, R. B., Hammer, L., Casper, L. M., Okechukwu, C. A., Hanson, G., & McHale, S. M. (2015). Parents' daily time with their children: A workplace intervention. *Pediatrics, 135*(5), 875–882. https://doi.org/10.1542/peds.2014-2057

Department of Health and Human Services, Centers for Disease Control and Prevention, & National Institute for Occupational Safety and Health. (2016). *A national agenda to advance Total Worker Health research, policy, and capacity*. Publication 2016–114. https://www.cdc.gov/niosh/docs/2016-114/pdfs/nationaltwhagenda2016-1144-14-16.pdf

Ellis, A. M., Crain, T. L., & Stevens, S. C. (2021). Is it my job? Leaders' family-supportive role perceptions. *Journal of Managerial Psychology.* https://doi.org/10.1108/JMP-09-2020-0493

Ferragina, E. (2020). Family policy and women's employment outcomes in 45 high-income countries: A systematic qualitative review of 238 comparative and national studies. *Social Policy and Administration, 54*(7), 1016–1066. https://doi.org/10.1111/spol.12584

French, K. A., & Shockley, K. M. (2020). Formal and informal supports for managing work and family. *Current Directions in Psychological Science, 29*(2), 207–216. https://doi.org/10.1177/0963721420906218

Goh, J., Pfeffer, J., Zenios, S. A., & Rajpal, S. (2015). Workplace stressors & health outcomes: Health policy for the workplace. *Behavioral Science & Policy, 1*(1), 43–52. https://doi.org/10.1353/bsp.2015.0001

Golden, L. (2009). Flexible daily work schedules in U.S. jobs: Formal introductions needed? *Industrial Relations, 48*(1), 27–54. https://doi.org/10.1111/j.1468-232X.2008.00544.x

Goodstein, J. D. (1994). Institutional pressures and strategic responsiveness: Employer involvement in work-family issues. *Academy of Management Journal, 37*(2), 350–382. https://doi.org/10.5465/256833

Halbesleben, J. R., Neveu, J. P., Paustian-Underdahl, S. C., & Westman, M. (2014). Getting to the "COR": Understanding the role of resources in conservation of resources theory. *Journal of Management, 40*(5), 1334–1364. https://doi.org/10.1177/0149206314527130

Hammer, L. B., & Brady, J. M. (2021). Worker well-being and work-life issues. In L. Koppes Bryan (Ed.), *Historical perspectives in industrial and organizational psychology* (2nd ed., pp. 270–291). Routledge/Taylor and Francis Group.

Hammer, L. B., Brady, J. M., & Perry, M. L. (2020). Training supervisors to support veterans at work: Effects on supervisor attitudes and employee sleep and stress. *Journal of Occupational and Organizational Psychology, 93*(2), 273–301. https://doi.org/10.1111/joop.12299

Hammer, L. B., Demsky, C. A., Kossek, E. E., & Bray, J. W. (2016). Work–family intervention research. In T. D. Allen & L. T. Eby (Eds.), *The Oxford handbook of work and family* (pp. 349–361). Oxford University Press. https://doi.org/10.1093/oxfordhb/9780199337538.013.27

Hammer, L. B., Kossek, E. E., Anger, W. K., Bodner, T., & Zimmerman, K. L. (2011). Clarifying work–family intervention processes: The roles of work–family conflict and family-supportive supervisor behaviors. *Journal of Applied Psychology, 96*(1), 134–150. https://doi.org/10.1037/a0020927

Hammer, L. B., Kossek, E. E., Yragui, N. L., Bodner, T. E., & Hanson, G. C. (2009). Development and validation of a multidimensional measure of family supportive supervisor behaviors (FSSB). *Journal of Management, 35*(4), 837–856. https://doi.org/10.1177/0149206308328510

Hammer, L. B., Neal, M. B., Newsom, J. T., Brockwood, K. J., & Colton, C. L. (2005). A longitudinal study of the effects of dual-earner couples' utilization of family-friendly workplace supports on work and family outcomes. *Journal of Applied Psychology, 90*(4), 799–810. https://doi.org/10.1037/0021-9010.90.4.799

Hammer, L. B., & Perry, M. L. (2019). Reducing work–life stress: The place for integrated interventions. In H. L. Hudson, J. A. S. Nigam, S. L. Sauter, L. C. Chosewood, A. L. Schill, & J. Howard (Eds.), *Total Worker Health* (pp. 263–278). American Psychological Association. https://doi.org/10.1037/0000149-016

Hammer, L. B., & Sauter, S. (2013). Total worker health and work–life stress. *Journal of Occupational and Environmental Medicine, 55,* S25–S29. https://doi.org/10.1097/JOM.0000000000000043

Hammer, L. B., Truxillo, D. M., Bodner, T., Pytlovany, A. C., & Richman, A. (2019). Exploration of the impact of organisational context on a workplace safety and health intervention. *Work and Stress, 33*(2), 192–210. https://doi.org/10.1080/02678373.2018.1496159

Hammer, L. B., Truxillo, D. M., Bodner, T., Rineer, J., Pytlovany, A. C., & Richman, A. (2015). Effects of a workplace intervention targeting psychosocial risk factors on safety and health outcomes: Psychosocial factors and workers health and safety. *BioMed Research International, 2015,* 836967. https://doi.org/10.1155/2015/836967

Hammer, L. B., Wan, W. H., Brockwood, K., Bodner, T., & Mohr, C. D. (2019). Supervisor support training effects on veteran health and work outcomes in the civilian workplace. *Journal of Applied Psychology, 104,* 52–69. https://doi.org/10.1037/apl0000354

Haney, L. (2010). *Offending women: Power, punishment, and the regulation of desire.* University of California Press. https://doi.org/10.1525/9780520945913

Hobfoll, S. E. (1989). Conservation of resources: A new attempt at conceptualizing stress. *American Psychologist, 44*(3), 513–524. https://doi.org/10.1037/0003-066X.44.3.513

Hobfoll, S. E. (2002). Social and psychological resources and adaptation. *Review of General Psychology, 6*(4), 307–324. https://doi.org/10.1037/1089-2680.6.4.307

Hobfoll, S. E., Halbesleben, J., Neveu, J. P., & Westman, M. (2018). Conservation of resources in the organizational context: The reality of resources and their consequences. *Annual Review of Organizational Psychology and Organizational Behavior, 5*(1), 103–128. https://doi.org/10.1146/annurev-orgpsych-032117-104640

Hurtado, D. A., Okechukwu, C. A., Buxton, O. M., Hammer, L., Hanson, G. C., Moen, P., Klein, L. C., & Berkman, L. F. (2016). Effects on cigarette consumption of a work–family supportive organisational intervention: 6-month results from the work, family and health network study. *Journal of Epidemiology and Community Health, 70*(12), 1155–1161. https://doi.org/10.1136/jech-2015-206953

Karasek, R. A., Jr. (1979). Job demands, job decision latitude, and mental strain: Implications for job redesign. *Administrative Science Quarterly, 24*(2), 285–308. https://doi.org/10.2307/2392498

Kelly, E. L., & Moen, P. (2007). Rethinking the clockwork of work: Why schedule control may pay off at work and at home. *Advances in Developing Human Resources, 9*(4), 487–506. https://doi.org/10.1177/1523422307305489

Kelly, E. L., Moen, P., Oakes, J. M., Fan, W., Okechukwu, C., Davis, K. D., Hammer, L., Kossek, E., King, R. B., Hanson, G., Mierzwa, F., & Casper, L. (2014). Changing work and work-family conflict: Evidence from the work, family, and health network. *American Sociological Review, 79*(3), 485–516. https://doi.org/10.1177/0003122414531435

Kelly, E. L., Moen, P., & Tranby, E. (2011). Changing workplaces to reduce work-family conflict: Schedule control in a white-collar organization. *American Sociological Review, 76*(2), 265–290. https://doi.org/10.1177/0003122411400056

Kossek, E., & Distelberg, B. (2009). Work and family employment policy for a transformed work force: Trends and themes. In N. Crouter & A. Booth (Eds.), *Work-life policies that make a real difference for individuals, families, and organizations* (pp. 1–51). Urban Institute Press.

Kossek, E. E., & Lautsch, B. A. (2018). Work–life flexibility for whom? Occupational status and work–life inequality in upper, middle, and lower level jobs. *The Academy of Management Annals, 12*(1), 5–36. https://doi.org/10.5465/annals.2016.0059

Kossek, E. E., & Lee, K.-H. (2020). The coronavirus & work–life inequality: Three evidence-based initiatives to update U.S. work–life employment policies. *Behavioral Science & Policy.* https://behavioralpolicy.org/journal_issue/covid-19/

Kossek, E. E., Pichler, S., Bodner, T., & Hammer, L. B. (2011). Workplace social support and work–family conflict: A meta-analysis clarifying the influence of general and work–family-specific supervisor and organizational support. *Personnel Psychology, 64*(2), 289–313. https://doi.org/10.1111/j.1744-6570.2011.01211.x

Kossek, E. E., Thompson, R. J., Lawson, K. M., Bodner, T., Perrigino, M. B., Hammer, L. B., Buxton, O. M., Almeida, D. M., Moen, P., Hurtado, D. A., Wipfli, B., Berkman, L. F., & Bray, J. W. (2019). Caring for the elderly at work and home: Can a randomized organizational intervention improve psychological health? *Journal of Occupational Health Psychology, 24*(1), 36–54. https://doi.org/10.1037/ocp0000104

Livingston, G., & Thomas, D. (2019, August 7). *Among 41 countries, only U.S. lacks paid parental leave.* Pew Research Center. https://www.pewresearch.org/fact-tank/2019/12/16/u-s-lacks-mandated-paid-parental-leave/

Masterson, C., Sugiyama, K., & Ladge, J. (2021). The value of 21st century work-family supports: Review and cross-level path forward. *Journal of Organizational Behavior, 42*(2), 118–138. https://doi.org/10.1002/job.2442

McHale, S. M., Lawson, K. M., Davis, K. D., Casper, L., Kelly, E. L., & Buxton, O. (2015). Effects of a workplace intervention on sleep in employees' children. *The Journal of Adolescent Health, 56*(6), 672–677. https://doi.org/10.1016/j.jadohealth.2015.02.014

Moen, P., Kelly, E. L., Fan, W., Lee, S.-R., Almeida, D., Kossek, E. E., & Buxton, O. M. (2016). Does a flexibility/support organizational initiative improve high-tech employees' well-being? Evidence from the work, family, and health network. *American Sociological Review, 81*(1), 134–164. https://doi.org/10.1177/0003122415622391

Mohr, C. D., Hammer, L. B., Brady, J., Perry, M., & Bodner, T. (2021). Can supervisor support improve daily employee well-being? Evidence of supervisor training effectiveness in a study of veteran employee moods. *Journal of Occupational and Organizational Psychology, 94*(2), 400–426. https://doi.org/10.1111/joop.12342

Murphy, L. D., Thomas, C. L., Cobb, H. R., & Hartman, A. E. (2021). A review of the LGBTQ+ work–family interface: What do we know and where do we go from here? *Journal of Organizational Behavior, 42*(2), 139–161. https://doi.org/10.1002/job.2492

Nieuwenhuis, R., & Van Lancker, W. (2020). Introduction: A multilevel perspective on family policy. In *The Palgrave handbook of family policy* (pp. 3–24). Palgrave Macmillan. https://doi.org/10.1007/978-3-030-54618-2_1

Olson, R., Crain, T. L., Bodner, T. E., King, R., Hammer, L. B., Klein, L. C., Erickson, L., Moen, P., Berkman, L. F., & Buxton, O. M. (2015). A workplace intervention improves sleep: Results from the randomized controlled Work, Family, and Health Study. *Sleep Health, 1*(1), 55–65. https://doi.org/10.1016/j.sleh.2014.11.003

Ooms, T. (2019). The evolution of family policy: Lessons learned, challenges, and hopes for the future. *Journal of Family Theory & Review, 11*(1), 18–38. https://doi.org/10.1111/jftr.12316

Perrigino, M. B., Dunford, B. B., & Wilson, K. S. (2018). Work–family backlash: The "dark side" of work–life balance (WLB) policies. *The Academy of Management Annals*, *12*(2), 600–630. https://doi.org/10.5465/annals.2016.0077

Perry-Jenkins, M., & Gerstel, N. (2020). Work and family in the second decade of the 21st century. *Journal of Marriage and Family*, *82*(1), 420–453. https://doi.org/10.1111/jomf.12636

Quick, J. C. (1999). Occupational health psychology: The convergence of health and clinical psychology with public health and preventive medicine in an organizational context. *Professional Psychology, Research and Practice*, *30*(2), 123–128. https://doi.org/10.1037/0735-7028.30.2.123

Robles-Saenz, F., Brossoit, R. M., Crain, T. L., Hammer, L. B., & Wong, J. R. (2021). Understanding the role of family-specific resources for immigrant workers. *Occupational Health Science*, *5*(4), 541–562. https://doi.org/10.1007/s41542-021-00099-0

Rousseau, D. M., Ho, V. T., & Greenberg, J. (2006). I-deals: Idiosyncratic terms in employment relationships. *Academy of Management Review*, *31*(4), 977–994. https://doi.org/10.5465/amr.2006.22527470

Scalia, E., & Beach, W. W. (2020, March). *National Compensation Survey: Employee benefits in the United States*. U.S. Bureau of Labor Statistics. https://www.bls.gov/ncs/ebs/benefits/2020/employee-benefits-in-the-united-states-march-2020.pdf

Schill, A. L., & Chosewood, L. C. (2013). The NIOSH Total Worker Health™ program: An overview. *Journal of Occupational and Environmental Medicine*, *55*, S8–S11. https://doi.org/10.1097/JOM.0000000000000037

Shifrin, N. V., & Michel, J. S. (2021). Flexible work arrangements and employee health: A meta-analytic review. *Work and Stress*, *36*(1), 60–85. https://doi.org/10.1080/02678373.2021.1936287

Shockley, K. M., Clark, M. A., Dodd, H., & King, E. B. (2021). Work–family strategies during COVID-19: Examining gender dynamics among dual-earner couples with young children. *Journal of Applied Psychology*, *106*(1), 15–28. https://doi.org/10.1037/apl0000857

Sinclair, R. R., Allen, T., Barber, L., Bergman, M., Britt, T., Butler, A., Ford, M., Hammer, L., Kath, L., Probst, T., & Yuan, Z. (2020). Occupational health science in the time of COVID-19: Now more than ever. *Occupational Health Science*, *4*(1–2), 1–22. https://doi.org/10.1007/s41542-020-00064-3

Stepler, R. (2017, March 23). *Key takeaways on Americans' views of and experiences with family and medical leave*. Pew Research Center. https://www.pewresearch.org/fact-tank/2017/03/23/key-takeaways-on-americans-views-of-and-experiences-with-family-and-medical-leave/

Tamers, S. L., Chosewood, L. C., Childress, A., Hudson, H., Nigam, J., & Chang, C. C. (2019). *Total Worker Health®* 2014–2018: The novel approach to worker safety, health, and well-being evolves. *International Journal of Environmental Research and Public Health*, *16*(3), 321. https://doi.org/10.3390/ijerph16030321

Tetrick, L. E., & Quick, J. C. (2011). Overview of occupational health psychology: Public health in occupational settings. In J. C. Quick & L. E. Tetrick (Eds.), *Handbook of occupational health psychology* (2nd ed., pp. 3–20). American Psychological Association.

Vaziri, H., Casper, W. J., Wayne, J. H., & Matthews, R. A. (2020). Changes to the work–family interface during the COVID-19 pandemic: Examining predictors and implications using latent transition analysis. *Journal of Applied Psychology*, *105*(10), 1073–1087. https://doi.org/10.1037/apl0000819

Williams, W. (2021, July 16). *Paid family and medical leave (PFML) by state*. Investopedia. https://www.investopedia.com/paid-family-and-medical-leave-by-state-5089907

Wiß, T., & Greve, B. (2020). A comparison of the interplay of public and occupational work-family policies in Austria, Denmark, Italy and the United Kingdom. *Journal of Comparative Policy Analysis*, *22*(5), 440–457. https://doi.org/10.1080/13876988.2019.1582151

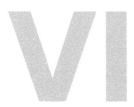

VI

METHODS AND
EVALUATION

INTRODUCTION: METHODS AND EVALUATION

Part VI of the handbook contains two chapters that are essential for understanding methodological approaches relevant not only for OHP but for the science and practice of other occupational health fields as well. The purpose of this part is to provide readers with a clear background about epidemiology and program evaluation. Chapter 27 is a primer about epidemiology with definitions of common terms used in epidemiological approaches and a summary of common research designs. This chapter provides readers an understanding of epidemiology to facilitate digesting occupational health research and/or applying these methods to their own research. Chapter 28 summarizes the importance of and approaches for conducting effective program evaluation. This process is critical for evaluating policies, programs, and/or practices for relevance, effectiveness, and impact and is particularly relevant given the advances in occupational health interventions over the past decade.

27

Epidemiology for Occupational Health Psychology Research

Understanding the Approach

Amanda Sonnega and John Sonnega

A s the study of diseases in populations, epidemiology falls squarely within the purview of occupational health psychology (OHP). For some occupational health psychologists, the methods and content of an epidemiological approach to research questions will be well understood. For others, whose scholarship deals more in the clinical or experimental domains, the methods and approach will be less familiar. The purpose of this chapter is to provide a primer of sorts for the latter audience and perhaps serve as a refresher for the former.

WHAT IS EPIDEMIOLOGY?

The derivation of the word *epidemiology* is from the Greek *epi* (upon), *demos* (people), and *logos* (the study of). A fairly technical and broad definition of *epidemiology* is "the study of the distribution and determinants of health-related states or events in specified populations and the application of this study to control health problems" (Porta, 2008, cited in Celentano & Szklo, 2019, p. 2). A basic premise of epidemiology is that diseases and health are not randomly distributed in populations (Celentano & Szklo, 2019). We can use epidemiological methods to learn about these population differentials and use that information to inform interventions to improve health outcomes and help eliminate disparities. Who gets sick, who stays well, and why? And what might

https://doi.org/10.1037/0000331-027
Handbook of Occupational Health Psychology, Third Edition, L. E. Tetrick, G. G. Fisher, M. T. Ford, and J. C. Quick (Editors)

we do about it? These questions form the foundation upon which the discipline is built.

The model shown in Figure 27.1, known as *the epidemiological triad* or triangle, is part of that foundation. Originally developed for understanding infectious disease, the model has clear relevance for chronic disease as well. The *agent* is the exposure that leads to disease. The agent can be a microbe but can also be a chemical agent (e.g., smoking) or a psychosocial factor (e.g., work stress). The *host* is the individual who gets the disease. Characteristics of the host, such as genetics or health behaviors, can influence their vulnerability to the agent. The *environment* brings the agent and the host together. Thus, disease results when an individual (host) is exposed to a deleterious agent in a given environment, characteristics of which can influence both agent exposure and host vulnerability. Understanding this framework is a good starting point for developing an epidemiological approach to research in OHP.

We note that this chapter is, of course, not an exhaustive review of topics in epidemiology, but rather represents a selection of subjects that are likely to be relevant to the scientific questions with which occupational health psychologists may engage. This chapter will familiarize the reader with the terminology used in epidemiology to describe and understand population health. We begin with topics within the area of descriptive epidemiology, providing basic definitions of incidence and prevalence and why it is important to differentiate between these terms accurately. We turn to topics in analytical epidemiology and describe three observational study designs (i.e., cross-sectional, case-control, and cohort), advantages and disadvantages of each, and sources of bias that can arise. We discuss causal inference and the measures of association we can derive from epidemiological studies.

We then highlight the implications and relevance of an epidemiological approach for OHP and provide several content-based examples to illustrate some of the concepts outlined in the chapter. Finally, we point the reader toward several valuable data resources for potential use. Although the aegis of OHP can include infectious as well as chronic disease, this chapter does not directly address the investigation of infectious disease outbreaks but acknowledges it as a major part of the work of epidemiology.

There are several fine introductory textbooks on epidemiology, but for definitions in this chapter, we utilize *Gordis Epidemiology*, sixth edition, by David D. Celentano and Moyses Szklo as the primary source. This excellent introductory text represents the thinking and approach of the late Leon Gordis,

FIGURE 27.1. The Epidemiological Triangle

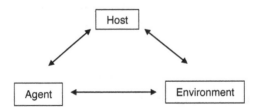

from whom we both first learned epidemiology in a yearlong course at the Johns Hopkins School of Hygiene and Public Health. While we were students in his class in 1985–1986, Dr. Gordis provided extensive handouts, which later served as the basis for this introductory text. Following his death in 2015, his colleagues continued the tradition, updating the materials as needed to ensure their relevance.

RELEVANCE FOR OHP

OHP and epidemiology share a common goal of fostering positive health outcomes through prevention and health promotion. Part of the National Institute of Occupational Safety and Health (NIOSH)–recommended core curricula for OHP graduate programs is coursework in public health and epidemiology. The COVID-19 pandemic has highlighted the role of epidemiology, particularly in terms of surveillance but also in terms of application. Epidemiologists and occupational health psychologists often work together to address health outcomes. Occupational health psychologists should be able to interpret epidemiologic findings that warrant implementing preventive efforts. Epidemiology conducts the public health surveillance of morbidity and mortality that often provides guidance for OHP interventions and evaluations. The work world is being challenged by the global pandemic, technological changes, distance working, and economic upheavals. All of these aspects contribute to the emergence of work-related risk factors for health and well-being. Epidemiological methods provide a useful tool for occupational health psychologists to monitor the health and well-being of a population and explore the effects of changes in the work environment that may point practitioners toward interventions.

DESCRIPTIVE EPIDEMIOLOGY: INCIDENCE AND PREVALENCE

Tracking diseases in the population, or disease surveillance, is at the heart of epidemiologic work and is a large part of the work of public health officials. As such, descriptive epidemiology aims to discern patterns of diseases in a population by focusing on elements of person, place, and time (i.e., who, where, when). Any health dimension can be part of epidemiologic investigation, including psychosocial factors like work stress. To identify cases of disease, epidemiologists can use a variety of data sources, including interviews, community screenings, and medical records. For some diseases, mandatory reporting to health departments is an additional source. Two key metrics used to track disease morbidity are incidence and prevalence.

Incidence

Incidence is the occurrence of disease in a given population at a given time. Incidence is the number of new events in a population during a specified time period. If we choose to express this as a rate per 1,000 people, we would define the incidence rate per 1,000 as

$$\frac{\text{\# of } \textit{new} \text{ cases of disease occurring in the population during a specified period of time}}{\text{\# of persons in the population at that specified time}} \times 1,000$$

One implication of this definition is that the individuals in the denominator have to be at risk of contracting the disease. Another significant concept underlying the task of surveillance is that risks unfold in individuals and in populations over time. Thus, it is important to consider the duration for which the individuals in the denominator are observed. We can specify a duration of observation and require that everyone in the denominator be present in our study during that time. In that case, we would likely keep the duration fairly short. It is not always possible to observe everyone for the same length of time, especially if we specify a longer duration such as months or years: in some cases, individuals attrite from the study during follow-up or die from other causes.

A helpful concept in this instance is *person-time*, which is the sum of the time that each person was observed, usually indicated as *person-months* or *person-years*. The denominator, in this scenario, is expressed as the total person-time. For many OHP applications, the period of follow-up is likely to be lengthy, so the concept of person-time is key in thinking about identifying incidence or new cases of disease. For example, in a study of workers at sea (an occupation with high rates of mortality and injury), there were 78 new injuries over a 4-year time period (Sagaro et al., 2021). The incidence *rate* was 6.31 per 1,000 seafarer-years (person-time) over the 4-year period.

Prevalence

Prevalence is the amount of disease in a given population at a given time. It includes the number of existing cases, both new and old. Again, expressing it as a rate per 1,000, prevalence can be defined as

$$\frac{\text{\# of cases of disease present in the population at a given time}}{\text{\# of persons in the population at that given time}} \times 1,000$$

Time, again, is important. Although we think of prevalence as a *point prevalence* (i.e., the exact prevalence at a specific point in time), in practice it is difficult to pinpoint without reference to some period of time. Thus, epidemiologists distinguish point prevalence from *period prevalence*, where the latter is the prevalence over some specified period of time. For example, in a national sample investigating mood disorders in the United States, the 12-month prevalence (specified time period) of workplace major depressive disorder was 6.4% (Kessler et al., 2006). At any particular point in the time frame (past year), prevalence may be higher or lower, depending on the course of illness. A related concept is *cumulative incidence*, which is the proportion of individuals who develop the disease during a specified period of time.

The Prevalence Pot

It may be clear at this point that these two basic indicators of disease in populations are related to each other but are important to distinguish. As graduate students, we worked as staffers on the 1988 Presidential Commission on the Human Immunodeficiency Virus Epidemic in Washington, D.C. On our first day, the medical director urgently asked us, "Quick, do you know the difference between incidence and prevalence?" We acknowledged we did, and he replied, "Well, go explain it to the admiral; he has to go out and explain it to the media." Admiral James D. Watkins was the head commissioner, and we were about to hold a press conference ahead of the first set of expert hearings on the incidence and prevalence of the disease. Luckily, we had learned from Dr. Gordis about the *prevalence pot*, a simple but highly effective graphic illustration that virtually guarantees clear understanding of the difference between incidence and prevalence.

Figure 27.2 depicts the prevalence pot. In A we see a baseline level of prevalence of a disease depicted by beads in a flask. B shows how new cases of disease (incidence) fill the pot, leading to increased prevalence. In C we see that either recovery or death from the disease/infection empties the pot and

FIGURE 27.2. The Dynamic Prevalence Pot

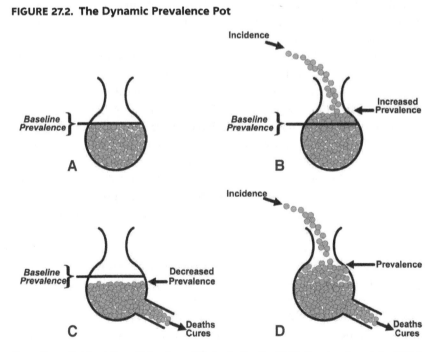

Note. From *Epidemiology* (5th ed., p. 53), by L. Gordis, 2013, Elsevier. Copyright 2013 by Elsevier. Reprinted with permission.

leads to decreased prevalence. D depicts the dynamic relationship among incidence, prevalence, and death or cure.

The admiral was impressively quick to apprehend the implications of the distinction—notably, that incidence primarily speaks to *risk of disease* and prevalence primarily speaks to the *burden of disease*. If we develop a treatment or intervention for a disease that keeps individuals alive or well longer but does not cure them, we are necessarily increasing the prevalence, which could be costly for health care financing but decidedly beneficial for individuals and for society in terms of those individuals' contributions. This helps illustrate a final important point about the relationship between incidence and prevalence: in the dynamic equilibrium depicted in D in Figure 27.2, we see that:

$$\text{Prevalence} = \text{Incidence} \times \text{Disease Duration}$$

This has important implications for understanding patterns of disease. If we compare the prevalence of a disease in two populations, it is important to have some information on the duration of disease. Even with a similar risk of disease, one population may have higher prevalence of the disease simply because they are likely to survive longer with it.

Crude and Adjusted Rates

A final important distinction epidemiologists commonly make is between crude and adjusted (prevalence or incidence) rates. *Crude rates* are the straightforward dividing of the total number of cases in a particular time frame by the total population. Crude rates provide a basic way to compare two or more populations on a disease outcome of interest. Such a simple comparison could be very misleading, however, as crude rates do not account for potentially confounding factors. To consider other factors, we calculate specific or *adjusted rates*. A simple illustration of this point would be that if we compared the prevalence of heart disease in the population of country A to country B, and found B to be much higher, we would have a hard time explaining why the countries differed. A first question would be: What is the age structure of the two populations? Is country B "older"? If yes, when we adjusted the prevalence estimates in each country for age, we would find that the difference between the two countries narrowed simply because the prevalence of heart disease increases with age. In other words, with an older population age structure, country B has a higher prevalence of heart disease.

Adjusted rates for specific occupations, age groups, or work environments may provide important information that reveals why we may be seeing a difference in disease rates between two groups. For example, in a report on nonfatal, violent workplace crimes, the crude rate of violent workplace crimes was 8 per 1,000 workers over a 3-year time period (Siegel et al., 2020). Adjusted rates for various occupations, however, revealed that workers in protective services displayed the highest rates—101 crimes per 1,000 workers—compared with 19 crimes per 1,000 community and social services workers and 17 crimes per 1,000 health care workers. High-risk occupations involve contact with people in what may be vulnerable situations. In this instance, information using adjusted rates would inform the tailoring of workplace violence prevention programs accordingly.

RESEARCH DESIGNS FOR ANALYTICAL EPIDEMIOLOGY

Next we turn to what is known as *analytical epidemiology*, which is concerned with determining whether there is an association between a given exposure and an outcome. In OHP the exposure is often a psychosocial dimension, like stress or lack of supervisor support, rather than a microbe or toxin. The same principles apply, however, regardless of the specific nature of the exposure. We discuss three epidemiological study designs that serve the purpose of collecting information to study an association between an exposure and a disease outcome: cross-sectional, case-control, and cohort studies. Specifically, the aim of these three observational study designs is to "elucidate the etiology of and risk factors for disease" (Celentano & Szklo, 2019, p. 147). We discuss the basic concepts of each study design, some of the relative advantages and disadvantages, as well as potential sources of bias that can arise.

Cross-Sectional Studies

Cross-sectional studies are often used to provide information on an exposure and a disease of interest to help generate hypotheses that merit further study. In a cross-sectional design, the exposure and the outcome are measured at the same point in time. We start with a population of interest and conduct a study that allows us to obtain information on exposure and disease. This information then allows us to generate a 2×2 table with exposure on the y-axis, disease on the x-axis, and four relevant groups, as shown in Figure 27.3.

Quadrant a contains those who were exposed and have the disease, b contains those who were exposed and have no disease, c contains those who were not exposed but have disease, and d contains those who were not exposed and have no disease. As Celentano and Szklo (2019) noted, we can consider two approaches to determining whether or not there is an association between the exposure and the disease. We can either analyze the prevalence of disease among those exposed ($a/a + b$) compared with disease prevalence among those not exposed ($c/c + d$), or we can calculate the prevalence of exposure among those with disease ($a/a + c$) and compare it with the prevalence of exposure among those without disease ($b/b + d$). Since temporal ordering is not strictly possible, either approach offers some insight into a possible association between exposure and outcome.

The major advantage of a cross-sectional design is that it is relatively inexpensive. It also can provide data that allow estimation of prevalence. The major drawbacks relate to various sources of bias that can arise with this design. The mantra in epidemiology and statistics is "correlation does not imply causation,"

FIGURE 27.3. Design of Hypothetical Cross-Sectional Study

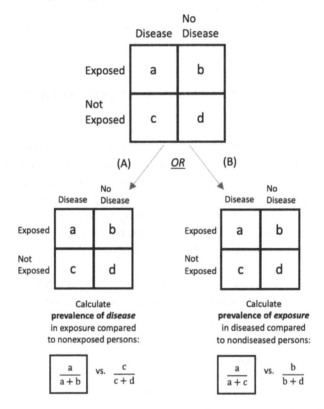

Note. From *Epidemiology* (5th ed., p. 155), by L. Gordis, 2013, Elsevier. Copyright 2013 by Elsevier. Reprinted with permission.

and yet our human nature urges us to attribute causality. Cross-sectional designs can only tell us whether two things are related to each other, not whether one causes the other. The classic example often cited in introductory epidemiology classes is the striking association between the population of storks and babies in European cities in the early 20th century. Storks did not bring babies; rather, the increasing birth rate led to more dwellings and toasty chimneys that storks often chose for their own nesting.

When we do not have temporal ordering, *reverse causation* is a concern. Sometimes common sense can help us discern a likely direction. For example, it is unlikely that lung cancer caused someone to smoke. But other associations are less obvious, such as those in the workplace, and may in fact involve a bidirectional causal connection. For example, we may observe an association between work stress and depression, but are they causally linked? If so, in what direction? Note that the survey (questionnaire or interview) can introduce temporality by, for example, asking *retrospectively* about the timing of exposures. This kind of retrospective information has been shown to be reasonably valid (Smith et al., 2021), although exact timing of events and exposures is often less so. An event history calendar is one method of data collection that can be used in any study design, but it may be especially useful when longitudinal follow-up is not possible. An event history calendar is a valuable research design that uses information across multiple life domains to prompt better recall for the timing of a specific event (Belli at al., 2007)—for example, asking about the timing of beginning a new job in relation to the timing of a marriage around the same time.

Other sources of bias that can arise with cross-sectional study designs are selection and survival. *Selection bias* is when the sample is not randomly obtained. Respondents, therefore, may not be representative of the population of interest. *Survival bias* is likely to occur when the exposed group is less likely to survive compared with the unexposed. This implies that potential respondents in the cross-sectional study must have lived long enough to participate, and therefore the unexposed would be overrepresented in our sample relative to the exposed, leading us to an inaccurate representation of the risk of exposure to disease.

Case-Control Studies

Case-control studies provide another methodology for investigating the relationship between an exposure and a health outcome. In this epidemiological study design, we identify the study groups based on the outcome; *cases* are those with the disease, and *controls* are those without the disease. Then we ascertain retrospective information on an exposure of interest. Like cross-sectional study designs, this method is especially useful in hypothesis generation.

Cases can be identified from a number of sources, from hospital records to survey data that have been collected on disease outcomes. Exposure information can likewise be obtained from interviews and surveys, or even by reviewing medical or employment records that contain exposure information. Typically, cases are "matched" with controls to make them similar or comparable. Thus, controls might be selected to be similar with regard to age, race, sex, or other characteristics. Because variables that are used for matching cannot be studied as potential risk factors, it is important to select controls carefully and not "overmatch." Note that with information on disease status and exposure status, a similar 2 × 2 table as that generated from a cross-sectional study can be created here, where a is exposed cases, b is exposed controls, c is unexposed cases, and d is unexposed controls. The interpretation of these conditions is slightly different, however. In a case-control study, we are identifying the proportion of the cases who were exposed ($a/a + c$) compared with the proportion of the controls who were not exposed ($d/b + d$). If an exposure is associated with the disease, we would find that the proportion of cases who were exposed is greater than the proportion of controls who are not exposed.

Like cross-sectional studies, case-control studies can be relatively inexpensive to conduct. Case-control studies are especially appropriate in the study of rare diseases and/or those with a very long *latency period*, which is the duration of time from exposure to a given risk and the manifestation of disease. They also depend on the availability of disease information that either contains or can be linked to exposure information. In occupational settings, this can come from employee health records and employment information. Case-control studies are less useful, however, when an exposure is very rare.

An especially significant source of bias in case-control designs is *recall bias*, which arises when exposure information is obtained through interviews with or survey of cases and controls. Those with a disease may be more likely than controls to recall exposures that they think may have been the reason for their illness. In addition, as with cross-sectional designs, selection may be a problem, especially with reference to identifying cases and controls if the putative exposure is indeed related to survival. Similarly, as with cross-sectional designs, it is not possible to infer causation. Finally, it is important to note that information collected for use in a case-control study does not allow us to calculate incidence or prevalence since we are starting with prevalent cases and not surveilling over time to identify new (incident) cases.

Cohort Studies

Cohort studies are an epidemiological design that offers a potentially more rigorous method for understanding a connection between an exposure and an outcome. Cohort studies begin with an at-risk (exposed) group and follow them concurrently over time to assess outcomes. Other terminology for this type of design includes *concurrent cohort design* or *longitudinal cohort design*. The most significant implication of this design is that it is possible to identify new, that is, incident, cases of disease. Again, referencing our 2×2 table, in this design, a represents exposed individuals who develop disease, b are those who are exposed but do not develop disease; c are not exposed who develop disease, and d are those who are not exposed and do not develop disease. We can calculate the *incidence* or *risk* of disease among the exposed as $a/a + b$ and among the unexposed as $c/c + d$. If there is an association between the exposure and the outcome, we expect the incidence in the exposed to be greater than the incidence in the unexposed.

One downside to the cohort design is that the length of follow-up may be considerable in order to collect enough information on exposures and outcomes to investigate an association. An alternative is to obtain exposure information retrospectively through, for example, examination of health or employment records. This shortens the duration of time that it takes to gather information on exposure risk. This alternate design is known as a *retrospective cohort* or *historical cohort study*, in contrast to a *prospective cohort design* in which both exposure and outcome information are obtained concurrently. The basic design of both prospective and retrospective cohort study is the same, however, in that we are still comparing exposed and unexposed individuals and following them forward to ascertain disease outcomes. The difference is in how we obtain our exposure information. Note that the temporality between exposure and outcome can be defined in either design but is likely to be more accurate in a prospective cohort design. Thus, cohort studies are an efficient design for studying relatively rare exposures but not for studying rare outcomes.

As we discuss in the next section, the design of a cohort study allows researchers to determine the relative risk of disease. Moreover, with temporal ordering of exposures and outcomes more clearly delineated, a stronger case can be made for a causal connection between an exposure and an outcome. Furthermore, longitudinal data provide opportunities for researchers to conduct advanced modeling methods such as growth-curve modeling, Cox regression, survival analysis, and fixed and random effects models. Cohort designs do not eliminate the risk of bias, especially the potential for selection and information bias.

In summary, with a case-control design, we are contrasting the proportion of cases who were exposed with the proportion of controls who were exposed. Whereas with a cohort design, we are comparing the proportion of exposed individuals in whom disease develops with the proportion of unexposed individuals in whom disease develops (Celentano & Szklo, 2019, p. 245). We discuss the implications of this in the section Measures of Risk.

Confounding

Implied in the foregoing discussion is the goal of making a causal inference between an exposure and a disease outcome. We have suggested that a design that allows us to establish temporal ordering, such as in a cohort design, moves us further in the right direction. Regardless of study design, however, the problem of confounding is of paramount concern. *Confounding* is when we observe an association between A and B and infer that A caused B, when in fact a third factor, a confounder, is responsible for the observed association. *Confounders* are characteristics associated with both the outcome and the putative causative element under study. Knowing what the confounders are and measuring them allows the researchers to take them into account in statistical analyses. A careful choice of comparison groups can help limit the effects of unknown confounders.

MEASURES OF RISK

Having collected the data, how do we now use those data to make statements about the risk of disease? Three measures of risk are commonly used: absolute risk, relative risk, and odds ratio. In the following sections, we discuss each of these measures of risk in relation to the study designs just described. In the next section, then, we are concerned with determining the strength of an association between exposures and outcomes, and whether or not there is *excess risk* associated with the exposure.

Absolute Risk

Another way to think about the incidence of disease is as the *absolute risk* of that disease in a population (Celentano & Szklo, 2019, p. 240). It is the probability of that disease developing in a population at risk. Although absolute risk does not specify a comparison with a reference group, it can nonetheless be useful as an indication of the *magnitude of the risk* in a given population. For example, it may be important for the occupational health psychologist in a particular clinical practice or in setting policy for a workplace.

Relative Risk

With data collected from a well-designed cohort study, we can take the concept of absolute risk to the next level by assessing the *relative risk*, which is defined as the "probability of an event (developing disease) occurring in exposed individuals compared with the probability of the event in unexposed individuals" (Celentano & Szklo, 2019, p. 242). Relative risk can be expressed as the ratio of the risk in the exposed group to the risk in the unexposed. Thus, it is also referred to as the *risk ratio*. If we return to the basic crosstab depicted in Figure 27.3, we can add elements to make it relevant to a cohort study; namely, the y-axis would represent the selection of exposed and unexposed individuals, and the x-axis would represent the probability (risk) of disease developing (yes or no). We can then express the incidence in the exposed as $a/a + b$ and the incidence in the unexposed as $c/c + d$. The relative risk is

$$\frac{a/a+b}{c/c+d}$$

For example, imagine a workplace with 250 workers, 100 of whom are working under conditions of high demand (exposed). A cohort study follows these workers over several years and reveals that 20 workers develop clinical depression. Our cohort study includes a comparison group of 150 (unexposed) whose work conditions can be characterized as low demand. In this group, 30 workers develop depression over the same period. The *absolute risk* for developing depression in both groups of workers is 20% (20/100 and 30/150). The relative risk (RR) comparing the two groups of workers is calculated as 0.20/0.20, or 1. Workers from the exposed working conditions are no more likely to develop depression than the workers from the unexposed working conditions. If the RR is 1, the risk in the exposed is equal to the risk in the unexposed, so there is no association. If the RR is greater than 1, then the risk in the exposed is greater than the risk in the unexposed. Conversely, an RR of less than 1 suggests that the risk in the exposed is less than the risk in the unexposed, possibly suggesting that the exposure might actually confer protection.

Perhaps the study collected information on other working conditions and found that part of the reason for there being no higher risk of depression in the exposed workers was that they also experienced high levels of supervisor support, which mitigated the effects of stress. Let us imagine that the supervisor of the high-demand group takes notice of these high rates of depression and implements further measures to combat stress by allowing the workers greater control over their work process. After 12 months of these measures, a study finds that eight of the 100 workers in the exposed group developed depression. The unexposed group (who had no additional stress management) remained the same, with 20 workers developing depression. The absolute risk for depression in the high-demand group of workers is now 0.08. The RR for depression now changes to $0.08/0.20 = 0.40$. The RR of developing depression in the workers in the high-demand condition is now 40% of the risk in the workers in the low-demand working conditions. Relative risk reduction is often utilized to evaluate an intervention.

Odds Ratio

As noted, calculation of the relative risk requires measures of incidence, which, as we have shown, we cannot obtain with a case-control study design. The case-control study design, however, does provide information on the probability of an event, which we can use to calculate the odds ratio. While it is a measure of the risk of the association between exposure and disease, the odds ratio frames the association differently. Because in the case-control study, we start with cases and then determine exposures, the *odds ratio* considers the odds that a case was exposed and that a control was exposed. Referring to Figure 27.3, we can express this as a/c and b/d, respectively. The odds ratio in a case-control study is

$$\frac{a/c}{b/d}$$

Notice that we can also derive information on probability from a cohort study design, and can therefore also use information from a cohort study to calculate an odds ratio. In this case, however, it takes the form of the ratio of the odds that an exposed person develops disease to the odds that a nonexposed person develops disease, or

$$\frac{a/b}{a/d}$$

Notice that we can also calculate the odds ratio as a cross-products ratio:

$$\frac{ad}{bc}$$

Thus, whether the data on exposure and disease come from a cohort study or a case-control study, the *cross-product odds ratio* is the same. The odds ratio can be interpreted the same as the relative risk ratio in that an odds ratio of 1 indicates no association between. An odds ratio greater than 1 indicates increased risk of disease associated with exposure, and an odds ratio less than 1 suggests a protective function.

As Celentano and Szklo (2019) noted, there are conditions when the odds ratio derived from a case-control design is a good approximation of the risk ratio of a specific exposure-disease in the population. Specifically, the odds ratio approximates the risk ratio when the sample cases selected for the study are representative of the population of cases and when the controls are representative of the population of those without disease, with reference to exposure status. A third condition that is required is what is known as the *rarity assumption*, in which the disease has a low incidence in the population. For many diseases we study, this assumption is easily met. Thus, when disease is infrequent, a + b approximates b and c + d approximates d, allowing us to calculate the relative risk as

$$\frac{a/b}{c/d}$$

This is the same as ad/bc.

A final conception of risk that is especially useful for estimating the potential for prevention is *attributable risk*. Whereas relative risk and odds ratios speak to etiology and, ultimately, causal inference, the concept of attributable risk is valuable for thinking about prevention. In particular, population attributable risk tells us how much of an impact the elimination of a particular exposure will have on the disease outcome of interest in a population.

ILLUSTRATIVE EXAMPLES OF OHP RESEARCH

Several different epidemiological designs of interest to occupational health psychologists have been outlined. The classical occupational epidemiological tradition (Kasl & Jones, 2011) continues to be a foundational methodology and has improved over the last decade with better measurement of the work environment. The use of epidemiology also continues to clarify psychosocial work factors and foster better evaluation. We briefly outline examples of occupational and psychosocial epidemiology to illustrate how researchers are using an epidemiological approach to study connections between work and health.

Occupational Epidemiology and Health Examples

Using data from the Health and Retirement Study (HRS), an ongoing longitudinal cohort design, Burgard and Sonnega (2018) explored occupational risk for unhealthy weight across a range of occupations. Body mass index was tracked over time, and potential confounding factors were considered. The longitudinal cohort design allowed the researchers to calculate trajectories of weight gain across a set of occupations. Professionals (across all occupations) of both genders displayed less risk of weight gain compared with their counterparts in sales, clerical, and production work. Adjustment for socio-demographic and lifestyle factors reduced this association more for men than women.

The longitudinal cohort design also allows for the examination of disease impairment on occupation. With advancing treatment and worksite wellness screening (often developed by occupational health psychologists), there is a growing population of disease survivors. Also using HRS data, Ekenga et al. (2020) examined long-term employment outcomes in female cancer survivors, comparing those with disease to those without. While there was no difference at baseline, cancer survivors were more likely to be employed than those without cancer (odds ratio = 1.33). Among long-term survivors (> 6–10 years), professional occupations were less likely to be employed than manual or service occupations (odds ratio = 0.40). The impact of cancer on employment may differ by occupation type. Again, these findings allow for more targeted interventions by occupational health psychologists.

Single Occupation

The occupational health literature has long contained studies of *single occupations* (Kasl & Jones, 2011). Single occupation studies may allow greater explication of the hazards of particular work. Recently, there have been many investigations of the effects of the global COVID-19 pandemic on the health of individuals in particular occupations, from grocery store employees to physicians (Lan et al., 2021). Work environments during the pandemic were often substantially altered due to public health interventions in response to COVID-19. These studies were often cross-sectional surveys exploring occupational stressors and challenges within a particular profession. One large cross-sectional study of health care workers in the United States (e.g., physician, nurses, emergency medical technicians EMTs, and nonclinical staff) surveilled COVID-19 risk and mental health outcomes. This study was a convenience sample that recruited participants through the internet. HCWs in emergency departments were more likely to report contracting COVID-19 compared with other departments. Those who contracted COVID-19 also reported high depression, anxiety, and burnout symptomatology (Firew et al., 2020).

A longitudinal study of nurses conducted in Wuhan, China, the epicenter of the pandemic, explored psychological symptomatology and occupation factors. Nurses from COVID-19 shelter hospitals were more likely to present psychological problems than those nurses from other frontline or non-frontline units. Severe insomnia was a particularly prevalent symptom in this group (38.3%). Examining a single occupation (nurses) can help elucidate symptomology related to occupational exposures (Cai et al., 2020).

Psychosocial Workplace

Social epidemiology aims to identify social characteristics, such as work stress and social inequalities, that impact the pattern of diseases and health (von dem Knesebeck, 2015). Surveillance of the psychosocial work environ-ment is a mainstay of occupational epidemiology and is central to models of work stress, such as the job demand–control model (Karasek, 1979) or the effort–reward imbalance model (Siegrist et al., 2009). A vast literature has documented the impact of occupational characteristics on a variety of physical and mental health outcomes (Bonde, 2008; Gilbert-Ouimet et al., 2014). Chronicling adverse psychosocial risk factors in various occupations is conducted with a range of epidemiological designs, including cross-sectional studies, case-control studies, and cohort studies.

A study of workers in Alberta, Canada, compared three job stress models in relation to the risk of anxiety and depression disorders (Wang et al., 2012). The researchers employed a longitudinal study design, recruiting 4,305 workers by random-digit dialing by telephone and collecting data about job stress, effort–reward, work–family conflicts, and depression. The 2-week prevalence of major depression was 3.2%. The baseline results revealed that all three models showed associations between job-related stress and depression and were equally important in predicting depression. Further, the constructs from the models interacted. Occupational health psychologists may utilize this type of workplace epidemiology to design more nuanced ways to improve work environments and employees' mental health.

Health Disparities

As previously noted, the coronavirus pandemic has brought to the fore the importance of work as a determinant of health. The pandemic has also high-lighted health disparities related to occupation, particularly between those who could work at home and those who could not (Eisen et al., 2022). Occupational epidemiology can help elucidate where and how work contributes to disparities for vulnerable populations. Although the differential spread of disease often focuses on behaviors, occupational environment is a central component of these disparities (McClure et al., 2020). Utilizing data from the Current Population Survey, Hawkins (2020) examined occupational segregation by race and eth-nicity. These data were combined with information about the essential nature of the occupation, the frequency of exposure to infections, and whether the work was conducted in proximity to others. Racial minorities were more likely to be working in occupations that were in essential industries and in occupations with more exposure to infections. Differential employment by race likely contributes to health disparities in COVID-19 outcomes.

RELEVANT EPIDEMIOLOGICAL DATA RESOURCES

In this section, we provide information on several epidemiological studies that offer exceptional research opportunities for OHP. They feature measurements of respondents' work histories, jobs, and job characteristics, along with rich multidisciplinary content in a wide range of other domains. Note that all the studies we describe here have searchable bibliographies accessible through their websites, where researchers can learn more about how others have used these data to study the (potentially reciprocal) impacts of work on health.

The Health and Retirement Study

The HRS is a nationally representative longitudinal cohort study of adults over age 50 in the United States. With the rapid aging of the population and the looming retirement of the baby boomer generation, the study's primary aim was to provide data to study retirement transitions and factors that influence successful aging through retirement (Sonnega et al., 2014). The study began in 1992 with an initial cohort of men and women born 1931–1941 with biennial data through 2020. The study content includes familial connections, health and health services, finances, cognition, and psychosocial and physical functioning. Sources of information on working conditions come from self-reported job characteristics in the core survey (1992–2020) and more detailed self-reported working conditions in the psychosocial questionnaire, both collected concurrently. The Life History Mail Survey was fielded as a sub-study of the HRS to obtain retrospective information on the early life experiences of HRS respondents, including detailed job histories. Occupation data in the HRS are coded using U.S. Census occupation and industry codes. The detailed codes are available as restricted data to preserve respondent confidentiality. Mullen (2021) supplied a detailed summary of the occupational data resources in the HRS. The data are available through the HRS website (https://hrs.isr.umich.edu/about).

Panel Study of Income Dynamics

Growing out of the War on Poverty in the 1960s, the Panel Study of Income Dynamics (PSID) began as a study of income and poverty and is now the longest running longitudinal household survey in the world (McGonagle et al., 2012). The study began in 1968 with a nationally representative sample of over 18,000 individuals living in 5,000 families in the United States. These individuals and their descendants were interviewed, creating an intergenerational study of more than 82,000 respondents with approximately 9,500 families still enrolled. The interviews included employment, income, wealth, expenditures, health, and many other topics. As in the HRS, the information collected on jobs is coded using Census codes and available as a restricted data product. Through linkages to external sources of information on occupational characteristics, the power of more than 50 years of panel data makes the PSID a rich and underutilized resource for OHP. The data are available through the study's website (https://psidonline.isr.umich.edu/).

Midlife in the United States

Midlife in the United States (MIDUS) began in 1995 as a nationally representative cross-sectional study aimed at providing in-depth information across a wide range of multidisciplinary topic areas in order to understand more about the behavioral, psychological, and social factors that influence health and well-being at midlife. The sample included 7,189 adults between the ages of 25 and 74. Data were collected through telephone and self-administered questionnaires. The expansive topical focus includes a wide range of occupational history information, including job characteristics and employment history. A second longitudinal follow-up of the 1995 sample was conducted beginning in 2004, with 4,963 respondents eventually completing a follow-up interview and questionnaire. In 2011–2016, MIDUS conducted a third wave of longitudinal data collection, including a sample refresh. The occupation information is coded using Census codes. Data from all three waves are archived with the University of Michigan Inter-university Consortium for Political and Social Research, through the MIDUS website (https://www.midus.wisc.edu).

Biosocial Surveys

All three longitudinal studies are also biosocial surveys in the sense that they include direct biological measurements from participants, including biomarkers and genetics. The addition of this kind of biological information provides exceptional opportunities to investigate biological mechanisms underlying potential connections between work conditions and later-life health outcomes.

External Linkages

As noted, these studies all contain detailed Census occupation and industry codes. These codes provide researchers with the means to link the survey data to external sources of information on job characteristics. OHP has long been interested in distinguishing subjective and objective measurements of the work environment (Kasl & Jones, 2011). To meet the need for more objective measurement and to expand the characterization of the work environment, researchers have begun linking the Census occupation codes in the HRS, the PSID, and MIDUS to the Occupational Information Network (O*NET) database. A project of the U.S. Department of Labor/Employment and Training Administration, the O*NET database provides standardized, occupation-specific measures related to approximately 1,000 occupations. It includes measures that describe work and worker characteristics. Details about the O*NET database can be found on the O*NET website (https://www.onetcenter.org). HRS researchers have recently released a user-friendly version of O*NET 26.1 database data covering nine content domains, including knowledge, skills, abilities, interests, work values, work styles, work context, job zone, and work activities. They have also provided these data linked to the HRS 2010 Census occupation codes covering 2010–2020 as a restricted data product (Carpenter et al., 2022). The O*NET data linked to the HRS data are available as a restricted data product on the HRS website. The stand-alone O*NET data that are ready to be linked are available from Florida State University's Claude Pepper Center.

A relatively new source of objective occupational information is now available through the Occupational Requirements Survey (ORS). The ORS is a joint project of the U.S. Bureau of Labor Statistics and the Social Security Administration. As with O*NET data, data in the ORS database can be linked to survey information at the individual level. The ORS data provide detailed information on the requirements of specific job titles in terms of education, training, and experience; cognitive and mental demands; physical demands; as well as environmental conditions.

Both of these sources of occupational information greatly expand on the content available in the studies described greatly expanding the content and therefore the scope of OHP investigation that is possible.

RAND American Life Panel American Working Conditions Survey

A final epidemiological survey data resource that should be of great interest is the American Working Conditions Survey (AWCS), which was conducted in 2015 as part of the RAND American Life Panel, a nationally representative sample of individuals living in the United States who have agreed to be participants in an online survey. The aim of the AWCS was to collect information using a cross-sectional design on a broad range of working conditions in American workplaces, especially conditions related to work sustainability (Maestas et al., 2017). Importantly, the survey also contains detailed health information to evaluate the associations between working conditions and health. The data are available through the study website.[1]

CONCLUSION

This chapter has provided some foundational information for occupational health psychologists who may be new to an epidemiological approach to research. We have focused on descriptive and analytical epidemiology, but there are other topics that are highly relevant. For example, Sarpy et al. (2013) provided important background information on sampling from an epidemiological perspective that is essential when designing a study and in understanding the complex sample designs of the data resources described in this chapter. Furthermore, Sinclair et al. (2013) offered a valuable set of recommendations to enhance progress in the field of OHP. To this we add that future strides in scientific discovery within the field will also come in a large degree through the use of longitudinal survey data resources, including those we have described here, and the application of an epidemiological approach to leverage the power of these resources.

---

[1]See the study website (https://www.rand.org/education-and-labor/projects/american-working-conditions.html).

REFERENCES

Belli, R. F., Smith, L., Andreski, P., & Agrawal, S. (2007). Methodological comparisons between CATI event history calendar and conventional questionnaire instruments. *Public Opinion Quarterly*, 71, 603–622.

Bonde, J. P. (2008). Psychosocial factors at work and risk of depression: A systematic review of the epidemiological evidence. *Occupational and Environmental Medicine*, 65(7), 438–445. https://doi.org/10.1136/oem.2007.038430

Burgard, S. A., & Sonnega, A. (2018). Occupational differences in BMI, BMI trajectories, and implications for employment status among older U.S. workers. *Work, Aging and Retirement*, 4(1), 21–36. https://doi.org/10.1093/workar/waw038

Cai, Z., Cui, Q., Liu, Z., Li, J., Gong, X., Liu, J., Wan, Z., Yuan, X., Li, X., Chen, C., & Wang, G. (2020). Nurses endured high risks of psychological problems under the epidemic of COVID-19 in a longitudinal study in Wuhan China. *Journal of Psychiatric Research*, 131, 132–137. https://doi.org/10.1016/j.jpsychires.2020.09.007

Carpenter, R., Carr, D., Chen, Q., Hafeez. A., Helppie-McFall, B., & Sonnega, A. (2022). Health and Retirement Study core 2004–2010 linkage to Occupational Information Network 5.0 and 10.0 Data: Data description and usage, Version 1. https://hrs.isr.umich.edu/data-products/restricted-data/available-products/12500

Celentano, D. D., & Szklo, M. (2019). *Gordis epidemiology* (6th ed.). Elsevier.

Claude Pepper Center. (2022). *FSU-UM Census Occupation Code-Occupational Information Network (O*NET) Data Project*. Florida State University. https://claudepeppercenter.fsu.edu/onet/

Eisen, E. A., Elser, H., & Picciotto, S. (2022). Working: The role of occupational epidemiology. *American Journal of Epidemiology*, 191(2), 237–240. https://doi.org/10.1093/aje/kwab243

Ekenga, C. C., Kwon, E., Kim, B., & Park, S. (2020). Long-term employment outcomes among female cancer survivors. *International Journal of Environmental Research and Public Health*, 17(8), 2751. https://doi.org/10.3390/ijerph17082751

Firew, T., Sano, E. D., Lee, J. W., Flores, S., Lang, K., Salman, K., Greene, M. C., & Chang, B. P. (2020). Protecting the front line: A cross-sectional survey analysis of the occupational factors contributing to healthcare workers' infection and psychological distress during the COVID-19 pandemic in the USA. *BMJ Open*, 10(10), e042752. https://doi.org/10.1136/bmjopen-2020-042752

Gilbert-Ouimet, M., Trudel, X., Brisson, C., Milot, A., & Vézina, M. (2014). Adverse effects of psychosocial work factors on blood pressure: Systematic review of studies on demand–control–support and effort–reward imbalance models. *Scandinavian Journal of Work, Environment & Health*, 40(2), 109–132. https://doi.org/10.5271/sjweh.3390

Gordis, L. (2013). *Epidemiology* (5th ed.). Elsevier.

Hawkins D. (2020). Differential occupational risk for COVID-19 and other infection exposure according to race and ethnicity. *American Journal of Industrial Medicine*, 63(9), 817–820. https://doi.org/10.1002/ajim.23145

Karasek, R. A. (1979). Job demands, job decision latitude, and mental strain: Implications for job redesign. *Administrative Science Quarterly*, 24(2), 285–308. https://doi.org/10.2307/2392498

Kasl, S., & Jones, B. A. (2011). An epidemiological perspective on research design, measurement, and surveillance strategies. In J. C. Quick & L. E. Tetrick (Eds.), *Handbook of occupational health psychology* (2nd ed., pp. 375–394). American Psychological Association. https://psycnet.apa.org/record/2010-06010-020

Kessler, R. C., Akiskal, H. S., Ames, M., Birnbaum, H., Greenberg, P., Hirschfeld, R. M., Jin, R., Merikangas, K. R., Simon, G. E., & Wang, P. S. (2006). Prevalence and effects of mood disorders on work performance in a nationally representative sample of U.S. workers. *The American Journal of Psychiatry*, 163(9), 1561–1568. https://doi.org/10.1176/ajp.2006.163.9.1561

Lan, F.-Y., Suharlim, C., Kales, S. N., & Yang, J. (2021). Association between SARS-CoV-2 infection, exposure risk and mental health among a cohort of essential retail workers in the USA. *Occupational and Environmental Medicine, 78*(4), 237–243. https://oem.bmj.com/content/78/4/237

Maestas, N., Mullen, K. J., Powell, D., von Wachter, T., & Wenger, J. B. (2017). *The American Working Conditions Survey Data: Codebook and data description.* RAND Corporation. https://doi.org/10.7249/TL269

McClure, E. S., Vasudevan, P., Bailey, Z., Patel, S., & Robinson, W. R. (2020). Racial capitalism within public health—How occupational settings drive COVID-19 disparities. *American Journal of Epidemiology, 189*(11), 1244–1253. https://doi.org/10.1093/aje/kwaa126

McGonagle, K. A., Schoeni, R. F., Sastry, N., & Freedman, V. A. (2012). The Panel Study of Income Dynamics: Overview, recent innovations, and potential for life course research. *Longitudinal and Life Course Studies, 3*(2), 188. https://doi.org/10.14301/llcs.v3i2.188

Mullen, K. J. (2021). *Using the Health and Retirement Study for research on the impact of the working conditions on the individual life course.* https://hrs.isr.umich.edu/publications/biblio/12203

Porta, M. (2008). *A dictionary of epidemiology* (5th ed.). Oxford University Press.

RAND American Life Panel. (2015). *American Working Conditions Survey (AWCS).* https://www.rand.org/education-and-labor/projects/american-working-conditions.html

Sagaro, G. G., Dicanio, M., Battineni, G., Samad, M. A., & Amenta, F. (2021). Incidence of occupational injuries and diseases among seafarers: A descriptive epidemiological study based on contacts from onboard ships to the Italian Telemedical Maritime Assistance Service in Rome, Italy. *BMJ Open, 11*(3), e044633. https://doi.org/10.1136/bmjopen-2020-044633

Sarpy, S. A., Rabito, F., & Goldstein, N. (2013). Sampling in occupational health psychology. In R. R. Sinclair, M. Wang, & L. E. Tetrick (Eds.), *Research methods in occupational health psychology: Measurement, design, and data analysis* (pp. 229–247). Routledge/Taylor & Francis Group. https://psycnet.apa.org/record/2012-25946-014

Siegel, M., Johnson, C. Y., Lawson, C. C., Ridenour, M., & Hartley, D. (2020). Nonfatal violent workplace crime characteristics and rates by occupation—United States, 2007–2015. *Morbidity and Mortality Weekly Report, 69*(12), 324–328. https://doi.org/10.15585/mmwr.mm6912a2

Siegrist, J., Wege, N., Pühlhofer, F., & Wahrendorf, M. (2009). A short generic measure of work stress in the era of globalization: Effort–reward imbalance. *International Archives of Occupational and Environmental Health, 82*(8), 1005–1013. https://doi.org/10.1007/s00420-008-0384-3

Sinclair, R. R., Wang, M., & Terick, L. (2013). Looking toward the future of OHP research. In R. R. Sinclair, M. Wang, & L. E. Tetrick (Eds.), *Research methods in occupational health psychology: Measurement, design, and data analysis* (pp. 395–414).

Smith, J., Hu, M., & Lee. H. (2021) Measuring life course events and life histories. In K. F. Ferraro, D. Carr, & E. Idler (Eds.), *Handbook of aging and the social sciences* (9th ed.). Academic Press.

Sonnega, A., Faul, J. D., Ofstedal, M. B., Langa, K. M., Phillips, J. W., & Weir, D. R. (2014). Cohort profile: The Health and Retirement Study (HRS). *International Journal of Epidemiology, 43*(2), 576–585. https://doi.org/10.1093/ije/dyu067

von dem Knesebeck, O. (2015). Concepts of social epidemiology in health services research. *BMC Health Services Research, 15*(1), 357. https://doi.org/10.1186/s12913-015-1020-z

Wang, J., Smailes, E., Sareen, J., Schmitz, N., Fick, G., & Patten, S. (2012). Three job-related stress models and depression: A population-based study. *Social Psychiatry and Psychiatric Epidemiology, 47*(2), 185–193. https://doi.org/10.1007/s00127-011-0340-5

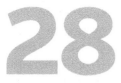

Program Evaluation

The Bottom Line in Organizational Health

Joyce A. Adkins, Susan Douglas, Patrick Voorhies, and Leonard Bickman

The practice of occupational health psychology (OHP) has continued to gain increasing acceptance across the few short decades since it was specifically recognized, meeting if not exceeding the expectations of the academic and scientific foundations from which it evolved. The rapidly growing popularity of the policies and practices advanced by OHP serves to validate the value perceived by the organizational community. OHP was conceived and continues to develop as a holistic approach to advance the health and well-being of the organization itself, the processes included in the activities and management of work, as well as the people within those organizations. While this comprehensive worldview is appealing, it can also be seen as overwhelming and idealistic by organizational leaders who are concerned about costs, time, and resource utilization as compared with associated results or benefits. In a highly competitive global market, organizations have become increasingly attuned to the need for evidence-based or evidence-informed decision making to increase the likelihood that scarce resources are appropriately targeted to the areas that provide the most bang for the buck. Therefore, resources are allocated to strategies and actions that have demonstrated utility for cost containment and improved productivity along with risk abatement and control. As a result, OHP practitioners must continue to ensure that their practices demonstrate value in addressing the needs of their organizational clients while also maintaining solid roots in a scientific and ethical foundation. Program evaluation serves a vital role in addressing that objective.

https://doi.org/10.1037/0000331-028
Handbook of Occupational Health Psychology, Third Edition, L. E. Tetrick, G. G. Fisher, M. T. Ford, and J. C. Quick (Editors)

Unfortunately, challenges in program evaluation arise out of the inherently applied nature of the activity. The dynamic context, numerous uncontrolled variables, and time-sensitive pressures in an occupational environment create challenges to the effective measurement of OHP interventions, whether those interventions come as policies, practices, or programs. When confronted with these complex issues, practitioners may be tempted to avoid the situation by neglecting to design or implement an evaluation plan, choosing instead to just try it and see if it works. But with trial and error, there is little ability to accurately identify the active components associated with success or failure. If a program is effective, the organization will lose the ability to know clearly what key component or practice led to the outcome, reducing the ability to replicate the results in the future. If the program is not effective, the organization can only guess what caused the failure, and future efforts will be curtailed or eliminated in total because of the error, which may have been modifiable. Others may choose to complete a cursory or nominal effort by focusing on more easily obtained data such as program activity levels, utilization rates, or customer satisfaction ratings compared with implementation costs. In using these strategies, these practitioner sacrifice the opportunity to actively demonstrate the effectiveness of their work and to make a valuable contribution to the future operations of the organization as well as to the science and practice of the profession. In point of fact, the gaps in published participatory and applied evaluation research and technical practice reports leave organizations and professionals with no other choice but to reinvent the wheel over and over again and stymies progress in this important area. Without practitioners who are willing to methodically plan, implement, evaluate, and report on the results of policies, practices, and programs, the ability to successfully improve the health and well-being of people and organizations will fail to flourish, and the collective wisdom of our efforts will be lost to future generations. Therefore, despite the obstacles, thorough and effective program evaluation strategies are vital to sustain the acceptance of OHP in the workplace and its growth as a professional discipline.

This chapter addresses program evaluation strategies within an OHP environment. Basic concepts along with a step-by-step guide for evaluation design and implementation will be discussed first, followed by a consideration of value, utility, and ethics associated with the use of program evaluation procedures.

STRENGTHENING PROGRAM EVALUATION

Program evaluation involves the intentional use of specific methods to collect and analyze information about a policy, program, or practice to determine its relevance, progress, efficiency, effectiveness, outcomes, or impact. The strategies and procedures are derived from a diverse set of social, behavioral, health, and managerial sciences, and their utility is central to the managerial process (Barends & Rousseau, 2018; Issel et al., 2021), making evaluation a natural fit for OHP.

The form and scope of an evaluation depend on its purpose, the interests of the relevant stakeholders, the maturity of the program, and the context in which the evaluation is being conducted (Rossi et al., 2018). An evaluation's purpose may be internally derived for organizationally specific purposes, externally derived from upper layers of management or external funding sources, or some combination. This group of stakeholders may have both shared and competing interests that must be negotiated to determine appropriate methods for the situation. The program's maturity in terms of how dynamic or evolving the associated activities may be, or the determination of what level or dose of intervention is required to achieve sufficient outcomes, may influence what type of evaluation is most suitable. The organizational and political contexts in which the evaluation occurs must be explicitly acknowledged to enhance the actual use of evaluation findings.

Types of Program Evaluation

Program evaluation is a multidimensional process that can focus on different facets of program design and implementation. The types of evaluation range along a continuum from formative (i.e., intended to inform the need for or implementation of a program) to summative (i.e., intended to evaluate a program's outcomes or impact).

Prior to beginning an evaluation, an *evaluability assessment* can help determine whether a meaningful evaluation is possible. A program's readiness for evaluation is informed by the clarity and plausibility of program goals, the agreement on criteria or standards to judge performance, the availability of relevant data that can be feasibly collected, and the agreement among stakeholders about how evaluation results will be used (Davies & Payne, 2015; Leviton et al., 2010). Evaluability assessments can help determine needed modifications to a program arising from an ill-defined target population, poor or underpowered program delivery, or other potential flaws so that they can be corrected or modified prior to beginning an evaluation process.

A *needs assessment*, also known as a *design evaluation*, asks questions related to the relevance of the program as determined by the nature and extent of the problem to be addressed. This function focuses on defining the problem, the target population, and how the program fits into the organization's overall strategic or operational plan. By determining needs based on the gap in the current situation and the desired future state (Watkins & Kavale, 2014), decision makers can consider alternative approaches and the amount of resources necessary to solve a problem or even whether it should be solved at all.

Process evaluations may be used at any stage of program development but are especially helpful early in a program's life cycle when implementation decisions are still being made in terms of how to deliver program activities so they are sufficient to impact outcomes of interest. In fact, implementation procedures are so critical that implementation has become a science in itself.[1] Process evaluation methods used within an implementation plan are critical

[1]See the University of Washington's Implementation Science Resource Hub (https://impsciuw.org/implementation-science/learn/implementation-science-overview/).

to understanding issues of program integrity and fidelity, such as what constitutes program drift away from the original plan for efficacy as well as successful adaptations that strengthen effectiveness (Hagermoser Sanetti & Kratochwill, 2014). In addition, process evaluation is useful in exploring the mechanisms of action underlying a program's strategies and any factors that influence how the program is realized in a given context (Moore et al., 2015).

An *outcome evaluation* looks at program results that include planned outcomes as defined by the objectives of the program as well as unintended outcomes that may help rule out alternative explanations. Outcomes differ from simple quantitative outputs, such as quantity of activity, and are associated with results or effects of that activity. In a program evaluation plan, *outcomes* is a term used to refer to those variables that are proximal to the program, whereas *impacts* (i.e., ultimate or distal outcomes) is a term typically used for results more distant from but related to the purpose of the program or policy. For example, a drug treatment program may include outputs (e.g., number of participants), outcomes (e.g., reduction of drug use for those who complete the program), and impacts (e.g., a reduction in burglaries).

Not only is it important to consider the effectiveness of the program, but we must also consider whether the program is the best alternative to other interventions that could be implemented with similar resources. In conducting a *cost analysis*, the evaluator must identify, measure, and compare costs of the program with competing programs. For example, de Oliveira and colleagues (2020) reviewed 56 studies of mental health and substance-use interventions in the workplace, finding that programs to prevent or treat depression are cost-saving but not necessarily cost-effective, whereas programs that target smoking cessation with medication and therapy and those dealing with mental health sick leave to encourage return to work are both cost-saving and cost-effective.

There are three main types of *cost evaluations*: cost–effectiveness analysis, cost–benefit analysis, and cost–utility analysis. The most common approach is *cost–effectiveness analysis*, which is used to compare programs with the same or similar outcomes. A *cost–utility analysis* makes comparisons across programs by using a common metric such as *quality adjusted life-years* (QALYs). Common outcome metrics are not shared outcomes across programs but rather a result of transformations of program outcomes to provide a single indicator of usefulness or value of those varied outcomes. Once values have been assigned to varying health outcomes, this approach is similar to cost–effectiveness analysis. The third type of cost evaluation is the most difficult to conduct. *Cost–benefit analysis* converts all outcomes into a common metric of dollars. It is most often used to compare programs that have very different outcomes, such as physical health and mental health outcomes.

The types and configurations of program evaluation strategies used depend on programmatic and organizational needs. Each provides important information and can be combined to good effect. For example, effectiveness-implementation hybrid designs allow a dual focus on outcomes and implementation strategies (Curran et al., 2012). Choosing an effective program evaluation strategy will ultimately provide valuable data for decision makers to answer the when, who, what, how, and—importantly—why questions of program success or failure. Indeed, placing a high priority on program evaluation and measurement of relevant health and work outcomes has been associated with more promising health and productivity management efforts (Goetzel et al., 2019; Grossmeier et al., 2020; Tamers et al., 2018).

Critical Role of Program Theory

The need for a clearly defined program theory is well established in evaluation practice and provides the foundation necessary to formulate the questions, design the evaluation, select the measures, and interpret the results (Bickman, 1987; Chen & Rossi, 1983; Rogers & Weiss, 2007). *Program theory* refers to a plausible, sensible, or logical conceptualization of how a program is expected or presumed to work (Bickman, 1987). When fully developed and articulated, the program theory allows for increased certainty that the results of the evaluation accurately represent the program. A clearly specified theory or model also allows for either program replication or adjustment of the conditions to achieve a different result. This is opposed to black-box evaluations that examine only the inputs and outputs of a program, without a clear understanding of how the program works. Identifying or constructing program linkages moves the evaluation "inside the box," and resulting data allows increased visibility into potential levers of action for implementing programs or explaining outcomes.

Unfortunately, many evaluations lack a clear theoretical and conceptual underpinning. The assumptions underlying the work often remain implicit and unspecified, providing little in the way of explanation and rendering the results less meaningful to decision makers. Limitations arising from the evaluation methodology are often cited as critical factors associated with the lack of demonstrated long-term effectiveness of OHP interventions, although it is certainly acknowledged that field-based research is challenging (Bickman & Rog, 2009). Program planners and evaluators who clearly identify, fully develop, and explicitly describe their guiding theory produce evaluation strategies that yield more satisfying and useful results. In addition, context-specific evaluations provide a useful framework for assessing contextual factors throughout the planning, implementation, and use of evaluation (Conner et al., 2012).

An established strategy to graphically represent how a program is intended to work, including the underlying program theory, is the logic model. *Logic models* vary but generally include standard elements such as program inputs (e.g., financial costs and personnel time incurred in program implementation), specific program activities, mediating variables or processes that may influence how the program works, and program results ranging from proximate to distal outcomes. As depicted in Figure 28.1, inputs and outputs constitute only the beginning of the process in evaluating OHP programs. These variables are then linked to expected program outcomes and ultimately to desired or targeted organizational goals or outcomes.

FIGURE 28.1. Program Evaluation Process Elements

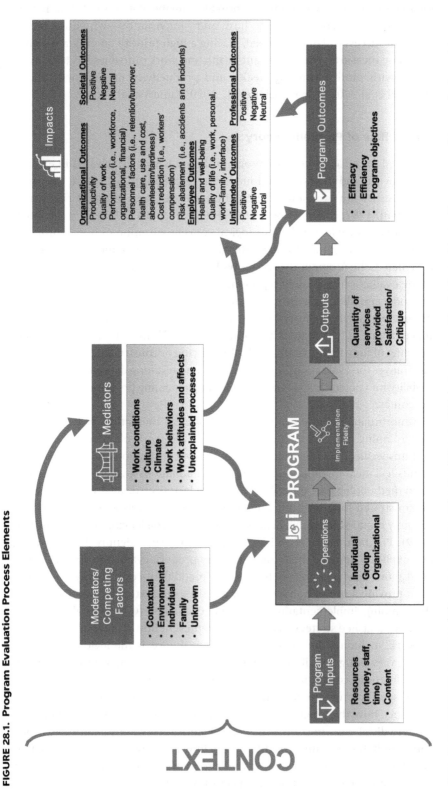

Note. Arrows represent processes, links, or assumptions, either implicit or explicit, known or hypothesized, consistent with a program theory or logic model.

To effectively develop a logic model, the program theory specific to that intervention identifies the inputs, outputs, outcomes, and the expected role of extraneous or contextual variables. In addition, the "glue" that is often missing in program models is represented by the underlying theories of social phenomena, which are nonspecific to that program and serve to link components together and unearth assumptions held by the program developers (Bickman, 1987). Involvement of the program stakeholders is key to developing a high-quality logic model to uncover unstated assumptions, clarify potential relationships among variables, and, importantly, build consensus and collaboration in the overall evaluation process (Taylor et al., 2020; West, 2014). Logic models can serve a crucial communication function and contribute to shared understanding and ownership of an ensuing evaluation. Both qualitative (e.g., case studies, observations, semi-structured interviews) and quantitative (e.g., standardized questionnaires, surveys) methods are recommended as systematic approaches to elucidate stakeholder views, with the actual development of the logic model as an iterative process of correction and enhancement (Frechtling, 2007; Goldman & Schmalz, 2006; Gugiu & Rodríguez-Campos, 2007; Porteous et al., 2002; Unrau, 2001).

Because programs are not implemented in a vacuum, mediating, moderating, or competing variables can exert a substantial influence. Organizational intervention programs that are multifaceted rather than focused on a single, isolated process have been found to be more effective in meeting organizational objectives (Adkins & Davidson, 2012; Sorensen et al., 2016; Taylor et al., 2020). For example, Sorensen and colleagues (2016) provided a comprehensive logic model of integrated approaches to the protection and promotion of worker health and safety that was rooted in theory and addressed both contextual factors and multiple levels of outcomes, from individual to organizational. Evaluation strategies, therefore, often look at the combined effect of various programs and tease out individual program effects whenever practical through clear designs, specific measures, and strategic data analysis.

EVALUATION PLANNING

Clearly, evaluation procedures enable organizations to document the initial need, ongoing implementation process, and subsequent impact of new programs as well as changes in existing practices, policies, or procedures. Evaluation strategies—especially those developed as an integral part of the initial program design and refined through a continuous quality improvement cycle, informing development, implementation, and effectiveness—also contribute to organizational learning (Barends & Rousseau, 2018). However, analysis cannot fix what design bungles, as so aptly stated by Light et al. (1990, p. viii). Evaluation plans are rarely taken directly from a standard manual or blueprint. Although reviews of previous evaluations on similar programs can be of assistance, the specific programs, the stakeholders, and the overall environment or context often have unique features that merit individualized planning.

Clarify the Question, Problem, or Issue

To begin any process, a clear purpose, target, or question is fundamental. Ambiguity in the beginning will only lead to vague results. An initial design evaluation or needs assessment can provide relevant information that would lead to the development of an evaluation plan during program development. In an ideal world, an evaluation component would be program-generated as a natural part of new program development. However, the world is not always ideal, and externally conducted evaluations designed after program initiation are frequently encountered. In such cases, the evaluator will likely need to assist in clarifying the evaluation question and operationalizing constructs to develop meaningful measures and assessment strategies.

Participatory approaches to evaluation planning improve relevance, credibility, and meaningfulness, and are critical to crafting useful evaluations (Cousins et al., 2014; Patton, 2008; Rossi et al., 2018). However, stakeholder participation does not automatically equate to positive impact on evaluation use, and can even have negative effects when program staff are included in some aspects of the evaluation but not in decision making about how the evaluation will affect the program (Froncek & Rohmann, 2019). The role of the evaluator is a key component in these cases. Evaluators must be skilled in facilitation (Patton, 2018), which enables a collaborative process with key stakeholders to determine the evaluation focus, make decisions about methods, interpret findings, and enhance the use of results. Moreover, involvement of stakeholders is particularly critical to better understand and mitigate the cultural and racial framing embedded in the organizations, programs, and theories that constitute the working arena of evaluation (Gill et al., 2016; House, 2017). Evaluation is not a value-free exercise, and attention to issues of diversity, equity, and inclusion as they affect the development, execution, and evaluation of programs and policies in OHP is an ethical imperative (Chatterjee & Leong, 2020; Sinclair et al., 2020).

Conceptualize the Program Theory

Each discipline approaches a situation differently and will likely explain the outcomes and assumptions based on their own conceptual viewpoint. OHP, as an interdisciplinary field, draws measures and methods from multiple fields. Each component discipline holds a different piece of the strategic puzzle. OHP efforts attempt to integrate the pieces into a single picture (Quick et al., 2013; Sorensen et al., 2016, 2021). However, many of the underlying foundations still lie within each puzzle piece. It is up to the practitioner to collect the puzzle pieces and fit them together in a way that makes sense to the organization and is in line with the program logic model. Furthermore, evaluators are encouraged to go beyond the objectives identified by the program staff to look for both positive and negative effects that may not be expected by either the designers or implementers, so that an effective and comprehensive program theory can be developed (Bickman, 1987).

In addition to attending to program theory in evaluation planning, monitoring of program implementation during operations is essential. Nielsen et al. (2006) provided an excellent example of an instance when the inclusion of both process and outcomes evaluation allowed the interpretation of unexpected results of an organizational-level health promotion intervention as likely due to implementation failure rather than theory failure. Although the program may work well in theory, if it is not implemented with fidelity, the expected results may not be forthcoming. Yet not all programs succeed even when implemented precisely as planned. Lack of success may also occur when the underlying assumptions of the program model, even those supported by scientific theory and empirical evidence, fail to hold true. Measuring implementation procedures can better explain null or even negative outcome results, or, alternatively, identify potential programmatic levers to increase impact when effect sizes are small (Douglas, 2020).

Pretesting or piloting is often helpful to illuminate black-box or implicit assumptions in the program design and can serve the same purpose in the evaluation design. If the assumptions of the program theory associated with the evaluation design are faulty, the evaluation results can be questionable. If the evaluation fails to find successful outcomes, it may be a result of the program, or it may be a result of a flawed theory or flawed assumptions. In a classic example, Rog and Bickman (1984) reported an evaluation of a stress management program that assumed employees experienced stress primarily associated with home and family. They designed their program around that assumption and implemented the program with fidelity. Unfortunately, the evaluation data found that employees experienced stress on the job, not at home.

The program theory also drives the selection of measures and the assessment strategy used. Individually oriented models hold that improving organizational health is achieved through assisting employees to expand personal resources through training or to manage strain through increased support. Criteria for success would likewise rely on individual changes that are presumed to ultimately lead to overall organizational benefits. More organizationally based models rely on making changes in organizational structure, culture, or processes and focus on organizationally based measures that ultimately are assumed to improve individual employee well-being. Most contemporary OHP-based models take a broader systems view and seek to examine an integrated measure of both individual and organizational predictors and outcomes. In fact, the concept of OHP as a discipline hinges on the intersection of organizational effectiveness and personal well-being, with research and practice aims focused on identifying integrated factors that predict both individual and organizational health outcomes (Adkins, 1999; Adkins et al., 2000; Quick et al., 2007; Sorensen et al., 2018, 2021). As a result, multiple theories can be used and even merged to guide data collection, which is particularly useful in cases where there are multiple and/or competing assumptions about how a program works (Weiss, 2000).

Select and Apply Assessment Measures

The crux of the evaluation process lies in the collection and analysis of data used to evaluate the program. The measures selected and applied as part of this assessment procedure represent key components of the evaluator's toolkit. A carefully crafted measurement strategy is an essential part of a comprehensive, integrated organizational assessment and serves as the functional core of an overall organizational intervention and evaluation plan. A comprehensive measurement strategy provides a thorough needs assessment and paints a detailed picture of the organization preintervention. It then pinpoints targets of high-leverage opportunity, populations at risk, and level of risk and provides meaningful outcome measures matched with organizational goals and objectives. As a general strategy, a combination of quantitative; qualitative; self-report; historical; and current, documented factual information provides a rich data set. In addition, using multiple measures from several sources establishes a means of building convergent validity. Results can provide insight into both the design and the ongoing implementation of change programs and policies. Repeated measures across time can be used to assess the direction and magnitude of the change in relevant indicators.

The act of measurement itself may in some cases create the beginning ripples of change. Therefore, taking preintervention measures whenever possible creates a foundation from which the direction and magnitude of change or program impact can be assessed. In terms of process, data are collected throughout the evaluation and analyzed according to the evaluation design, which relies on the program theory for functional linkages. In consultation with organizational and program leaders, the assessment begins with the evaluation question(s). A strategy is then formulated to identify standardized measures from the literature that will illuminate the question together with supplemental questions targeted at the particular population(s) and issue.

Mixed-methods approaches, including quantitative and qualitative strategies, produce more complete results (Tamers et al., 2018). The use of standardized measures provides an opportunity to benchmark or compare with established norms, and targeted questions fill in specific information that may be unique to the population or issue. Self-report data can provide a baseline snapshot of the preintervention organization and assist in exploring changes that take place over time and across employment groups. Qualitative data from interviews and focus groups can add depth and detail to the numerical data. Behavioral observations and review of relevant organizational records can add important context to better understand results. To minimize the potentially myopic view of a single practitioner, a multidisciplinary team that is inclusive of stakeholders with diverse views is useful to collect and analyze the data and develop recommendations.

The complex system of interlinking factors that influence assessment and analysis procedures in OHP encompasses structural and process measures, with outcomes measures that span both organizational and individual worker categories. For example, the Workplace Integrated Safety and Health (WISH) assessment (Sorensen et al., 2018) is a questionnaire directed toward middle managers designed to assess formal policies and informal practices related to leadership commitment, participation, organizational and environmental working conditions, collaboration, adherence, and data-driven approaches.

Measurement planning not only includes current state organizational assessment and program implementation metrics but also requires effective, business-driven outcome measures (Barends & Rousseau, 2018; Quick et al., 2007). Planning outcome measures can be a challenge to evaluators, and the process often drives the need for novel problem-solving, reflection on the logic model, and collaboration with organizational stakeholders. Monetary outcomes, improved productivity, decreased costs, and risk abatement are effective in the organizational environment and often lead to risk-benefit-oriented evaluation data sets. Measures such as health care cost containment, decreased safety mishaps, presenteeism or unplanned absenteeism, workers' compensation claims, turnover, civil misbehavior, improved worker engagement, and lost person-years or even loss of life to illness or injury have found effective placement in OHP program evaluations. It is important to consider different perspectives when estimating costs since they can be measured from several points of view, including the evaluation sponsor, the program recipient, the company in which the program is being conducted, or society at large. For example, Gaillard and colleagues (2020) found strong yet varied economic evidence for return-to-work interventions for mental illness from the employer's and society's perspectives, with some studies showing that the cost effectiveness was favorable for society but not for the company. Another important perspective that influences measurement in economic analysis is who benefits or who loses in the implementation of a program. A program may appear to save costs not by changing the actual costs of the intervention but by shifting costs to some other entity. In contrast, a program may not save money but may offset the costs of some other entity (Foster & Bickman, 2000).

Design the Analysis Methodology

Despite the complex, applied nature of the evaluation process, scientific rigor is critical to drawing valid conclusions. Programs that can affect individual and organizational health and well-being should be evaluated using the highest standards possible. Therefore, technical issues associated with design and analysis require concentrated attention in program evaluation efforts.

The context of evaluation necessitates the consideration of all valid and practical designs for applied and participatory research in addition to randomized experiments, quasi-experiments, qualitative studies, mixed-methods approaches, and research synthesis such as meta-analysis (for a more thorough discussion, see Bickman & Rog, 2009). The use of multiple methods and attention to a number of issues that often influence research in real-world settings (e.g., selection bias, attrition, unanticipated or unequal changes in the work environment) can strengthen the design of program evaluation. Tamers and colleagues (2018) provided a thorough review of research methodologies relevant to the OHP context, with an emphasis on participatory and mixed-methods approaches and detailed data reporting processes for multicomponent interventions.

Analyze Program Usefulness

Although basic and evaluation research share the same design objective of maximizing confidence in causal inferences, that similarity should not hide the important differences between their broader objectives. Basic research serves the master of theory. Its structure is deduction and its aim is examining the credibility of theoretical propositions. Program evaluation serves the decision maker, who is interested in the usefulness of a specific program or intervention, particularly as compared with alternative courses of action. Therefore, the basic research criterion of statistical significance is not enough to provide information to decision makers about usefulness and efficacy. Evaluation results must be able to assess the strength of the effects of programs, look at multiple outcomes, and judge gains against costs to compare programs in cost-effectiveness and/or cost–benefit terms.

Focusing on the importance of technical issues is not intended to discourage program evaluation efforts. The OHP practitioner must balance the perspectives of multiple disciplines, and the program evaluator must similarly balance the practical constraints of the program with the technical requirements of scientific inquiry. An evaluation team with strong stakeholder consultation blends strengths of practice and science that serve to build a technically sound and practically useful evaluation strategy.

VALUE ADDED USING EVALUATION RESULTS

The value of an evaluation lies primarily in the utility of the results in informing policy or improving programs (Leviton & Hughes, 1981; Weiss, 1993). Use can take many forms. While the stated purpose is to provide information for decision making or problem solving to validate or change the program under review, evaluation information is often used less for concrete decision making than for its capacity to empower users of the information (Henry & Mark, 2003; Patton, 2008). Insights from the evaluation feed the program evolution. Resultant information can reduce uncertainty, confirm results from other sources, control implementation schedules, or trigger modifications in implementation or direction of an existing program or policy.

The emphasis on evidence-based practices is an example of evaluation use that has influenced the field of translational research in OHP (Dugan & Punnett, 2017; Punnett et al., 2020; Schulte et al., 2017). For example, Punnett et al. (2020) reviewed the literature related to the integration of workforce health promotion and health protection for the purpose of establishing a clear definition of the term *integration* that could be used for program evaluation. They found that integration spanned both program content and process variables, and that the implementation of workplace health programs requires both structural support and culture-building across functional areas. In a classic meta-analysis of evaluation research, Leviton and Hughes (1981) identified a number of factors still applicable today that increase the probability of use of program evaluation results. The following sections describe these factors in detail.

Relevance

Information that is perceived as relevant to policy or program concerns and that addresses decision-maker needs is more likely to be used. Developing relevant information requires a partnership of the OHP evaluator with the program being evaluated. The OHP practitioner is grounded in both organizational operations and behavioral science, creating an important role as a knowledge broker and translator of psychosocial or behavioral science information to organization and program managers. To be effective in that role, the practitioner may be required to formulate the findings from the evaluation in language that is practical and actionable and to integrate seemingly contradictory pieces of information that may arise from the process. Development of an effective program logic model aids in this process (e.g., Taylor et al., 2020; West, 2014). A needs assessment affords practitioners the opportunity to become familiar with the business objectives, culture, and language of the organization. Both the goals of the program and the objectives of the evaluation can then be tied to the overall organizational short-term and long-term goals and objectives, increasing the likelihood that evaluative products will be perceived as a part of and therefore relevant to the business plan. In addition, relevance is affected by the timing of results. Windows of opportunity in decision-making processes occur in every organization and in every program. Data that are realized in the window become imminently more useful. Increasing knowledge of organizational processes will likewise increase awareness of windows of opportunity.

Communication and Involvement

A flow of undistorted and unbiased communication between the potential user of information and the producer of that information throughout an evaluation process results in both a better understanding of initial needs and a greater likelihood of use. As the level of user involvement increases, so, too, does ownership of the process and the resultant information. Information flow in organizations tends to be impeded by those who may feel threatened by potentially negative findings. Identifying and involving those individuals with a stake in the outcome of the evaluation can help minimize resistance and facilitate the crafting of results in a format that is palatable.

Presentation of the information is also critical. Clearly established goals, explicit recommendations, and easily understood written and verbal communication will obviously enhance the probability that the information will be used (Evergreen, 2017). Clarity and specificity can also assist in reducing potential misuse. Qualitative information can provide relevant examples to help users understand quantitative findings. Sensitive communication of negative or unanticipated findings and direct communication with organizational leaders and managers can reduce the amount of organizational censorship or distortion that can take place when program personnel or other affected groups feel threatened by the evaluation process, as may be the case in any evaluation but perhaps most significantly in evaluations that are either externally required or imposed from higher levels within the organization.

Credibility and Quality

An evaluation is not the only source of information available to decision makers, occurring in the context of existing preconceptions and day-to-day experiences. Issues of power and resources within organizations will influence the entire evaluation process, from whether one occurs at all to whether and how findings are used. Knowledge of the context will assist in developing information that fills informational gaps. While the results of the evaluation cannot be predicted in advance, information that is completely misaligned with expectations or with other sources of information is likely to be met with skepticism. Such information would require extensive explanation and justification of the quality of the work. Even high-quality evaluations may not be used in decision making if not perceived as credible (Weiss et al., 2008).

Credibility, although highly subjective, acknowledges the place of evaluation as a source of knowledge among other types of information and also accounts for issues of organizational power and resources as well as aspects of quality. The quality of evaluation findings is determined by several factors, including the evaluator's role related to the program, evaluation questions, evidence gathered to answer those questions, depth and breadth of the evaluation, design and methods, analytic plan, and context (Bickman & Reich, 2009). The importance of quality increases when findings must be persuasive or in situations posing a high risk of information misuse. Credibility of information increases when the source is seen as fair and impartial with no specific stake in the outcome. Therefore, for practitioners who develop evaluation components for their own programs, high methodological quality and well-developed perceptions of credibility in the organization will become increasingly important.

Commitment, Advocacy, and Politics

Evaluations are conducted in the political context of an organization. Advocates of multiple positions battle over issues that correspond with their own interests. Understanding that context is critical. In the end, results generally are used by specific individuals rather than a group or an organization as a whole. The presence of a champion for the evaluation will increase the likelihood of the results being heard and used. The emotional investment of that champion and their position in the organization can have a substantial impact on the advocacy of both OHP programs and evaluations. To ensure effectiveness, advancing marketing and building solid relationships in the planning and implementation phase will set the stage for a receptive attitude once the results of the evaluation are completed. Building relationships within the organization is a critical but often neglected activity of both program managers and evaluators. Targeting information to key users and marketing the importance of that information to decision makers promotes the meaningful use of evaluation results.

ETHICAL CONSIDERATIONS

Evaluators have obligations to diverse groups, including the client organization, stakeholders in the program, program managers and staff, program beneficiaries, and other professionals in their discipline. These obligations include conducting evaluations with fairness, objectivity, and professionalism (Galport & Azzam, 2017; Garcia & Stevahn, 2019). Evaluations must begin with realistic objectives and questions that the evaluator or evaluation team is capable of answering. Valid constructs and measures followed by skilled and unbiased data collection and thoughtful analysis lead to results that can be relied upon to guide policy or program decisions. In the process, it is important that individuals and the organization are protected from harm. Protection involves a respect for confidentiality and may require informed consent from those who participate (O'Flynn et al., 2016). Ethical challenges arise when it appears that the project cannot be accomplished as defined. There may be questions about how much information is enough to answer the question, how much analysis is required as opposed to straight presentation of the information, or when causal inferences are appropriate to the data and methodology of the evaluation. Requests may be made from a variety of factions to present the findings in the best possible light. Information can be misused by clients or by individuals within the organization to support their own ideas or interests. Finally, findings can result in harmful action taken against participants in the evaluation, participants in the program, or employees in the organization if the findings fail to support health-engendering practices. Because of the potential for harm, it is incumbent on practitioners to consider the possible consequences of the evaluation process and to ensure that a process is established that will protect the participants, the organizational client, and the professional integrity of the evaluation itself.

CONCLUSION

The landscape of OHP practice continues to evolve and expand. To continue to grow and adapt to a dynamic workplace, it is important to understand the details of what and why practices, policies and programs have the desired results, creating effective core technologies and procedures. It is critical for practitioners to envision the future and to find, acquire, and develop skills to implement alternative strategies to meet the needs of their client organizations. Effectively designed, conducted, and well-documented program evaluations provide the cornerstone for continued success in this important field of practice.

REFERENCES

Adkins, J. A. (1999). Promoting organizational health: The evolving practice of occupational health psychology. *Professional Psychology, Research and Practice, 30*(2), 129–137. https://doi.org/10.1037/0735-7028.30.2.129

Adkins, J. A., & Davidson, B. M. (2012). Large-scale trauma: Institutionalizing pre- and post-trauma prevention, intervention, and treatment. In R. Hughes, A. Kinder, & C. L. Cooper (Eds.), *International handbook of workplace trauma support* (pp. 30–47). Wiley-Blackwell. https://doi.org/10.1002/9781119943242.ch3

Adkins, J. A., Quick, J. C., & Moe, K. O. (2000). Building world class performance in changing times. In L. R. Murphy & C. L. Cooper (Eds.), *Healthy and productive work: An international perspective* (pp. 107–132). Taylor & Francis. https://doi.org/10.4324/9780203305645

Barends, E., & Rousseau, D. M. (2018). *Evidence-based management: How to use evidence to make better organizational decisions.* Kogan Page.

Bickman, L. (1987). Using program theory in evaluation. *New Directions for Program Evaluation, 1987*(33), 5–18. https://doi.org/10.1002/ev.1443

Bickman, L., & Reich, S. M. (2009). Randomized controlled trials: A gold standard with feet of clay? In S. I. Donaldson & C. A. Christie (Eds.), *What counts as credible evidence in applied research and evaluation practice?* (pp. 51–77). SAGE. https://doi.org/10.4135/9781412995634.d10

Bickman, L., & Rog, D. (2009). *The SAGE handbook of applied social research methods* (2nd ed.), https://doi.org/10.4135/9781483348858

Chatterjee, D., & Leong, F. T. L. (2020). Occupational health disparities among racial and ethnic minorities: Lessons from diverse research frameworks. *Occupational Health Science, 4*(3), 215–237. https://doi.org/10.1007/s41542-020-00067-0

Chen, H.-T., & Rossi, P. H. (1983). Evaluating with sense: The theory-driven approach. *Evaluation Review, 7*(3), 283–302. https://doi.org/10.1177/0193841X8300700301

Conner, R. F., Fitzpatrick, J. L., & Rog, D. J. (2012). A first step forward: Context assessment. *New Directions for Evaluation, 2012*(135), 89–105. https://doi.org/10.1002/ev.20029

Cousins, J. B., Goh, S. C., Elliott, C. J., & Bourgeois, I. (2014). Framing the capacity to do and use evaluation. *New Directions for Evaluation, 2014*(141), 7–23. https://doi.org/10.1002/ev.20076

Curran, G. M., Bauer, M., Mittman, B., Pyne, J. M., & Stetler, C. (2012). Effectiveness-implementation hybrid designs: Combining elements of clinical effectiveness and implementation research to enhance public health impact. *Medical Care, 50*(3), 217–226. https://doi.org/10.1097/MLR.0b013e3182408812

Davies, R., & Payne, L. (2015). Evaluability assessments: Reflections on a review of the literature. *Evaluation, 21*(2), 216–231. https://doi.org/10.1177/1356389015577465

de Oliveira, C., Cho, E., Kavelaars, R., Jamieson, M., Bao, B., & Rehm, J. (2020). Economic analyses of mental health and substance use interventions in the workplace: A systematic literature review and narrative synthesis. *The Lancet Psychiatry, 7*(10), 893–910. https://doi.org/10.1016/S2215-0366(20)30145-0

Douglas, S. (2020). An innovator and a disruptor: Leonard Bickman on program theory, null findings, and advice to future child mental health services researchers.

Administration and Policy in Mental Health, 47(5), 788–794. https://doi.org/10.1007/s10488-020-01043-0

Dugan, A. G., & Punnett, L. (2017). Dissemination and implementation research for occupational safety and health. *Occupational Health Science*, 1(1–2), 29–45. https://doi.org/10.1007/s41542-017-0006-0

Evergreen, S. (2017). *Presenting data effectively* (2nd ed.). SAGE Publications.

Foster, E. M., & Bickman, L. (2000). Refining the costs analyses of the Fort Bragg evaluation: The impact of cost offset and cost shifting. *Mental Health Services Research*, 2(1), 13–25. https://doi.org/10.1023/A:1010139823791

Frechtling, J. A. (2007). *Logic modeling methods in program evaluation*. Jossey-Bass.

Froncek, B., & Rohmann, A. (2019). "You get the great feeling that you're being heard but in the end you realize that things will be done differently and in others' favor": An experimental investigation of negative effects of participation in evaluation. *The American Journal of Evaluation*, 40(1), 19–34. https://doi.org/10.1177/1098214018813447

Gaillard, A., Sultan-Taïeb, H., Sylvain, C., & Durand, M.-J. (2020). Economic evaluations of mental health interventions: A systematic review of interventions with work-focused components. *Safety Science*, 132, 104982. https://doi.org/10.1016/j.ssci.2020.104982

Galport, N., & Azzam, T. (2017). Evaluator training needs and competencies: A gap analysis. *The American Journal of Evaluation*, 38(1), 80–100. https://doi.org/10.1177/1098214016643183

Garcia, G. L., & Stevahn, L. (2019). Situational awareness and interpersonal competence as evaluator competencies. *The American Journal of Evaluation*. https://doi.org/10.1177/1098214018814941

Gill, S., Kuwahara, R., & Wilce, M. (2016). Through a culturally competent lens: Why the program evaluation standards matter. *Health Promotion Practice*, 17(1), 5–8. https://doi.org/10.1177/1524839915616364

Goetzel, R. Z., Berko, J., McCleary, K., Roemer, E. C., Stathakos, K., Flynn, P. R., Moscola, J., & Nevola, G. (2019). Framework for evaluating workplace health promotion in a health care delivery setting. *Population Health Management*, 22(6), 480–487. https://doi.org/10.1089/pop.2018.0177

Goldman, K. D., & Schmalz, K. J. (2006). Logic models: The picture worth ten thousand words. *Health Promotion Practice*, 7(1), 8–12. https://doi.org/10.1177/1524839905283230

Grossmeier, J., Johnson, S. S., O'Donnell, M. P., Goetzel, R. Z., Snow, S., Kelly, R., Kullar, J., Simons, B., Mancuso, M., Dee, M., Faulkner, A., Fries, R., Hall, D., Johnson, S. S., & Grossmeier, J. (2020). The art of health promotion: Linking research to practice. *American Journal of Health Promotion*, 34(1), 105–118. https://doi.org/10.1177/0890117119887857

Gugiu, P. C., & Rodríguez-Campos, L. (2007). Semi-structured interview protocol for constructing logic models. *Evaluation and Program Planning*, 30(4), 339–350. https://doi.org/10.1016/j.evalprogplan.2007.08.004

Hagermoser Sanetti, L. M., & Kratochwill, T. R. (2014). *Treatment integrity: A foundation for evidence-based practice in applied psychology*. American Psychological Association. https://doi.org/10.1037/14275-000

Henry, G. T., & Mark, M. M. (2003). Beyond use: Understanding evaluation's influence on attitudes and actions. *The American Journal of Evaluation*, 24(3), 293–314. https://doi.org/10.1177/109821400302400302

House, E. R. (2017). Evaluation and the framing of race. *The American Journal of Evaluation*, 38(2), 167–189. https://doi.org/10.1177/1098214017694963

Issel, L. M., Wells, R., & Williams, M. (2021). *Health program planning and evaluation: A practical systematic approach to community health*. Jones & Bartlett Learning.

Leviton, L. C., & Hughes, E. F. X. (1981). Research on the utilization of evaluations: A review and synthesis. *Evaluation Review*, 5(4), 525–548. https://doi.org/10.1177/0193841X8100500405

Leviton, L. C., Khan, L. K., Rog, D., Dawkins, N., & Cotton, D. (2010). Evaluability assessment to improve public health policies, programs, and practices. *Annual Review of Public Health, 31*(1), 213–233. https://doi.org/10.1146/annurev.publhealth.012809.103625

Light, R. J., Singer, J. D., & Willett, J. B. (1990). *By design: Planning research on higher education.* Harvard University Press. https://doi.org/10.4159/9780674040267

Moore, G. F., Audrey, S., Barker, M., Bond, L., Bonell, C., Hardeman, W., Moore, L., O'Cathain, A., Tinati, T., Wight, D., & Baird, J. (2015). Process evaluation of complex interventions: Medical Research Council guidance. *BMJ, 350,* h1258. https://doi.org/10.1136/bmj.h1258

Nielsen, K., Fredslund, H., Christensen, K. B., & Albertsen, K. (2006). Success or failure? Interpreting and understanding the impact of interventions in four similar worksites. *Work and Stress, 20*(3), 272–287. https://doi.org/10.1080/02678370601022688

O'Flynn, P., Barnett, C., & Camfield, L. (2016). Assessing contrasting strategies for ensuring ethical practice within evaluation: Institutional review boards and professionalisation. *Journal of Development Effectiveness, 8*(4), 561–568. https://doi.org/10.1080/19439342.2016.1242643

Patton, M. Q. (2008). *Utilization-focused evaluation* (4th ed.). SAGE Publications.

Patton, M. Q. (2018). *Facilitating evaluation: Principles in practice.* SAGE Publications. https://doi.org/10.4135/9781506347592

Porteous, N. L., Sheldrick, B. J., & Stewart, P. J. (2002). Introducing program teams to logic models: Facilitating the learning process. *The Canadian Journal of Program Evaluation, 17*(3), 113–141. https://doi.org/10.1093/annweh/wxaa003

Punnett, L., Cavallari, J. M., Henning, R. A., Nobrega, S., Dugan, A. G., & Cherniack, M. G. (2020). Defining 'integration' for Total Worker Health®: A new proposal. *Annals of Work Exposures and Health, 64*(3), 223–235. https://doi.org/10.1093/annweh/wxaa003

Quick, J. C., Macik-Frey, M., & Cooper, C. L. (2007). Managerial dimensions of organizational health: The healthy leader at work. *Journal of Management Studies, 44*(2), 189–205. https://doi.org/10.1111/j.1467-6486.2007.00684.x

Quick, J. C., Wright, T. A., Adkins, J. A., Nelson, D. L., & Quick, J. D. (2013). *Preventive stress management in organizations* (2nd ed.). American Psychological Association. https://doi.org/10.1037/13942-000

Rog, D. J., & Bickman, L. (1984). The feedback research approach to evaluation: A method to increase evaluation utility. *Evaluation and Program Planning, 7*(2), 169–175. https://doi.org/10.1016/0149-7189(84)90042-9

Rogers, P. J., & Weiss, C. H. (2007). Theory-based evaluation: Reflections ten years on: Theory-based evaluation: Past, present, and future. *New Directions for Evaluation, 2007*(114), 63–81. https://doi.org/10.1002/ev.225

Rossi, P. H., Lipsey, M. W., & Henry, G. T. (2018). *Evaluation: A systematic approach.* SAGE Publications.

Schulte, P. A., Cunningham, T. R., Nickels, L., Felknor, S., Guerin, R., Blosser, F., Chang, C.-C., Check, P., Eggerth, D., Flynn, M., Forrester, C., Hard, D., Hudson, H., Lincoln, J., McKernan, L. T., Pratap, P., Stephenson, C. M., Van Bogaert, D., & Menger-Ogle, L. (2017). Translation research in occupational safety and health: A proposed framework. *American Journal of Industrial Medicine, 60*(12), 1011–1022. https://doi.org/10.1002/ajim.22780

Sinclair, R. R., Allen, T., Barber, L., Bergman, M., Britt, T., Butler, A., Ford, M., Hammer, L., Kath, L., Probst, T., & Yuan, Z. (2020). Occupational health science in the time of COVID-19: Now more than ever. *Occupational Health Science, 4*(1–2), 1–22. https://doi.org/10.1007/s41542-020-00064-3

Sorensen, G., Dennerlein, J. T., Peters, S. E., Sabbath, E. L., Kelly, E. L., & Wagner, G. R. (2021). The future of research on work, safety, health and wellbeing: A guiding conceptual framework. *Social Science & Medicine, 269,* 113593. https://doi.org/10.1016/j.socscimed.2020.113593

Sorensen, G., McLellan, D. L., Sabbath, E. L., Dennerlein, J. T., Nagler, E. M., Hurtado, D. A., Pronk, N. P., & Wagner, G. R. (2016). Integrating worksite health protection and health promotion: A conceptual model for intervention and research. *Preventive Medicine, 91*, 188–196. https://doi.org/10.1016/j.ypmed.2016.08.005

Sorensen, G., Sparer, E., Williams, J. A. R., Gundersen, D., Boden, L. I., Dennerlein, J. T., Hashimoto, D., Katz, J. N., McLellan, D. L., Okechukwu, C. A., Pronk, N. P., Revette, A., & Wagner, G. R. (2018). Measuring best practices for workplace safety, health and well-being: The Workplace Integrated Safety and Health Assessment. *Journal of Occupational and Environmental Medicine, 60*(5), 430–439. https://doi.org/10.1097/JOM.0000000000001286

Tamers, S. L., Goetzel, R., Kelly, K. M., Luckhaupt, S., Nigam, J., Pronk, N. P., Rohlman, D. S., Baron, S., Brosseau, L. M., Bushnell, T., Campo, S., Chang, C.-C., Childress, A., Chosewood, L. C., Cunningham, T., Goldenhar, L. M., Huang, T. T.-K., Hudson, H., Linnan, L., . . . Sorensen, G. (2018). Research methodologies for Total Worker Health®: Proceedings from a workshop. *Journal of Occupational and Environmental Medicine, 60*(11), 968–978. https://doi.org/10.1097/JOM.0000000000001404

Taylor, W. C., Das, B. M., Paxton, R. J., Shegog, R., Suminski, R. R., Johnson, S. R., Akintola, O. A., Hammad, A., & Guidry, M. K. (2020). Development and implementation of a logic model: Occupational stress, physical activity, and sedentary behavior in the workplace. *Work, 67*(1), 203–213. https://doi.org/10.3233/WOR-203266

Unrau, Y. A. (2001). Using client exit interviews to illuminate outcomes in program logic models: A case example. *Evaluation and Program Planning, 24*(4), 353–361. https://doi.org/10.1016/S0149-7189(01)00029-5

Watkins, R., & Kavale, J. (2014). Needs: Defining what you are assessing. *New Directions for Evaluation, 2014*(144), 19–31. https://doi.org/10.1002/ev.20100

Weiss, C. H. (1993). Where politics and evaluation research meet. *Evaluation Practice, 14*(1), 93–106. https://doi.org/10.1177/109821409301400119

Weiss, C. H. (2000). Which links in which theories shall we evaluate? *New Directions for Evaluation, 2000*(87), 35–45. https://doi.org/10.1002/ev.1180

Weiss, C. H., Murphy-Graham, E., Petrosino, A., & Gandhi, A. G. (2008). The fairy godmother—and her warts: Making the dream of evidence-based policy come true. *The American Journal of Evaluation, 29*(1), 29–47. https://doi.org/10.1177/1098214007313742

West, J. F. (2014). Public health program planning logic model for community engaged Type 2 diabetes management and prevention. *Evaluation and Program Planning, 42*, 43–49. https://doi.org/10.1016/j.evalprogplan.2013.09.001

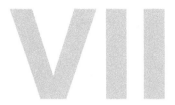

ALLIED DISCIPLINES

INTRODUCTION: ALLIED DISCIPLINES

Occupational health psychology (OHP) is an interdisciplinary field. As explained in Chapter 2, the field of OHP has origins in occupational medicine and overlaps with other fields, such as occupational ergonomics, industrial hygiene, public health, and occupational medicine. Part VII has been added as a new section to this edition of the handbook to provide readers with a primer on four occupational health fields that overlap with OHP and to broaden readers' knowledge of occupational health beyond solely OHP.

Chapter 29 describes occupational ergonomics, which considers interactions between people and the design of workspaces, products, systems, and processes to maximize capabilities and understand limitations to protect and promote worker health and well-being. Although Chapter 17 also discusses work-related musculoskeletal disorders (WMSDs, also abbreviated in the literature as WRMSDs), Chapter 29 provides additional information about skeletal structure and injury prevention based on workspace design and movement. This chapter concludes with a summary of recent literature about the ergonomics climate. Chapter 30 describes the field of industrial hygiene, which aims to anticipate, recognize, evaluate, and control physical workplace hazards that may pose risks for workers' health and well-being. This chapter describes the history as well as the common methods and approaches used by industrial hygienists, including the hierarchy of controls as a common framework for preventing and addressing workplace hazards. Chapter 31 describes public health practice for the prevention of occupational illnesses and injuries and for the promotion of worker health and well-being. More specifically, this chapter describes key principles and approaches to public health practice and summarizes how public health overlaps with OHP. Many chapters throughout the handbook describe *Total Worker Health*® (TWH) as an approach for protecting and promoting worker health and well-being. Chapter 31 also underscores the benefits of a TWH approach. Chapter 32 describes the field of occupational medicine. This chapter is particularly important for readers to understand more about this medical specialty focused on the prevention and treatment of occupational illnesses and injuries given its influence on the field of OHP. The authors of Chapter 32 describe some of the challenges they face in their medical practice and suggest ways in which OHP professionals may benefit from the clinical experience and practice of occupational medicine physicians.

It is our hope that increased knowledge and understanding of these fields may lead to more collaborative research opportunities, improved occupational health practice among a variety of occupational health professionals, and advancement not only in OHP but in occupational health more generally to protect and promote worker safety, health, and well-being.

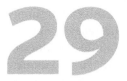

Occupational Ergonomics

David Gilkey

*E*rgonomics is the science of work and is central to the design of systems, workspaces, products, and processes where people are intended to be users, employees, supervisors, managers, and/or executives. Understanding the capabilities and limitations of the user population supplies the opportunity to design features that compliment users' capabilities, increase efficiency and productivity, and decrease errors. Ergonomic designs enhance productivity and quality of the work system as well as safety, employee health, and worker well-being. Having a clear understanding of the intended goals and audience is the optimal starting place. Who is the user, what are the requirements of the task, and what is the purpose?

The inclusion of occupational ergonomics and human factors in this book is of value to occupational health psychology (OHP) professionals, industrial engineers, industrial hygienists, occupational therapists, and other occupational safety and health (OSH) professionals. Most problems in the workplace are multifactorial, and no single practitioner is fully trained with the adequate depth of knowledge, skills, and abilities to comprehensively address complex problems and optimize outcomes. Therefore, collaboration across disciplines is more likely to maximize positive health impacts in the workplace and modern work systems.

This past decade has moved OSH compliance in the transformational direction of *Total Worker Health*® to optimize worker health and well-being by including prevention with protection using a public health model (Lee et al.,

https://doi.org/10.1037/0000331-029
Handbook of Occupational Health Psychology, Third Edition, L. E. Tetrick, G. G. Fisher, M. T. Ford, and J. C. Quick (Editors)

2016). The multidisciplinary or integrated approach to optimize or maximize worker health and well-being is far more effective and inclusive than simply reducing and/or eliminating hazards to reduce costs and relieve pain and suffering associated with worker exposures, accidents, injuries, or illnesses (National Institute for Occupational Safety and Health [NIOSH], 2017). I strongly encourage OHP students and professionals to learn about their allied OSH professionals and the benefits of collaborating to optimize business practices, worker health, and well-being. The multidisciplinary approach will achieve maximum performance, efficiency, productivity, and worker health and well-being.

A BRIEF HISTORY OF ERGONOMICS

The word *ergonomics* is derived from the Greek words *Ergon*, meaning "work," and *Nomos*, meaning "laws" (Jastrezebowski, 1857). Thus, *ergonomics* literally translates to "the laws of work." Although there are many definitions of the term, I prefer the following: "Ergonomics (or human factors) is the scientific discipline concerned with the understanding of interactions among humans and other elements of a system, and the profession that applies theory, principles, data and methods to design in order to optimize human well-being and overall system performance" (Helander, 2006, p. 6).

The discipline of ergonomics and human factors has evolved with contributions from many disciplines. Knowing the history of that evolution gives great insight into the integration of several disciplinary contributions, including those of psychologists. Early physicians learned about ergonomics by making observations and recognizing the relationship between workplace exposures and adverse health outcomes. Although OHP also has roots in occupational medicine, psychologists initially used scientific investigation methods to study, evaluate, and understand human behaviors. Psychologists developed new methods to evaluate and improve the worker–work interface and experience. The contributions of psychologists led to many improved outcomes such as reduced injury and increased productivity, efficiency, quality, worker satisfaction, and well-being. Ergonomics did not become the allied health discipline it is today without the significant contributions of psychologists, who became human factors engineers, and, more recently, occupational health psychologists.

Bernardino Ramazzini, an Italian physician, described the account of work-related diseases in 1713 in his famous book *De Morbis Artificum Diatriba*, meaning "diseases of workers" (Franco and Fusetti, 2004). His work earned him recognition as the "Father of Ergonomics and Occupational Health." As a physician, he made observations about various ailments associated with workplace exposures to diseases, including musculoskeletal conditions apparently caused by poor or unnatural postures (Franco & Fusetti, 2004).

Ergonomics continued to evolve as a discipline, becoming more prominent with the industrial revolution and the need to maximize human power in rapidly expanding industries (Pandve, 2017). Frederick W. Taylor's seminal work to improve productivity at Bethlehem Steel resulted in a dramatic increase in production and wages using ergonomic principles that paired the best tool for specific tasks (Baumgart & Neuhauser, 2009; Pandve, 2017). Frank and Lillian Gilbreth, other early ergonomists, are credited with developing the time and motion study methods leading to increasing efficiency of work by examining and breaking work tasks down into subparts. They measured the time it took to complete jobs and tasks by dividing them into major and minor steps, identifying more efficient and satisfying ways to carry out work and bringing the concept of worker fulfillment into industry. Frederick W. Taylor and the Gilbreths are early advocates of scientific management of work. The Gilbreths took their interests a step further to consider worker satisfaction in the overall enhancement of performance (Baumgart & Neuhauser, 2009; Pandve, 2017).

World War II brought human factors engineering and ergonomics front and center. The U.S. military leadership needed ways to enhance the performance of humans when using complex machines for battle. Human factors engineers and ergonomists studied collaboratively with other experts in anatomy, physiology, and psychology to better understand the human–machine interface (Waterson, 2011). Research groups were formed that represented government, industry, and the armed forces. Their work focused on improving information displays, placement of controls, types and shapes of controls, signal transmission, comprehension, and reaction times (Waterson, 2011). Significant advances in ergonomics were made during this time period and into the present day.

Modern ergonomics took yet another leap forward with the invention and proliferation of computers (Pandve, 2017). Today's ergonomic practices draw from not only anatomy, physiology, and psychology but other disciplines, as well, including engineering, design, and management (Waterson, 2011). The three broad disciplines of psychology, engineering, and health dominate the research and practice of ergonomics. Three major themes or concepts continue to underlie occupational ergonomics: human variability, homeostasis, and systems approach. The contemporary view of ergonomics has been described in terms of human interactions including organizational interactions, logistic interactions, setting interactions, task interactions, interface interactions, contextual interactions, temporal and spatial interactions, and co-operations interactions (Wilson, 2000).

The role of ergonomics in work systems has been described differently by various stakeholders. Perspective and need create a variety of descriptions, roles, and purposes (Wilson, 2000). One major role is the intention to purposefully understand the interaction between humans and objects such as tools, equipment, and displays (Wilson, 2000). To do so, we must consider the capabilities, needs, desires, and limitations of the people who interact with the wide array of stimuli and options in the workplace. Another major role is the contribution to the design of objects, tools, tasks, and environments that are used by people both inside and outside the workplace (Wilson, 2000).

Occupational ergonomics will play major collaborative roles in adjusting to the ongoing work system evolution, technology revolution, globalization, and trade liberalization; accommodating a demographic shift of workers; designing new organizational forms and ways of working; and implementing green ergonomics in response to political, economic, social, technological, and environmental pressures (Bentley et al., 2021). The fundamental goal of human factors and occupational ergonomics is to optimize the interactions for the maximum efficiency, productivity, quality, and worker health and well-being.

WORKER WELL-BEING

Worker well-being is more than the absence of injury or illness or the protection from occupational hazards and risks; it addresses other factors such as work–life balance, life satisfaction, vitality, mood, work-related stress, and mental health (Richardson et al., 2017). Workplace well-being has six essential features: (a) resources to do the job and communication, (b) some control of the work process and environment, (c) a balanced workload, (d) job security and change, (e) positive work relationships, and (f) satisfying job conditions (British Safety Council, 2018). Worker well-being is only achieved through an integrated approach including health promotion, positive organizational leadership, and active engagement of positive lifestyle choices.

Occupational ergonomists fully embrace the newer concepts of *Total Worker Health*® (TWH) practice advocated by NIOSH (Lee et al., 2016). The framework for TWH now includes prevention as well as protection using public health practices. The TWH model is integrated by design and requires OSH professionals, company leaders, human resource professionals, and other employees to work together to achieve optimal outcomes. Key to the success of TWH health programs and worker well-being is fitting the work environment to the worker (Bentley et al., 2021). Fitting the worker to the work environment is poor ergonomics (Pheasant, 1991). Ergonomics has long advocated the design of work systems based upon fitting the job to the person rather than fitting the person to the job (Pheasant, 1991). Fitting the environment to the person involves using both objective specifications such as anthropometric measurements, push, pull, or lifting limits, as well as subjective perceptions including worker satisfaction and preference. The design of work determines the best fit; therefore, adjustability is core to ergonomics. Adjustability of workstations allows individual workers to personalize their work environments, maximize their mechanical advantages, work with their preferred interface characteristics, and improve job satisfaction. To support worker safety, health, and wellness, OHP and OSH professionals, including ergonomists, must work together to maximize the fit and experience that achieves wellness.

ANATOMY, PHYSIOLOGY, AND BIOMECHANICS

Occupational ergonomics is concerned with the structure and function of humans and strives to support optimal fit and function by designing work systems that complement user capacities. How a human is designed directly influences their capabilities and establishes limitations. These limitations and capabilities change as humans change their posture. Human variability is nearly infinite when considering genetic variation in addition to humans' many body parts.

The Human Skeleton

The skeletal bone structure creates the framework for the human form. It comprises approximately 206 bones and divided into two major areas: the axial and appendicular skeletons (Hall, 2015). The axial skeleton is made up of the head, neck, rib cage, and spine. The appendicular skeleton is made up of the appendages and shoulder and pelvic girdles. The spinal vertebrae make up 75% of the vertebral column height, with 23 disc structures interposed between segments in the cervical, thoracic, and lumbar areas only. The discs initially make up the remaining 25% of total vertebral column height and thin over time related to aging and injury. The sacrum and coccyx do not have functional discs.

The Intervertebral Disc

The disc is a unique, avascular structure made of strong ligamentous outer rings called the annulus fibrosis, with a gelatinous center called the nucleus pulposus (Hall, 2015). It is the disc that allows us the freedom to move in the many directions required for activities. The cervical, thoracic, and lumbar verte-brae have facets or joints that also give us the ability to move. The facets are oriented differently in each area of the spine, and thus we can move differently in each area (Hall, 2015).

Keeping the disc healthy and free from injury is of paramount concern to occupational ergonomists. The disc structure is healthiest when we are young, until we are about 25 years old, and tends to dry out and thin over time. The loss of disc height brings the facet joints closer together as we age, resulting in accentuated curves (flexion deformity) in the cervical, thoracic, and lumbar areas, which causes us to get shorter in the seventh and eighth decades of life. Ultimately, gravity wins, and many spinal segments become ankylosed or fused, causing significantly reduced spinal motion in later decades of life. In essence, we give up mobility for stability of spinal segments.

Muscles and Movement

The body has approximately 650 muscles of three different types: skeletal, smooth, and cardiac (Library of Congress, 2019). The largest percentage of our muscles, the skeletal muscles, enable us to move. Smooth muscles are in the digestive tract and glands, and they function without our thinking. The cardiac or heart muscle is unique and always works, never tiring throughout one's lifetime (Library of Congress, 2019). Skeletal muscles are anchored at bony origins and cross joints to insert onto other bones (Hall, 2015). A muscle has only one action: contraction. The muscle contracts concentrically, the origin and insertion move closer together, and the joint angle is reduced; thus, we achieve movement (Hall, 2015).

Spinal motion is unique in that many layers of muscles work together to accomplish global movements such as bending forward or backward, leaning sideways, twisting and turning, or stooping to lift an object from one location and bending to place the object in an entirely new location (Hall, 2015). The physical demands of work can challenge spinal capacity; thus, protecting spinal health is paramount.

The Shoulder

The shoulder is one of the most flexible structures of the musculoskeletal system (Hall, 2015). It is designed as a ball (head of the humerus) and shallow socket (glenoid fossa), with multiple muscles (rotator cuff) anchored on the anterior and posterior axial skeleton. Shoulder stability depends upon soft tissues and is vulnerable to excessive stress to the upper extremity.

Extremities

The arm, forearm, wrist, and hand compose the upper extremity, and the thigh, leg, ankle, and foot compose the lower extremity (Hall, 2015). Each extremity has skeletal bones, joints, and muscles that act together, resulting in movement (Hall, 2015). The unique design of extremities gives us a wide range of movements and power for work and play. The upper extremities are used in reaching, grasping, handling, manipulating, carrying, and placing objects (Hall, 2015). The upper extremities allow us to drive cars, type on computers, and operate machinery, for instance. The lower extremities give us mobility and power to manage our body weight in addition to external loads that must be lifted, carried, and placed in new locations (Hall, 2015). We often coordinate upper and lower extremity movements when accomplishing tasks at work, especially in industries such as construction, manufacturing, and agriculture. Sedentary workers often work their upper extremities more than lower extremities. In other industries, both upper and lower extremities work together to accomplish tasks.

ANTHROPOMETRY

Anthropometry addresses the measurement of humans (Kroemer, 2017). Ergonomists use anthropometric data in the design of workplaces and systems to optimize the physical fit, interface, and functional performance (Kroemer, 2017). Common anthropometric dimensions used by ergonomists are in relation to design of devices, tools, equipment, furniture, buildings, factories, and other items to be used by humans or workspaces with human–work interface.

Three-dimensional scanning of the human body is the modern standard for body measurement (Heymsfield et al., 2018). This type of scanning allows for volumetric measurements in addition to simple dimensions between landmarks, such as the average length of body parts or a girth. Body measurements are used for other purposes, such as sizing of clothing and garments, tools, or common interfaces (e.g., a typical automobile) and custom fit (e.g., a race car).

Manufacturing companies may use anthropometric specifications for the design of access points, repairs and/or maintenance space requirements, assembly line heights, hand tool dimensions, container dimensions for manual materials handling, and workstation workspace envelops. If humans will occupy workspaces and use objects to complete work tasks, their physical fit is important. The wrong fit has been linked to increased physical and mental stress, work-related musculoskeletal disorders, errors, decreased productivity, and reduced product quality.

Data tables are available for various populations and provide a quick reference for most common dimensions, such as stature and reach (Haslegrave, 2018). When applying anthropometry to design, ergonomists decide what range of population is to be accommodated or excluded. For example, it is common to use the 95th percentile when designing for access and 5th percentile for reach (e.g., access through a doorway or reaching the steering wheel of a car). By using these percentiles, most of the population is accommodated. Adjustability is a major theme in design, allowing the optimal fit for function and comfort on an individual basis. Although the "average person" does not really exist, we use "average" dimensions as well in design. For example, when designing the height of a countertop, it is important to know the user.

MUSCULOSKELETAL DISORDERS

We cannot discuss occupational ergonomics without addressing work-related musculoskeletal disorders (WMSDs), which are also covered thoroughly in Chapter 17. Work systems designed with human limitations in mind or ergonomics stressors and risk factors may prevent WMSDs. We have seen that human anatomy, physiology, and biomechanics have inherent limitations related to size, shape, age, disease status, and fitness level of the individual. Common WMSDs that may be associated with work-related stressors and risk factors include excessive force, repetition, awkward posture, contact pressure, vibration, drastic temperatures, and a combinations of other risk factors (Bernard & Putz-Anderson, 1997; Hollnagel, 1997; National Research Council, 1998). Common conditions include tendonitis, tenosynovitis, disc herniation, neck tension syndrome, muscle spasm, or nerve entrapment such as carpal tunnel syndrome (median nerve) and thoracic outlet syndrome (brachial plexus; Bernard & Putz-Anderson, 1997; National Research Council, 1998).

COGNITIVE ERGONOMICS

Cognitive ergonomics (CE), also called human factors engineering, originated in the field of cognitive psychology (Hollnagel, 1997). CE is a specialization within occupational ergonomics dedicated to the optimization of human well-being and the performance of the work system (Dittmar et al., 2021). It has been stated that classical ergonomics addresses the physical interface and CE addresses how work affects the mind in addition to how the mind affects work (Bridger, 2018; Hollnagel, 1997). Many CE researchers and practitioners are concerned with mental loads and processes including perception, memory, reasoning, and motor responses (Dittmar et al., 2021) as well as skilled performance, human reliability, error, diagnosis, cognitive control, memory heuristics, modeling, and training (Hollnagel, 1997).

To design optimal usability in work, investigators study complex systems, cognition, task analysis, decision making, information presentation, mental workload, work stress, context, and collaboration (Dittmar et al., 2021). The European Union (EU) established the European Association of Cognitive Ergonomics in 1982. Since the beginning, EU countries have developed programs focused on specific areas of CE.

France established programs to investigate psychological analysis of thinking in complex process controls and task evaluation as seen in aviation (Dittmar et al., 2021). Scandinavian investigators have been working on ergonomics in safety, interactive systems, and the value of people. The United Kingdom has focused on user-centered design, cognitive behavior, and mental models. Dutch researchers are working on the psychology of programming languages and how to think about how to think. Germany is working on programming languages and the design of user interface management systems. Spain and Italy are working on standards development for CE. The EU has taken this diverse approach knowing that knowledge will be presented at conferences to grow their overall understanding of CE and work systems. Additional goals are to address socio-technical systems and expand into other areas, including virtual reality and other work environments (Dittmar et al., 2021).

Specific projects were aimed at addressing human needs, such as technical support systems specifying what protective equipment is needed to protect firefighters during responses to chemical spills (Dittmar et al., 2021). Another application of CE included the development of health care information technologies (HIT) to lessen medical treatment errors and pharmaceutical mistakes, decrease inefficiencies, and reduce costs (Lawler et al., 2011). Many HIT initiatives and projects have led to significant positive improvements in health care safety, efficiencies, and reduced costs. Another example was a group of investigators who used CE to evaluate drivers' responses to three different types of speedometers (François et al., 2017). The research team measured viewing time, task completion time, response time, usability, and user preference.

The integration of CE and human–computer interaction (HCI) has been underway for some time and has led to proving cross-discipline relationships with professionals interested in product design and usability. The collaborative view has worked to unify the understanding about well-designed interfaces through high-value knowledge sharing, focused research, and translated applications (Dittmar et al., 2021). Classical occupational ergonomics laid the foundations for the evolution of CE and HCI, which now address socio-technical systems as a whole.

DISPLAYS AND CONTROLS

Displays are a common interface for human work. Well-designed displays increase efficiency, accuracy, and quality of work. Many industries, jobs, and tasks require monitoring and control through the integration of visual cues displayed on a screen. The user may execute a task by interacting with a device such as a computer or cell phone via the display. The interface has input keys, buttons, icons, voice controls, or other features to start a process or command (Bridger, 2018). Displays and controls vary widely between products, equipment, and consoles, depending on their purpose and function. Displays may be visual, touch, auditory, olfactory (smell), and gustatory (taste) sensors to supply information on the status of a work process for the human operator and to supply input. Additionally, the layout of the display must complement the human operator's abilities. To do so, the designer must know something about the user population, for instance: What are the gender and ethnicity of the users? What are the anthropometric characteristics? What are the cultural norms, characteristics, and expectations? What information is routinely given? What information is needed in an emergency? What input device or method is best for the user to supply correct adjustments and infrequent or frequent use, and will reduce physical, psychological, and emotional stress? What position will the operators engage? Seated, standing, or both? What environmental conditions exist? Much information may be needed to optimally design displays and controls for specific work systems.

Perception is how we interpret the world around us. How cues are designed and organized greatly influences the accuracy of choices and outcomes. Standard perceptual principles dominate display designs (Bridger, 2018). Organizing into a common area on the display such as calculator numbers on a computer keyboard to the right of the alphabet allows the user to at once go to the location for performing calculations (Bridger, 2018). Organizing the display by proximity is also a principle to ease of use for commands that may be in sequence, such as the numeric keys at the top of the computer keyboard, which are organized in horizontal proximity (Bridger, 2018). Command or input similarity principle may be the priority for a display layout such as scientific notation keys on a calculator, grouped by purpose (Bridger, 2018). It is common to use color for grouping command keys, icons, or buttons. In American culture, green means go, yellow means caution, red means stop, and white means on or operational. Other similarities for grouping might be the size and/or shape of input controls (Bridger, 2018). The symmetry principle may also be used to design display layout (e.g., a clock or watch, and the location of numbers on the dial). The principle of closure is the ability to see and understand the complete target when presented with partial information (e.g., many icon commands that represent a whole function with a partial view of the desired outcome; Bridger, 2018). The continuity principle dictates that all command options follow a smooth line to the target (e.g., an arrow on the backspace key). The visual apprehension principle requires that the user counts their way to the desired target (e.g., the top row of numeric keys on the computer keyboard; Bridger, 2018).

Complex displays can be confusing and even dangerous. Common features of three catastrophic accidents were the result of poorly designed control displays (Meshkati, 1991; Pheasant, 1991). The complex nature of nuclear power controls failed at Chernobyl and Three Mile Island in part because of the displays. When the Three Mile Island event was unfolding on March 28, 1979, the 8-foot-by-100-foot display console had more than 3,000 unique displays that "lit up like a Christmas tree," which confused the operators (Pheasant, 1991). The Bhopal accident and release of poisonous gas was also due in part to poorly designed controls and displays.

Because of catastrophic disasters and lessons learned, design criteria have become increasingly important and have been developed to reduce chances of error when designing displays for complex systems (Bridger, 2018). Examples of design criteria include: (a) eliminating the need for unnecessary or complex movements that encourage muscle memory by keeping movements simple, (b) locating the controls and displays optimally to lessen postural stress and strain, (c) avoiding control actions that might obscure critical display areas, and (d) avoiding spatial transformations to ensure spatial proximity for controls and displays used frequently (Bridger, 2018). These basic principles enhance effective communication between human operators, displays, and controls.

Fitts's law helps with the design of displays and controls as well (MacKenzie, 1992). Fitts's law supplies a model to predict activation success and error based on the size of the target and the distance from the operator. This becomes especially important in complex displays (MacKenzie, 1992). Additional design guidelines for both displays and controls include (a) using dials to display rates of change, (b) using alphanumeric displays when discrete values are important, (c) using color when absolute judgment is needed, (d) using varied shapes for differential functions, (e) use lights and sounds to alert operator when system status has changed, (f) reduce glare when possible to support viewing accuracy and reducing eye fatigue, (g) using illumination when ambient lighting is low to enhance contrast, (h) consider using trend displays if changes are slow and historical readings are important, and (i) using pictorial displays if data from subsystems is being integrated (Bridger, 2018).

Control design guidelines also include recommendations for using pushbutton activation for binary or singular high-frequency use (Bridger, 2018). Use of foot-activated buttons should be limited to when the hands are occupied or for noncritical activations. Toggle switches may be used when single or multiple settings are needed and clear toggle values are given (Bridger, 2018). Push/pull controls are good for on and off actions such as using a handbrake. Pedals and levers may be used when larger forces are needed to activate commands. Rotary switches are good when three to 24 selections are offered (Bridger, 2018). Thumb wheels are recommended for occasional use only. Knobs are recommended for precision and adjustment for continuous scales (e.g., a dimmer switch). Handwheels are proper for two-handed operations (e.g., operation of valves; Bridger, 2018).

INDUSTRIAL DESIGN

Designing work systems calls upon knowledge of anthropometry and physiology to accommodate physical characteristics and capacities of users, whereas knowledge of CE helps designers understand how the mind works for mental loads, signal perception, processing, evaluation, and response. More recently, ergonomics has included the social aspects of work design that impact worker satisfaction and quality of work life. The integrated approach to design is most effective when addressing all domains of human performance. Designers interact and collaborate with systems engineers, design engineers, product engineers, OHP professionals, safety professionals, and industrial hygiene experts.

Industrial design methods include a variety of approaches and specifications. One approach is the design for manufacturing (DFM; Helander, 2006; Konz & Johnson, 2016). The DFM approach is intended to create workflow with the greatest efficiency and lowest cost. DFM goals are to design optimal workflow and worker interface for ease of visibility and feedback, manipulations, handling, tactile and auditory feedback, spatial similarity, mental load, transferable training, and job satisfaction (Helander, 2006). To optimize worker satisfaction, designers, supervisors, and managers should support social interaction and job autonomy by allowing workers to speak with each other, collaborate where appropriate, receive constructive feedback, control the work pace, exercise judgment, be decision makers in their work, and have opportunities to learn new skills to enhance their capacities (Helander, 2006).

Computer Workstation Design

Workstation design varies depending on the environment, purpose, and work system. The workspace envelope defines the immediate work area and supplies guidance on placement of computer, devices, equipment, and activities based on frequency of use. Well-designed workstations optimize worker productivity, efficiency, quality, safety, health, and well-being. Computer workstation design has been shaped by extensive investigation and experience over the past 40 years. General guidelines and optimal HCI designs for the human–computer interface (HCI) have been recommended, including (a) adjustability to meet the comfort needs of the user and/or multiple users; (b) designs that agree with the users' mental model and expectations; (c) stability and consistency of the interface that will lead to mastery, improved productivity, and quality; (d) minimizing mental loads of users to reduce stress and fatigue; (e) providing immediate feedback so users know what the status of any project or operation is at any time; and (f) allowing users to manipulate information and simplify information access, use, and control (Helander, 2006).

The American National Standards Institute and the Human Factors and Ergonomics Society published updated standards (ANSI/HFES 100-2007) for computer workstations (ANSI/HFES, 2007). Their guiding principles were to enhance usability by improving ease of use and learning; to support optimal efficiency; accomplish error recovery; to accommodate a wide range of users with varied expertise and morphological features; and to embrace user preference as well as worker satisfaction, health, and well-being (ANSI/HFES, 2007). Workstation designs include basic features to optimize perception, including labeled keys, clearly identified key locations, device feedback for user, and status of toggle keys that are locked (e.g., capital key). General guidelines for operation include adaptability of assistive devices for users needing accommodation, designs that reduce accidental activation, features that support error correction and recovery, and designs that accommodate varied rates of user input. General guidelines for optimal outcomes also include appropriate software that is easily understood by the user and can be quickly used and mastered (ANSI/HFES, 2007).

Workstation Postures

The optimal posture for work is one where the body segments are closest to neutral. Neutral postures are the least stressful position to the user. Moving in any direction changes the balance of forces and creates stress as muscles work to support the body parts away from the midline. In most cases, deviations of 20 to 30 degrees are tolerable unless for a sustained period or in combination with high forces and/or repetitions. For knowledge, office, and seated workers, the chair is the most important piece of equipment. A chair should have at minimum features that support the spine, buttock, and thighs. Some chairs have armrests as well. The common parts of the chair include the seat pan, seat back, armrests, stem, and base. A well-designed chair is adjustable to maximize user support, preference, and comfort. The well-designed computer workstation should include full-range adjustability to facilitate sitting or standing postures, optimal placement of monitor(s), computer keyboard, and mouse platform to support neutral postures of the upper extremity during work.

Organizing the Workstation

Occupational ergonomics offers guidelines for organizing workstations to optimize efficiency, accuracy of work, and conservation of user energy (Pheasant, 1991). The following principles apply to both industrial and office environments. The workspace envelope is organized to meet the needs of the operators and/or users to maximize their performance by keeping commonly used items within easy reach. Several advantages of efficient design and layout include greater capability and improved quantity, quality, and lower costs per unit of product or service (Pheasant, 1991). Reach, frequency of use, importance, movement, and ease of use are all considerations that influence workstation organization. Organizing the workstation to encourage natural movement that is smooth and fluid will reduce errors, conserve energy, and provide greater worker satisfaction (Pheasant, 1991). Organizing for ease of use is fundamental to ergonomics. This overriding concept translates to designs and practices that conserve energy, minimize errors, reduce unnecessary motions, and increase job satisfaction.

MANUAL MATERIALS HANDLING

Manual materials handling (MMH; e.g., lifting heavy objects) is not value added and should be avoided whenever possible. MMH is a leading cause of low back injury and other WMSD (Ferguson et al., 2019). Despite the efforts by occupational ergonomists to eliminate MMH, most companies have circumstances, jobs, and processes where it is required. It is important to recognize that the design of humans carries both advantages and disadvantages for MMH. Loads that are handled close to the body at waist height provide the best mechanical advantage for MMH. Many employers establish weight limits to be lifted manually at 15.9 kg (35 lb.) to protect workers. This is advisable practice but remember that lighter is better.

Using the hierarchy of controls provides a host of options to reduce or eliminate the need for MMH and risk for injury (Lyon & Popov, 2019). Good designs and interventions should increase efficiency, productivity, quality, job satisfaction, worker health, and well-being. The hierarchy of controls includes

- elimination: Design out the need to manually handle objects from the beginning;
- substitution: Replace heavy objects with lighter materials or repackage to lighter loads;
- engineering: Design out MMH or add assistive engineering devices;
- administrative: Establish "safer" weight limits for MMH;
- personal protective equipment (PPE): Not routinely advised. Using back belts may be considered in an MMH program; and
- training: All employees should be trained in "safer" MMH practices.

The first and most effective option to improve the work process is to avoid MMH and the associated risks altogether by automating receiving, transfer, and handling of materials, parts, or objects. This can be accomplished several ways by designing the production process so that it is free of MMH (e.g., using conveyor systems and/or robotics to move materials free of manual handling).

Substitution may be possible by selecting reduced weights of objects handled. For example, if supplies are delivered in 80 lb. (36 kg) boxes, consider requesting that the supplier repackage the products into two 40 lb. (18 kg) boxes that can be handled easier and reduce MMH risks. Another alternative is to have objects repackaged into heavier loads that cannot be handled manually and can only be handled using engineering. The design of containers can be altered as well to reduce risk by adding cutouts or handles for improved grip and stability when handling.

Engineering controls are preferred when redesigning to improve a production process. The best engineering intervention results in the elimination of

MMH using conveyors, robotics, pallet jacks, or other mechanical devices and methods to handle objects. Assistive engineering controls have been developed that support the workers' capability when performing MMH to reduce stresses and associated risks rather than eliminate handling. For example, lift assist devices have proliferated over recent decades because of the significant benefits seen in the workplace. A basic manually controlled device (e.g., a dolly or hand truck) that workers can use to move objects significantly reduces the need to lift and carry loads. Pneumatic lift devices transfer worker interface to object and load control while moving materials rather than lifting. Pallet lift devices raise the load to the optimal mechanical advantage area and/or tilt the load to improve access and reduced bending. Most recently, exoskeletons are being adapted to industry to enhance workers' strength and stability for handling objects (Howard et al., 2020).

Administrative controls may include establishing weight limits for MMH, required training in lifting and handling techniques, using two-person lifts, and/or job rotation. The weight of the object lifted is only one factor in the causal chain that leads to increased stress, strain, and WMSD. Total compressive forces to the spine are a product of the load lifted, the weight of the person, the position of the body and load, and muscle-reactive forces that stabilize the joints and support the body (Gilkey et al., 2007). Compressive forces on the joints evaluated with biomechanical modeling by qualified ergonomists are a better estimate of the risk of injury than just looking at the weight of load handled.

Training is an essential part of the comprehensive occupational health, safety, and ergonomics program. It is important to train workers on how to lift and handle heavy objects and to ensure that workers can lift loads without undue stress to their shoulders and/or spine. If needed, workers should perform stretching exercises to prepare muscles for work, and they should test the load to assess the actual weight. Injury may occur if the worker is not aware of the weight being lifted and thus is unprepared. Workers should evaluate the shape and size of the object to be lifted and should avoid bulky loads that cannot be managed without taking a significant risk of loss of control and injury. In addition:

- Bulky loads may require two people to manage.
- Inspect the object for its weight and good coupling.
- Loads that have good coupling are better managed and safer to handle.
- It is best to have cutouts or handles for lifting.
- Plan the lift and know the origin and destination.
- Be confident that the worker can safely lift and transfer the object from one point to another.
- MMH is preferred without bending, leaning, twisting, or stooping.
- If the load is placed on the floor, use a squat lift to protect the back and spine.

The squat lift maximizes leg strength and spinal stability. Move close to the load and keep the back as straight as possible before beginning the lift. Jerking loads can be dangerous as well as loads with shifting centers of gravity or lack of handholds (e.g., as in carrying a bag of fertilizer). Maintain stability of the contracting muscles while lowering a load. Eccentric contraction carries the risk of injury to the weaker muscles, tendon units, and ligaments. If the load is in tight quarters, clear the path for lifting and handling so that the worker is not prevented from practicing good lifting techniques. Remind workers to be aware of their surroundings, clean up spills, and clear debris that could cause a slip, trip, or fall. If engineering lifts assist devices are used in the workplace, train workers on correct and safe use and ensure that preventative maintenance programs are in place.

ERGONOMICS CLIMATE

For the past 4 decades, safety climate has become a major consideration for companies wishing to improve workers' commitment to safety, reduce losses, and become more competitive (Zohar, 2010). Ergonomics climate assessment was conceptualized by a team of OHP professionals and occupational ergonomists who developed and validated a tool to assess ergonomics climate assessment (Hoffmeister et al., 2015). This is a novel approach to measuring company climate by measuring commitment and practices that support worker well-being as well as performance. More recent research (e.g., at two power plants in Iran; Faez et al., 2021) found that worksites with higher ergonomics climate scores were reported to have more favorable management practices that fostered collaboration, participation, and employee involvement in decision making related to ergonomics, safety, and training (Faez et al., 2021). This tool can be used cross-culturally and supplies valuable information to employers for resource prioritization to address production goals and employees' well-being.

CONCLUSION

Occupational ergonomics is an OSH discipline striving to optimize the human fit to maximize productivity, efficiency, quality, safety, and worker well-being. It has a rich history and evolution that demonstrates its contributions and benefits to both employers and workers. Occupational ergonomists also strive to identify and eliminate risk factors for WMSDs by designing work systems that complement the human capacities. Ergonomists are trained in the use of tools and methods to conduct the worker–work interface and guide design interventions to reduce stressors and improve the bottom line. Occupational ergonomists are ready to collaborate with OHP professionals and other OSH disciplines to comprehensively address workplace challenges. I encourage OHP students and professionals to learn more about occupational ergonomics and seize the opportunity for collaborative work.

REFERENCES

ANSI/HFES. (2007). *Human factors engineering of computer workstations*. HFES.
Baumgart, A., & Neuhauser, D. (2009). Frank and Lillian Gilbreth: Scientific management in the operating room. *Quality & Safety in Health Care, 18*(5), 413–415. https://doi.org/10.1136/qshc.2009.032409

Bentley, T., Green, N., Tappin, D., & Haslam, R. (2021). State of science: The future of work–ergonomics and human factors contributions to the field. *Ergonomics, 64*(4), 427–439.

Bernard, B. P., & Putz-Anderson, V. (1997). *Musculoskeletal disorders and workplace factors: A critical review of epidemiologic evidence for work-related musculoskeletal disorders of the neck, upper extremity, and low back* (Publication No. 97BB141). National Institute for Occupational Safety and Health. https://certisafety.com/pdf/mdwf97-141.pdf

Bridger, R. S. (2018). *Introduction to human factors and ergonomics* (4th ed.). CRC Press.

British Safety Council. (2018). *Future risk: The impact of work on health, safety and well-being: A literature review.* British Safety Council.

Dittmar, A., Murray, D. M., van der Veer, G. C., & Witchel, H. J. (2021). Cognitive ergonomics: A European take on HCI. *Interaction, 28*(2), 88–92. https://doi.org/10.1145/3447792

Faez, E., Zakerian, S. A., Azam, K., Hancock, K., & Rosecrance, J. (2021). An assessment of ergonomics climate and its association with self-reported pain, organizational performance and employee well-being. *International Journal of Environmental Research and Public Health, 18*(5), Article 2610. https://doi.org/10.3390/ijerph18052610

Ferguson, S. A., Merryweather, A., Thiese, M. S., Hegmann, K. T., Lu, M. L., Kapellusch, J. M., & Marras, W. S. (2019). Prevalence of low back pain, seeking medical care, and lost time due to low back pain among manual material handling workers in the United States. *BMC Musculoskeletal Disorders, 20*(1), Article 243. https://doi.org/10.1186/s12891-019-2594-0

Franco, G., & Fusetti, L. (2004). Bernardino Ramazzini's early observations of the link between musculoskeletal disorders and ergonomic factors. *Applied Ergonomics, 35*(1), 67–70. https://doi.org/10.1016/j.apergo.2003.08.001

François, M., Crave, P., Osiurak, F., Fort, A., & Navarro, J. (2017). Digital, analogue, or redundant speedometers for truck driving: Impact on visual distraction, efficiency and usability. *Applied Ergonomics, 65*, 12–22. https://doi.org/10.1016/j.apergo.2017.05.013

Gilkey, D. P., Keefe, T. J., Bigelow, P. L., Herron, R. E., Duvall, K., Hautaluoma, J. E., Rosecrance, J. S., & Sesek, R. (2007). Low back pain among residential carpenters: Ergonomic evaluation using OWAS and 2D compression estimation. *International Journal of Occupational Safety and Ergonomics, 13*(3), 305–321. https://doi.org/10.1080/10803548.2007.11076731

Hall, S. J. (2015). *Basic biomechanics.* McGraw-Hill Education.

Haslegrave, C. M. (2018). *Bodyspace: Anthropometry, ergonomics and the design of work.* CRC Press.

Helander, M. (2006). *A guide to human factors and ergonomics.* CRC Press.

Heymsfield, S. B., Bourgeois, B., Ng, B. K., Sommer, M. J., Li, X., & Shepherd, J. A. (2018). Digital anthropometry: A critical review. *European Journal of Clinical Nutrition, 72*(5), 680–687. https://doi.org/10.1038/s41430-018-0145-7

Hoffmeister, K., Gibbons, A., Schwatka, N., & Rosecrance, J. (2015). Ergonomics Climate Assessment: A measure of operational performance and employee well-being. *Applied Ergonomics, 50*, 160–169. https://doi.org/10.1016/j.apergo.2015.03.011

Hollnagel, E. (1997). Cognitive ergonomics: It's all in the mind. *Ergonomics, 40*(10), 1170–1182. https://doi.org/10.1080/001401397187685

Howard, J., Murashov, V. V., Lowe, B. D., & Lu, M. L. (2020). Industrial exoskeletons: Need for intervention effectiveness research. *American Journal of Industrial Medicine, 63*(3), 201–208. https://doi.org/10.1002/ajim.23080

Jastrezebowski, Wojciech. (1857). *The science of nature.* Central Institute for Labour Protection.

Konz, S., & Johnson, S. (2016). *Work design occupational ergonomics.* CRC Press.

Kroemer, K. H. (2017). *Fitting the human: Introduction to ergonomics/human factors engineering* (7th ed.). CRC Press. https://doi.org/10.1201/9781315398389

Lawler, E. K., Hedge, A., & Pavlovic-Veselinovic, S. (2011). Cognitive ergonomics, socio-technical systems, and the impact of healthcare information technologies. *International Journal of Industrial Ergonomics*, *41*(4), 336–344. https://doi.org/10.1016/j.ergon.2011.02.006

Lee, M. P., Hudson, H. L., Richards, R., Chang, C., Chosewood, L. C., & Schill, A. L. (2016). *Fundamentals of Total Worker Health approaches: Essential elements for advancing worker safety, health, and well-being* (DHHS [NIOSH] Publication No. 2017-112). U.S. Department of Health and Human Services, Centers for Disease Control and Prevention, National Institute for Occupational Safety and Health.

Library of Congress. (2019). *What is the strongest muscle of the body?* https://www.loc.gov/everyday-mysteries/biology-and-human-anatomy/item/what-is-the-strongest-muscle-in-the-human-body/

Lyon, B. K., & Popov, G. (2019). Risk treatment strategies: Harmonizing the hierarchy of controls and inherently safer design concepts. *Professional Safety*, *64*(05), 34–43.

MacKenzie, I. S. (1992). Fitts' Law as a research and design tool in human-computer interaction. *Human-Computer Interaction*, *7*(1), 91–139. https://doi.org/10.1207/s15327051hci0701_3

Meshkati, N. (1991). Human factors in large-scale technological systems' accidents: Three Mile Island, Bhopal, Chernobyl. *Industrial Crisis Quarterly*, *5*(2), 133–154. https://doi.org/10.1177/108602669100500203

National Research Council. (1998). *Work-related musculoskeletal disorders: A review of the evidence*. National Academies Press.

National Institute for Occupational Safety and Health. (2017). *What is Total Worker Health®?* https://www.cdc.gov/niosh/twh/totalhealth.html

Pandve, H. T. (2017). Historical milestones of ergonomics: From ancient human to modern human. *Journal of Ergonomics*, *7*(4), Article e169. https://doi.org/10.4172/2165-7556.1000e169

Pheasant, S. (1991). *Ergonomics, work and health*. Macmillan International Higher Education. https://doi.org/10.1007/978-1-349-21671-0

Richardson, M., Maspero, M., Golightly, D., Sheffield, D., Staples, V., & Lumber, R. (2017). Nature: A new paradigm for well-being and ergonomics. *Ergonomics*, *60*(2), 292–305. https://doi.org/10.1080/00140139.2016.1157213

Waterson, P. (2011). World War II and other historical influences on the formation of the Ergonomics Research Society. *Ergonomics*, *54*(12), 1111–1129. https://doi.org/10.1080/00140139.2011.622796

Wilson, J. R. (2000). Fundamentals of ergonomics in theory and practice. *Applied Ergonomics*, *31*(6), 557–567. https://doi.org/10.1016/S0003-6870(00)00034-X

Zohar, D. (2010). Thirty years of safety climate research: Reflections and future directions. *Accident Analysis and Prevention*, *42*(5), 1517–1522. https://doi.org/10.1016/j.aap.2009.12.019

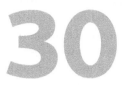

Industrial Hygiene and the Physical Work Environment

Jennifer Cavallari, Len Zwack, and Cora Roelofs

Industrial hygiene, also referred to as occupational hygiene, is the practice of the anticipation, recognition, evaluation, and control of workplace hazards that may result in injury or impaired health or well-being among workers. Industrial hygiene is a part of the larger field of occupational health that addresses the recognition, diagnosis, treatment, and prevention of illnesses, injuries, and threats to well-being resulting from hazardous exposures in the workplace. The practice of occupational health requires multidisciplinary skills and knowledge, including both health and exposure assessment and control, which is the expertise of an industrial hygienist. The broader field of occupational health also encompasses workplace safety (Chapter 5) as well as ergonomics (Chapter 29) in addition to occupational medicine.

THE HISTORY OF INDUSTRIAL HYGIENE

The link between work and health has long been recognized. Hippocrates (ca. 460–370 BC) provided the first record of occupational diseases, linking lead poisoning to work in the mines. In 1713, Bernardino Ramazzini published what is considered to be the first book on occupational diseases—*De Morbis Artificum Diatriba* (Disease of Workers)—based on his observations of workers, their exposures, and resulting diseases. Ramazzini is known as the "father of industrial medicine" (Anna, 2011).

https://doi.org/10.1037/0000331-030
Handbook of Occupational Health Psychology, Third Edition, L. E. Tetrick, G. G. Fisher, M. T. Ford, and J. C. Quick (Editors)

While the link between workplace exposures and the health of workers has been historically recognized, the field of prevention and hazard control was slow to develop. Legislation controlling hazardous workplace conditions can be traced back to England in 1802, although these early laws were seen as ineffective due to lack of inspection or enforcement. It is not until the British Factories Act of 1901, requiring the creation of regulations to control dangerous trades, that industrial medicine and hygiene began to influence workplace conditions.

Around that same time in the United States, Dr. Alice Hamilton, an American physician, began her study of occupational illness and the effects of industrial metal and chemical exposures. After receiving her doctor of medicine degree from the University of Michigan in 1893, Hamilton moved to Chicago and became a member and resident of Hull House, a settlement house focused on providing education and recreational facilities for European immigrant women and children founded by social reformer Jane Addams (Hamilton, 2013). In living side by side with workers at Hull House, Hamilton observed firsthand the problems that workers faced. As a champion of social responsibility, in addition to presenting substantial evidence between workplace exposures and disease, Hamilton also proposed concrete solutions. In this way, she advanced the field of industrial medicine to include not only the recognition of occupational disease but also the evaluation of the work environment and control of hazardous exposures, earning her the title of the "mother of U.S. occupational medicine" and a pioneer of industrial hygiene (Baron & Brown, 2009).

In response to growing public concern over workplace hazards, in 1970 the first comprehensive federal law addressing occupational safety and health for general industry, the U.S. Occupational Safety and Health (OSH) Act, was passed. The OSH Act allowed the U.S. Occupational Safety and Health Administration (OSHA) to develop and enforce regulations and the National Institute for Occupational Safety and Health (NIOSH) to be established as a separate entity to conduct research and provide OSHA with scientifically based recommendations. The Act states that standards shall be set that

> most adequately assure, to the extent feasible, on the basis of the best available evidence, that no employee will suffer material impairment of health or functional capacity even if such employee has regular exposure to the hazard dealt with by such standard for the period of his [*sic*] working life.

Since its creation over 50 years ago, the OSH Act has been both successful and has had its shortcomings (Michaels & Barab, 2020). Worker deaths and injuries have decreased dramatically over the last 50 years. Yet the U.S. Bureau of Labor and Statistics reports that in the United States in 2019 more than 5,000 workers were killed and nearly 3 million experienced a work-related injury or illness. These numbers are likely a gross underestimation due to widespread and well-documented underreporting of occupational injury and illnesses (Spieler & Wagner, 2014), in which employers or employees choose not to report a worker injury or illness to OSHA. Many factors may influence worker injury or illness underreporting. For example, lung cancer due to occupational exposure to diesel may be attributed to nonoccupational exposures (e.g., cigarette smoking) and is difficult to associate with work due to the long latency period between workplace exposure and the onset of the disease.

One of the primary tools that OSHA has to protect worker health is through the enforcement of *permissible exposure limits* (PELs). PELs are legally enforceable maximum pollutant levels that employers must strive to achieve within the workplace through control of their work processes. These were originally adopted during the formation of OSHA in 1971. Since that time, OSHA has had difficulty in updating these PELs to reflect the current state of the science. Many of the PELs were set largely on the bases of industry consensus standards that were determined in the 1960s and what was deemed achievable at that time (OSHA, 2014). In 1989, OSHA tried to simultaneously update outdated limits as well as set new PELs for over 300 chemicals. However, this rulemaking was subject to legal challenges and the courts eventually forced them to return to the original values (Rappaport, 1993). Since that time, OSHA has been able to update some of its PELs (e.g., respirable crystalline silica was updated in 2016) and to make a few new ones, but OSHA has not been able to update the vast majority of them. For the vast majority of chemicals used in today's workplaces, there are no OSHA chemical exposure standards. Additionally, there are currently no OSHA standards related to musculoskeletal hazards, heat exposure, nor workplace violence, which are among the most common workplace hazards. Some employers choose to follow voluntary guidelines produced through consensus processes such as the *Threshold Limit Values*® (TLVs) of the American Conference of Governmental Industrial Hygienists (ACGIH®), the American National Standards Institute (ANSI), or through "local limits" established within an organization to best protect worker health, safety, and well-being beyond what is required by OSHA.

Some OSHA standards—for example, the hearing conservation amendment to reduce noise exposure hazards—require periodic exposure monitoring, training including hazard communication, health monitoring, exposure control procedures, and record keeping (OSHA, 1983). The industrial hygienist plays a large role in implementing the components of OSHA standards and assuring compliance.

THE ROLE AND APPROACH OF INDUSTRIAL HYGIENISTS

Industrial hygienists play a critical role in ensuring the health and safety of workers. Most industrial hygienists have earned a bachelor's or master's degree in science and/or engineering, which they combine with additional training and experience to perform their duties. Industrial hygienists examine the workplace environment and the hazards posed to workers. At the core of the industrial hygienist's role is the anticipation, recognition, evaluation, prevention, and control of workplace hazards.

Anticipation and Recognition

Industrial hygienists investigate work processes and how workers interact with their work environment in order to anticipate and recognize work hazards. Industrial hygienists may work with production or process engineers in the development of new work processes to anticipate, and potentially prevent, hazards. Occupational medicine and public health surveillance plays an important role in recognizing emerging disease clusters related to occupational exposures. For example, in 2000 an occupational physician alerted NIOSH to a cluster of eight cases of fixed obstructive lung disease among workers at a microwave popcorn facility (Kreiss et al., 2002). These initial cases precipitated the recognition of hazardous exposure to flavoring chemicals, specifically diacetyl, that can cause flavorings-related lung disease.

Evaluation

Depending on the type of hazard, an industrial hygienist may perform sampling to quantify exposure by estimating the concentration of an airborne contaminant to which the workers are exposed. A thorough understanding of the work processes and worker activities allows the industrial hygienist to evaluate the potential exposures and exposure routes, which, when combined with the knowledge of the toxicity of a substance or agent, allows for a characterization of risk or hazard.

Prevention and Control

The primary goal of an industrial hygienist is to prevent occupational disease and injury. The most effective means of controlling risk is preventing a hazard at the source, either by eliminating the exposure or by reducing it through exposure control. This is a guiding principle of the industrial hygienist's hierarchy of control, as discussed in more detail in the following section. Regulations also play an important role in guiding the prevention and control of workplace hazards.

CHARACTERIZING HAZARDS COMMONLY ENCOUNTERED IN OCCUPATIONAL SETTINGS

Understanding the exposure route, or the way in which a worker comes into contact with a physical or chemical agent, is a key part of evaluating and ultimately controlling a hazard. Traditionally, the hazards encountered by industrial hygienists in occupational settings are categorized as chemical, biological, or physical (related to the movement of energy or matter) in nature. Workers may also be exposed to psychosocial/psychological or safety hazards, but these are typically covered by professionals in the fields of occupational health psychology (see Chapter 3 as well as many other chapters in this book) and safety (see Chapter 5).

Importantly, there is a difference between a *hazard*, which is the potential for a substance to cause harm, and a *risk*, which is the degree of likelihood that harm will be caused. The industrial hygienist seeks to understand the hazard and limit the risk. For example, paint may include high levels of toxic volatile organic chemicals. The paint presents less risk of an injury or illness when it is mixed using a closed mechanical system versus when mixed by hand. The risk of that paint causing harm to an individual through exposure to volatile organic chemicals is reduced to almost zero after the paint has been applied and dried; however, the risk of exposure may be dramatically different if applied by a spray applicator versus a brush and if the paint container is open or closed.

Exposure Routes

Industrial hygienists evaluate four *exposure routes*: inhalation, ingestion, dermal, or injection. In general, the most common exposure route that industrial hygienists encounter is the inhalation exposure route. The exposure route is an important factor to consider when conducting an industrial hygiene evaluation because the route of exposure can determine the extent of the hazard. Many chemicals are harmful if inhaled. They may impact the health of the worker through systemic effects as the chemical enters the bloodstream through the lungs, directly within the lungs, or in other areas of the respiratory system. However, they may be less harmful if they deposit in the skin or are ingested. Additionally, the exposure route is very important when considering what types of controls are most appropriate to control the exposure. As an example, if the exposure is a respiratory irritant with primary exposure via the inhalation route, improved ventilation controls may capture the chemical at the source and reduce worker exposures. Protective gloves may reduce the risk of developing allergic contact dermatitis resulting from skin exposure to chlorothalonil during manufacture of pesticides (Milam et al., 2020).

Chemical Hazards

Chemical hazards are typically the hazards that first come to mind when a person thinks about an occupational hazard. These hazards can take many forms and span a wide breadth of chemicals. Some of the most common chemical hazards that an industrial hygienist is likely to encounter include respirable crystalline silica, asbestos, metals (e.g., lead), or classes of chemicals such as degreasers and cleaners, paint and paint removers, food additives, and pharmaceuticals. Many of these are chemical mixtures with components of different toxicities and exposure potential. These are all well-studied hazards, where much is known about their toxicity and the ways to properly control them. However, new and emerging chemical hazards present challenges to the industrial hygienist. In recent years, new topics such as exposure to emissions from electronic cigarettes (vaping) and exposure to perfluoroalkyl and polyfluoroalkyl substances (PFAS) have received great interest in the scientific literature. Research indicates that PFAS may cause cancer and have cardiovascular and immune effects (Agency for Toxic Substances Disease Registry, 2021). PFAS-exposed workers include chemical manufacturing workers, firefighters, and ski wax technicians.

Biological Hazards

Biological hazards can come from a wide variety of sources. Bacteria, viruses, plants, fungi, animals, and insects are just a few of the sources of potential biological hazards. Indoor exposure to mold is one of the most common ways in which workers are exposed to biological hazards. Industrial hygienists play an important role in responding to mold exposure due to flooding, such as after hurricanes. Industrial hygienists can identify mold-related damage, initiate remediation, and suggest strategies to protect workers and occupants from mold exposures (e.g., ventilation).

Many industries have potential exposure to biological hazards. Health care workers are required to have bloodborne pathogen training to prevent exposure to potentially infectious materials in blood. Outdoor workers, such as agricultural workers, involved in activities that disturb soil may need to be trained on how to avoid exposure to the fungi (*Coccidioides*) found in the soil in parts of the Western United States that cause valley fever. Since 2020, a biological hazard has been one of the main focuses of industrial hygienists; the COVID-19 pandemic is caused by a respiratory virus (SARS-CoV-2). The COVID-19 pandemic has drawn attention to biological hazards in the workplace.

Physical Hazards

A physical hazard is characterized by the ability to cause harm upon contact. Common physical hazards encountered in workplaces include ergonomic hazards, heat and cold stress, radiation, noise, and vibration. Similar to chemical hazards, occupational exposure limits have been set for some of these hazards. For example, OSHA has set limits on the amount of ionizing radiation, or the amount of noise, that a worker can be exposed to in the workplace. Yet there are no occupational standards to prevent or control ergonomic hazards despite the fact that musculoskeletal disorders comprise a third of reported work-related nonfatal injuries (Reeves et al., 2019). In recent years, more and more attention has been paid to these physical issues. As an example, heat stress has been implicated as a cause of chronic kidney disease in sugarcane workers (Glaser et al., 2016).

Notable Occupational Diseases

An *occupational disease* is defined as an ailment that is caused or aggravated by a work-related exposure. The health consequences of work exposures include both acute and reversible impacts on bodily systems, such as headaches and lacerations, as well as chronic and progressive/irreversible diseases such as allergic sensitivity and cancers. Occupational exposures have been

TABLE 30.1. Notable Occupational Diseases

Exposure(s)	Worker population	Disease(s)
Coal dust	Miners	Black lung disease (coal miners pneumoconiosis; Leonard et al., 2020)
Latex gloves	Health care providers	Allergic hypersensitivity: skin rash, asthma (Raulf, 2020)
Formaldehyde/combustion products/mold/organic solvents/carbon dioxide mix	Office workers	Sick building syndrome (Brightman et al., 2008)
Dust, debris, trauma from 9/11 terrorist attacks on the World Trade Center in New York City	First responders to the 9/11 terrorist attacks	Chronic rhinosinusitis, gastroesophageal reflux disease, asthma, sleep apnea, cancer, posttraumatic stress disorder, chronic respiratory disease, chronic obstructive pulmonary disease, depression, and anxiety disorders (Yu et al., 2021)
Pesticides	Agricultural workers	Cancers, skin and respiratory irritation, nausea, neurological disorders, headache, death (Curl et al., 2020)
Noise	Construction workers	Hearing loss (Suter, 2002)
Ticks	Foresters	Lyme disease (Schotthoefer et al., 2020)
Multiple mixed chemicals	Semiconductor manufacturing workers	Spontaneous abortion and other reproductive health effects (Kim et al., 2019)

linked to every major body part and function, including the skin, soft tissues, neurological pathways, reproductive function, and the respiratory and cardiovascular systems. Some notable occupational diseases as well as the affected worker populations and exposures are presented in Table 30.1.

INDUSTRIAL HYGIENE EVALUATION

An *industrial hygiene evaluation* is the primary tool that an industrial hygienist has at their disposal to try to improve worker health and safety. The evaluation typically consists of a walkthrough survey at the facility or location of interest, the creation of a sampling and evaluation plan, the actual sampling itself, data analysis, and, finally, the creation of actionable recommendations to fix the identified issues.

Walkthrough Survey

A *walkthrough survey* should be undertaken as the first step of any industrial hygiene evaluation. This is a key step that allows the industrial hygienist to get a sense of the company's processes and workflow. It also gives them time to engage with employees and hear about issues at the facility as well as employee concerns. The walkthrough survey typically includes a short visit to the facility where the industrial hygienist will do a walkthrough of the entire facility, asking questions of both the management and the employees, and observing exactly what occurs at the facility. They will be on the lookout for things such as hazards, identifying work processes or tasks for further investigation, and observing personal protective equipment (PPE) use that may not have been described to them when they first learned of the problem. They will also use their professional judgment to see whether other potential hazards may exist. This walkthrough will help them form a sampling and analysis plan, which is often challenging to create when an industrial hygienist is not very familiar with a site.

Sampling Design and Execution

The collection of samples is one of the main tools that an industrial hygienist uses to address an occupational health problem. To do this well, the industrial hygienist needs to know what to sample for, how to properly collect and store the samples, how many samples to collect, and where to collect samples. It is very important that the industrial hygienist comes up with a comprehensive sampling and analysis plan that is specific to the site they are working at and addresses the specific problem that they are trying to solve. One of the key considerations that every industrial hygienist faces when creating a sampling plan is determining which workers to sample and determining how many workers should be sampled. While it may be ideal from an industrial hygienist's perspective to sample all workers, that approach is not often feasible due to logistics and the cost involved. One approach to sampling workers is to separate them into similar exposure groups (SEGs) based on various workplace factors (e.g., work location, type of work done, which shift they work). For example, if exposure to lead is a problem, one simple way to create SEGs would be to acquire a roster of employees at the site and conduct a detailed job-hazard analysis of each position to determine whether the employees work with lead or not. Then, a subset of those employees expected to be exposed to lead could be selected for sampling. It may also be necessary to collect some samples among workers in the nonlead SEGs to ensure that these individuals are not being exposed as well.

 Understanding worker exposure patterns and variability is key to sampling workers and ultimately controlling exposures. Data from the walkthrough survey, combined with information on production and prior exposure monitoring, allows the industrial hygienist to better understand what a worker is exposed to, how a worker is exposed (the exposure routes), and when worker exposures occur. The exposure parameters including the frequency, duration, and intensity are combined with an understanding of the substance's toxicity to assess risk. *Frequency* refers to how often an exposure occurs and can be characterized on a variety of time scales (e.g., minutes, days, weeks, years). *Duration* refers to how long the exposure period lasts, and, like frequency, it can occur across a range of time scales. Intensity is a measure of the magnitude of the exposure, which for a chemical is its concentration. While the frequency, duration, and intensity all help characterize workers' exposure, variability within and between workers also plays a role. *Within worker variability* refers to the range of exposures a single worker may experience from day to day or even task to task. *Between worker variability* refers to the differences between workers performing the same task or working on the same day. Exposure patterns and variability are an important part of fully characterizing worker exposure.

In addition, exposure sampling is largely governed by *occupational exposure limits* (OELs), which often dictate exposure sampling protocols. For OELs reported as an 8-hour time-weighted average (8-hr), 8-hour samples over a work shift are collected; for short-term exposure limits (STEL) or ceiling standards, 15-minute or instantaneous samples are collected.

The types of samples that an industrial hygienist can collect typically fall into a few categories. *Personal air samples* are commonly collected to estimate worker inhalation exposure to chemicals of interest. Typically, these samples are collected by a device that includes a small pump to pull air through sampling media (typically a filter or sorbent tube), specifically designed to capture the pollutant of interest. These samplers are typically worn by a worker over the course of a full work shift. At the end of the work shift, the worker removes the sampling equipment, and the sampling media is sent to a laboratory for analysis. Depending on the pollutant, data can sometimes be collected in real time, with equipment that can provide the industrial hygienist with continuously updated air concentrations.

In addition to air samples, other types of samples can also be collected. Wipe samples are commonly used to determine whether work surfaces are being adequately cleaned and are free of contamination, and to assess the likelihood of dermal exposure to the workers. These are commonly used to look for surface contamination due to metals in a workplace. Noise samples are collected using noise dosimeters, which provide information on how much noise a worker is exposed to during their work shift. Mold samples (via tape lift) are often collected from surfaces to determine whether a stain on a surface is due to mold.

Often, an industrial hygienist will need to send out air samples, as well as other media that have been collected at a site, to an analytical laboratory for analysis. These samples can often be analyzed in a relatively short period of time (a few days), but certain samples may take longer due to their complexity or the lab's availability. Care must be taken when collecting the sample to ensure that it is properly collected, stored, and shipped to the laboratory in the proper manner, so that the sample is not contaminated or otherwise tampered with, prior to analysis. The analytical laboratory will typically report the sample concentrations along with the quality assurance and quality control results back to the industrial hygienist.

Data Interpretation

Once the industrial hygienist receives the laboratory report, they must analyze and interpret this data and transform the results into actionable recommendations for the facility. If OELs are present for the exposure of interest, the industrial hygienist will typically compare their sampling results to these limits to determine whether the exposure exceeds regulatory and/or recommended OELs set by various organizations. The most common OELs used by industrial hygienists in the United States are OSHA's PELs, the National Institute of Occupational Safety and Health's (NIOSH's) Recommended Exposure Limit (REL), and the American Conference of Governmental Industrial Hygienists' (ACGIH®) Threshold Limit Value (TLV®). The OSHA PEL is a regulatory standard that, if exceeded, can result in fines or citations for a company. The NIOSH REL and the ACGIH TLV are not regulatory limits and do not have the force of law behind them. The industrial hygienist will compare their sampling results with these or other limits to help determine what types of actions to take to reduce worker exposure. For certain exposures, there may be no OELs for the industrial hygienist to compare with their results. In these situations, professional judgment is often used to help determine how to control the exposure. Information about an exposure's toxicity and how well it is absorbed by the body, among many other factors, may play a role in controlling the exposure.

It is important to note that the OELs do not represent a dividing line between safe and unsafe exposures. This is particularly true with exposure to allergens, carcinogens, or indoor air irritants (e.g., formaldehyde) for which any exposure may result in a health effect in a susceptible worker. Furthermore, exposure can occur through multiple routes—respiratory and dermal, or at low levels, but in mixtures whose components target the same organs. For example, nail salon workers are exposed to combinations of chemicals that target the central nervous system. Thus, while chemical-by-chemical exposure levels may be below the OELs, the exposure to multiple chemicals is associated with reports of health effects (Roelofs & Do, 2012).

CONTROLLING HAZARDS

One of the most important jobs of the industrial hygienist is to make sound, science-based recommendations on how to control the hazards identified during their survey. The traditional way of organizing and implementing potential controls is through the hierarchy of controls, pictured in Figure 30.1.

In general, the controls at the top of the hierarchy are preferred to the controls at the bottom. The concepts at the top of the hierarchy (e.g., elimination and substitution) can completely eliminate the hazard, while the controls at the bottom of the hierarchy (e.g., PPE) reduce but do not eliminate the hazard. The controls at the bottom are used to help protect workers from hazards that have not been eliminated or sufficiently controlled through

FIGURE 30.1 Hierarchy of Controls

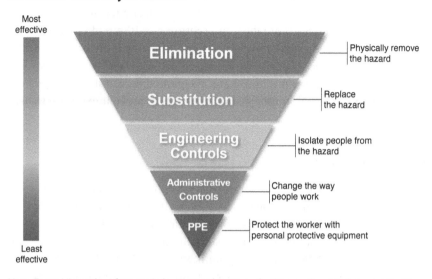

Note. From *Hierarchy of Controls*, by National Institute for Occupational Safety and Health, 2023a (https://www.cdc.gov/niosh/topics/hierarchy/default.html). In the public domain.

engineering interventions. We will now briefly discuss each of the various types of controls.

Elimination and Substitution

These two categories of control are the most desirable and are best able to protect workers. The process producing the hazard is eliminated, or the hazard is substituted for something that is nonhazardous or less hazardous. For elimination, an example of this type of control could include stopping or altering an unnecessary process that causes harmful exposures to employees.

An example of substitution could be replacing a chemical with known toxicity in a process with a less or nontoxic chemical. For example, perchloroethylene (or "perc"), a solvent used in dry cleaning garments, poses numerous health hazards, and is a probable human carcinogen. Substitution of perc with wet cleaning methods has been shown to be a safer alternative (National Institute for Occupational Safety and Health, 1999). Great care must be taken to ensure that the newly substituted chemical is not toxic itself. This was the case when n-Hexane replaced perc as a degreasing cleaning solvent in brake cleaner. Subsequently, exposure to n-Hexane among automotive technicians resulted in peripheral neuropathy (Centers for Disease Control and Prevention, 2001).

Engineering Controls

Engineering controls are typically mechanical interventions that prevent a worker from coming into contact with a hazardous agent. These interventions are usually designed to prevent the worker from being exposed in the first place or reducing the amount of contaminant to safer levels. One of the most common types of engineering controls encountered in industrial hygiene is ventilation. When workers are exposed to airborne hazards, ventilation controls (such as down-draft tables and capture hoods) are often an effective way of preventing workers from coming into contact with the hazardous substance. Other examples of engineering controls could include machine guarding to prevent safety hazards from mechanical equipment, lead shields to prevent radiation exposure, and soundproofing materials to prevent exposure to high levels of noise.

Administrative Controls

Administrative controls are employed when substitution, elimination, or engineering controls are not sufficient to prevent harmful employee exposure. The most common administrative control, effective hazard communication, is seen as the cornerstone of an occupational safety and health program and forms the basis of OSHA's Hazard Communication or "Right to Know" Standard. Hazard communication includes worker training, material labeling, and the use of Safety Data Sheets (SDS), which include information on chemical hazards and how to safely handle them. Administrative controls may also consist of workplace rules to help reduce employee exposure. For example, employers could implement policies to mandate that employees wash their hands when starting lunch or taking breaks. This would help prevent potential dermal and ingestion exposure to the chemicals that employees are working with.

One final type of administrative control involves reducing the time an employee can perform a hazardous task. The company could create safety plans that involve job rotations or limiting the time an employee may spend doing this specific, hazardous task that cannot be controlled via engineering controls. For example, in the manufacturing industry, workers often rotate jobs to reduce highly repetitive movements—although the success of this intervention strategy for reducing musculoskeletal injuries is weak (Padula et al., 2017). While preferable to the next level of controls in the hierarchy (e.g., PPE), administrative controls do not typically prevent worker exposures, which is why they are lower down in the hierarchy of controls.

Personal Protective Equipment

PPE is considered the last resort when it comes to the hierarchy of controls because it places the burden of protection on the worker and does not actually reduce the hazard in the workplace. Typically, exposures are not well controlled, and placing workers in PPE is the only way to reduce their exposures.

PPE can take many forms. One of the most common, and important, types of PPE is respiratory protection. In order for respirators to effectively reduce a worker's exposure, they must be properly selected, fit-tested, maintained, and used by trained workers. There are many different respirators available to choose from and include two main types: air-purifying respirators and supplied-air respirators. Air-purifying respirators purify the air by filtering out particulates (e.g., dusts, metals, fumes) or by adsorbing gas or vapor by passing through a cartridge or canister. Respirators are tight-fitting and offer a variety of coverage, ranging from quarter-masks that cover the nose and mouth to full-face pieces that cover the face from above the eyes to below the chin.

One of the most common types of respirators encountered in occupational settings are filtering face-piece respirators. These respirators are designed to be disposable and are commonly found in N95 or P100 varieties. These respirators filter particles, such as dusts and viruses, out of the air and are not designed to provide protection against vapors or gases. The letter and number code of the product provides information about what it protects against and its filtration efficiency. The "N" means that the respirator is not oil resistant, while the "P" designation means that the mask is strongly resistant to oil (sometimes called oil-proof). The numerical value tells you how much of the airborne particulate the mask can filter out. For an N95, it filters out at least 95% of the airborne particles at the size most difficult to filter (0.3 micron). Similarly, a P100 filters out at least 99.97% of these 0.3-micron airborne particles.

While properly chosen and properly worn respirators can provide protection to workers, some common pitfalls need to be avoided when asking workers to wear them. First, respirators can be uncomfortable to wear for long periods of time. It is not uncommon to see employees either not wearing them at all or not wearing them properly. Sometimes employees are not properly trained on their use, which is why OSHA has issued regulations for how they should be worn. Respirators should fit tight to the face with no air gaps. Employees should not have facial hair that interferes with the respirator's fit to the face. The straps need to be properly positioned on the head, and they need to be worn at all times when working with the hazard they are designed to protect the worker from.

In addition to respirators, other types of PPE are commonly used every day in workplaces across the country. PPE items such as hearing protection (ear plugs or muffs), gloves, hard hats, work clothes and coverings, and eye protection are all commonly required in many types of industries.

PROGRAM MANAGEMENT

In addition to ensuring compliance and handling the technical aspects of worker exposure monitoring and control, industrial hygienists often lead occupational health safety programs at the company level. Industrial hygienists work as part of a larger team including production staff, human resources, ergonomists, physicians, and occupational health psychologists who come together to understand and control a workplace hazard. For example, an industrial hygienist may work with an occupational physician to investigate how workplace exposures are contributing to an employee's symptoms or health condition. In addition to hazard identification and assessment as well as hazard prevention and control, core occupational safety and health program practices include management leadership, worker participation, education and training, as well as communication and coordination for employers, contractors, and staffing agencies (OSHA, 2016).

As occupational safety and health program leaders, industrial hygienists must integrate worker protection into the larger company goals and advocate for the organization's commitment to worker safety, health, and well-being. To be successful in protecting workers, industrial hygienists must understand the larger organization and provide their expertise to anticipate and prevent hazards. For example, in a manufacturing facility, industrial hygienists play a critical role when implementing production changes to anticipate and prevent new hazards that may be introduced.

THE INDUSTRIAL HYGIENE PROFESSIONAL

Many industrial hygienists become certified through the American Board of Industrial Hygiene, Board for Global EHS (environment, health, and safety) Credentialing. A certified industrial hygienist (CIH) must meet the minimum requirements for education and experience and through the successful completion of an exam demonstrate a minimum level of knowledge and skills across the areas considered essential to the practice of industrial hygiene. In order to maintain their certification, CIHs must comply with the code of ethics and demonstrate continuing competence through education and practice activities.

Due to the changing nature of work and the hazards that workers face, continuing education through professional learning is a core practice of industrial hygienists. U.S.-based professional societies for industrial hygienists include the American Industrial Hygiene Association (AIHA) and the American Conference of Governmental Industrial Hygienists (ACGIH).

CURRENT ISSUES IN INDUSTRIAL HYGIENE

The industrial hygienist needs to be prepared to address novel workplace and worker issues that impact worker well-being. Following is a collection of current issues that impact the field of industrial hygiene.

Total Worker Health®

NIOSH defines *Total Worker Health* (TWH) as "policies, programs, and practices that integrate protection from work-related safety and health hazards with promotion of injury and illness-prevention efforts to advance worker well-being"

(National Institute for Occupational Safety and Health, 2023b, para. 2). The occupational safety and health fields, including industrial hygiene, have been called upon to expand their practice to include a TWH approach (Schulte et al., 2019). TWH encourages industrial hygienists to consider both work and nonwork risk factors for safety and health. Rather than taking a siloed approach to risk, the TWH approach urges industrial hygienists to recognize that risk factors accumulate and may interact. This includes addressing disorders influenced by combined workplace and other environment factors, as well as the traditional industrial hygienist concerns relating to chemical, physical, and biological exposures. For example, noise exposures may occur at work and at home, and can contribute to hearing loss when excessively loud. The TWH approach recognizes that hearing loss prevention efforts should emphasize both work and nonwork exposures. For example, a study of transportation construction workers used a TWH approach to hearing conservation, emphasizing the use of hearing protection devices at work and home through training and hazard identification, and found increases in both work and nonwork hearing protection device use (Cavallari et al., 2021).

The TWH approach also encourages industrial hygienists to consider worker well-being, which is more than just the absence of disease and includes physical and mental health as well as social connection. In order to implement a TWH approach, an industrial hygienist collaborates with a broad range of individuals supporting worker well-being across the institution, including occupational health psychologists.

Industrial Hygienists and the COVID-19 Pandemic

Industrial hygienists have a broad mandate to respond to the ever-changing hazards within the workplace. In response to the COVID-19 pandemic, industrial hygienists have served many roles. They have provided their expertise on preventing exposure to airborne hazards via ventilation, physical distancing, and respirator and face mask selection. They have also provided information on training. The AIHA's Back to Work Safely initiative (https://www.backtoworksafely.org) was launched in 2020 to provide industry-based guidance documents to help businesses and consumers implement science-based procedures for limiting the spread of SARS-CoV-2 in the workplace.

CONCLUSION

The role of the industrial hygienist is to evaluate and control job hazards from chemical, biological, and physical risks. Industrial hygienists are one member of a team of broader professionals that seek to protect and improve worker health and well-being. The occupational health psychologist is a necessary partner in achieving this goal. Exhibit 30.1 provides a summary of recommended resources for occupational health psychologists who would like to learn more about industrial hygiene.

EXHIBIT 30.1. Recommended Resources for Industrial Hygiene

Books

Anna, D. H. (2011). *The occupational environment: Its evaluation, control, and management.* American Industrial Hygiene Association.

American Conference of Governmental Industrial Hygienists. (2021). *Threshold Limit Values and biological exposure indices* [Booklet].

American Conference of Governmental Industrial Hygienists. (2019). *Industrial ventilation: A manual of recommended practice for design* (30th ed.).

Clayton, G. D., Clayton, F. E., Allan, R. E., & Patty, F. A. (1991). *Patty's industrial hygiene and toxicology.* Wiley.

Ficklen, C. B. (2019). *Industrial hygiene reference and study guide.* American Industrial Hygiene Association.

Jahn, S. D., Bullock, W. H., & Ignacio, J. S. (2015). *A strategy for assessing and managing occupational exposures* (4th ed.). American Industrial Hygiene Association.

Journals

American Journal of Industrial Medicine

Annals of Work Exposures and Health

Occupational and Environmental Medicine

Journal of Occupational and Environmental Hygiene

Journal of Occupational and Environmental Medicine

The Synergist

Organizations

American Conference of Governmental Industrial Hygienists (acgih.org)

American Industrial Hygiene Association (aiha.org)

Board for Global EHS Credentialing/American Board of Industrial Hygiene (abih.org)

National Institute of Occupational Safety and Health (cdc.gov/niosh)

Occupational Safety and Health Administration (osha.gov)

U.S. Bureau of Labor Statistics (bls.gov)

REFERENCES

Anna, D. H. (2011). *The occupational environment: Its evaluation, control and management.* American Industrial Hygiene Association.

Baron S. L., & Brown T. M. (2009). Alice Hamilton (1869–1970): Mother of US occupational medicine. *American Journal of Public Health, 99*(Suppl. 3), S548. https://doi.org/10.2105/AJPH.2009.177394

Brightman, H. S., Milton, D. K., Wypij, D., Burge, H. A., & Spengler, J. D. (2008). Evaluating building-related symptoms using the US EPA BASE study results. *Indoor Air, 18*(4), 335–345. https://doi.org/10.1111/j.1600-0668.2008.00557.x

Cavallari, J. M., Suleiman, A. O., Garza, J. L., Namazi, S., Dugan, A. G., Henning, R. A., & Punnett, L. (2021). Evaluation of the HearWell Pilot program: A participatory *Total Worker Health®* approach to hearing conservation. *International Journal of Environmental Research and Public Health, 18*(18), 9529. https://doi.org/10.3390/ijerph18189529

Centers for Disease Control and Prevention. (2001). n-Hexane-related peripheral neuropathy among automotive technicians—California, 1999–2000. *Morbidity and Mortality Weekly Report, 50*(45), 1011–1013. https://www.cdc.gov/mmwr/preview/mmwrhtml/mm5045a3.htm

Curl, C. L., Spivak, M., Phinney, R., & Montrose, L. (2020). Synthetic pesticides and health in vulnerable populations: Agricultural workers. *Current Environmental Health Reports, 7*(1), 13–29. https://doi.org/10.1007/s40572-020-00266-5

Glaser, J., Lemery, J., Rajagopalan, B., Diaz, H. F., García-Trabanino, R., Taduri, G., Madero, M., Amarasinghe, M., Abraham, G., Anutrakulchai, S., Jha, V., Stenvinkel, P., Roncal-Jimenez, C., Lanaspa, M. A., Correa-Rotter, R., Sheikh-Hamad, D., Burdmann, E. A., Andres-Hernando, A., Milagres, T., . . . Johnson, R. J. (2016). Climate change and the emergent epidemic of CKD from heat stress in rural communities: The case for heat stress nephropathy. *Clinical Journal of the American Society of Nephrology, 11*(8), 1472–1483. https://doi.org/10.2215/CJN.13841215

Hamilton, A. (2013). *Exploring the dangerous trades–The autobiography of Alice Hamilton, MD*: Read Books Ltd.

Kim, K., Sung, H. K., Lee, K., & Park, S. K. (2019). Semiconductor work and the risk of spontaneous abortion: A systematic review and meta-analysis. *International Journal of Environmental Research and Public Health, 16*(23), 4626. https://doi.org/10.3390/ijerph16234626

Kreiss, K., Gomaa, A., Kullman, G., Fedan, K., Simoes, E. J., & Enright, P. L. (2002). Clinical bronchiolitis obliterans in workers at a microwave-popcorn plant. *The New England Journal of Medicine, 347*(5), 330–338. https://doi.org/10.1056/NEJMoa020300

Leonard, R., Zulfikar, R., & Stansbury, R. (2020). Coal mining and lung disease in the 21st century. *Current Opinion in Pulmonary Medicine, 26*(2), 135–141. https://doi.org/10.1097/MCP.0000000000000653

Michaels, D., & Barab, J. (2020). The Occupational Safety and Health Administration at 50: Protecting workers in a changing economy. *American Journal of Public Health, 110*(5), 631–635. https://doi.org/10.2105/AJPH.2020.305597

Milam, E. C., Nassau, S., Banta, E., Fonacier, L., & Cohen, D. E. (2020). Occupational contact dermatitis: An update. *The Journal of Allergy and Clinical Immunology: In Practice, 8*(10), 3283–3293. https://doi.org/10.1016/j.jaip.2020.08.004

National Institute for Occupational Safety and Health. (1999). Control of exposure to perchloroethylene in commercial drycleaning (substitution). *Applied Occupational and Environmental Hygiene, 14*(7), 433–435. https://doi.org/10.1080/104732299302611

National Institute for Occupational Safety and Health. (2023a, January 17). *Hierarchy of controls*. https://www.cdc.gov/niosh/topics/hierarchy/default.html

National Institute for Occupational Safety and Health. (2023b). *NIOSH Total Worker Health Program*. https://www.cdc.gov/niosh/twh/default.html

Occupational Safety and Health Administration. (1983). *Occupational noise exposure: Hearing Conservation Amendment; Final rule*. 48 Fed. Reg.

Occupational Safety and Health Administration. (2014). Chemical management and permissible exposure limits (PELs). *Proposed Rule, 79*, 61383–61438.

Occupational Safety and Health Administration. (2016). *Recommended practices for safety and health programs* (OSHA 3885).

Padula, R. S., Comper, M. L. C., Sparer, E. H., & Dennerlein, J. T. (2017). Job rotation designed to prevent musculoskeletal disorders and control risk in manufacturing industries: A systematic review. *Applied Ergonomics, 58*, 386–397. https://doi.org/10.1016/j.apergo.2016.07.018

Rappaport, S. M. (1993). Threshold limit values, permissible exposure limits, and feasibility: The bases for exposure limits in the United States. *American Journal of Industrial Medicine, 23*(5), 683–694. https://doi.org/10.1002/ajim.4700230502

Raulf, M. (2020). Current state of occupational latex allergy. *Current Opinion in Allergy and Clinical Immunology, 20*(2), 112–116. https://doi.org/10.1097/ACI.0000000000000611

Reeves, H., Stephens, S., Pegula, S., & Farrell, R. (2019). 25 years of worker injury, illness, and fatality case data. U.S. Bureau of Labor Statistics. https://www.bls.gov/spotlight/2019/25-years-of-worker-injury-illness-and-fatality-case-data/home.htm

Roelofs, C., & Do, T. (2012). Exposure assessment in nail salons: An indoor air approach. *International Scholarly Research Notices, 2012*, Article 962014. https://doi.org/10.5402/2012/962014

Schotthoefer, A., Stinebaugh, K., Martin, M., & Munoz-Zanzi, C. (2020). Tickborne disease awareness and protective practices among U.S. Forest Service employees from the upper Midwest, USA. *BMC Public Health, 20*(1), Article 1575. https://doi.org/10.1186/s12889-020-09629-x

Schulte, P. A., Delclos, G., Felknor, S. A., & Chosewood, L. C. (2019). Toward an expanded focus for occupational safety and health: A commentary. *International Journal of Environmental Research and Public Health, 16*(24), 4946. https://doi.org/10.3390/ijerph16244946

Spieler, E. A., & Wagner, G. R. (2014). Counting matters: Implications of undercounting in the BLS survey of occupational injuries and illnesses. *American Journal of Industrial Medicine, 57*(10), 1077–1084. https://doi.org/10.1002/ajim.22382

Suter, A. H. (2002). Construction noise: Exposure, effects, and the potential for remediation; a review and analysis. *AIHA Journal, 63*(6), 768–789. https://doi.org/10.1080/15428110208984768

U.S. Agency for Toxic Substances and Disease Registry. (2021). *Toxicological profile for perfluoroalkyls.* https://stacks.cdc.gov/view/cdc/59198

Yu, S., Alper, H. E., Nguyen, A. M., Maqsood, J., & Brackbill, R. M. (2021). Stroke hospitalizations, posttraumatic stress disorder, and 9/11-related dust exposure: Results from the World Trade Center Health Registry. *American Journal of Industrial Medicine, 64*(10), 827–836. https://doi.org/10.1002/ajim.23271

31

Public Health Practice for Prevention

Liliana Tenney, Carol Brown, and Natalie V. Schwatka

Public health practice is central to occupational safety and health (OSH) and is crucial for enhancing engagement in the field across research, translation, education, and partnerships. Advancing the identity of public health practice, specifically in the role that occupational health psychology (OHP) plays, is important in preventing work-related injury and illness. Fundamental to public health practice is the acknowledgment that work is a social determinant of health. Work is also impacted by other social determinants of health, including economic status, education, and access to health care (World Health Organization, 2010). The problems of public health today include obesity, mental health, substance use disorders (e.g., drug abuse, alcoholism), suicide, heart disease, and sedentary lifestyles. These health concerns are influenced by the work environment, challenging employers and occupational health professionals to identify ethical and effective ways to promote health through workplace interventions. Experts in infectious and chronic disease epidemiology have provided evidence for the modifiable health risk factors that could be targeted in the workplace to aid in disease prevention and management. Major achievements of public health practice in workplace settings have been seen with influenza, and most recently COVID-19, vaccines that have protected workers so that they can stay healthy and stay on the job.

In this chapter, we address how public health practice and OHP can synergistically apply to enhance OSH interventions and how OHP serves to benefit by considering a broader context to disease prevention and health promotion. This chapter provides examples of how the principles of public

https://doi.org/10.1037/0000331-031
Handbook of Occupational Health Psychology, *Third Edition*, L. E. Tetrick, G. G. Fisher, M. T. Ford, and J. C. Quick (Editors)

health practice can inform workplace interventions, and specifically how they can apply to strategies used in the practice of OHP to design and deliver effective and scalable interventions.

UNDERSTANDING PUBLIC HEALTH PRACTICE

In the past decade, public health practice professionals have expanded their focus on primary prevention efforts that go "beyond the clinic" to elevate the role employers play as agents of well-being in the workplace (Golden & Timberlake, 2013). The definition of *well-being* in the occupational realm is used to describe a worker who benefits from a workplace that is safe and supportive, who is engaged in meaningful work, and who enjoys health benefits as part of the work experience (Schulte et al., 2015). National guidance has proposed how workplaces play an important role in disease prevention. For instance, the Healthy People Initiative started in 1979 when Surgeon General Julius Richmond issued the report titled "Healthy People: The Surgeon General's Report on Health Promotion and Disease Prevention." Beginning in 1980, and occurring every decade since, the Office of Disease Prevention and Health Promotion has released 10-year measurable objectives for improving health and well-being nationwide. Public health practice in the workplace is a key area that defines how to reach these objectives by encouraging employers to take on an active role in promoting health and preventing disease through workplace initiatives. Finally, the National Institute for Occupational Safety and Health (NIOSH) Strategic Plan for 2019–2023 outlines seven goals related to advancing worker well-being through public health practice. Goal 7 is to promote safe and healthy work design and well-being (NIOSH, 2023). This goal specifically attributes translational and intervention science as the mechanism to deliver on the goals of increasing the use of safety and health interventions in addition to developing new cost-effective interventions that contribute to worker safety, health, and well-being (i.e., *Total Worker Health*®). *Total Worker Health* (TWH) was created by NIOSH as a holistic methodology to improve the well-being of the U.S. workforce and the community (NIOSH, 2023). As presented in this handbook, TWH strategies focus on identifying policies, programs, and practices that integrate protection from work-related safety and health hazards with health promotion. We describe how TWH approaches are implemented in a workplace setting that applies key principles of public health practice.

Distinguishing public health practice activities from public health research activities is important because the primary purpose of each is different. Research is primarily conducted to create generalizable knowledge, and practice is meant to prevent disease and improve population health through community-based efforts (Otto et al., 2014). Public health practice spans many different domains. One example is occupational health surveillance through a state health department to track and record work-related injuries and fatalities. Another example is training health educators to engage employers or develop a communications campaign to increase awareness about the importance of offering diabetes prevention and/or management programs at the workplace. Common elements of public health practice and public health research include the application of evidence, the use of systematic methods, the use of study designs, the use of hypothesis testing, and the collection and use of data. Notably, the beneficiaries of public health research versus practice also tend to be different. Public health practice in most cases is intended to benefit stakeholders in a defined community, whereas research typically benefits those beyond the participating community (Otto et al., 2014).

Public health practice principles coupled with OHP approaches aim to benefit employers and workers to improve health, safety, and well-being. In this chapter, we will discuss an approach that we used to distinguish practice from research and discuss the fixed factors for dissemination and implementation. Figure 31.1 illustrates concepts of *evidence-based public health* (EBPH) and how the primary purpose of an activity defines whether it is considered research or practice (Brownson et al., 2009). If the primary purpose is to either enhance and/or scale an intervention, the concepts of public health practice apply. These include leveraging existing resources, such as researchers, practitioners, and partner organizations. In the context of a workplace intervention, it involves understanding the needs of the employer, management, and individual workers to identify core values and contextual factors in designing implementation strategies to deliver the intervention. Evidence-based practices are applied in the process of designing the intervention and adapting it to meet the needs of stakeholders. Dissemination involves fixed factors measured by readiness to change, adoption, implementation, and sustainability of the intervention. For example, if an employer is providing supervisor training with the primary goal of improving safety climate, it would be beneficial to understand how supervisors valued safety and the differences in their readiness to change behavior to design the intervention in a way that encouraged positive adoption. Once implemented, the fixed factors become measures that can be used to evaluate the uptake and effectiveness of interventions (i.e., public health practice).

Public health models provide different approaches to addressing health promotion and disease prevention, each having different goals (Tengland, 2010). For example, health promotion efforts implemented in workplaces to encourage physical activity for workers that spend most of their day sitting can lead to increased motivation, productivity, and physical health status (Pronk, 2021). In contrast, disease prevention efforts in workplaces can focus on lifestyle management programs for higher risk individuals. The following case study demonstrates that by offering both health promotion and disease prevention in the workplace, many individuals who would otherwise lack access to health care, specifically primary prevention services, can live healthier lives.

There are several models that support public health practice. They are commonly used in program planning to understand health behavior and to guide the development, delivery, and implementation of interventions. One

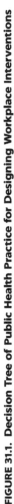

FIGURE 31.1. Decision Tree of Public Health Practice for Designing Workplace Interventions

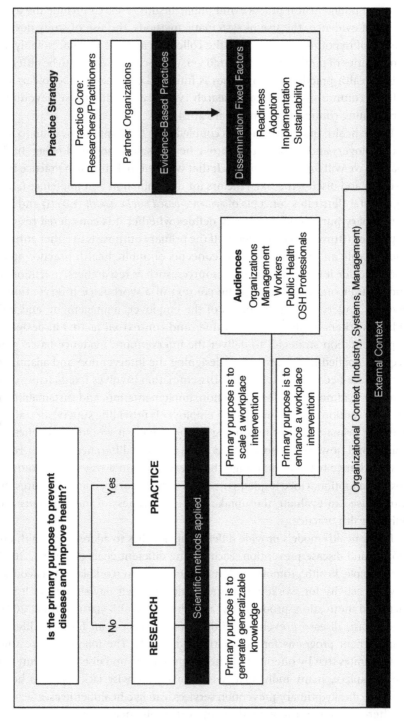

Note. Based on concepts of evidence-based public health (EBPH) from Brownson et al. (2009). OSH = occupational safety and health.

model is the Health Impact Pyramid, which is a five-tier pyramid that provides a scale of impact for the different types of public health practice interventions (Frieden, 2010). The model illustrates how interventions that have broader reach and require less effort tend to be more effective at scale. This applies to public health practice in that the design of intervention aimed at improving worker health should consider what level would be most appropriate to target, a process that involves looking outside the walls of an organization. External factors such as access to health care and social norms are associated with how people respond to public health interventions. Intervention Mapping has been developed as a public health practice protocol for guiding the design of multilevel health promotion interventions and implementation strategies (Fernandez et al., 2019). This process lends itself to designing effective workplace interventions that are guided by the following five key principles of public health practice. Public health practice

1. builds on the strengths of communities to address key health concerns. In the workplace, this involves identifying existing resources, social networks, and structures that are set to assist in the delivery of health and safety programs.

2. facilitates participation in the process. Stakeholders need to have a say in the process to provide their perspectives and opinions about public health priorities. In the workplace, this means involving stakeholders (i.e., managers, supervisors, employees) early and often. Administering surveys to understand needs and interests, to pinpoint concerns and barriers to safety and health participation, and to bridge shared values is critical to establishing social justice and an equitable process. Involving individuals in the process also helps build collaboration and empowerment in decision making among stakeholders. Stakeholders also grow from participating in the process collectively. It provides them with an opportunity to find shared values instead of feeling like safety and health is something that just comes from the top down. Interventions that are built on participation tend to last longer because of the sense of ownership the organization has to support sustainability.

3. designs programs based on proven theories and evidence-based practices to strengthen interventions in both effectiveness and efficiency. In the workplace, this involves being devoted in the time it takes to work with all stakeholders in the organization to learn and build programs that are based on needs assessments. It also involves considering the unique factors among management, business structures, and individuals. This approach leads to better results because it enhances a broader and better uptake among workplaces and workers.

4. evaluates intervention accessibility and acceptability to understand the way communities respond to public health interventions. In the workplace, this means identifying gaps in access to safety and health protections and services. It also means testing the appropriateness of interventions by looking at the costs, burdens, and barriers to participation.

5. ensures equity in all efforts. In the workplace, this means that all are able to benefit from public health interventions. Programs focus on the reach of interventions to all workers regardless of position, job duties, location, or personal health status. Considering the needs of all group members, especially the most vulnerable, helps gather diverse perspectives that are important in informing how worker safety and health is valued and improved in the workplace.

It is important to note that the study of health disparities spans across workplace settings (Souza et al., 2010). Occupational health inequalities occur when factors associated with work across the spectrum of communities, organizations, and individuals are ignored. Public health practice provides an opportunity to design interventions in ways that are effective at addressing common barriers to health in the workplace, such as disproportionate employment, workplace injustice, workplace restructuring, workplace protections, and differential vulnerability (Landsbergis et al., 2014).

PUBLIC HEALTH INFORMS OHP

OHP emerged from the fields of public health and preventive medicine as well as health and clinical psychology. As such, OHP recognized the legitimacy of both approaches—environmental or population-wide interventions and individual-level interventions—to improve the health and safety of workers. Prior to the establishment of OHP as a discipline, health psychology mostly focused on individual-level characteristics and interventions. Since the field of OHP was established, there has been interest in drawing theories of psychology closer to public health to apply methods for improving worker health (Sauter & Hurrell, 1999). There are numerous ways in which public health practice informs OHP, from epidemiologic practices of building surveillance systems to the design and implementation of evidence-based interventions. This section discusses the ways in which public health practice impacts OHP and, conversely, the ways in which OHP impacts the field of public health practice.

Since its inception, OHP has focused both on addressing individual behaviors and creating healthy work environments. Individual characteristics include career stage, age, individual health status, self-reliance, and concepts such as how individuals experience anger and commit to work. The work environment consists of factors that influence how work is experienced by individuals, such as workload, pace, job control, and the physical environment. Finally, OHP has recognized that people do not inhabit only one environment, and that work affects family/life outside work and vice versa. The field of OHP was built upon the idea that designing healthy work environments for workers would maximize the fit between work environment, individual characteristics, and the work–family interface (Quick, 1999a). It is in the design of interventions to create healthy work environments that OHP has most drawn upon public health practice concepts.

The focus of public health practice, on the other hand, has been to prevent disease or injury and improve the health of entire populations, such as states, communities, or workplaces. Public health practice strategies are likely to be more successful in keeping populations healthy than traditional medical interventions that seek to treat illnesses (Braveman & Gottlieb, 2014). First, the health-related problem should be identified. Second, the population's resistance to the health-related problem should be strengthened. Finally, the population's risk of transmitting the health-related problem should be lessened.

The concepts of prevention were built into OHP, starting with primary prevention, which focuses on intervening before health effects occur. In public health practice, primary prevention takes the form of vaccinations, improving healthy diet, and decreasing tobacco use, among many other examples. In OHP, this public health concept has been translated to interventions that enhance the design of the work environment, the health of the individual, or the work–family interface (Quick, 1999a). Specific examples of primary prevention at the environmental level include job design or redesign, addressing organizational culture, and mitigating organizational demands (Quick, 1999a). At the individual level, primary prevention in OHP may focus on time management and learned optimism. Finally, OHP interventions that address the work–family interface may include primary prevention areas such as flexible schedules, child or elder care, and increasing family supportive supervisor behaviors (Allen & Martin, 2017). These primary prevention intervention areas in OHP can help reduce stress, decrease work–family conflict, decrease physical injuries such as musculoskeletal disorders, and increase resilience (Allen & Martin, 2017; Sauter & Hurrell, 1999; Quick, 1999a, 1999b).

In public health, primary prevention—addressing health challenges before they manifest into illnesses or injuries—is the optimal goal. When interventions that address primary prevention goals have been exhausted or are not feasible, public health practitioners turn to secondary or tertiary prevention measures. In public health, secondary prevention measures are lower intensity and lower cost. Examples of secondary prevention measures include screening to identify disease at early stages, such as mammography to detect breast cancer or A1C testing to identify diabetes. In OHP, secondary prevention interventions address social supports and team building (environmental), physical fitness or relaxation training (individual), and family leave policies (work–family; Quick, 1999b). With secondary prevention interventions, it is acknowledged that all stress cannot be eliminated from a job and that some jobs are mentally and physically demanding. The role of OHP, then, is to implement secondary prevention interventions that can help mitigate the effects of job demands that cannot otherwise be eliminated through primary prevention (Quick, 1999a).

Tertiary prevention measures occur when dealing with diagnosed disorders and diseases and are higher intensity and higher cost. This prevention process focuses on slowing or stopping disease progression through measures such as rehabilitation or screening for complications. In OHP, tertiary prevention interventions at the work environment level focus on task revision or implementing employee assistance programs (EAPs; e.g., counseling or legal assistance), which help employees address problems that affect their job. At the individual level, OHP interventions may focus on career counseling and may assist at the level of the work–family interface; interventions for tertiary prevention may include changes to health insurance and counseling with family systems (Quick, 1999a).

In its infancy, OHP focused on fixing existing workplace health hazards versus designing workplaces to be healthy from the start (Schaufeli, 2004). If occupational health psychologists want to design healthy workplaces, they should draw upon some key public health concepts and move upstream. Upstream interventions may involve changes to regulation that impact many individuals (e.g., increasing tobacco taxes as a method of decreasing smoking rates), whereas midstream interventions may target a single site, such as a workplace (e.g., implementing smoke-free workplace policies). Finally, downstream interventions focus on individual-level behavioral changes (e.g., individual smoking cessation program participation). An occupational public health example would be a national mental health standard (upstream), a workplace mental health policy (midstream), and EAPs offered through individual employers. Public health practice interventions often occur at multiple levels (McKinlay, 1998).

Public health practitioners have long highlighted structural factors that must be addressed before effective interventions can be put into place. These upstream elements are discussed in terms of social determinants of health and include factors such as poverty, food insecurity, access to education, employment opportunities, and systemic racism (Seligman & Hamad, 2021). Upstream factors in occupational settings may include regulations, working conditions, and management practices that must be considered before interventions can be implemented in the workplace (Eakin et al., 2010). Work is experienced differently by people across populations based on their individual characteristics and underlying social determinants of health. A strength of OHP is its focus on protective factors, such as social support, self-esteem, and self-efficacy, that may mitigate negative workplace experiences (Braveman & Gottlieb, 2014; Quick, 1999b).

In the field, there is an important focus on EBPH, which has touted benefits such as access to higher quality information (evidence) about what works best, increased likelihood of successful program implementation, as well as more efficient use of public and private resources (Brownson et al., 2009). These concepts are important for OHP practitioners to consider as well. Programmatic (i.e., intervention) decisions are often made based on short-term opportunities, have limited evidence about best practices, and lack systematic planning. One study reported that only 58% of public health practitioners reported using EBPH interventions (Dreisinger et al., 2008), a number that mirrors the medical field, where only 55% of medical care was based on best practices in the medical literature (McGlynn et al., 2003). Brownson and colleagues (2009) identified ways that public health practitioners, and by extension OHP practitioners, can increase their use of evidence-based interventions. The first step is to rely on scientific information about programs and policies that are most likely to achieve health outcomes. Second, there must be a greater effort to translate scientific findings into the real world so that what works in controlled "lab" settings (effectiveness) also works in messy occupational or clinical settings where factors such as limited time and resources impact how work gets accomplished (efficacy). Finally, there must be more effort made toward the dissemination of interventions that have proved effective (Brownson et al., 2009).

The field of *dissemination and implementation* (D&I) science is increasingly important in both medical and public health domains to design interventions that can be implemented in the real world and are sustainable. D&I science has grown considerably over the past 2 decades and has built upon the recognition that many new discoveries of successful interventions and products are never implemented (Glasgow et al., 2012). While initially centered on the medical field, D&I science has expanded its focus on many public health concerns such as tobacco cessation, cancer education, and healthy diet. This was a natural evolution based on the emphasis that public health practitioners have placed on addressing the systems that underlie health outcomes (Estabrooks et al., 2018). These same concepts translate to the field of OHP.

Applying concepts of public health practice to OHP broadens the focus of prevention outside the walls of an organization and beyond the teams and individuals who form functioning workplaces. Considering how to address social determinants of health, community, workplace, and economic factors in the process of designing interventions can enhance OHP practice to improve both organizational practices and individual behaviors.

OHP INFORMS PUBLIC HEALTH

OHP, in turn, contributes to primary prevention through health protection (e.g., reducing exposure to workplace risk factors for illness and injury by improving working conditions) and health promotion (e.g., equipping workers with the knowledge and resources to improve their own health and resist contact with hazards in the work environment; Sauter & Hurrell, 1999). The foundation of OHP is stress management and mental health (Quick, 1999a). There are also many concepts within the field of OHP that inform the work of public health practitioners, including concepts related to motivation, engagement, and leadership practices. Incorporating these ideas into more traditional public health interventions can increase the success of OSH interventions in workplace settings.

The history of OHP has helped inform how we address health promotion and well-being in the workplace. Much of the early OHP work focused on negative consequences of work, such as burnout, disease, and injury (Shimazu

& Schaufeli, 2009), while more recent foci have been on positive aspects of health and well-being at work. *Work engagement* is defined as "a positive, fulfilling, affective-motivational state of work-related well-being that can be seen as the antipode of job burnout" (Bakker et al., 2008, 187–88). For instance, engaged employees put more effort into their job because they strongly identify with their work, and this produces positive outcomes at both an individual level (e.g., personal development) and an organizational level (e.g., productivity). The field of OHP has developed well-validated work engagement measures. Previous research in the field has consistently demonstrated a relationship between work engagement and job resources, including social support, feedback, autonomy, and opportunities for development. As public health practitioners continue to design workplace interventions, a focus on the ideas developed by OHP will help ensure that the workplace context is well addressed.

OHP has contributed to public health practitioners' understanding of the importance of motivation. OHP research has evaluated the motivational processes involved in areas such as workload, performance, and recovery (Schaufeli, 2004). *Self-determination theory* posits that individuals are growth oriented and strive to reach their full potential (Van den Broeck et al., 2008). In particular, concepts of intrinsic and extrinsic motivation are relevant for public health practitioners. Intrinsic motivation is the act of participating in an activity for the satisfaction and enjoyment one receives, whereas extrinsic motivation relies on outcomes that are separate from the activity, such as monetary compensation (Van den Broeck et al., 2008). Motivation has been applied in general OSH as well, particularly within the safety literature. Researchers have found consistent relationships between motivation and safety climate and safety performance (Griffin & Neal, 2000). Other research has demonstrated the relationship between safety and health climates, safety and health behaviors, and the mediating role of different types of motivation (Schwatka et al., 2021).

Public health practitioners who are implementing workplace health and safety interventions may particularly focus on learning more about the different roles of intrinsic and extrinsic motivations and how they may impact participation in programming. A common practice in the field is for employers to offer incentives for participating in health and safety programs. Numerous OHP studies demonstrated that verbal rewards (e.g., positive feedback) enhanced intrinsic motivation while monetary rewards (e.g., cash incentives, gym memberships) decreased intrinsic motivation, particularly when tied to task completion, such as participating in a worksite health program (Deci et al., 1999, 2001). The evidence around incentives in OSH is mixed (Tenney et al., 2019; Verbeek, 2010).

The importance of leadership interventions in OHP is well established (Kelloway & Barling, 2010) and is another area in which OHP can inform the field of public health, regarding public health interventions in the workplace. The effects of good leadership on positive outcomes, including psychological well-being (Arnold, 2017; Arnold et al., 2007) and organizational safety climate (Zohar, 2002, 2010), are well documented. Poor leadership can also have negative impacts on employees, such as increased stress (Kelloway & Barling, 2010) and workplace injuries (Barling et al., 2002; Kelloway et al., 2006). One of the challenges of conducting workplace leadership interventions has been that the outcomes of interest are indirect—researchers and practitioners are interested in the effect of leadership training on employee outcomes, such as safety behaviors or well-being, and not the effect on the people who actually participate in the leadership intervention (Kelloway & Barling, 2010). Further, the relationship between leadership and employee outcomes is mediated by a number of factors that may impact how leadership interventions affect employees (Arnold, 2017).

The role leadership plays in OHP is also directly related to how public health practice approaches goals related to participant engagement and intervention effectiveness overall. Areas of focus on the importance of leadership in OHP include abusive leadership, which is linked to reduced job satisfaction, increased stress, burnout, feelings of helplessness, and reduced self-efficacy, as well as employee commitment to the organization (Kelloway & Barling, 2010). The field has also focused on the positive aspects of leadership—transformational leadership—discussed in previous editions of this handbook. Transformational leadership has a positive impact on several employee outcomes, including well-being, decreased job-related stress, greater optimism, happiness, and enthusiasm. Finally, the field has established the importance of leadership practices related to health and safety outcomes, including lower blood pressure, reduced risk of heart disease, and health behaviors such as increased uptake of influenza vaccinations. On the safety side, safety climate perceptions are strongly related to supervisory practices (Zohar, 2010), and leadership is associated with safety compliance and safety behaviors (Mattson Molnar et al., 2019). There is an identified need to develop interventions in the workplace that are effective at increasing leadership skills (Nielsen & Taris, 2019); this is true for OHP practitioners and is an area where public health practitioners can take note. If public health practice interventions are to be successful, they must account for the role that organizational leadership plays in workplace safety and health.

Finally, researchers and practitioners in OHP can contribute their expertise to public health practitioners, such as knowledge in areas including psychometrics, intervention design, and interpretation of results (Fisher et al., 2016; Sauter & Hurrell, 1999; Tetrick, 2017). These areas highlight the need for OHP to move in the direction of D&I science to not only increase the number of intervention studies that are conducted but also ensure that the research translates into practice. OHP has developed and used advanced statistical methods and analyses, which often require large samples of people. Public health practice is focused on the real-world application of interventions to improve health. Working together, OHP and public health can advance both fields in terms of developing, implementing, and evaluating EBPH interventions.

CASE STUDIES

We present three case studies that demonstrate the key principles of public health practice and OHP applied to OSH. These examples share three common goals: (a) identifying and delivering evidence-based programs to employers, (b) preventing disease and improving health among employees, and (c) demonstrating the application of public health practice to tailor and scale existing interventions aimed at improving organizational and individual health and safety outcomes.

Scaling a TWH Intervention to Help Small Businesses

Designing workplace interventions requires finding ways to ensure they are both effective and scalable. Reaching and engaging small enterprises to address health and safety has been challenging as small enterprises face common barriers, including competing priorities, lack of time, knowledge of where to start and how to implement changes, and lack of access to resources (McCoy et al., 2014; Newman et al., 2015). We started Health Links™ as an intervention aimed at helping organizations of all types, specifically small and midsized businesses, with adopting evidence-based TWH approaches to worker health, safety, and well-being (Tenney et al., 2019, 2021). The approach we took involved several key frameworks and concepts of public health practice: community-based participatory research (CBPR), Intervention Mapping, Designing for Dissemination, and RE-AIM (Bartholomew et al., 2006; Israel et al., 1998). These models provided the process for involving stakeholders early, identifying the appropriate channels for dissemination, tailoring messaging, and executing all intervention strategies. Specifically, Intervention Mapping is commonly used as a guide to planning health promotion programs because it provides a theory- and evidence-based interactive process that links needs assessment with program planning in a way that can add efficiency and feasibility and improve outcomes. As we applied key principles of Intervention Mapping and CBPR, we identified three core components to the Health Links intervention: (a) an organizational-level assessment of TWH policies and practices across six benchmarks, (b) certification to recognize businesses in one of four levels based on their assessment scores, and (c) advising to provide guidance and action planning for improving TWH adoption and sustainability.

Through the initial stages of program implementation, we met with employers, employees, chambers of commerce, and workers' compensation teams to solicit feedback about what motivated them, what words resonated with them, and what they would find most valuable for a TWH-based program. As a result, we discovered that most organizations are committed to improving the health and safety of working people (Tenney et al., 2019). We observed that there are differences in how businesses implemented TWH approaches based on their size, with smaller organizations doing less for both wellness and safety. We used mixed methods to evaluate the public health impact of Health Links with a focus on RE-AIM to measure Reach, Effectiveness, Adoption, Implementation, and Maintenance of Health Links (Glasgow et al., 2019; Tenney et al., 2021). We collected and tracked participation rates, changes in outcomes related to TWH policies and programs, and the impact that advising had on measures of organizational-level change year over year. We also evaluated the quality of advising sessions to understand how participants were applying the recommendations in practice. While Health Links requires a strategy aimed at engaging health and safety champions within an organization, the program aims to have a multiplied effect across changes in individuals' health and safety behaviors, economic growth through business performance, and community-level interest and investing in workplace initiatives.

Health Links has demonstrated the importance of engaging stakeholders throughout the process to find practical solutions for implementing TWH approaches. Each component of the intervention was developed to meet the unique needs of organizations and the teams that are responsible for health and safety. The action plan was built to be digestible and universal, meaning the goal was to ensure that the recommendations that are made are relevant and useful for all participants, whether they were implementing TWH approaches in a construction company or a hospital.

Partnering With Public Health to Engage Employers in Diabetes Prevention and Management

With chronic disease rates increasing, public health has a strong agenda to identify ways to deliver the National Diabetes Prevention Program (DPP) to more individuals through DPP program providers, insurers, and employers. At the Center for Health, Work & Environment, one of six national Centers of Excellence for *Total Worker Health*®, we partnered with the Colorado Department of Public Health and Environment on a project to engage employers in chronic disease prevention and management programs to improve the health and well-being of working adults. The primary goal of the project was to increase awareness and adoption of evidence-based diabetes and cardiovascular disease prevention and management programs as a covered benefit among Colorado employers.

The project focused on providing DPP options through existing providers and programs for employers and their at-risk employees in different industries as well as across urban and rural areas of Colorado. Through public health practice efforts aimed at serving employers, the project increased access to the National DPP, a proven lifestyle-change program that reduces the risk of Type 2 diabetes. Over 1.5 million adults in Colorado have prediabetes and are at risk for developing Type 2 diabetes; therefore, increasing access to the National DPP will result in fewer cases of Type 2 diabetes over time. The adult working population also benefited from this project because it resulted in increased access and employer coverage of the National DPP.

To enact the program, we convened representatives from employers across a range of industries to provide education on the National DPP; worked with community partners in public health, business coalitions, and health care to identify outreach strategies; and conducted direct outreach to employers through our network of organizations committed to workplace health and safety. We provided technical assistance to answer questions about options and to help employers make the decision to offer the National DPP as a covered benefit. We worked with public health agencies and business partners to develop communication materials that educated employers about the DPP program and provided information about the benefits to organizations and at-risk individuals.

A key part of our outreach to encourage employers to add the National DPP as a covered health benefit included helping them navigate the options of National DPP providers and assisting them in determining effective employee engagement strategies. To do this, we conducted follow-up outreach through emails, phone calls, and meetings to encourage employers who needed more information about the benefits of providing coverage to attend the virtual breakfast events to learn more about DPP. We provided advising sessions to respond to any specific questions from employers. Over the project period, we conducted a total of 32 advising sessions with employers representing a range of sectors and sizes. The advising sessions offered guidance on the importance of helping employees prevent and manage chronic disease, specifically diabetes. At each initial advising session, we discussed the evidence-based efficacy of DPP and asked questions about whether the DPP was a covered benefit. These sessions also served to gather input on values and motivations in delivering the DPP. Most interested employers noted that preventing chronic disease was a priority of their larger efforts to promote health in the workplace. As a result of the advising sessions, we were able to tailor specific resources that addressed their key concerns, including providing business case studies and access to cost calculators.

We tailored our messaging to each of our audiences during advising. For those employers already offering DPP as a covered benefit, the conversation focused on how to best promote program engagement among employees. For advising sessions with local municipalities, the conversation generally steered toward offering DPP to the community at large. During advising sessions with towns and cities, we recommended reserving spots in the DPP for municipal employees while opening the program to the wider community to build additional capacity.

This project identified future opportunities for employer engagement in offering chronic disease prevention and management programs as a covered benefit to employees. We were successful in leveraging an existing network of organizations through a trusted program, Health Links, described previously, to offer educational opportunities and advising to help employers navigate the decision-making process. We learned that employers were interested in diabetes prevention as a workplace-based program for improving worker health. Applying concepts of public health practice, we identified ways to engage stakeholders early in the process and establish partnerships with groups that have established relationships with employers, specifically aside from insurers or vendors. This involved training local public health agencies on how to better communicate with employers and establishing new partnerships with business groups.

Training Business Leaders at Scale

Leadership can be a means of primary prevention in the workplace. As stated previously, prevention is a core component of public health, and public health practitioners prioritize primary prevention in their efforts to influence health. Organizational leadership practices can be an effective mechanism to achieve primary prevention in the workplace as they play a major role in the development and implementation of workplace health and safety policies and programs (Kelloway & Barling, 2010). Leaders allocate resources, role model, communicate, recognize, and hold people accountable. Indeed, recommendations for health and safety programs always call for management buy-in and support as a prerequisite for program success (Sorensen et al., 2013). The existing literature on health and safety leadership training offers promising evidence that such interventions can influence the working environment and workforce health. However, the literature does not describe how to train business leaders at scale to achieve broad public health impact.

Focusing on leadership as a means of protecting and promoting workforce health allows us to tackle all the key principles of public health practice described previously. Leaders play a key role in understanding the strengths and challenges of achieving good health among their organization and the teams they manage. Involving these individuals in the intervention process can lead to a greater understanding of shared values for health, a focus on needs and interests of all team members, collaboration and empowerment, and a vested interest in workforce health. Leaders are key decision makers that can help us evaluate interventions for accessibility and acceptability within their business—they know what works. At the same time, when leaders have data on health and safety along with evidence-based recommendations, they are better positioned to make informed decisions and execute them in collaboration with their employees. Importantly, these data should include a focus on workplace health and safety culture as well as employers' own well-being practices to ensure broader and better uptake of interventions and equity in who benefits across the organization.

Several steps must be taken to achieve broad workforce health impact with a leadership intervention (Schwatka et al., 2021). First, the intervention must focus on leadership skills (e.g., inspirational motivator) while also giving the leader a chance to develop their business strategy for workforce health in the context of employees' needs. This combined approach results in tangible changes to business policies and programs while giving the leader the skills to implement the policies and programs successfully. Second, the intervention must be evaluated for implementation in addition to effectiveness. This means that we must understand whether the intervention was implemented as planned, participant reactions, and barriers to training transfer, among other factors. Third, the intervention must be tested with a diverse audience (e.g., among organizations of different industries or sizes). A leadership intervention for one company may not translate well to another company. Importantly, we must focus on leadership interventions that fit with small-business needs. These businesses face unique challenges due to resource constraints, such as time and expertise. Given that the majority of businesses are small, a leadership training approach focused on small-business needs can provide an opportunity for broad public health impact.

Several years ago, we recognized a need to help small businesses implement TWH approaches. We started by initially offering those responsible for worker well-being in their organization a TWH assessment and advising through the Health Links program, which was designed to fit the needs of small businesses from any industry. While this program demonstrated a method to help businesses develop safety and health policies and programs, it did not provide businesses with the leadership training needed to ensure the new policies and programs were effective. Next, we describe a leadership focused TWH intervention, and our evaluation of it, that sought to address each of the five principles of public health impact.

As a complement to Health Links, we developed and evaluated a TWH leadership development program that could be implemented at scale (Schwatka et al., 2021). The program included 10 hours of self-paced reflection, in-person training, and virtual training transfer support over 4 months. It was applicable to businesses in any industry, geared toward small businesses, and could be implemented with cohorts of leaders from different companies. While the training was primarily delivered in person, our assessment and training transfer strategy was implemented virtually. The goal of the program was to help small-business leaders change their behaviors around workforce health protection and promotion. It followed the theory of transformational leadership as well as Burke and Litwin's (1992) organizational change theory, which accounts for the transactional and transformational changes that organizations can undergo.

Given that our focus was on leader behavioral change, we needed to create a leadership development program focused on action. The first way we accomplished this was through a data-driven training approach. Leaders received results from three assessments: (a) business TWH policies and programs, (b) employee health and safety culture perceptions, and (c) the TWH leadership practices and health of the leader. For many of the small businesses that participated, this was the first time they had had access to these kinds of data. It gave them the opportunity to identify their business and employee needs. Second, we invited a small-business key decision maker as well as someone from their TWH team (e.g., safety manager) to attend the training together to facilitate shared leadership and peer support. The final way we facilitated behavioral change was through virtual training transfer activities. Leaders set goals for themselves in each of the three assessment areas and inputted them into an online goal-setting platform during the training. For 3 months following the in-person training, leaders were asked to track their goals online and to participate in up to three 30-minute one-on-one coaching sessions with experts from our center.

It was clear from our program evaluation data that the intervention was successful at improving self-reported TWH leadership behaviors, but it suffered from some implementation challenges. The small-business leaders reported a lack of time to engage in the transfer of their training to their workplaces due to time pressures and competing demands. Importantly, they reported increased work-related stress. These findings highlight the real-world challenges of implementing occupational health and safety interventions in small businesses. It requires us to consider how to develop interventions that are rigorous enough to influence change. This study, in particular, sheds light on how a 10-hour leadership program with both in-person and virtual components may be too much for a small-business leader to engage in.

It is critical for the small-business leader to practice behaviors that demonstrate a commitment to workforce health, but it may also be important for them to share responsibly and influence over workforce health. Indeed, this may help alleviate stress for them. This is akin to participatory approaches to workforce health; however, the focus would be on building a culture in which influence over workforce health is shared (Punnett et al., 2013). In contrast, a larger organization may have a position or a team dedicated to workforce health; the small business likely does not have this full-time support. A shared leadership approach would ensure that small-business workforce health initiatives are developed and implemented effectively.

FUTURE DIRECTIONS

As the field of OHP evolves to address the future of work priorities, there will be an increasing need to identify synergies between workplace interventions and public health practice approaches to leverage shared goals for improving workplace and worker health and safety. The case studies discussed in this chapter illustrate ways that public health and OSH professionals are collaborating to design interventions that engage stakeholders in the process, enhance access and acceptance among workers and employers, and ensure equity to benefit all workers. The examples demonstrate the importance of needs assessments and targeting motivation, leadership, and employee engagement as primary ways to change organizational behavior and increase the adoption and implementation of programs. Future training in OHP must consider principles of public health practice as a guide for increasing reach to employers and to ensure occupational health equity.

REFERENCES

Allen, T. D., & Martin, A. (2017). The work-family interface: A retrospective look at 20 years of research in *JOHP*. *Journal of Occupational Health Psychology, 22*(3), 259–272. https://doi.org/10.1037/ocp0000065

Arnold, K. A. (2017). Transformational leadership and employee psychological well-being: A review and directions for future research. *Journal of Occupational Health Psychology, 22*(3), 381–393. https://doi.org/10.1037/ocp0000062

Arnold, K. A., Turner, N., Barling, J., Kelloway, E. K., & McKee, M. C. (2007). Transformational leadership and psychological well-being: The mediating role of meaningful work. *Journal of Occupational Health Psychology, 12*(3), 193–203. https://doi.org/10.1037/1076-8998.12.3.193

Bakker, A. B., Schaufeli, W. B., Leiter, M. P., & Taris, T. W. (2008). Work engagement: An emerging concept in occupational health psychology. *Work and Stress, 22*(3), 187–200. https://doi.org/10.1080/02678370802393649

Barling, J., Loughlin, C., & Kelloway, E. K. (2002). Development and test of a model linking safety-specific transformational leadership and occupational safety. *Journal of Applied Psychology, 87*(3), 488–496. https://doi.org/10.1037/0021-9010.87.3.488

Bartholomew, L. K., Parcel, G. S., Kok, G., & Gottlieb, N. H. (2006). *Planning health promotion programs: An intervention mapping approach* (2nd ed.). Jossey-Bass.

Braveman, P., & Gottlieb, L. (2014). The social determinants of health: It's time to consider the causes of the causes. *Public Health Reports (1974), 129*(Suppl. 2), 19–31.

Brownson, R. C., Fielding, J. E., & Maylahn, C. M. (2009). Evidence-based public health: A fundamental concept for public health practice. *Annual Review of Public Health, 30*(1), 175–201. https://doi.org/10.1146/annurev.publhealth.031308.100134

Burke, W., & Litwin, G. (1992). A causal model of organizational performance and change. *Journal of Management, 18*(3), 523–545. https://doi.org/10.1177/014920639201800306

Deci, E. L., Koestner, R., & Ryan, R. M. (1999). A meta-analytic review of experiments examining the effects of extrinsic rewards on intrinsic motivation. *Psychological Bulletin, 125*(6), 627–668. https://doi.org/10.1037/0033-2909.125.6.627

Deci, E. L., Koestner, R., & Ryan, R. M. (2001). Extrinsic rewards and intrinsic motivation in education: Reconsidered once again. *Review of Educational Research, 71*(1), 1–27. https://doi.org/10.3102/00346543071001001

Dreisinger, M., Leet, T. L., Baker, E. A., Gillespie, K. N., Haas, B., & Brownson, R. C. (2008). Improving the public health workforce: Evaluation of a training course to enhance evidence-based decision making. *Journal of Public Health Management and Practice, 14*(2), 138–143. https://doi.org/10.1097/01.PHH.0000311891.73078.50

Eakin, J. M., Champoux, D., & MacEachen, E. (2010). Health and safety in small workplaces: Refocusing upstream. *Canadian Journal of Public Health* [*Revue canadienne de sante publique*], *101*(Suppl. 1), S29–S33. https://doi.org/10.1007/BF03403843

Estabrooks, P. A., Brownson, R. C., & Pronk, N. P. (2018). Dissemination and implementation science for public health professionals: An overview and call to action. *Preventing Chronic Disease, 15*, 180525. https://doi.org/10.5888/pcd15.180525

Fernandez, M. E., Ten Hoor, G. A., van Lieshout, S., Rodriguez, S. A., Beidas, R. S., Parcel, G., Ruiter, R. A. C., Markham, C. M., & Kok, G. (2019). Implementation mapping: Using intervention mapping to develop implementation strategies. *Frontiers in Public Health, 7*, 158. https://doi.org/10.3389/fpubh.2019.00158

Fisher, G. G., Matthews, R. A., & Gibbons, A. M. (2016). Developing and investigating the use of single-item measures in organizational research. *Journal of Occupational Health Psychology, 21*(1), 3–23. https://doi.org/10.1037/a0039139

Frieden, T. R. (2010). A framework for public health action: The health impact pyramid. *American Journal of Public Health, 100*(4), 590–595. https://doi.org/10.2105/AJPH.2009.185652

Glasgow, R. E., Harden, S. M., Gaglio, B., Rabin, B., Smith, M. L., Porter, G. C., Ory, M. G., & Estabrooks, P. A. (2019). RE-AIM planning and evaluation framework: Adapting to new science and practice with a 20-year review. *Frontiers in Public Health, 7*, 64. https://doi.org/10.3389/fpubh.2019.00064

Glasgow, R. E., Vinson, C., Chambers, D., Khoury, M. J., Kaplan, R. M., & Hunter, C. (2012). National Institutes of Health approaches to dissemination and implementation science: Current and future directions. *American Journal of Public Health, 102*(7), 1274–1281. https://doi.org/10.2105/AJPH.2012.300755

Golden, R. N., & Timberlake, K. (2013). Population health improvement: Moving beyond the clinic and into the community. *WMJ: Official Publication of the State Medical Society of Wisconsin, 112*(4), 181–182. https://wmjonline.org/112-4/

Griffin, M. A., & Neal, A. (2000). Perceptions of safety at work: A framework for linking safety climate to safety performance, knowledge, and motivation. *Journal of Occupational Health Psychology, 5*(3), 347–358. https://doi.org/10.1037/1076-8998.5.3.347

Israel, B. A., Schulz, A. J., Parker, E. A., & Becker, A. B. (1998). Review of community-based research: Assessing partnership approaches to improve public health. *Annual Review of Public Health, 19*(1), 173–202. https://doi.org/10.1146/annurev.publhealth.19.1.173

Kelloway, E. K., & Barling, J. (2010). Leadership development as an intervention in occupational health psychology. *Work and Stress, 24*(3), 260–279. https://doi.org/10.1080/02678373.2010.518441

Kelloway, E. K., Mullen, J., & Francis, L. (2006). Divergent effects of transformational and passive leadership on employee safety. *Journal of Occupational Health Psychology, 11*(1), 76–86. https://psycnet.apa.org/doi/10.1037/1076-8998.11.1.76

Landsbergis, P. A., Grzywacz, J. G., & LaMontagne, A. D. (2014). Work organization, job insecurity, and occupational health disparities. *American Journal of Industrial Medicine, 57*(5), 495–515. https://doi.org/10.1002/ajim.22126

Mattson Molnar, M., Schwarz, U. V. T., Hellgren, J., Hasson, H., & Tafvelin, S. (2019). Leading for safety: A question of leadership focus. *Safety and Health at Work, 10*(2), 180–187. https://doi.org/10.1016/j.shaw.2018.12.001

McCoy, K., Stinson, K., Scott, K., Tenney, L., & Newman, L. S. (2014). Health promotion in small business: A systematic review of factors influencing adoption and effectiveness of worksite wellness programs. *Journal of Occupational and Environmental Medicine, 56*(6), 579–587. https://doi.org/10.1097/JOM.0000000000000171

McGlynn, E. A., Asch, S. M., Adams, J., Keesey, J., Hicks, J., DeCristofaro, A., & Kerr, E. A. (2003). The quality of health care delivered to adults in the United States. *The New England Journal of Medicine, 348*(26), 2635–2645. https://doi.org/10.1056/NEJMsa022615

McKinlay, J. B. (1998). Paradigmatic obstacles to improving the health of populations—Implications for health policy. *Salud Pública de México, 40*(4), 369–379. https://doi.org/10.1590/S0036-36341998000400010

National Institute for Occupational Safety and Health. (2023). NIOSH *Total Worker Health®* Program. https://www.cdc.gov/niosh/twh/default.html

Newman, L. S., Stinson, K. E., Metcalf, D., Fang, H., Brockbank, C., Jinnett, K., Reynolds, S., Trotter, M., Witter, R., Tenney, L., Atherly, A., & Goetzel, R. Z. (2015). Implementation of a worksite wellness program targeting small businesses: The Pinnacol Assurance health risk management study. *Journal of Occupational and Environmental Medicine, 57*(1), 14–21. https://doi.org/10.1097/JOM.0000000000000279

Nielsen, K., & Taris, T. W. (2019). Leading well: Challenges to researching leadership in occupational health psychology–and some ways forward. *Work and Stress, 33*(2), 107–118. https://doi.org/10.1080/02678373.2019.1592263

Otto, J. L., Holodniy, M., & DeFraites, R. F. (2014). Public health practice is not research. *American Journal of Public Health, 104*(4), 596–602. https://doi.org/10.2105/AJPH.2013.301663

Pronk, N. P. (2021). Implementing movement at the workplace: Approaches to increase physical activity and reduce sedentary behavior in the context of work. *Progress in Cardiovascular Diseases, 64*, 17–21. https://doi.org/10.1016/j.pcad.2020.10.004

Punnett, L., Warren, N., Henning, R., Nobrega, S., Cherniack, M., & the CPH-NEW Research Team. (2013). Participatory ergonomics as a model for integrated programs to prevent chronic disease. *Journal of Occupational and Environmental Medicine, 55*(12, Suppl.), S19–S24. https://doi.org/10.1097/JOM.0000000000000040

Quick, J. C. (1999a). Occupational health psychology: The convergence of health and clinical psychology with public health and preventive medicine in an organizational context. *Professional Psychology, Research and Practice, 30*(2), 123–128. https://doi.org/10.1037/0735-7028.30.2.123

Quick, J. C. (1999b). Occupational health psychology: Historical roots and future directions. *Health Psychology, 18*(1), 82–88. https://doi.org/10.1037/0278-6133.18.1.82

Sauter, S. L., & Hurrell, J. J., Jr. (1999). Occupational health psychology: Origins, content, and direction. *Professional Psychology, Research and Practice, 30*(2), 117–122. https://doi.org/10.1037/0735-7028.30.2.117

Schaufeli, W. B. (2004). The future of occupational health psychology. *Applied Psychology, 53*(4), 502–517. https://doi.org/10.1111/j.1464-0597.2004.00184.x

Schulte, P. A., Guerin, R. J., Schill, A. L., Bhattacharya, A., Cunningham, T. R., Pandalai, S. P., Eggerth, D., & Stephenson, C. M. (2015). Considerations for incorporating "well-being" in public policy for workers and workplaces. *American Journal of Public Health, 105*(8), e31–e44. https://doi.org/10.2105/AJPH.2015.302616

Schwatka, N. V., Brown, C. E., Tenney, L., Scott, J. G., Shore, E., Dally, M., & Newman, L. S. (2021). Evaluation of a Total Worker Health® leadership development program for small business. *Occupational Health Science, 5*(1–2), 1–26. https://doi.org/10.1007/s41542-021-00086-5

Schwatka, N. V., Sinclair, R. R., Fan, W., Dally, M., Shore, E., Brown, C. E., Tenney, L., & Newman, L. S. (2020). How does organizational climate motivate employee safe and healthy nehavior in small business?: A self-determination theory perspective. *Journal of Occupational and Environmental Medicine, 62*(5), 350–358. https://doi.org/10.1097/JOM.0000000000001839

Seligman, H. K., & Hamad, R. (2021). Moving upstream: The importance of examining policies to address health disparities. *JAMA Pediatrics, 175*(6), 563–564. https://doi.org/10.1001/jamapediatrics.2020.6985

Shimazu, A., & Schaufeli, W. B. (2009). Towards a positive occupational health psychology: The case of work engagement. *Japanese Journal of Stress Science, 24*(3), 181–187.

Sorensen, G., McLellan, D., Dennerlein, J. T., Pronk, N. P., Allen, J. D., Boden, L. I., Okechukwu, C. A., Hashimoto, D., Stoddard, A., & Wagner, G. R. (2013). Integration of health protection and health promotion: Rationale, indicators, and metrics. *Journal of Occupational and Environmental Medicine, 55*(12, Suppl.), S12–S18. https://doi.org/10.1097/JOM.0000000000000032

Souza, K., Steege, A. L., & Baron, S. L. (2010). Surveillance of occupational health disparities: Challenges and opportunities. *American Journal of Industrial Medicine, 53*(2), 84–94. https://doi.org/10.1002/ajim.20777

Tengland, P. A. (2010). Health promotion or disease prevention: A real difference for public health practice? *Health Care Analysis, 18*(3), 203–221. https://doi.org/10.1007/s10728-009-0124-1

Tenney, L., Dexter, L., Shapiro, D. C., Dally, M., Brown, C., Schwatka, N., Huebschmann, A. G., McMillen, J., & Newman, L. S. (2021). Impact of Advising on Total Worker Health Implementation. *Journal of Occupational and Environmental Medicine, 63*(8), 657–664. https://doi.org/10.1097/JOM.0000000000002212

Tenney, L., Fan, W., Dally, M., Scott, J., Haan, M., Rivera, K., Newman, M., & Newman, L. S. (2019). Health Links™ assessment of Total Worker Health® practices as indicators of organizational behavior in small business. *Journal of Occupational and Environmental Medicine, 61*(8), 623–634. https://doi.org/10.1097/JOM.0000000000001623

Tetrick, L. E. (2017). Trends in measurement models and methods in understanding occupational health psychology. *Journal of Occupational Health Psychology, 22*(3), 337–340. https://doi.org/10.1037/ocp0000076

Van den Broeck, A., Vansteenkiste, M., & De Witte, H. (2008). Self-determination theory: A theoretical and empirical overview in occupational health psychology. In S. Leka & J. Houdmont (Eds.), *Occupational health psychology: European perspectives on research, education, and practice* (Vol. 3, pp. 63–88). Nottingham University Press. https://www.researchgate.net/publication/281605739_Self-determination_theory_A_theoretical_and_empirical_overview_in_occupational_health_psychology

Verbeek, J. (2010). How do we know if monetary incentives are effective and efficient for controlling health and safety risks at work? *Scandinavian Journal of Work, Environment & Health, 36*(4), 269–271. https://doi.org/10.5271/sjweh.3032

World Health Organization. (2010). *A Conceptual Framework for Action on the Social Determinants of Health*. https://www.who.int/publications/i/item/9789241500852

Zohar, D. (2002). Modifying supervisory practices to improve subunit safety: A leadership-based intervention model. *Journal of Applied Psychology, 87*(1), 156–163. https://doi.org/10.1037/0021-9010.87.1.156

Zohar, D. (2010). Thirty years of safety climate research: Reflections and future directions. *Accident Analysis and Prevention, 42*(5), 1517–1522. https://doi.org/10.1016/j.aap.2009.12.019

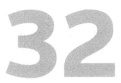

Occupational and Environmental Medicine and the Occupational Health Psychology Interface

Richard Pompei, Brian Williams, and Lee S. Newman

Occupational and environmental medicine (OEM) is a clinical branch of medicine dedicated to the diagnosis, treatment, and prevention of injuries and illnesses resulting from exposures to hazards in the workplace. In the United States, OEM physicians provide much of their medical care through the workers' compensation insurance system. The OEM physician essentially works as the primary care physician limited to that portion of patient care related to work injury or illness. In addition to direct clinical care of workers, the OEM physician is trained to serve as a consultant, helping employers prevent occupational injuries and illnesses and promote health and well-being. Physicians receive training in public health and receive OEM board certification as one of the preventive medicine specialties. The spectrum of research conducted in OEM is vast, including epidemiology, hazardous exposure-related health effects, medical surveillance, substance use disorder treatment, injury prevention, health promotion, *Total Worker Health*®, clinical trials, observational studies, and intervention science, among other fields.

With growing numbers of workers, an aging workforce, and an increasing prevalence of chronic health conditions among workers, OEM physicians have begun to broaden their scope to address how personal health conditions contribute to work-related injuries and delayed recovery and affect a worker's ability to return to work. Reciprocally, researchers increasingly address how

https://doi.org/10.1037/0000331-032
Handbook of Occupational Health Psychology, Third Edition, L. E. Tetrick, G. G. Fisher, M. T. Ford, and J. C. Quick (Editors)

the conditions of work can both negatively and positively impact workers' lives outside of work, not just while they are on the job.

In OEM practice, occupational illness and injury prevention efforts usually take the form of secondary prevention, through medical surveillance and/or medical screening programs. Many such programs fulfill one of four purposes: (a) to identify and diagnose work-induced or work-aggravated health conditions that result from exposures to various physical and chemical hazards in the workplace (e.g., occupational lung disease screening for silicosis) at early or more treatable stages; (b) to help organizations comply with governmental regulations (e.g., lead surveillance); (c) to determine whether workers meet health qualifications for certain forms of work (e.g., assessing firefighters' physical abilities); and (d) to identify and treat workers who may pose a risk to themselves or others—for instance, those working in so-called safety-sensitive positions (e.g., workplace drug testing). In medical screening, the goal is to identify a problem at its earliest stage, allowing timely intervention and thereby preventing further injury, disease, and disability. *Medical surveillance* describes activities that target a health event or a change in a biological function of an exposed person or persons (Nasterlack, 2011). Medical surveillance usually involves recurrent medical examinations and data analysis over an extended period. Although some long-standing medical surveillance programs are well defined, such as those mandated for identifying lung disease due to exposure to silica, asbestos, or beryllium, the process of medical surveillance is not always clear cut (Nasterlack, 2011). For some working populations, such as firefighters, first responders, and agricultural workers, exposures cannot be easily measured or quantified given the variability of exposure conditions in the occupational setting. Psychological factors present an added challenge.

An interdisciplinary approach has become customary for optimal care of injured workers. OEM physicians frequently engage with other professionals in occupational and environmental health specialties such as industrial hygienists, ergonomics and safety professionals, occupational health nurses, and, increasingly, with experts in the fields of psychology, psychiatry, addiction medicine, social work, and others.

While OEM specialists are predominantly practitioners, many also serve as consultants, act as internal (in-house) or external (contract) corporate medical directors, conduct occupational health surveillance programs, monitor workplace drug monitoring programs, or serve in other roles in organizations' health and safety departments and human resources departments. Like occupational health psychologists, OEM practitioners who have consulting or corporate medical director roles may address organizational and other work environment factors that affect workers' health, safety, and well-being. Here is where one of the greatest opportunities exists for OEM and occupational health psychology (OHP) to learn from each other. In this chapter we provide clinical cases that illustrate some of these opportunities for collaboration in response to many of the greatest emerging challenges facing employers and employees. However, the points of intersection between these fields are even broader, ranging from shared interests in occupational stress and its relation to mental health and burnout of workers; the impact of changes in work itself, such as mechanization's effects on psychological well-being as well as novel forms of physical injury; the impacts of shift work and fatigue on job performance and injury risk; the blurring of the work–nonwork interface; the increasing diversity of the workforce, calling for a revisiting of cross-cultural considerations needed to better prevent and treat injuries and mitigate occupational injustice; the ways in which organizational climates affect worker health; substance use disorders and pain management; the opioid epidemic; factors affecting return to work; and worksite health interventions, among others.

The remainder of this chapter offers an OEM physician perspective by focusing on some of the greatest challenges we face in practice. We hope these examples will trigger insights into ways that OHP may benefit from the clinical experience and practice of OEM for collaboration in the discovery and solutions of new, unaddressed challenges. There is untapped potential for OHP approaches to contribute to injury and illness prevention through partnership with OEM researchers and practitioners.

OEM ROLES IN TREATMENT, RETURN TO WORK, AND WORKERS' COMPENSATION SYSTEMS

The field of OEM plays a crucial role in helping people fulfill basic needs, by helping workers continue to work, even in the face of hardship. Getting workers back to work at the highest possible level of function is the primary goal of OEM physicians and allied health professionals. In addition to the obvious loss of income, common consequences of limited employment include mental health risks such as anxiety and depressed mood, poor sleep, financial stress, interpersonal stress between employee and employer and between employee and family; poorer health behaviors and worsening chronic health conditions, such as weight gain from inactivity; and dependence on unhealthy coping skills like smoking and consumption of illicit drugs and alcohol. While some workers feel overly pressured to return to work by their health care providers, employers, families, and themselves, studies have shown that injured workers recover faster and more completely when they return to work sooner. Statistics have shown that once an injured worker has been out of work for 6 months, the odds of them returning to any work is 50%, and at one year out of work, the odds decrease further to around 35% (Orslene, 2017). While workers' compensation insurance programs may provide financial support (e.g., wage replacement) for work-related illnesses, this is often at a reduced rate or is capped and varies widely by state and even by the type of employer. Thus, an injured worker can have significant financial incentive to return to work. An injured worker who was previously healthy may be suddenly faced with frequent visits to doctors, therapists, and diagnostic centers for radiological imaging or labs. They must manage the medical side of a work-related injury/illness claim along with the administrative side of the claim with human resources at their employer and the adjuster or claim representative with the workers' compensation insurance carrier. Legal representation is sometimes necessary to help the worker navigate these systems or advocate for benefits denied by the insurer, adding further stress—particularly for those with low educational attainment, second-language speakers or those without English proficiency, and those with low socio-economic status. Many small businesses do not have dedicated human resources staff, so the company's representative handling the injured worker's claim may not be familiar with the complexities of the workers' compensation system. Poor or incomplete advice can contribute to animosity between the injured worker and the company.

Care for the injured worker focuses on return to function. An OEM practitioner makes both temporary and permanent recommendations about work ability, depending on the worker's degree of recovery from occupational illness or injury and the practitioner's medical opinion about the likelihood that additional treatment may result in further improvement. At the end of an occupational injury or illness, the treating physician makes the determination that the claim is closed, decides whether there is any permanent impairment or the need for permanent restrictions, and will assess the residual extent of the injury or illness. As such, OEM practitioners must have knowledge of the type of work being performed, including insight into both the physical and cognitive demands of the job, and help match workers' occupational ability with job demands. While most workers fully recover from their injuries, some may not. In this case the OEM physician must determine whether the worker's injury has resulted in a permanent disability. When a physician determines and documents that the worker has reached the point of *maximum medical improvement*, the patient is not expected to achieve any improvement in function with additional care. This often means the patient has fully returned to their pre-injured state or that the patient is not continuing to improve back to their baseline, despite adequate medical care. This determination can and often does cause the patient to lose the job they held prior to the time of the injury. These permanent restrictions may also limit the type of future employment the injured worker is able to secure. Notably, OEM physicians consider whether the patient's occupational injury has resulted in psychological as well as physical or cognitive harm and impairment. Depression is a frequent consequence of work-related injuries and illnesses, especially when recovery is prolonged, complicated, or fails to return the patient to their baseline level of function. In some cases, depression may be considered work-related, secondary to the original injury.

MUSCULOSKELETAL INJURIES

Musculoskeletal (MSK) *injuries* to bone and surrounding soft tissues, which include muscles, joints, ligaments, nerves, and skin, represent the largest category of work-related injury types and thus the largest proportion of most OEM practices and claims for compensation. In the United States there are an estimated 400,000 MSK injuries yearly, with a direct cost of $45 billion to $54 billion. There are also large indirect costs, such as lost productivity and added pressures on coworkers. A common example would be an ankle sprain, which, when severe, can cause injury to the bones of the lower leg and foot, including the articulation of the ankle joint, ligaments, tendons, and small blood vessels. Such MSK injuries can occur at almost any anatomic site. Hazards in the workplace such as slips, trips, and falls; being struck by a moving object; lifting; overhead work; and repetitive trauma are all common causes of MSK injuries. Most MSK injuries are minor and resolve themselves with little to no medical intervention. Others are more substantial, requiring conservative care from a physician or advanced medical care provider such as a nurse practitioner or physician assistant, ranging from the application of ice and/or heat; relative rest; prescription and over-the-counter medications; and manual therapies such as physical therapy, massage therapy, chiropractic care, and acupuncture. Relative rest may require that the worker stay physically active but limit certain, more strenuous activities. In these instances, the physician issues work restrictions as well as recommendations for the patient to modify their activities both in and outside of work.

Beyond conservative care, some MSK injuries are severe enough to require interventional care. This can include more invasive procedures like injections or surgery. As the severity of the MSK injury and the complexity of the treatment increases, so does the risk of psychological as well as psychosocial consequences, including but not limited to depression, anxiety, and substance use disorders.

MANAGEMENT OF ACUTE AND CHRONIC PAIN

For context, consider the following OEM clinical scenario. A 45-year-old male truck driver arrives at the clinic for evaluation and treatment of a back injury that occurred 1 week ago while he was climbing into the cab of his truck. It is determined that the mechanism of injury involved no heavy lifting, pushing, or pulling. It appears to be a minor strain. He says his pain is "unbearable" and nothing has helped relieve his pain so far. He has a prior history of back injuries at work, the most recent being 6 months ago from a similar situation. He requests an opioid pain medication, stating that "it is the only thing that takes the edge off." Upon review of the state's prescription drug monitoring program (PDMP) database, in which prior and current filled prescriptions are documented, it is evident that the patient has filled multiple past prescriptions for narcotics from multiple different providers. Conservative management is recommended, including nonsteroidal anti-inflammatory drugs (NSAIDs) and physical therapy. It is explained to the patient that opioids are not considered to be an appropriate form of treatment according to medical treatment guidelines. The patient becomes visibly upset and frustrated, despite an explanation about how this is the appropriate course of action for a mild injury. He responds, "That won't work for me! I need something stronger." Further investigation into the patient's medical history reveals anxiety and depression for which he is no longer taking medication or receiving therapy.

This all-too-common scenario is part of the regular practice of OEM in the United States. Acute and chronic pain are conditions that are frequently encountered in management of MSK injury, most commonly lower back pain. *Acute pain* is defined as pain lasting up to 3 months, whereas *chronic pain* is defined as lasting beyond 3 months and may persist for years (Hegmann et al., 2014). Strategies for treatment and management of acute and chronic pain have evolved, especially with the rising awareness of the potential for dependency, evidence of the efficacy of opioids for treatment of pain, the prevalence of other forms of therapy, and recognition of the potential for misuse and drug diversion contributing to the opioid epidemic. Opioid prescriptions, including those written by OEM physicians for acute and chronic pain, contribute to the current public health epidemic of prescription opioid misuse and prescription opioid–related deaths in the United States. While the extent of medication misuse and the potential for diversion have become more recognizable, OEM physicians' practices are placed in a challenging position; physicians must continue to need to treat patients who have become dependent on these drugs and cannot simply be weaned off. Additionally, physicians have learned to recognize that there are workers in marginalized populations, such as people of color, who suffer from pain but have been undertreated for their symptoms due to conscious or unconscious bias, lack of cultural competency, language barriers, and other contributing factors.

The opioid epidemic presents issues and barriers to care in OEM. Ongoing efforts to curb the contribution of prescribed opioids to the epidemic are improving OEM physicians' ability to improve treatment and mitigate the risk of harm in the workplace. In the health care environment, PDMP systems are now incorporated into electronic health records and often include data from neighboring states' PDMPs. This step has changed prescribing patterns and has decreased prescription opioid abuse (Rhodes et al., 2019). Concurrently, there are increasingly restrictive policies and prescription guidelines issued by federal, state, and professional medical associations to limit opioid prescribing to only those cases in which these medications have been proven to be efficacious (Hegmann et al., 2014). There has also been a shift in provider education, instructing OEM practitioners to follow more effective pain management and opioid-prescribing guidelines. In terms of patient education, the implementation of so-called provider–patient pain contracts has become more frequent in clinical practice. These contracts often include provisions for urine drug testing to assess patient compliance as well as to identify if the patient is using illicit substances (McAuliffe Staehler & Palombi, 2020).

Use of opioids for management of acute and chronic pain in the worker translates to concerns spanning outside of the clinical setting and into the workplace. The issue of substance use within the workplace can be detrimental to workplace safety and productivity. The U.S. Substance Abuse and Mental Health Services Administration (SAMHSA) recommends five types of employer-related interventions (SAMHSA, 2021). These interventions include (a) the establishment of a clear written workplace policy on substance use within the workplace; (b) employee education to improve knowledge about opioids and other potentially addictive substances; (c) the training of supervisors to keep updated with the most recent workplace drug policies, identification of signs of impairment, and reintegration of employees into the workplace after receiving preventive and treatment services; (d) employee assistance programs to support confidential treatment of affected workers; and (e) conducting drug testing to aid in compliance with federal regulations or insurance carrier requirements. Employee drug testing programs necessitated the development of another branch of practice for many OEM physicians, as the medical review officer (MRO).

If a company conducts tests to detect substance use in employees, a positive drug result reported by the laboratory does not automatically mean that an individual is misusing the medication, unless it is an illegal drug or one for which the worker has no prescription. The MRO is a physician who wears essentially two hats. They review lab results, and if a test is positive, they document whether the worker has a legal prescription. Following strict rules for ensuring confidentiality, they communicate information back to the employer. They also play a role in workplace safety by way of considering job duties, reviewing medications, assessing safety risks, and reporting concerns (Smith et al., 2002). The increase in the use of prescription drugs for legitimate medical diagnoses has created a challenge for the MRO, who is responsible for determining whether a valid prescription is causing serious impairment of the worker's ability to perform their job duties safely. The MRO must be especially knowledgeable of pharmacology of drugs being screened for, causes of false positive and false negative results, specificity of various laboratory techniques using drug testing, and, importantly, the legal issues surrounding drug testing and whether the drug will compromise job performance and safety (Huston & Heidel, 2014).

Over the past 2 decades, OEM providers have come to understand and apply the biopsychosocial model of injury/pain management (Bruns et al., 2012). This has resulted in a paradigm shift in practice norms away from solely relying on physical and pharmacotherapy treatment of injury and adding an extremely effective tool to the treatment toolbox. Pain is complex in nature and is not just a by-product of a physical injury; it has deeper psychological roots. In the case of chronic pain, sensations and emotions can lead to catastrophizing, which then perpetuates thoughts and emotions that worsen the perception of pain. Therefore, when managing a patient with acute or chronic pain, it is imperative to consider the psychosocial aspect of their condition. The goal of implementing the biopsychosocial model of care is to improve understanding of the patient's condition with greater diagnostic clarity, identify other rehabilitation methods that may be beneficial, and identify psychosocial factors that may be contributing to a patient's disability (Bruns et al., 2012). One type of model that has proven effective in implementing a biopsychosocial approach to care is referred to as *functional restoration programs*. The workers' compensation system stresses setting functional outcomes and return-to-work goals for the worker as opposed to leading a completely pain-free existence, recognizing that the eradication of pain is often an unrealistic goal. Functional restoration programs are multidisciplinary treatment protocols for chronic pain patients that heavily rely on the biopsychosocial model of care. A number of recent studies of patients with chronic MSK injuries have demonstrated the effectiveness of identifying psychosocial risk factors and incorporating the bio-psychosocial model of care into treatment to improve functionality and help restore a worker to their livelihood (K. J. Howard et al., 2017). The importance of recognizing this paradigm shift cannot be stressed enough. This model has led to and will continue to lead to improvements in management strategies for patients suffering from acute and chronic pain.

MENTAL HEALTH AND WORK

Globally, the prevalence of mental illness was increasing among the working-age population prior to the COVID-19 pandemic and has accelerated since 2020. For a variety of reasons, mental illness can be a barrier to employment. Yet, obtaining and maintaining meaningful employment has been used as an indicator of recovery for adults with mental illness, underscoring the value of employment from a psychosocial standpoint (Gmitroski et al., 2018). Although employment fosters recovery in mental illness, there are instances where it can exacerbate or result in various degrees of mental health strain and injury. With many factors in a growing workforce, such as long working hours, shift work, lack of job control, high job demands, changes in work arrangements including hybrid and remote work, occupation-related stress and mental health issues are becoming an increasingly recognized source of disability and economic loss in the workplace. Overall, rates of depression and anxiety have been increasing over the past decade and have clearly been reflected by shifts in OEM practice. Their prevalence has spiked significantly, along with other adverse mental health symptoms, suicide, and substance use disorders during the COVID-19 pandemic (Cénat et al., 2021).

Before the pandemic, workplace stressors had been shown to account for more than $190 billion in excess health care costs. Depressive disorders among employees alone cost an estimated $44 billion in lost productivity, not including labor costs or cost associated with short- and long-term disability (Fragala et al., 2021). Although staggering, these costs are likely to be substantially underestimated and will be compounded by the effects of the pandemic. It is therefore imperative in OEM to understand the impact that workplace stress has on worker health and well-being. Stress in general can have multiple deleterious physical and mental effects on an individual, as everyone experiences stress differently. Effects of stress that are commonly observed in OEM clinics include both exacerbating or contributing to psychiatric conditions. Other apparent effects are related to productivity (e.g., absenteeism, presenteeism), job burnout and attrition, and strained home relationships. The following case examples highlight the importance of recognizing how mental health issues can manifest in the workplace and affect work life, home life, and injury recovery from an OEM perspective.

1. A 23-year-old woman who works at a grocery store arrives at the clinic for evaluation of a minor wrist sprain that occurred while removing some frozen

goods from a freezer shelf for a customer. She shares that she has not had a good working relationship with her coworkers and employer since she started her job a year ago. She is open about her past medical history and states she has been treated for anxiety and depression with medications alone for several years, conditions that are now exacerbated by her current working conditions. Over the ensuing weeks, she progresses well with physical therapy and NSAIDs; however, she feels she cannot return to full-duty work status. Upon further questioning, it is revealed that her complete recovery is delayed by her current work environment, which she perceives as "hostile." Her anxiety has increased on questionnaires completed during each clinic visit, and she states that she "does not feel supported at work." She is referred for cognitive behavior therapy and medication management under her workers' compensation claim to aid in her physical recovery, and she ultimately improves.

2. A 45-year-old man who works at a merchandise distribution facility comes to the clinic to claim workplace stress from high job demands producing mental injury and decreased productivity. He states that he cannot cope at work given the stress of having to increase his workload beyond his perceived physical and mental capabilities. He is visibly upset, stating, "I really need this job to support my family, but I cannot keep up anymore." There has been high employee turnover, leaving many positions unfilled at his place of employment, thereby increasing the workload. Given his increased stress at work, he notes a strained family relationship, lack of enjoyment of hobbies, decreased appetite, and whole-body aches that worsen on his way to work and throughout the workday. He did not experience symptoms like these in the past and has never been diagnosed with anxiety, depression, or any mental health issues. He notes an overwhelming sense of despair in feeling that he cannot provide for his family. The case of this worker represents a gray area within the U.S. workers' compensation system that is discussed in the following section.

3. A 38-year-old guard at a local corrections facility arrives at the clinic complaining of work-related stress. He states that a few weeks prior, an inmate experienced a seizure and became unconscious. The guard panicked and began performing cardiopulmonary resuscitation. Ultimately, the inmate recovered, but this experience rattled the guard. He states that since the incident he has not been sleeping well and experiences flashbacks of the event. He has had difficulties even driving to work and expresses a feeling of impending doom when he arrives at the gates to the facility. He is ultimately referred to a mental health practitioner and is diagnosed with posttraumatic stress disorder (PTSD). His claim is covered under the workers' compensation system due to meeting criteria for workplace incident–induced PTSD. He has since decided to change jobs as he feels he cannot go back to his prior place of employment.

Although there are workplace interventions purporting to improve employee mental health and access to care, many models have been unsuccessful (Goetzel et al., 2018). However, on the individual patient level, OEM practitioners utilize a variety of screening tools in the outpatient occupational medicine setting that help identify workers struggling with mental health conditions. Ultimately, identifying mental issues early in a worker's care can accelerate treatment and recovery, reduce health care resource utilization, and increase worker productivity. Screening is an important preventive tool in the occupational health practitioner's care repertoire. Even more so, connection with appropriate mental health services in a timely manner following screening has shown to be very effective in terms of workers' symptom reduction and occupational outcomes. For example, studies have shown that screening workers for depression and referral for follow-up support resulted in lower self-reported depression scores, higher job retention, and more hours worked by employees (Wang et al., 2007).

Screening for mental health concerns/illness in the outpatient setting follows recommendations put forth by the United States Preventive Services Task Force. Commonly used depression-screening tools include the Patient Health Questionnaire (PHQ), Generalized Anxiety Disorder Scale (GAD-7), and Hospital Anxiety and Depression Scale (HADS), to name a few. When patients' scores on these scales indicate a form of mental distress, prompt referral is usually made to a mental health professional. Exemplified in case #1, many mental health issues experienced by workers are preexisting conditions that can be exacerbated by several factors (such as the aforementioned work conditions and injury) and act as a multiplier in terms of perceived injury severity and delayed recovery times. Therefore, timely recognition and referral can shorten case lengths and hasten functional recovery with prompt return to work. The worker in case #1 had an initial physical injury that exacerbated underlying mental health conditions. As such, the treatment for mental health was covered under her insurance claim because it was exacerbated by her physical work injury. The case of worker #2 without a physical injury is less clear cut.

Workers' compensation insurance coverage for mental health conditions in the United States varies widely. Currently, nine states cover mental only injury, with 28 that offer limited treatment coverage under circumscribed circumstances, and 13 where mental only injuries are not covered at all (Gerber & Holder, 2019). As such, if the worker in case #2 were to file a claim for mental health–related treatment, acceptance of that claim will depend on the state in which the worker filed the claim. To add to difficulty arising from state coverage variability, filing a claim can be stressful within itself. In a study performed by Kyron et al. (2021), an anonymous first responder was quoted saying, "The process of seeking support and compensation is sometimes more stressful and damaging than the original event." There is also an unfortunate stigma underlying claiming mental injury as being perceived as weak. These sentiments act as a deterrent to ultimately seeking appropriate care.

Other countries handle work-related mental health problems quite differently. In Canada, for example, a worker is entitled to compensation for a mental disorder alone if it arises out of and during employment, or if a mental condition arises because of a work injury, if certain criteria apply. These criteria include a reaction to one or more traumatic events that occurred during the worker's employment or were predominantly caused by a significant work-related stressor (as in case #2). Understandably, for the claim to be compensable there also needs to be a diagnosis of a mental health condition made by a psychiatrist or psychologist in accordance with the most updated criteria in the *Diagnostic and Statistical Manual of Mental Disorders, Fifth Edition.*

There have been recent modifications and headway in the U.S. system for coverage of mental health issues arising from the workplace in terms of expansion of coverage for PTSD as seen in case #3. It is increasingly recognized that responses to trauma vary widely, including those traumas often associated with PTSD. Such traumas include, for example, experiencing a severe injury, near-death experience, physical or sexual assault, or other extreme social or natural events. Any number of these can manifest in the workplace, especially in populations such as police officers, firefighters, and first responders. Many states' workers' compensation statutes have expanded coverage for these populations and are working toward covering other working populations as well.

Since the beginning of the COVID-19 pandemic, mental injury or illness issues arising from the workplace have gained greater attention. Numerous uncertainties arose from the global pandemic in terms of the impact on people's ability to return to work. These uncertainties stem in part from instances of PTSD, such as those seen in health care professionals, arising from overwhelming mortality numbers of COVID-19 patients, fear of contracting the virus, hesitancy of returning to the workplace after an injury due to concern for personal and family safety, in addition to workplace and interpersonal conflicts over the use of personal protective equipment and vaccination requirements, among others. This has sparked recognition of the need for broader compensation coverage of mental health issues stemming from the workplace in the U.S. workers' compensation system. In a model heavily geared toward treating physical injury, the increasing recognition of the importance of mental health and prevalence of work-related mental health injury demands systemic change. The heavy economic impact of these conditions in terms of lost productivity, job attrition, and increased health care costs will likely continue to promote more research, spark policy change and legislation, and hopefully lead to increased prevention efforts and better mental health care coverage.

WORKPLACE VIOLENCE

OEM practitioners often see patients who have been victims of workplace violence. Many may initially be seen in emergency departments, but if a link to the workplace is identified, OEM physicians often become involved. In the United States, workplace violence is endemic and takes many forms. Incidents can occur between workers, between workers and their supervisors and business owners, or between employees and customers, clients, or patients, depending on the work setting. Workplace violence can include intimidation, bullying, harassment, verbal or physical assaults, and altercations that have led to deaths. There are unfortunately common examples of workplace shootings that serve as the most extreme cases of workplace violence, but lesser forms are pervasive.

Occupational Safety and Health Administration (OSHA) defines *workplace violence* as "any act or threat of physical violence, harassment, intimidation, or other threatening disruptive behavior that occurs at the work site," and it is cited as the third most common cause of occupational-related death in the United States. Harassment is a form of workplace discrimination under Title VII of the Civil Rights Act of 1964 and the Americans with Disabilities Act of 1990. Harassment in the workplace is generally regarded as conduct toward a coworker that is considered unwelcome, particularly if the actions or speech are based on the recipient's race, color, national origin, age, sexual identity, or physical/mental disabilities. Intimidation usually involves creating a sense of fear that some harm may occur. This can be a physical or emotional threat that is considered an intentional act. Bullying tends to be a pattern of behavior where the victim is subjected to physical, emotional, or psychological harms. Bullying can be verbal or physical and can include intimidation and humiliation.

Workplace violence can occur in any setting. Some factors that create higher risk include working late at night, working with mentally unstable or volatile clients, working in high-crime areas, working alone, or working where money is directly exchanged. These factors and others mean that certain workers—including bartenders and food-service workers, police officers and first responders, health care workers, delivery drivers, and customer service agents—are at greater risk for being victims of workplace violence.

Assault in the workplace is a disturbingly common cause of occupational injuries that are severe enough to require treatment for physical and mental health effects. Consider the following examples from our clinical practice.

- A landscaper and his supervisor argue over the quality of work being done. As the landscaper turns away, he is punched in the face by the supervisor, leading to transient vision loss with subsequent posttraumatic glaucoma, cataract, and nasal bone fractures.

- A saleswoman is berated by her boss after asking to leave early due to a headache that resulted from a work-related motor vehicle accident that was not her fault. She felt powerless to ask for additional time off for medical appointments and self-care.

- A delivery man is mauled by dogs when a young child left home alone released them into the courtyard as he attempted a delivery, causing loss of muscle mass and strength in his arms in addition to significant residual scarring from defensive wounds. These scars serve as a daily reminder of the attack. He leaves the job he loves and begins driving a truck, resulting in more time away from his family.

- A store clerk is beaten and kicked following a robbery. He locks up his store early and refuses to let his family members cover the store for him for fear of another attack.

- A special needs teacher is punched and slapped by a student. She is given the day off from work but is expected to return the following day, knowing that the student will still be in class since he is not subject to the same disciplinary structure because of his mental disability.

- A security guard is punched by an irate and intoxicated customer who was asked to leave the store. The security guard suffers an eye injury, requiring multiple surgeries. After his workers' compensation carrier only agrees to cover the standard implantable lens, his employer raises additional money for an implantable lens that will fully correct his vision. His vision is better than it was before the accident, but he now has a deformity around his eye socket and upper eyelid. He leaves his job in security.

In OEM practice, we observe firsthand what research has shown: Workplace violence and reporting workplace violence take a toll on workers. It has a negative impact on a worker's mental health and function outside of the workplace. Many injured workers fear entry into the workers' compensation system. For example, investigators have found that after experiencing workplace violence, workers reported feelings such as "depressed, anxious, and drained" along with "occasionally getting panic attacks" and "taking stress out on others" (Brown et al., 2020). These researchers showed that workers of all ages failed to report at least one episode of workplace violence to their managers "out of fear of retaliation" and "fear of not being taken seriously." There was also note of a concern for a power differential in terms of managerial staff firing workers, economic withholding, verbal abuse, and having workers perform job tasks they were not comfortable performing. Fear of entering the workers' compensation system also plays a role in underreporting due to concerns of ongoing financial strain, family tensions, claim denial, and stigma from managers and fellow employees, to name a few factors (Gewurtz et al., 2018). Workplace violence significantly affects workers both inside and outside of the workplace. There is a great need for research on workplace programs that create safer work conditions and psychologically safe reporting systems so that workers who experience workplace violence can report incidents without fear of retaliation.

WORKPLACE HEALTH PROMOTION

For nearly 50 years, OEM physicians have played pivotal roles in the development and management of workplace health promotion programs. "Wellness" programs adopted by employers as early as the 1970s were touted as means of improving worker productivity that would generate a return on the investment. Early efforts focused largely on health behavioral change tended to prioritize the health needs of managers and were not well supported by evidence of sustained benefit on either economics or health. Over time, several factors helped wellness programs take root and spread in U.S. industry, including the need of employers to address the rising cost of health care and pharmaceuticals, increases in the number of chronic health conditions among workers, and the prevalence of an aging workforce. Increasingly, wellness programs added chronic disease management to their offerings, reinforced by a small number of studies showing that, at least in large enterprises, such programs reduced business costs (Song & Baicker, 2019). Despite mixed results, ethical concerns, potential for discriminatory practices, and a paucity of data to suggest efficacy in smaller enterprises (McCoy et al., 2014), the workplace wellness industry has grown exponentially. OEM physicians play numerous roles, including in the design, supervision, and provision of care. Components of wellness programs may include clinical screening programs for health conditions, like diabetes mellitus, chronic respiratory illnesses such as chronic obstructive lung disease and asthma, hypertension and other cardiovascular disease, as well as depression and cancer, calling upon OEM physicians to engage in both diagnosis and prevention. Such health-screening programs are analogous to other types of screenings conducted by OEM practitioners, including mandatory workplace-screening programs for substance use and as medical examiners providing screening/certification of workers in safety-sensitive positions, such as pilots, air traffic controllers, and commercial vehicle operators.

OEM AND EMERGENCY RESPONSE: THE COVID-19 PANDEMIC

The COVID-19 pandemic placed unprecedented pressures on the global workforce. As a result, OEM physicians have needed to help workers address symptoms of psychological strain and burnout at unprecedented rates and from a variety of different workplace settings. *Burnout* is a multifaceted syndrome characterized by depersonalization (negative attitude about one's job and/or clientele), emotional exhaustion, and sense of low personal accomplishment, which may persist after a period of recovery from work. If affected by burnout, the worker may experience absenteeism, increased health problems, and reduced performance on the job (Maslach et al., 2001). Burnout in the setting of COVID-19 became especially prevalent in fields with high job demands such as health care, public health, and public safety. In general, health care workers are very susceptible to job burnout, especially in those working in high-acuity settings such as the emergency department or intensive care unit. Factors contributing to burnout in these settings include high mortality rate of patients, variable shift work, long working hours, constant job-related pressures with little time for worker recovery (Dyrbye et al., 2019). Firefighters, first responders, and police officers are subject to similar job-related stressors such as the frequent witnessing of traumas resulting in PTSD, sleep deprivation due to shift work, hazardous working conditions, and long working hours. Compounding the already stressful nature of these jobs in addition to the uncertainties of a global pandemic has been a recipe for increased job-related burnout.

Increasing worker burnout represents a unique challenge for OEM practitioners. The spectrum of clinical presentations ranges from an increased demand for clinicians to conduct so-called fitness for duty exams to evaluating and managing patients experiencing compassion fatigue. The following clinical case from our academic OEM practice exemplifies the challenges discussed with worker burnout among health care professionals, although it is applicable to the firefighter/first responder community as well.

A 34-year-old nurse is called for a return-to-work evaluation after she contracted COVID-19 while caring for patients on an inpatient unit, pre-vaccination. She has been out of work for several weeks, with lingering post-COVID symptoms of headaches, fatigue, and cough. She is emotionally distraught. She lives alone. Work provides her with a sense of social connectedness and a sense of purpose. She states that her fatigue prevents her from keeping up with her normal job demands. For health reasons, her supervisor recommended that she stay home. She is concerned about how her coworkers now perceive her, since she is not contributing to the increasing workload caused by the COVID-19 pandemic. She also states that due to her ongoing symptoms, she has not been able to engage in physical exercise and has been spending more time inside and inactive. She expresses frustration and at one point during the interview she places blame on the carelessness of patients she was taking care of, accusing them of not practicing appropriate hygiene measures.

This scenario unfortunately became an all-too-common presentation among health care workers during the pandemic and highlights some of the difficulties that OEM physicians have faced when determining whether a patient is fit to return to work. In this case, the patient exhibited hallmarks of burnout and compassion fatigue brought about by her current illness contracted from a high-stress work environment. These conditions significantly limit her ability to function at work as well as her activities of daily living. The compassion fatigue manifests in this situation as emotional distress and avoidance behavior in professional/patient relationships, ultimately diminishing the quality of care provided (Ruiz-Fernández et al., 2020).

As part of the return-to-work evaluation, the OEM physician's role is to identify hallmarks of emotional distress and provide avenues to mitigating stressors. If left unchecked, patients may require a prolonged period to return to their occupations, or it may even be recommended that they leave their employment and profession. This particular patient was referred to a mental health provider (through telehealth), eventually returning to work four months after developing her initial symptoms. She benefited from cognitive behavior therapy, which she continued after she returned to work during the ongoing pandemic. This case offers just one of many examples of how OEM practitioners have engaged in COVID-19 pandemic responses. While the principles and roles are similar to OEM participation in other emergency response situations that impact workers, none have compared to the massive scale of response necessitated by the COVID-19 pandemic.

OEM ROLE IN ADDRESSING HEALTH DISPARITIES IN VULNERABLE POPULATIONS

The social conditions under which the human population lives and works comprise social determinants of health (SDH; Moure-Eraso et al., 2007). SDH are implicated in *health inequities*, defined as health conditions that affect certain socioeconomic, ethnic, and gender population subgroups disproportionately (Forst et al., 2020; G. Howard et al., 2014).

Worker health inequities and disparities in relation to vulnerable populations span cultures and present unique issues experienced by occupational health professionals in the patient care setting. The increasingly diverse and multi-cultural workforce of the 21st century is transforming the provider–patient relationship in occupational health practice. In forging a therapeutic relation-ship, OEM practitioners must understand and take into consideration the chal-lenges experienced by women; lesbian, gay, bisexual, transexual, and queer/questioning (LGBTQ+); Black, Indigenous, people of color (BIPOC); and Latinx working populations. People working with disabilities, as well as new, young workers, and aging workers who are staying in the job market past traditional retirement age all face work-related vulnerabilities. Not uncommonly, an OEM physician encounters patients with language and cultural barriers that affect their understanding of how to safely perform work, how the workers' compen-sation system functions, and OEM practitioner's role in their care. Language and cultural barriers also influence understanding, ability, and willingness to form a collaborative relationship leading to successful medical intervention.

Historically, racial/ethnic minority groups have faced many of the worst working conditions, increasing their hazardous exposures and health risks. For example, in the steel industry, coke oven workers had the highest lung cancer mortality rates, with Black workers' risk being higher than that of white workers' (Lloyd, 1971). More than half a century later, the accumulated evidence continues to suggest that members of minority populations face higher workplace injury risks compared to white workers with an increased injury pattern similar in both men and women (Seabury et al., 2017). Being the largest minority group in the United States, both native- and foreign-born Hispanic/Latinx workers are subject to health disparities and are highly vulner-able to mistreatment in the workplace. The Hispanic population in the United States includes many migrant and temporary foreign-born workers. Undocu-mented immigrant workers play an important role in the economy. Often, undocumented migrant workers are employed in high-risk jobs with hazardous occupational exposures and limited or no health insurance (Velasco-Mondragon et al., 2016). Tackling these issues while ensuring respect for cultural norms is an important goal within OEM. The following case is illustrative of the clinical setting often encountered by OEM physicians who care for the Hispanic/Latinx working population.

A 63-year-old Hispanic male construction worker who is employed by his son-in-law visits the clinic because of an injury sustained to his right eye more than 6 months ago while working on the job. His visit is conducted with an interpreter present. He initially appears hesitant to discuss events that resulted in his injury or to say why he has waited so long to report it. As it turns out, he got into an altercation with his son-in-law (who is also his supervisor) on the jobsite and was struck in the eye, resulting in significantly decreased vision. His family had pressured him to not report this as a work-related injury. Upon further review of his medical history, it is noted that he had a prior injury to his other eye, significantly affecting his vision. He has poorly controlled diabetes mellitus, due to lack of health insurance, and limited insight into the need for proper treatment. Additionally, his vision has worsened to the point of significantly affecting his quality of life at work and home, and he desperately wants treatment under the workers' compensation system as he does not have primary insurance. He also states he was unsure of the reporting process for workers' compensation claims or how to navigate the system.

This case highlights a few of the many barriers met by the Hispanic working population in the workplace and health care setting. First, the worker's home and work environment, along with fear of repercussions reporting his incident, have delayed his care and worsened his clinical outcomes. Second, the delayed recognition of a work-related condition plus a poorly controlled underlying chronic health condition for which he lacks adequate access to health care (Velasco-Mondragon et al., 2016) have converged, resulting in tragic loss of vision. Recognizing and navigating the barriers to care experienced by vulnerable populations such as the Latinx workforce are integral to the practice of OEM. They must understand SDH such as environmental and employment conditions, social environment, and homelife in order to improve care of vulnerable populations.

BRINGING OEM AND OHP TOGETHER: THE POTENTIAL OF *TOTAL WORKER HEALTH*® (TWH) APPROACHES

Many of the examples provided in this chapter illustrate that OEM physicians are in a strong position to contribute to, and benefit from, the field of OHP. The two fields' shared interest in TWH (NIOSH, 2020; Tamers et al., 2019) illustrates the opportunity. Physicians, nurses, advanced care professionals, and others who work directly with injured workers and with employers are beginning to embrace core concepts that bridge worker health, safety, and well-being (Newman et al., 2020). All the clinical cases described in this chapter share two common features: Workers were impacted by SDH, and their injuries and illnesses were preventable. TWH approaches are defined by the CDC and NIOSH as policies, programs, and practices that integrate protection from work-related safety and health hazards with promotion of injury and illness-prevention efforts to advance worker well-being (NIOSH, 2020). TWH approaches embrace the importance of SDH, taking into consideration many of the issues that OEM practitioners address with workers, their families, and their employers, including considerations such as workload, workability, supervisor–worker interactions, substance use disorders, health promotion, hazard recognition and reduction (including psychological and physical stressors), to name just a few of the points of intersection. We share common goals of preventing occupational illness and injury and improving the physical, cognitive, and psychological outcomes for all workers, including those who become our patients.

REFERENCES

Brown, B., Myers, D., Casteel, C., & Rauscher, K. (2020). Exploring differences in the workplace violence experiences of young workers in middle and late adolescence in the United States. *Journal of Safety Research, 74,* 263–269. https://doi.org/10.1016/j.jsr.2020.06.008

Bruns, D., Mueller, K., & Warren, P. A. (2012). Biopsychosocial law, health care reform, and the control of medical inflation in Colorado. *Rehabilitation Psychology, 57*(2), 81–97. https://doi.org/10.1037/a0028623

Cénat, J. M., Blais-Rochette, C., Kokou-Kpolou, C. K., Noorishad, P.-G., Mukunzi, J. N., McIntee, S.-E., Dalexis, R. D., Goulet, M.-A., & Labelle, P. R. (2021). Prevalence of symptoms of depression, anxiety, insomnia, posttraumatic stress disorder, and psychological distress among populations affected by the COVID-19 pandemic: A systematic review and meta-analysis. *Psychiatry Research, 295,* 113599. https://doi.org/10.1016/j.psychres.2020.113599

Dyrbye, L. N., Shanafelt, T. D., Johnson, P. O., Johnson, L. A., Satele, D., & West, C. P. (2019). A cross-sectional study exploring the relationship between burnout, absenteeism, and job performance among American nurses. *BMC Nursing, 18*(1), 57. https://doi.org/10.1186/s12912-019-0382-7

Forst, L., Grant, A., & Hebert-Beirne, J. (2020). Work as a social determinant of health: A landscape assessment of employers in two historically disinvested urban communities. *American Journal of Industrial Medicine, 63*(11), 1038–1046. https://doi.org/10.1002/ajim.23174

Fragala, M. S., Hunter, J. L., Satish, A., Jelovic, N. A., Carr, S., Bailey, A. M., Stokes, M., Hayward, J. I., Kim, P. M., & Peters, M. E. (2021). Workplace mental health: Application of a population health approach of proactive screening to identify risk and engage in care. *Journal of Occupational and Environmental Medicine, 63*(3), 244–250. https://doi.org/10.1097/JOM.0000000000002116

Gerber, B., & Holder, T. (2019). *Which states offer workers' comp benefits for post-traumatic stress disorder and mental-only injuries?* https://www.gerberholderlaw.com/workers-comp-ptsd-by-state/

Gewurtz, R. E., Premji, S., & Holness, D. L. (2018). The experiences of workers who do not successfully return to work following a work-related injury. *Work, 61*(4), 537–549. https://doi.org/10.3233/WOR-182824

Gmitroski, T., Bradley, C., Heinemann, L., Liu, G., Blanchard, P., Beck, C., Mathias, S., Leon, A., & Barbic, S. P. (2018). Barriers and facilitators to employment for young adults with mental illness: A scoping review. *BMJ Open, 8*(12), e024487. https://doi.org/10.1136/bmjopen-2018-024487

Goetzel, R. Z., Roemer, E. C., Holingue, C., Fallin, M. D., McCleary, K., Eaton, W., Agnew, J., Azocar, F., Ballard, D., Bartlett, J., Braga, M., Conway, H., Crighton, K. A., Frank, R., Jinnett, K., Keller-Greene, D., Rauch, S. M., Safeer, R., Saporito, D., . . . Mattingly, C. R. (2018). Mental health in the workplace: A call to action proceedings from the mental health in the workplace—public health summit. *Journal of Occupational and Environmental Medicine, 60*(4), 322–330. https://doi.org/10.1097/JOM.0000000000001271

Hegmann, K. T., Weiss, M. S., Bowden, K., Branco, F., DuBrueler, K., Els, C., Mandel, S., McKinney, D. W., Miguel, R., Mueller, K. L., Nadig, R. J., Schaffer, M. I., Studt, L., Talmage, J. B., Travis, R. L., Winters, T., Thiese, M. S., Harris, J. S., & the American College of Occupational and Environmental Medicine. (2014). ACOEM practice guidelines: Opioids for treatment of acute, subacute, chronic, and postoperative pain. *Journal of Occupational and Environmental Medicine, 56*(12), e143–e159. https://doi.org/10.1097/JOM.0000000000000352

Howard, G., Peace, F., & Howard, V. J. (2014). The contributions of selected diseases to disparities in death rates and years of life lost for racial/ethnic minorities in the

United States, 1999–2010. *Preventing Chronic Disease, 11,* 140138. https://doi.org/10.5888/pcd11.140138

Howard, K. J., Castaneda, R. A., Gray, A. L., Haskard-Zolnierek, K. B., & Jordan, K. (2017). Psychosocial factors related to functional restoration treatment completion and return-to-function for patients with chronic disabling occupational musculoskeletal disorders. *Journal of Occupational and Environmental Medicine, 59*(3), 320–326. https://doi.org/10.1097/JOM.0000000000000953

Huston, M., & Heidel, S. (2014). Substance use disorders. In LaDou, J., & Harrison, R. *Current occupational & environmental medicine* (5th ed.). McGraw-Hill Education/Medical. https://accessmedicine.mhmedical.com/book.aspx?bookid=1186

Kyron, M. J., Rikkers, W., O'Brien, P., Bartlett, J., & Lawrence, D. (2021). Experiences of police and emergency services employees with workers' compensation claims for mental health issues. *Journal of Occupational Rehabilitation, 31*(1), 197–206. https://doi.org/10.1007/s10926-020-09909-8

Lloyd, J. W. (1971). Long-term mortality study of steelworkers. V. Respiratory cancer in coke plant workers. *Journal of Occupational Medicine: Official Publication of the Industrial Medical Association, 13*(2), 53–68. https://pubmed.ncbi.nlm.nih.gov/5546197/

Maslach, C., Schaufeli, W. B., & Leiter, M. P. (2001). Job burnout. *Annual Review of Psychology, 52*(1), 397–422. https://doi.org/10.1146/annurev.psych.52.1.397

McAuliffe Staehler, T. M., & Palombi, L. C. (2020). Beneficial opioid management strategies: A review of the evidence for the use of opioid treatment agreements. *Substance Abuse, 41*(2), 208–215. https://doi.org/10.1080/08897077.2019.1692122

McCoy, K., Stinson, K., Scott, K., Tenney, L., & Newman, L. S. (2014). Health promotion in small business: A systematic review of factors influencing adoption and effectiveness of worksite wellness programs. *Journal of Occupational and Environmental Medicine, 56*(6), 579–587. https://doi.org/10.1097/JOM.0000000000000171

Moure-Eraso, R., Flum, M., Lahiri, S., Tilly, C., & Massawe, E. (2007). A review of employment conditions as social determinants of health part II: The workplace. *New Solutions, 16*(4), 429–448. https://doi.org/10.2190/R8Q2-41L5-H4W5-7838

Nasterlack, M. (2011). Role of medical surveillance in risk management. *Journal of Occupational and Environmental Medicine, 53*(Suppl. 6S), S18–S21. https://doi.org/10.1097/JOM.0b013e31821b1d54

Newman, L. S., Scott, J. G., Childress, A., Linnan, L., Newhall, W. J., McLellan, D. L., Campo, S., Freewynn, S., Hammer, L. B., Leff, M., Macy, G., Maples, E. H., Rogers, B., Rohlman, D. S., Tenney, L., & Watkins, C. (2020). Education and training to build capacity in Total Worker Health®: Proposed competencies for an emerging field. *Journal of Occupational and Environmental Medicine, 62*(8), e384–e391. https://doi.org/10.1097/JOM.0000000000001906

NIOSH. (2020). *What is Total Worker Health®?* https://www.cdc.gov/niosh/twh/totalhealth.html

Orslene, L. (2017). *Accommodation and Compliance Series: Return to work programs.* https://askjan.org/topics/return.cfm?csSearch=3774130_1

Rhodes, E., Wilson, M., Robinson, A., Hayden, J. A., & Asbridge, M. (2019). The effectiveness of prescription drug monitoring programs at reducing opioid-related harms and consequences: A systematic review. *BMC Health Services Research, 19*(1), 784. https://doi.org/10.1186/s12913-019-4642-8

Ruiz-Fernández, M. D., Ramos-Pichardo, J. D., Ibáñez-Masero, O., Cabrera-Troya, J., Carmona-Rega, M. I., & Ortega-Galán, Á. M. (2020). Compassion fatigue, burnout, compassion satisfaction and perceived stress in healthcare professionals during the COVID-19 health crisis in Spain. *Journal of Clinical Nursing, 29*(21–22), 4321–4330. https://doi.org/10.1111/jocn.15469

Seabury, S. A., Terp, S., & Boden, L. I. (2017). Racial and ethnic differences in the frequency of workplace injuries and prevalence of work-related disability. *Health Affairs, 36*(2), 266–273. https://doi.org/10.1377/hlthaff.2016.1185

Smith, D. E., Glatt, W., Tucker, D. E., Deutsch, R., & Seymour, R. B. (2002). Drug testing in the workplace: Integrating medical review officer duties into occupational medicine. *Occupational Medicine, 17*(1), 79–90, v. https://pubmed.ncbi.nlm.nih.gov/11726338/

Song, Z., & Baicker, K. (2019). Effect of a workplace wellness program on employee health and economic outcomes: A randomized clinical trial. *Journal of the American Medical Association, 321*(15), 1491–1501. https://doi.org/10.1001/jama.2019.3307

Substance Abuse and Mental Health Services Administration. (2021). *The drug-free workplace toolkit.* U.S. Department of Health and Human Services. https://www.samhsa.gov/workplace/employer-resources#the-toolkit

Tamers, S. L., Chosewood, L. C., Childress, A., Hudson, H., Nigam, J., & Chang, C.-C. (2019). *Total Worker Health®* 2014–2018: The novel approach to worker safety, health, and well-being evolves. *International Journal of Environmental Research and Public Health, 16*(3), 321. https://doi.org/10.3390/ijerph16030321

Velasco-Mondragon, E., Jimenez, A., Palladino-Davis, A. G., Davis, D., & Escamilla-Cejudo, J. A. (2016). Hispanic health in the USA: A scoping review of the literature. *Public Health Reviews, 37*(1), 31. https://doi.org/10.1186/s40985-016-0043-2

Wang, P. S., Simon, G. E., Avorn, J., Azocar, F., Ludman, E. J., McCulloch, J., Petukhova, M. Z., & Kessler, R. C. (2007). Telephone screening, outreach, and care management for depressed workers and impact on clinical and work productivity outcomes: A randomized controlled trial. *Journal of the American Medical Association, 298*(12), 1401–1411. https://doi.org/10.1001/jama.298.12.1401

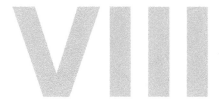

VIII

CONCLUSION

INTRODUCTION: CONCLUSION

The final chapter of this handbook discusses recent themes in OHP research and practice that cut across many of the other individual chapters, including more integrative and holistic approaches to worker health and safety; an increased emphasis on intervention research; research on individual responses and vulnerabilities to occupational stressors and hazards; the social and economic context of OHP; and new hazards, resources, and health outcomes in OHP research that had not been studied as frequently prior to the previous edition of the handbook.

In addition, this final chapter identifies some directions for future research, including advancing knowledge about how OHP constructs change over time, improving measurement of key constructs, better sampling practices, more intervention research, making theoretical progress, and attending to changes in the social context of work while incorporating the perspectives of historically underrepresented groups.

Finally, the chapter discusses graduate training in OHP, focusing on the need to teach the knowledge and skills that an OHP professional should have, along with recent developments in and potential directions for training in OHP.

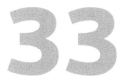

Occupational Health Psychology Today

Research Themes, Reflections, and Looking to the Future

Michael T. Ford, Gwenith G. Fisher, Lois E. Tetrick, and
James Campbell Quick

This edition of the handbook identifies many developments in occupational health psychology (OHP) research and practice over the past 10 years. Whereas some of these developments are specific to particular topics, several reflect broader themes that cut across content areas. The goal of this chapter is to highlight some of these broader developments, especially those that we have observed over the previous 10 years, and identify some potential directions for research in the coming years.

HOLISTIC AND INTEGRATIVE APPROACHES TO WORKER HEALTH AND SAFETY

One recurring theme across the chapters was a holistic approach to OHP topics that increasingly integrates both negative and positive contributions of working conditions to advance the science and practice to improve worker well-being and considers different levels of analysis and targets for intervention. This integration of positive and negative issues and experiences reflects a focus on both preventing ill-health effects of work and promoting health and well-being in the workforce. Research and intervention models incorporate several interrelated factors, balancing positive and negative factors, while acknowledging that some factors can and do have both positive and negative effects on worker health and well-being.

https://doi.org/10.1037/0000331-033
Handbook of Occupational Health Psychology, Third Edition, L. E. Tetrick, G. G. Fisher, M. T. Ford, and J. C. Quick (Editors)

Several chapters delved into positive and negative contributions of work to employee health and well-being. For example, scholarship in many topic areas draws from the job demands–resources (JD-R) model (Demerouti et al., 2001), which specifies job demands (e.g., workload) that contribute to job burnout alongside job resources (e.g., social support and feedback) that contribute to employee engagement. Balanced perspectives such as the JD-R model have had a major influence on the OHP field over the past 2 decades. Chapter 7 takes a similar approach to theory on the work–family interface, culminating in an integrative model of work–family balance. Other work (e.g., Chapters 3, 4, and 19) has focused on the multidimensional nature of stress and well-being, clarifying important distinctions between eustress and distress, as well as between hedonic and eudaimonic components of well-being. Chapter 21 reviewed recent developments in our understanding of meaningful work, attending to the benefits as well as the potential costs of work as a calling. These and other chapters point to a balanced approach to OHP that incorporates the potential costs and benefits of work and organizational practices for health and well-being.

Other chapters identified integrative approaches to OHP that bring together different hazards, points of intervention, and levels of analysis into a single, more holistic model. Chapter 6 brought together the individual, team, and organizational levels of analysis into an integrative approach to organizational well-being. Research on climate (see Chapter 9) in organizations has also focused on the measurement and outcomes of climate at different levels of aggregation. Chapter 16 highlighted the role of organizational and macro-level factors that contribute to cardiovascular disease (e.g., lean production, downsizing, and psychosocial safety climate). Chapter 28 described the need to integrate different levels of analysis into a systems view when evaluating initiatives. Chapter 23 discussed the interplay among parts of the organizational system and the need for multiple targets or levels of intervention. These are just some examples of how we are increasingly seeing approaches to OHP that consider the complex assortment of multiple individual, organizational, and contextual factors that are interrelated—in addition to causes and consequences of occupational health and health hazards across individuals, groups, organizations, and beyond—to shape and hopefully improve public health for communities and society in general.

INTERVENTION RESEARCH

A second recurring theme is that over the past decade there has been much more work on the translation of OHP knowledge into practice through interventions. We see continued scholarly emphasis on organizational interventions that address the changeable environmental causes of employee health and well-being. This is in keeping with the field's primary emphasis on the prevention of illness and injuries and the creation of safe and healthy workplaces. It is more effective to prevent hazards and stressors (i.e., primary prevention) than to reduce negative outcomes associated with existing stressors or other hazards or treat downstream poor health and well-being later on (i.e., tertiary prevention). At the same time, research has encompassed the whole spectrum of primary, secondary, and tertiary interventions. We recognize the important role that interventions have at each stage, as primary prevention, although most desirable, is not always feasible.

Several discussions of intervention work appear in this handbook. Specific examples of interventions include efforts to improve the physical work environment, furnishings, and layouts (Chapter 6); work group dynamics (Chapter 15); work organization flexibility (Chapter 16); legislative, regulatory, and contractual initiatives (Chapter 16); leadership (Chapters 12, 25, and 26); and participatory interventions that target and monitor multiple stressors based on employee input (Chapters 16 and 22). Other chapters (e.g., Chapters 15, 18, and 24) addressed the effectiveness of secondary interventions such as mindfulness and yoga, which affect employees' reactions to stressors, and tertiary interventions such as employee assistance programs, which help employees rehabilitate from health problems.

Another common theme was the challenges associated with intervention research and practice. For example, Chapter 15 described the difficulty in conducting randomized controlled trials to properly assess the causal effect of organizational interventions. Chapter 5 discussed several barriers to implementation of quality management, such as having large projects and teams dispersed across different locations as well as an emphasis on efficiency and cost reduction. Chapter 22 noted negative employee reactions and a lack of employee experiences with interventions as a potential barrier to intervention success. To overcome these barriers, several chapters (e.g., Chapters 5, 15, 22, and 28) considered the importance of employee participation throughout the intervention process.

INDIVIDUAL RESPONSES AND VULNERABILITIES

A third theme across the handbook is a more systematic consideration of individual differences in how employees respond to workplace stressors. This reflects an increasing recognition that workers are not passive recipients of working conditions, work experiences, and work stressors. Workers often react to and address their stressors in different ways. One burgeoning area of research along these lines is on the construct of job crafting (see Chapters 4 and 19), which refers to workers' attempts to change their own working conditions to fit their needs. Other work of this nature has focused on boundary management (Chapter 7), or the ways in which workers create and maintain boundaries between work and nonwork. There has also been major advancement in our understanding of sleep and recovery from work during off-work time through recovery experiences and activities, as highlighted in chapters on recovery, sleep, fatigue, and burnout (e.g., Chapters 12, 15, and 20).

Individuals differ in their vulnerability to specific types of work stressors. This handbook covers advancements in our understanding of these individual differences. For example, Chapter 10 discussed differences across age, gender, and chronotypes in how workers respond to shift work. Chapter 14 noted individual characteristics that are associated with being a target of workplace mistreatment. Chapter 17 discussed the considerable variation in workers' functional limitations, beliefs, and perceived need for accommodation as a challenge for managing pain and return to work. Chapter 18 noted several individual characteristics and beliefs that increase the likelihood of workers' alcohol use in response to work stressors.

Considering the emphasis on employee participation in recent intervention research and scholarship, it appears that the most effective interventions may be those that incorporate employee needs and perspectives in addition to the organization's general philosophy toward employee health (e.g., Chapter 23).

SOCIAL AND ECONOMIC CONTEXT

The macro-level social and economic context of work continues to receive growing scholarly attention in the field of OHP. This includes the study of differences in hazards, stressors, and reactions to stress across cultures and regions of the world (Chapter 8) as well as among worker populations that are at high risk for poor health and well-being for a variety of reasons, in addition to workers who are traditionally underrepresented in research, such as immigrant or LGBTQ+ workers (Chapter 26). Organizational approaches that provide an important contextual frame, such as attention to lean production processes (Chapters 5 and 16), also continue to be important. Organizational approaches shape the climate (Chapter 9) and have implications for the performance pressures that workers experience.

One rapidly growing area of OHP research has been nonstandard work arrangements that give employers more flexibility, often at the expense of employees' control, predictability, and job security. Nonstandard work arrangements (Chapter 11) include agency, contract, and gig arrangements in which workers do not expect to have a long-term or predictable relationship with the organization for which they are working. This can change the employee–organization relationship as well as the perceived and actual responsibility that employers may have for protecting the health and safety of their employees. Recent research has also delved into the broader issue of precarious work, which encompasses job insecurity, a lack of schedule control and predictability, and a lack of benefits (e.g., paid vacation) that are common in more standard work arrangements. This issue is addressed to some degree in several chapters (e.g., Chapters 10, 11, 16, 17, and 23). We expect and encourage continued growth in OHP research on these work arrangements and practices in the coming years, particularly as jobs, work arrangements, and employee–organization relationships continue to evolve.

NEW HAZARDS, RESOURCES, AND HEALTH OUTCOMES

Several stressors and working conditions have emerged in the OHP literature over the past 2 decades, with particular growth since the second edition of the handbook appeared. These include different forms of mistreatment (Chapters 8, 14, and 16); remote work environments that interface with several aspects of OHP (e.g., Chapters 10, 11, 14, 17, and 29); variable work schedules, which correspond with nonstandard work arrangements and employer flexibility (e.g., Chapters 10, 11, 16, and 17); and experiences with ethics, morality, diversity, and inequality in the workplace (e.g., Chapters 13, 14, and 26). Increased attention has also been given to resources that can help promote employee well-being and reduce negative responses to work stressors. This includes research on worker flexibility and giving workers more control over their time (e.g., Chapters 10 and 26). Several chapters also discussed the importance of effective leadership, leader support, and training in various contexts (e.g., Chapters 12, 14, 25, 26, and 31).

Although there is continued interest in many of the same psychological and physical health outcomes that have always been the focus of research in the field, there is further evidence for casting a broad net for conceptualizing and assessing worker health and well-being. In particular, we see a growing emphasis on a few particular outcomes, such as energy and related constructs. For example, research highlighted in this handbook has addressed feelings of fatigue, exhaustion, and depletion as unique health outcomes (e.g., Chapters 10, 12, and 15). Other work has focused on sleep and recovery experiences that contribute to energy replenishment (e.g., Chapters 12 and 20). Such experiences of fatigue may be distinct from other forms of distress. Collectively, these chapters highlighted important linkages between psychosocial work experiences, physical health, and mental health. Other work has noted the general diversity of well-being constructs, illustrating the multidimensional nature of worker health and well-being (e.g., Chapter 19). In addition, new research has been conducted on longer term health effects of work in recent years (e.g., Chapters 10, 13, 16, and 21), which is needed to understand fuller and longer term implications of occupational hazards for workers.

FUTURE DIRECTIONS FOR OHP RESEARCH

Although significant advancements in the field have been made over the past decade, there remain many topics for OHP researchers to pursue in the coming years. All chapters in the handbook identified several themes for future directions for research and practice. We highlight many of these suggestions for future research and practice based on our work in assembling this handbook, although this is by no means an exhaustive list of suggested future research topics.

Research Methods and Data

As in other areas of psychology and public health, OHP research methods have become increasingly sophisticated to capture more complex models and assess dynamic processes and changes over time. Research during the past decade has often used multilevel, experience sampling, longitudinal, and quasi-experimental designs to draw new insights into the effects of work on employee health.

Despite the increased variability and sophistication of research designs incorporated in OHP research, some particular methodological issues hold promise for further advancing the field. Perhaps one of the greatest needs in OHP is longitudinal research conducted over longer time frames than have been typical. Whereas much is known about how workers immediately or concurrently perceive and react to work stressors and resources, less is known about longer-term effects. This is particularly important for evaluating and understanding mediating mechanisms in models of work stress and worker well-being, and for assessing the extent to which beneficial intervention effects last over time.

Many dimensions of health and well-being show stability over time and appear resistant to sustained change. It is not clear to what extent this is due to artifacts of measures that are not very sensitive to detecting changes over time, the corresponding stability in the work context and workers' experiences of their work situations, or the ways in which workers adapt to work stressors and resources over time. As such, creating *sustained* improvement in worker health and well-being remains a topic of interest across many areas of OHP, theoretically and practically.

In addition to seeking sustainable benefits to improving worker health and well-being, there is a continued need to accumulate evidence across studies on longitudinal effects. The methods used to assess change over time vary across studies, with some using regression controlling for baseline or cross-lagged panel modeling, and others using more sophisticated analytic strategies (e.g., latent growth modeling, latent change score modeling, growth mixture modeling, and random-intercept cross-lagged panel modeling). These types of analyses can yield different results, making it challenging to integrate studies that use different analytical approaches. To gain a better understanding of the medium- and longer term relationships among work stressors, resources, and employee health and well-being, we hope for some integration and common understanding of results to emerge across these methods. This will hopefully build a stronger evidence base for how to improve employee well-being in a sustained manner.

In addition to a focus on longitudinal methods, there remains a need to continue improving measurement and surveillance of key constructs. Several chapters noted that scales in their area of study need refinement to make them more diagnostic. Other chapters (e.g., Chapters 11 and 16) discussed the need to conduct more research on the prevalence of exposures and/or ill-health effects of work, hopefully resulting in better surveillance of physical and psychosocial exposures as well as their effects on worker health over time. Incorporation and application of epidemiological approaches (e.g., Chapter 27), with careful attention to sampling to achieve precise measurement and generalizable samples representative of the population, represents an opportunity for advancement in the field, especially as work practices continue to evolve.

An additional theme that continues be dominant within OHP is a strong need for intervention research: developing, conducting, evaluating, and disseminating research as well as translating results to stakeholders to make use of the information. Intervention studies are difficult to conduct, as noted with respect to burnout interventions (see Chapter 15). Many of the difficulties with intervention research identified in Chapter 15 apply to other areas of intervention as well. Yet interventions, whether at the individual, organizational, or policy level, remain one of the key avenues through which research results can be translated into practical applications that improve worker health.

Theoretical Progress

Psychology is rich in theory, which is one characteristic that sets the science of psychology—and, in this case, OHP—apart from public health and medicine, which focus more on data and results with an absence of theory. It could be argued that theoretical progress has been slower in recent years for many OHP topics, and especially for the development of theories related to occupational stress (as described in Chapter 3). It may be that popular theories (e.g., the job demands–resources model) have qualities that make them useful and enduring. As such, much of the recent research has applied long-studied theories of stress and well-being to particular contexts and problems. However, some researchers have questioned how useful popular theories in OHP are for interventions and other practical concerns (e.g., Chapter 23). One approach to advance theory may be to identify ways in which theories compete with one another to make different predictions and test them against each other. This requires identifying the specific predictions that theories make about how work influences well-being. Rigorously testing theories may help increase their usefulness and precision. More recent research (e.g., Ganster & Rosen, 2013) has drawn attention to the allostatic load model. More empirical tests and applications of this model may serve to further advance the field. Going forward, we hope that the reliance upon continued development and empirical evaluation of theories will serve to advance the field of OHP. These theories can provide explanations for observations and results in occupational health that may be evident but not explained in the same manner in other, related disciplines.

Context

Finally, changes in the context of work and workers will yield many research needs and opportunities. The COVID-19 pandemic has brought about, and in some ways accelerated, changes in the workplace, and new OHP issues have emerged (Sinclair et al., 2020). Telework (i.e., remote work arrangements) has become more common than ever, raising new questions about benefits for worker health and safety when people work from home, as well as who is even responsible for health and safety in home offices. Additionally, COVID-19 has put the spotlight on sick leave policies that may encourage presenteeism (i.e., encouraging workers to attend work while ill, potentially spreading disease and delaying their own recovery; Lohaus & Habermann, 2019). Also needed is the continued study of the severe physical and emotional burden that COVID-19 has placed on frontline health workers, which may have immediate and longer term effects. Finally, high levels of turnover and staffing shortages in restaurants and other customer service industries have brought to light the stressful nature of dealing with abusive customers, which has reportedly driven some workers to exit these jobs.

In part resulting from the effects of the COVID-19 pandemic as well as other technological changes, forms of gig work such as food and package delivery have grown in prevalence as well, as consumers take advantage of the convenience offered by online food and shopping services. However, little is known about the types, prevalence, and effects of the working conditions experienced by these workers. This presents another important need and opportunity for future research.

The protests against racism and police brutality during the summer of 2020 throughout the United States also pointed to an urgent need to address and achieve diversity, equity, and inclusion throughout many areas of society, including the workplace. Some OHP research, as reviewed in Chapter 13, has delved into the effects of perceived discrimination on workers' health and well-being. However, to address pervasive health disparities, more efforts in research and practice are needed to study worker populations that have been traditionally underrepresented. There is a clear need for OHP research to more directly investigate the interface between employee health and diversity, equity, and inclusion in the workplace. We recommend that more research investigates and considers the perspectives of members of underrepresented groups.

GRADUATE TRAINING IN OHP

One important issue relevant to the field of OHP that has not been addressed elsewhere in the handbook pertains to the education and training of the next generation of OHP scientists and practitioners. The goal of graduate training in OHP is to prepare professionals for successful careers in research and practice. In 2005, the Society for Occupational Health Psychology organized a task force that conducted a job analysis and outlined an Occupational Health Psychologist Profile. The knowledge and skills described in the profile and our review suggest that an OHP professional should

1. acquire knowledge and skills in OHP; organizational psychology (including organizational structure, leadership, and work motivation); psychological testing and scale development; research design and quantitative methods; and allied occupational health fields such as public health, epidemiology, ergonomics and safety, and occupational medicine.

2. apply psychological principles, research methods and design, and quantitative and qualitative analytic skills to design and conduct research to investigate, evaluate, and solve occupational concerns. Examples of such concerns may include

   - identifying and classifying physical and psychosocial risk factors
   - prioritizing resources
   - developing validating, administering, and interpreting psychological tests and organizational surveys
   - designing and evaluating health and safety intervention/prevention programs, research, and practices

3. apply the scientific method to occupational health and safety challenges. This includes, for example:

   - leading employee and organizational change initiatives to create healthy, safe, and productive workplaces (e.g., safety management systems, training, safety culture, health promotion, and wellness)
   - conducting health services and health and productivity management
   - eliminating workplace mistreatment (e.g., violence prevention, harassment, incivility)
   - conducting work, job, and task design to improve workers' health and well-being
   - addressing work and family issues by improving balance between work and family life with nonwork life
   - understanding and reducing negative psychological and biological effects of work stress
   - designing effective and efficient work schedules to reduce sleep and fatigue problems at work
   - identifying and addressing mental health issues in the workplace
   - improving and managing human resources to maximize workers' potentials and well-being and reduce absenteeism, presenteeism, and turnover

4. reflect the values that are the underpinnings of OHP as an interdisciplinary science, and recognize the dynamics between human-related systems and physical-related systems

5. communicate effectively and intelligently in a variety of formats (e.g., written or verbal) with many audiences (e.g., research, technical, managerial, and public/lay audiences)

6. build a business case for workplace safety, health, and well-being

7. demonstrate knowledge and technological competence, including substantive knowledge and research skills

8. understand workplace diversity and inclusion, including minority and immigrant workers to reduce occupational health disparities

Chapter 2 described the history of the development of the field as well as the growth of graduate training programs specializing in OHP and funded by the American Psychological Association and the National Institute for Occupational Safety and Health, which have shaped and generously supported graduate training in OHP for multiple decades. Many of the current OHP graduate training programs are affiliated with and/or led primarily by faculty in graduate programs in industrial-organizational psychology, although they may also be accessible to students in other graduate programs. There are excellent opportunities to further broaden and strengthen approaches to OHP by bridging areas like clinical and counseling psychology to address mental health and substance use in the workplace or related to work, as well as build new collaborations or strengthen ties with other related disciplines. Over the past few years, the field has seen the establishment of new programs for *Total Worker Health*® that are interdisciplinary in nature and associated with public health programs. Based on the strong overlap between OHP and other occupational health disciplines, such as public health, epidemiology, ergonomics and safety, industrial hygiene, occupational medicine, and occupational health nursing, one suggestion is to foster more integration of these allied disciplines in future OHP graduate training. We hope and expect to see more interdisciplinary collaboration among occupational health professionals. We advocate for training the next generation so that these researchers can understand and appreciate various disciplines and approaches that are relevant to occupational health, safety, and well-being more broadly and are beyond the scope of traditional OHP.

CONCLUSION

This chapter highlights the many OHP research areas that have shown major progress over the past couple of decades, and particularly since the previous edition of this handbook. Across these areas has been a holistic perspective that considers the organization, the individual, and the society, as well as the various points of potential intervention to improve worker health and safety. The future promises many opportunities for researchers to advance the more mature OHP research areas while also taking on the challenge of investigating new workplace dynamics and emerging forms of work. There is much to be done on all fronts, and we look forward to what researchers in the field of OHP can accomplish in the years ahead.

REFERENCES

Demerouti, E., Bakker, A. B., Nachreiner, F., & Schaufeli, W. B. (2001). The job demands–resources model of burnout. *Journal of Applied Psychology, 86*(3), 499–512. https://doi.org/10.1037/0021-9010.86.3.499

Ganster, D. C., & Rosen, C. C. (2013). Work stress and employee health: A multidisciplinary review. *Journal of Management, 39*(5), 1085–1122. https://doi.org/10.1177/0149206313475815

Lohaus, D., & Habermann, W. (2019). Presenteeism: A review and research directions. *Human Resource Management Review, 29*(1), 43–58. https://doi.org/10.1016/j.hrmr.2018.02.010

Sinclair, R. R., Allen, T., Barber, L., Bergman, M., Britt, T., Butler, A., Ford, M., Hammer, L., Kath, L., Probst, T., & Yuan, Z. (2020). Occupational health science in the time of COVID-19: Now more than ever. *Occupational Health Science, 4*(1), 1–22. https://doi.org/10.1007/s41542-020-00064-3

INDEX

ABOUT THE EDITORS

Lois E. Tetrick, PhD, received her doctorate in industrial and organizational psychology from the Georgia Institute of Technology in 1983. Upon completion of her doctoral studies, she joined the faculty of the Department of Psychology at Wayne State University and remained there until 1995, when she moved to the Department of Psychology at the University of Houston. She joined the faculty at George Mason University as the director of the Industrial and Organizational Psychology Program in 2003.

Dr. Tetrick served as editor of the *Journal of Occupational Health Psychology* (2006–2010). She coedited the first and second editions of the *Handbook of Occupational Health Psychology* with James Campbell Quick and *Health and Safety in Organizations* with David A. Hofmann. She also coedited *The Employment Relationship: Examining Psychological and Contextual Perspectives* with Jacqueline A.-M. Coyle-Shapiro, Lynn M. Shore, and M. Susan Taylor; and *Research Methods in Occupational Health Psychology* with Robert R. Sinclair and Mo Wang.

Dr. Tetrick is a Fellow of the European Academy of Occupational Health Psychology, the American Psychological Association (APA), the Society for Industrial and Organizational Psychology (SIOP), and the Association for Psychological Science. She served as president of SIOP (2007–2008), chair of the Human Resources Division of the Academy of Management (2001–2002), SIOP representative on the APA Council of Representatives (2003–2005), and member of the APA Board of Scientific Affairs (2006–2009).

Her research interests are occupational health and safety, occupational stress, the work–family interface, and the psychological contracts and exchange relationships between employees and their organizations.

James Campbell Quick, PhD, is a Distinguished University Professor and Professor Emeritus at the University of Texas (UT) at Arlington, and Colonel, United States Air Force (Ret.) whose senior awards were the Legion of Merit and the Meritorious Service Medal. Colonel Quick served on the Defense Health Board (2008–2011) by appointment of SECDEF Robert Gates and was a member of the Society of Air Force Clinical Psychologists.

Dr. Quick is a Fellow of the American Psychological Association, the Society for Industrial and Organizational Psychology, and the Society of Antiquaries of Scotland (FSAScot). He was awarded the 2002 Harry and Miriam Levinson Award by the American Psychological Foundation. He and his brother Jonathan's signature work is the theory of preventive stress management (TPSM), and the term *preventive stress management* is included in the *APA Dictionary of Psychology*.

Dr. Quick has more than 130 publications in 10 languages and over 15,000 scholarly citations. He was elected to the University of Texas Arlington Academy of Distinguished Scholars in 2013 and won a UT System 2016 Regents Outstanding Teaching Award. He was honored with the Maroon Citation by Colgate University. He is married to the former Sheri Grimes Schember; both are members of the Chancellor's Council and the Ashbel Smith Circle of the University of Texas System and the Silver Society, American Psychological Foundation.

Michael T. Ford, PhD, is an associate professor of management at the University of Alabama's Culverhouse College of Business. Dr. Ford received a PhD in industrial–organizational psychology from George Mason University and worked for 9 years in the Psychology Department at the University at Albany, State University of New York, before joining the Department of Management at the University of Alabama.

Dr. Ford's research has appeared in several journals of interest to occupational health psychology, including the *Journal of Applied Psychology*, the *Journal of Occupational Health Psychology*, *Work & Stress*, and the *Psychological Bulletin*. He has also served as an associate editor for *Occupational Health Science* and the *Journal of Vocational Behavior* and has served on the Society for Occupational Health Psychology executive committee. Dr. Ford's research interests include the work–family interface, the employee–organization relationship, and employee health and well-being.

Gwenith G. Fisher, PhD, is an associate professor of psychology and director of the Industrial–Organizational Psychology program at Colorado State University. She is also the director of the Occupational Health Psychology training program, funded by the National Institute for Occupational Safety and Health (NIOSH) Mountain and Plains Education and Research Center, adjunct associate professor in the Colorado School of Public Health, and affiliate researcher with the Centre for Population Ageing and Research in Australia.

Dr. Fisher received her BA in psychology from Pennsylvania State University and MA and PhD degrees in psychology with a focus on industrial–organizational psychology and a minor in quantitative methods at Bowling Green State University. Prior to joining the psychology faculty at Colorado State University in 2013, she was an associate research scientist at the Survey Research Center at the University of Michigan Institute for Social Research.

Dr. Fisher is currently the president of the Society for Occupational Health Psychology. She has served on the editorial boards of the *Journal of Occupational Health Psychology, Occupational Health Science,* the *Journal of Business and Psychology,* and *Work, Aging and Retirement.* In 2015, Drs. Fisher and Tetrick received an award for the Best Article in the *Journal of Occupational Health Psychology* (2013–2014 Publications). Dr. Fisher's research interests include occupational health psychology, aging workforce issues with an emphasis on cognitive aging and worker health, work–nonwork issues, and research methods. When not working, she enjoys spending time with family and friends, skiing, hiking, ice hockey, traveling, cooking, and eating.